Rheumatology

Textbook Series

- *Acute Internal Medicine,* edited by Laurence B. Gardner, M.D.
- *Essential Neurology,* Second Edition, William Pryse-Phillips, M.D. and T. J. Murray, M.D.
- *Gynecology,* Ralph W. Hale, M.D. and John A. Krieger, M.D.
- *Infectious Diseases,* edited by Robert H. Waldman, M.D. and Ronica M. Kluge, M.D.
- *Nephrology,* edited by Marvin Forland, M.D.
- *Pediatric Allergy,* R. Michael Sly, M.D.
- *Pediatric Cardiology,* Courtney L. Anthony, M.D. and Rica G. Arnon, M.D.
- *Pediatric Endocrinology,* Wellington Hung, M.D., Gilbert P. August, M.D., and Allen M. Glasgow, M.D.
- *Pediatric Gastroenterology,* edited by Mervin Silverberg, M.D.
- *Rheumatology,* edited by Robert A. Turner, M.D. and Christopher M. Wise, M.D.
- *Sexual Development and Disorders in Childhood and Adolescence,* edited by Raymond M. Russo, M.D.

$ 48.25

Textbook of Rheumatology

Edited by

Robert A. Turner, M.D.
Professor of Medicine
Chief, Section on Rheumatology

Christopher M. Wise, M.D.
Assistant Professor of Medicine (Rheumatology)

Bowman Gray School of Medicine
Winston-Salem, North Carolina

MEDICAL EXAMINATION PUBLISHING CO.

Main entry under title:

Textbook of rheumatology.

Includes bibliographies and index.
1. Rheumatism. 2. Arthritis. I. Turner, Robert A., (date). II. Wise, Christopher M. [DNLM: WE 140 T355]
RC927.T49 1985b 616.7'23 85-15214
ISBN 0-87488-041-6

52 Vanderbilt Avenue
New York, New York 10017

Printed in the United States of America

To *Dr. Joseph E. Johnson,* whose support of rheumatology during his 13 years as Chief of Medicine at our institution, made this work possible

Contents

Contributors *ix*
Foreword *xi*
Preface *xiii*

Part I Fundamentals of Clinical Rheumatology

1. Introduction and Approach to the Patient with Musculoskeletal Complaints 3
   Christopher M. Wise, M.D.

2. Laboratory Testing in Rheumatology 36
   Henry Rothberger, M.D., Tung-Kwang Lee, M.D., and Maria P. McGee, M.D.

3. Diagnostic Radiology in the Rheumatic Diseases 58
   Alan Klein, M.B., B.Ch., and Wells Martin III, M.D.

4. Clinical Pharmacology of Antirheumatic Drugs 124
   Jack W. Strandhoy, Ph.D.

5. Arthritis Nursing and the Team Approach in the Management of Rheumatic Disease 153
   Nirma Perricone, B.S.N. and Jo Ann Fahey, B.S.N.

6. Psychological Aspects of Arthritis 178
   Karen O. Anderson, Ph.D., Laurence A. Bradley, Ph.D., Larry D. Young, Ph.D., and Lisa K. McDaniel, M.A.

7. The Surgical Management of Arthritis 214
   Anthony G. Gristina, M.D. and Lawrence X. Webb, M.D.

Part II Rheumatologic Diseases

8. Rheumatoid Arthritis 237
Robert A. Turner

9. Osteoarthritis 261
John F. Benson, M.D., Edward J. Pisko, M.D., and Christopher M. Wise, M.D.

10. Seronegative Spondyloarthropathies 287
Christopher M. Wise, M.D.

11. Crystal-Induced Arthritis 323
Carlos A. Agudelo, M.D.

12. Nonarticular Rheumatism 339
Christopher M. Wise, M.D.

13. Systemic Lupus Erythematosus 386
Carlos A. Agudelo, M.D.

14. Progressive Systemic Sclerosis (Scleroderma) 411
Edward J. Pisko, M.D.

15. Sjögren's Syndrome 445
Christopher M. Wise, M.D. and Elliott L. Semble, M.D.

16. Polymyositis and Dermatomyositis 458
Christopher M. Wise, M.D. and Carlos A. Agudelo, M.D.

17. Mixed Connective Tissue Disease 477
Edward J. Pisko, M.D.

18. Vasculitis 494
Elliott L. Semble, M.D.

19. Rheumatic Disease of Childhood 522
Sara H. Sinal, M.D.

20. Heritable and Metabolic Diseases of Connective Tissue and Bone 562
K. Patrick Ober, M.D. and John Hennessy, M.D.

21. Infectious Arthritis 591
Elliott L. Semble, M.D. and Carlos A. Agudelo, M.D.

22. Neoplasms of Bone and Joints 611
Ivan L. Holleman, M.D.

23. Rheumatic Manifestations of Systemic Disease 635
Elliott L. Semble, M.D. and Christopher M. Wise, M.D.

Index 667

Contributors

Carlos A. Agudelo, M.D., Associate Professor of Medicine (Rheumatology)

Karen O. Anderson, Ph.D., Instructor of Medical Psychology

John F. Benson, M.D., Clinical Assistant Professor of Medicine (Rheumatology)

Laurence A. Bradley, Ph.D., Associate Professor of Psychiatry and Behavioral Medicine, and Chief, Section on Medical Psychology

JoAnn Fahey, B.S.N., R.N., Arthritis Nurse Clinician, Section on Rheumatology

Anthony G. Gristina, Professor of Surgery, Chief, Section on Orthopedic Surgery

John Hennessy, M.D., Associate Professor of Medicine (Endocrinology)

Ivan L. Holleman, M.D., Associate Professor of Pathology

Alan Klein, M.B., B.Ch., Assistant Professor of Radiology

Tung-Kwang Lee, M.D., Research Associate in Medicine (Rheumatology)

Wells Martin III, M.D., Assistant Professor of Radiology

Lisa K. McDaniel, M.A., Data Coordinator, Section on Medical Psychology

Maria P. McGee, M.D. Research Assistant Professor in Medicine (Rheumatology)

K. Patrick Ober, M.D., Associate Professor of Medicine (Endocrinology)

Nirma Perricone, B.S.N., R.N., Arthritis Nurse Clinician, Division of Rheumatology

Edward J. Pisko, M.D., Associate Professor of Medicine (Rheumatology)

Henry Rothberger, M.D., Associate Professor of Medicine (Rheumatology)

Elliott L. Semble, M.D., Assistant Professor of Medicine (Rheumatology)

Sara H. Sinal, M.D., Assistant Professor of Pediatrics

Jack W. Strandhoy, Ph.D., Associate Professor of Pharmacology

Robert A. Turner, M.D., Professor of Medicine

Lawrence X. Webb, M.D., Assistant Professor of Orthopedic Surgery

Christopher M. Wise, M.D., Assistant Professor of Medicine (Rheumatology)

Larry D. Young, Ph.D., Assistant Professor of Psychology

Bowman Gray School of Medicine
Winston-Salem, North Carolina

Foreword

The ever-increasing scope and complexity of knowledge in medicine have necessitated more and more subspecialization as each aspect of medicine itself becomes more complex. There is no other division of internal medicine which has grown so much during my professional lifetime (nearly 50 years) as the field of rheumatology. When I entered the field there were very few who knew what rheumatology consisted of, so our textbook had to be called *Arthritis and Allied Conditions* until finally we could add the secondary title, *Textbook of Rheumatology,* nearly 20 years later. Now it has become such a complex field that the original textbook, after 10 editions, is literally an encyclopedia of rheumatology, which necessitates smaller texts for those starting their pursuit of knowledge in this aspect of medicine.

This *Textbook of Rheumatology* is truly a "pattern for learning" tailored to the student of the field, whether medical student, intern, resident in medicine or orthopedics, or practicing physician who wants to learn how to diagnose and treat arthritis in its many forms, as well as the many other conditions involving the musculoskeletal system so often misdiagnosed and inadequately treated.

The editors have done a splendid job in "cutting the pattern" by organizing the sequence and content of the chapters, and in their choice of authors expert in their subjects who have "trimmed the fat" to make the volume concise yet comprehensive. I predict great success for this book, and congratulate both authors and editors on their achievement.

Joseph Lee Hollander, M.D.

Preface

Rheumatology, in conjunction with the other medical subspecialties, is undergoing an ever-accelerating expansion. Tremendous advances have been made in understanding the normal function of the musculoskeletal and immune systems. Such advances have made possible the elucidation of the basic pathogenetic mechanisms responsible for the initiation and perpetuation of many rheumatologic disease processes. At the same time, increased interest in the clinical practice of rheumatology has resulted in the generation of more detailed and comprehensive information regarding the classification, clinical manifestations, complications, and therapeutic approaches to various rheumatic diseases.

The rapid expansion of the broad field of rheumatology has led to progress in the evaluation and care of patients with rheumatic diseases. However, this expansion has resulted in difficulty for medical students, physicians-in-training, family practitioners, and general internists in approaching this subject. To the medical student, recently exposed to the latest in basic immunology, rheumatic diseases constitute a peculiar array of conditions that seem to have no relationship to each other except for their immunologic abnormalities. To the physician- in-training, most of whom still have a heavily hospital-based experience, the rheumatic diseases are typically viewed as rare multisystem diseases that usually lead to crippling deformities or death. To the practicing family physician or internist, for whom musculosketletal complaints constitute a significant proportion of outpatient practice, recent advances in laboratory testing and therapy and lack of formal training in this area may result in a feeling of insecurity when dealing with rheumatic disease patients.

In this textbook, we have attempted to make the complicated field of rheumatology more understandable to students, house staff, and practitioners. This book is not designed as a reference for rheumatologists, and it not intended to supplement or replace any of the large major textbooks available in this subspecialty. The overall emphasis of the book is clinical, with elements of basic science covered in the context of their clinical applicability.

This book is organized into two major sections. The first seven chapters cover the fundamentals of clinical rheumatology. The first section stresses overall aspects of the clinical, laboratory, and radiographic evalulation of patients and covers the broad therapeutic areas of comprehensive care, and pharmacologic, psychological, and surgical management of rheumatic conditions. It is our hope that this section will serve as a reference for later parts of the book, as well as become a source of general information for the practitioner. The second section of the book, made up of Chapters 8-23, includes discussions of each of the major rheumatologic diseases. In addition to the classic rheumatologic disorders, we have included chapters on the rheumatic diseases of childhood, heritable and metabolic conditions, bone and joint neoplasms, and rheumatic manifestations of major systemic diseases.

This is a book with many authors, and we have attempted to capitalize on the expertise available within the Bowman Gray School of Medicine to make this a comprehensive yet concise text. We have drawn on the special interests of each of our authors, who have come primarily from the Section on Rheumatology, but also from the Sections on Endocrinology, Medical Psychology, Orthopedic Surgery, and from the Departments of Pathology, Radiology, and Pediatrics. Although the authors have retained their own styles in writing each chapter, we have attempted to utilize, where practical, a standardized format in order to provide cohesiveness and make the book easier to use as a practical reference.

Throughout the synthesis of this text, we have been greatly assisted by our associates at the Medical Examination Publishing Company, without whose patience and assistance this work would not have been possible. We are also greatly indebted to the Audio-Visual Resources Department, and secretaries in each of the contributing sections and departments at the Bowman Gray School of Medicine for their understanding and cooperation in bringing the many facets of this project together in what we hope is a useful new textbook.

notice

Part I

FUNDAMENTALS OF CLINICAL RHEUMATOLOGY

Chapter 1

INTRODUCTION AND APPROACH TO THE PATIENT WITH MUSCULOSKELETAL COMPLAINTS

Christopher M. Wise, M.D.

The rheumatic diseases, as we know them today, constitute a heterogeneous group of conditions in which pain and stiffness of some portion of the musculoskeletal system are prominent (1). The term rheumatism is derived from the Greek word "rheuma" which was first encountered in works on the humoral theory of disease. The word literally means "flowing" and was used to designate mucus as an evil humor which was thought to flow from the brain to the joints and other portions of the body, producing pain (2).

The field of rheumatology today encompasses a wide variety of conditions which are manifest by a multitude of clinical, immunologic, and metabolic abnormalities. Although specific causes are known for a relatively few of these conditions, a great deal has been learned about many of the others that may eventually allow us to uncover etiologic mechanisms.

The rheumatic diseases covered in this book are summarized in Table 1.1. Rheumatoid arthritis is a chronic inflammatory disease often accompanied by systemic and immunologic abnormalities, and is probably the best known of the rheumatic diseases. Osteoarthritis is a degenerative condition affecting primarily the joints and is probably even more common. The seronegative spondyloarthropathies represent a group of conditions which have in common low grade inflammatory periarticular and articular abnormalities and possible associations with infections. Crystal-induced arthropathies represent diseases that can often be attributed to underlying metabolic disturbance and result from deposition of inflammation-evoking crystals in and around joints. Nonarticular conditions are localized syndromes that must be differentiated from true arthritis and are generally noninflammatory. The diffuse connective tissue diseases include systemic lupus erythematosus, scleroderma, Sjögren's syndrome, polymyositis, dermatomyositis, and mixed connective tissue disease. These are all multisystem disorders that are manifest by a wide variety of immunologic, musculoskeletal, cutaneous, and

TABLE 1.1 The Rheumatic Diseases

Inflammatory Arthritis of Unknown Etiology
- Rheumatoid arthritis
- Seronegative spondyloarthropathies (ankylosing spondylitis, Reiter's syndrome, psoriatic arthritis, enteropathic arthritis)

Noninflammatory and Mechanical Conditions
- Osteoarthritis
- Nonarticular rheumatism

Crystal-Induced Arthritis
- Gout
- Pseudogout
- Others

Diffuse Connective Tissue Diseases
- Systemic lupus erythematosus
- Scleroderma
- Sjögren's syndrome
- Polymyositis and dermatomyositis
- Mixed connective tissue disease

Vasculitis

Rheumatic Diseases of Childhood

Heritable and Metabolic Diseases of Connective Tissue and Bone

Infectious Arthritis

Neoplasms of Bone and Joints

Systemic Diseases with Rheumatologic Manifestations

visceral organ abnormalities. The vasculitides constitute another heterogeneous group of multisystem diseases where inflammatory vascular changes are prominent. The rheumatic diseases of childhood include many of those seen in adults as well as several apparently unique to the pediatric population. Several diseases can be attributed to heritable and metabolic abnormalities of bone and connective tissue. Infectious agents have been directly implicated in causing arthritis in some situations, while neoplasms may also affect the bones and joints. Finally many systemic diseases may present with or be complicated by rheumatologic syndromes and should always be kept in mind when evaluating patients with musculoskeletal complaints.

Although several other classification systems for the rheumatic diseases have been suggested over the years, none have been entirely satisfactory. As additional knowledge is gained over the years in the field, further changes in terminology and classification will undoubtedly be made.

The magnitude of the problem of the rheumatic diseases to the practicing physician is large. It has been estimated that one in six visits by a patient to a health professional is for a musculoskeletal complaint (2). Although a great majority of these visits are for self-limited conditions, it has still been estimated as recently as 1975 that over 20 million people in the United States suffer from some form of arthritis or related condition (3).

Approach to the Patient

In spite of continued technologic advances in the diagnosis of rheumatic disorders, the practice of rheumatology continues to be primarily a clinical endeavor. The physician assessing patients with musculoskeletal complaints must rely heavily on elements of the history and physical exam and, for the most part, uses radiographic and other laboratory studies to confirm or deny what is already suspected. The main effort of the history and physical exam should be to categorize the patient's problem into one of four broad categories of disease: inflammatory, noninflammatory, functional (psychogenic), or unknown (4). With skill, experience, and a systematic approach, further categorization and sometimes even a specific diagnosis can be made on the basis of history and physical exam alone (5).

History

The physician's first encounter with the patient, the interview, is an invaluable tool in providing details about a patient's musculoskeletal symptoms. During the interview, the physician should be able to define the complaints as the patient perceives them. The history should suggest whether there are anatomically definable problems and also permit evaluation of the patient's cooperation, motivation, and goals (6). In general, the medical history as it relates to rheumatic disease is not appreciably different from standard history, but naturally focuses more on the musculoskeletal system, while history of conditions involving other organ systems may become important as the interview proceeds.

The Chief Complaint and Present Illness

The interview should begin with a focus on the reason the patient has presented to the physician at this time. The patient should be encouraged to tell the story of the illness in his own way. Even though this may result in a disjointed and incomplete story, a great deal can be learned from the way in which the patient emphasizes aspects of the history.

There are times when initial broad questions will not elicit a free-flowing, informative response and, at such times, the physician should begin to take a more active role and ask more specific questions, as for example, "What symptom bothers you the most?" In general, brief and simple questions, asked one at a time, will aid the flow of information, and the patient should be encouraged to go into more detail about specific problems, as he becomes more comfortable in the interview.

At some point in the interview, the chronology of events should be summarized and defined. The patient should be prompted to be as specific as possible about the overall pattern of symptoms, the order in which they occurred, and how rapidly they occurred. Other important features include the time of day when symptoms have their onset or when they are the worst. Severity of symptoms may be estimated by the extent to which they interfere with function, sleep, or work patterns. When symptoms are episodic and self-limited in nature, it should be determined how long episodes lasted, how frequently they occurred, and what, if any, therapeutic interventions provided relief. A migratory process is one in which the process has subsided completely in one joint before it crops up in another previously unaffected joint. Progressive involvement indicates that one joint has become affected initially, but that eventually additional joints are recruited while symptoms persist in the initial joint.

Information about specific anatomic regions and joints should be as as precise as possible. If there are any questions, the patient should be encouraged to point to the affected area.

Specific Symptoms

Pain

Pain is the most common symptom bringing patients with rheumatic disease to the physician. The phenomenon of pain is complex and often very difficult to define, measure, and explain. Pain may have different meanings to different people and even to the same person at different times. An analysis of pain should include attempts to define location, character, circumstances of occurrence, and associated factors.

The location of a pain provides an invaluable clue to the underlying pathologic process. Pain localized strictly to a joint region more often than not represents a primary process within the joint. Pain which is in areas between joints may suggest a variety of conditions, including those which affect bone and muscle, but may represent pain referred from a distant site. Pain can sometimes be localized to periarticular structures, such as bursae, fascial planes, tendons, tendon insertions, or ligaments and suggest pathology within these structures. Diffuse, migratory pain lacking anatomic correlation may suggest a functional disorder, fibrositis, or again may represent referred pain. When descriptions of pain are vague, the physician must take a more active role in getting the patient to localize this. A good example of this is pain in the region of the hip girdle. Most patients consider all pain in the buttocks, lateral thighs, and groin as "hip pain" while it is usually pain in the anterior region that implies a process within the acetabular joint itself. The pattern, distribution, and chronologic evolution of pain are very important in evaluating painful syndromes. Such information may be useful not only at the time of the first interview, but also much later.

The character of pain is sometimes very difficult for the patient to describe. Often it is best to allow the patient to use his own words, but sometimes the suggestion of certain terms may be necessary. Such terms as "steady," "crampy," or "throbbing" may be used to describe a pain within a joint or muscle, while "burning," "numbing," or "tingling" may suggest a neurogenic origin.

Circumstances associated with pain should be sought. The effects of body positions, movements, activity or inactivity, touch, pressure, and emotional stress can all provide important information. The relationship of pain to activity and rest is important. Pain that occurs only during movement can usually be attributed to a mechanical cause. Pain that occurs both at rest and with movement is more suggestive of an inflammatory condition. Other events of life, such as trauma, emotional stress, or changes in social situation can be important in the pathogenesis of pain.

Symptoms occurring at or near the same time of a joint complaint often provide important diagnostic information. Certain symptoms, such as muscle spasm, paresthesia, weakness, or Raynaud's phenomenon may easily explain localized pain. Constitutional symptoms, such as autonomic dysfunction, weight loss or gain, fever, chills, or interference with activities of daily living may suggest a more systemic process or even a nonarticular disease. Emotional aspects of a patient's pain should be evaluated. Depression, anxiety, and tension can all interact significantly with pain and may either be an underlying cause or a significant contributing factor to an existing pathologic process.

Swelling

A history of swelling should be sought during the evaluation of any patient with musculoskeletal complaints. Patients may describe swelling voluntarily, or may mention it only as an afterthought. An attempt should be made to make the patient be as specific as possible when describing swelling. Many patients may describe a vague or diffuse sense of swelling in an extremity, and the diagnostic significance of this is much different from the discrete localized swelling in a joint or bursal sac. Symmetry or asymmetry of swelling is important as is information regarding whether the onset of swelling was acute or gradual. The degree of pain associated with swelling is also helpful information. Certainly, symptoms of swelling are not specific for rheumatic disease, and other disorders, such as local infection or circulatory disturbance, may cause swelling. On the other hand, when musculoskeletal symptoms occur without any swelling, the symptoms are often due to nonarticular causes.

Stiffness

Stiffness is a subjective and nonspecific symptom which may have different meanings to different patients. It is important to differentiate the symptom of stiffness from pain, fatigue, aching, or weakness, since these terms are often confused. Stiffness is best defined as a discomfort or restriction which the patient perceives as he begins to move a joint after a period of inactivity. This may occur after only a few minutes of rest during the day, and the term "gelling" sometimes is used to describe this sort of daytime stiffness. When stiffness occurs after a long period of rest, such as a night's sleep, it carries much more diagnostic importance. It is thought that the duration of morning stiffness is directly proportional to the severity of an inflammatory process in an extremity. In general, noninflammatory, mechanical, or degenerative conditions cause morning stiffness of short duration, usually on the order of less than one-half hour. Inflammatory conditions, such as rheumatoid arthritis, ankylosing spondylitis, or polymyalgia rheumatica are usually accompanied by morning stiffness of at least one hour and sometimes up to several hours of duration. The mechanism by which this occurs is unclear, but there is some evidence that this phenomenon is related to localized tissue edema which is relieved by muscular activity and improved lymphatic flow and venous return. It is helpful to attempt to accurately quantitate the duration of morning stiffness for purposes of monitoring disease activity in inflammatory conditions. For this purpose, two questions should be asked: 1) At what time do you get up in the morning? and 2) When do you become as limber as you are likely to be for the day? This two-question technique is a relatively reproducible way of quantitatively assessing morning stiffness (4).

Weakness

Weakness may result from a variety of conditions, from primary disease of the joints to conditions affecting muscles or the nervous system. The historian should differentiate weakness from other similar symptoms, such as stiffness or fatigue. Weakness implies inability to perform voluntary actions with specific muscle groups. It is usually a persistent symptom. Localization of weakness often gives a clue to the underlying cause. Difficulty in using the hands or legs, when associated with a painful joint in the same region is most often attributable to an articular process. Weakness in the proximal muscles is a frequent symptom in myositis, and most patients with this sort of condition have little difficulty identifying muscle weakness as the cause of their problems. Distal or unilateral weakness is most often a symptom of a primary neurologic problem.

Associated Symptoms

Limitation of motion and loss of function are frequent complaints of patients with rheumatic disorders. These are usually expressed in terms of the patient's own activities of work and daily living. Most patients will volunteer that they are unable to do things they are accustomed to doing. This loss of function is often the most important aspect of a patient's complaint. The restoration of motion and function may serve as a valuable therapeutic goal and emphasis on this will enhance patient compliance and satisfaction with results.

Fatigue, like stiffness, is a subjective and imprecise term. The time frame over which fatigue develops can be a very helpful piece of information. Insidious and persistent fatigue which does not resolve over a very short period of time has a much greater effect on a patient's daily routine. When fatigue is the primary complaint, it may be an early or prominent symptom of a significant inflammatory illness or may represent an underlying functional or emotional problem. In rheumatoid arthritis, for example, fatigue usually develops as the day goes on. The patient with fibrositis, on the other hand, often notices fatigue immediately on arising in the morning.

A history of previous therapy should always be sought. This often provides a great deal of insight into the nature of the illness and its effect on the patient and is helpful in planning future therapy. The following questions should be asked: 1) What types of therapy have been tried? 2) How was previous therapy given? 3) Was previous therapy effective? 4) Were there side effects? 5) Why were previous forms of therapy abandoned? 6) Is the patient under treatment for any other condition? Careful attention to detail in eliciting a history of previous forms of therapy will often reveal simple correctable mistakes, such as inadequate salicylate dosage, poor compliance, too short a trial of a long-acting medication, or even medications given for other conditions which interfere with therapy.

Emotional and behavioral factors are assessed during the interview both by observation and direct questioning. Body movements, speech patterns, and facial expressions provide information about the patient's general mood and his reaction to illness. Insight into the effect of the present illness on the patient's interrelationships with others is often best elicited by direct questioning. The physician should also attempt to understand factors which have led to the consultation in the first place. Some patients come to a physician looking for relief of a symptom, while others are seeking reassurance that their symptom does not represent an underlying neoplasm or progressively disabling disease. Still others use symptoms as a vehicle to attain changes in job, more support or understanding from family members, or even monetary compensation. A careful history will often bring such things out and enable the physician to direct his diagnostic workup and therapeutic approach more appropriately.

Past Medical History

The past medical history is an important part of any medical evaluation. Previous musculoskeletal symptoms are obviously important but more subtle previous illnesses such as "growing pains," chorea, or joint swelling in childhood may help differentiate a subsequent illness in an adult. Past surgical procedures, psychiatric illnesses, obstetric history, and medical illnesses all may have potential diagnostic or therapeutic importance in evaluating and treating rheumatic diseases. A thorough knowledge of the association of rheumatic diseases with nonarticular symptoms and other diseases is obviously important in obtaining a thorough and meaningful review of past medical problems. Certainly, a history of ocular symptoms, renal stones, cutaneous disease, gastrointestinal or pulmonary disease, or previous venereal or nonvenereal infections can all have significance in certain settings.

A family history can be important in many respects. Certain rheumatic diseases have a genetic basis and the ever growing field of immunogenetics makes this of even more value. Certain conditions such as gout, pseudogout, ankylosing spondylitis, rheumatoid arthritis, and systemic lupus erythematosus have genetic components. Psychological factors can also be important in the family history. Attitudes towards illness, fears, and expectations can be based on previous illness within the family and must be dealt with by the physician along with other aspects of the disease.

Personal and social histories are meaningful as well. Specific questions should be asked about current living arrangements, family or other relationships, present occupation, economic status, and social commitments. Leisure activities, patterns of sleep, and dietary habits should be determined. Finally, information should be sought regarding drug intake and tobacco and alcohol use.

Physical Examination of the Joints

A basic knowledge of joint structure and function greatly facilitates the interpretation of the findings on physical examination. Joints, or articulations, are the connections between two or more bones, and provide various degrees of motion and stability between bones.

There are many different classifications of joints, but essentially two major types of joints are recognized: 1) Synarthroses are joints where the bones are held together by continuous intervening layers of fibrous tissue and fibrocartilage. Since the surfaces of the bones are in almost direct contact, these joints have little or no movement. Examples of synarthroses are the symphysis pubis, sternomanubrial joint, and the distal union of the tibia and fibia. 2) Diarthroses are joints in which the articulating ends of the bones are covered by cartilage and enclosed in a capsule of fibrous tissue. These joints are the most common ones found in the body and are essentially freely moveable. The joint capsule of these joints is lined by a mesenchymal tissue known as synovium and these joints are known as synovial joints. Synovial-lined joints usually contain various amounts of synovial fluid, secreted by cells lining the cavity, which provides lubrication for the inner surface of the joints as well as a medium for the transmission of nutrients to avascular tissue such as cartilage.

Examination of the patient actually begins as the patient enters the room. The general appearance of the patient, gross deformity, gait, and the performance of simple activities such as getting in and out of a chair may be observed before the physical examination formally begins.

Each observer should develop a systematic approach to the examination of the joints. A logical system might begin with the joints of the head, neck, and spinal column, proceeding to the joints of the upper extremity and then the lower extremity. Each examiner should develop his/her own routine, in order that a complete exam is performed and that relatively asymptomatic, but abnormal areas are not overlooked.

The Basic Physical Signs of Arthritis

The eyes and the hands are the chief tools used in examining the joints. Careful inspection and palpation should be carried out in each joint and the following should be evaluated: swelling, tenderness, range of motion, temperature and color, crepitus, deformity, and strength and function.

Swelling

The enlargement of a joint is a reliable and objective sign which may be one of the earliest signs of arthritis. A swollen joint may be the result of an intraarticular process such as synovial thickening or effusion, or may result from an extraarticular process, such as bursitis, tendonitis, bony enlargement, or extraarticular fat collections. It is important that these conditions be differentiated from one another. Joint effusions are usually easily palpated and can be balloted. Since synovial fluid lies within a closed sac, compression of one portion will cause fluid to shift within the sac and add to its distension elsewhere. Synovial thickening, on the other hand, is less distinct and has a doughy feeling. Synovial thickening and effusion frequently occur together, and reliable differentiation between the two processes is not always possible by physical examination. Fluid accumulation within bursae also causes discrete swelling, but is usually not accompanied by limited range of motion. Swelling of tendon sheaths or ligaments should be localized to their anatomic locations. Bony enlargement tends to be more firm and irregular in shape. Sometimes, interstitial edema of an extremity can be confused with joint swelling, but is recognized by its diffuse ill-defined border and by swelling in areas not related to the joint.

Tenderness

Tenderness is the most sensitive, but not always the most specific, sign of an ongoing intraarticular process. Most joints are not normally tender to palpation. The examiner should exert enough force over joints to blanch the thumbnail, or roughly 74 lb/square inch (7). The absence of local tenderness does much to exclude underlying pathologic change within the joint. Tenderness may signify either a pathologic process or a low pain threshold. In general, patients with low pain thresholds will exhibit tenderness localized to the so-called fibrositic areas which are mainly periarticular structures. Patients with arthritis will have tenderness directly over joints.

Range of Motion

Active and passive range of motion should be assessed in all joints. Obviously, the range and type of motion will depend on several things, including the type of joint, restraining ligaments and periarticular structures, and the control of muscles acting on the joint. Limitation of motion is common in articular disease. Active range of motion should be observed first and any abnormality in this should be followed up with passive range of motion. When active range of motion is restricted and passive range of motion is normal, this usually signifies pathology in periarticular structures such as muscles, tendons, or bursae. When only intraarticular structures are involved, active and passive motion should be approximately the same. Limitation of motion may be transient or permanent. Transient limitation may result from muscle spasm, periarticular inflammation, synovitis, intraarticular loose bodies, or fibrous proliferation. Permanent limitation may be the result of bony ankylosis, destruction of articular surface, subluxation, or contracture of periarticular structures.

Changes in Temperature and Color

Changes in temperature and color about the joints are best interpreted by comparison with the opposite joint and with structures nearby on the same extremity. Careful comparison of these areas to each other should allow the observer to differentiate even very small temperature differences. This is much easier to do over large joints, but it can also be done for small joints.

Crepitus

Crepitus is the palpable or audible crunching sensation produced by motion of a joint. Many normal joints exhibit some coarse crackling which is of no pathologic significance and is probably due to tendons snapping over bony prominences. In general, fine crepitus is much more significant than coarse crepitus, and is palpable as a fine vibratory sensation when a joint is moved. Crepitus can be caused by grating of cartilage surfaces against one another, as in osteoarthritis or in severe rheumatoid arthritis. Tendon crepitus may be observed in scleroderma or as a result of tendinitis.

Joint Deformity

Joint deformity is the malalignment of a joint. This may be caused by ligament destruction, contracture of surrounding soft tissue, bony enlargement, collapse of bone from erosive disease, and subluxation. Deformity is best described relative to the long axis of the body. Flexion deformities are defined as the inability to passively extend the joint to its full extension. Deformities in the coronal plane are described as varus and valgus. By convention, these are described with reference to the distal segment. Lateral deviation of the distal segment is designated valgus, as in genu valgus or knock-knees. Medial deviation is designated varus, as in genu varus or bow-legs.

Muscle Function

Muscle function and joint function are closely related and any examination of the joints should include a careful examination of muscle strength. This not only serves as an indirect assessment of the severity of articular disease, but may also be useful in differentiating an articular problem from a primary muscle problem. Various systems of grading have been described for assessing muscle strength. Table 1.2 summarizes the most commonly used system of grading muscle strength. This system grades muscle strength on the basis of the ability to overcome gravity and/or resistance. Other methods may be used for specific joints. In the hand, a measurement of grip strength not only reflects muscle strength but also periarticular stiffness, joint pain, deformity, and motivation. It is performed by using a folded blood pressure cuff. The cuff is partially inflated to a reading of 30 mm and the patient is asked to grip maximally on three attempts and a mean value of these attempts is recorded (8). Proximal muscle strength can be assessed by simple measures, such as the ability to resist downward pressure on the arms and the ability to rise from a low chair or perform a deep knee bend.

Specific Joint Examination

Temporomandibular Joint

This joint is formed by the fossa of the articular tubercle of the temporal bone and the condyle of the mandible. A fibrocartilage meniscus divides the joint and the joint cavities are lined with synovial membrane. Swelling in this joint is relatively common and must be moderate or marked before it is apparent on inspection. This will appear as a rounded bulge over the joint just anterior to the external auditory meatus.

The joint may be palpated by placing the forefinger just anterior to the external auditory meatus. As the patient opens his mouth, the fingertip will drop into a depressed area overlying the joint. Swelling in the joint will prevent this normal movement and marked swelling will be felt as a fluctuant mass. Local tenderness and warmth may also be detected here.

The temporomandibular joint has three types of motion: opening and closing, protrusion and retrusion of the mandible, and lateral motion. Vertical motion is best determined by measuring the space between the upper and lower incisor teeth

TABLE 1.2 Assessment of Muscle Strength

Grade	Adjective	Description
5	Normal	Complete motion against gravity and full resistance
4	Good	Complete motion against gravity with moderate resistance
3	Fair	Complete motion against gravity alone
2	Poor	Motion only with gravity eliminated
1	Trace	Muscle activity but no motion

with the patient's mouth opened maximally. Normally, this distance reaches 3-6 cm. Lateral motion is measured by having the patient partially open his mouth, protrude the lower jaw, and then move the lower jaw from side to side. This lateral motion is normally about 1-2 cm.

Cervical Spine

The cervical spine consists of seven vertebrae. Each contains a transverse process and posterior elements which articulate with adjacent vertebrae. The vertebral artery passes through the transverse foramen. The first, second, and seventh bodies have special modifications. The first cervical vertebra, the atlas, does not have a body, but instead consists of an anterior and posterior arch and thickened lateral masses. A transverse ligament stretches across the ring of the atlas, dividing the vertebral foramen into a smaller anterior portion and larger posterior portion. The posterior portion encloses the spinal cord, while the anterior portion encloses the odontoid process of the second cervical vertebra (axis). The axis is unique in being the only vertebra that has such a projection. The axis articulates with the atlas through a pair of lateral joints and a midline joint formed between the odontoid process and the ring of the anterior arch. The seventh cervical vertebra has a particularly long spine, and this makes this vertebra more prominently palpable in the midline at the base of the neck posteriorly. At the articulation of the skull with the atlas, several ligaments are present which limit motion to flexion, extension, limited lateral bending, and no rotation.

Examination of the neck begins with observation of the patient at rest. Normally, there should be a slight anterior curve (lordosis) to the contour of the cervical spine. The patient should be observed carefully for spasm or torticollis (tilting and rotation at rest). The normal cervical spine allows about 45° of flexion and 50-60° of extension, most of this taking place at the atlantooccipital joint. The patient should be able to bring the mandible within two finger breadths of the manubrium in flexion and extend the occiput to within two finger breadths of the spinous process of C7. There is normally about 60-80° of rotation in each direction and most of this occurs at the atlantoaxial joint. This is best assessed by having the patient touch the chin to both of his shoulders. About 40° of lateral flexion takes place in each direction. Most of this occurs below the atlas in the articulations between the second and seventh vertebrae. This can be assessed by having the patient attempt to touch his ear to each shoulder.

The location of neck pain elicited during range of motion will sometimes indicate the site of pathology. Pain felt on the side toward which the neck is tilted suggests involvement of the apophyseal joints on this side. Pain occurring on the side opposite the movement suggests muscle or ligamentous strain or injury. The head compression test is performed by applying gradual downward pressure on the top of the head. This can be useful in reproducing symptoms of nerve root irritation. The distraction test is done by placing gentle upward pressure under the chin and occiput and may result in relief of symptoms of nerve root compression or joint disease. The Adson test is performed by feeling the patient's radial pulse as he abducts, extends, and externally rotates his arm. The patient then is asked to take a deep breath and rotate his head maximally toward the side being tested. In patients with neurovascular compression syndromes related to a cervical rib or other abnormalities, this test will result in a decrease in volume or obliteration of the radial pulse.

The Thoracolumbar Spine

The exam should begin with observation of the patient from behind in a standing position, as in Figure 1.1. It should be noted whether or not there is abnormal curving of the spine to one side or the other (scoliosis), or whether there is exaggeration or loss of the normal lumbar lordosis or thoracic kyphosis. Observation of the levels of the iliac crests should be made to determine whether significant leg length discrepancy exists resulting in functional scoliosis.

Palpation and percussion of the back may produce pain or reveal tenderness of abnormal structures. Tenderness may result from a variety of causes, including abnormalities of the joints and bones, muscle spasm, referred nerve pain, or localized soft tissue structures, such as fat pads or ligaments.

Movement of the thoracic spine is limited by the relatively small size of the discs as well as the articulations of the ribs and sternum. Rotation can be assessed by having the patient rotate his trunk while his legs and pelvis are stabilized in a standing or sitting position. Usually about 30° of rotation is possible in each direction. Movement of the posterior articulation of the ribs with the thoracic vertebrae is determined by measuring chest expansion. This is best estimated by the use of a cloth measuring tape at the level of the nipples, and is usually around 5-6 cm.

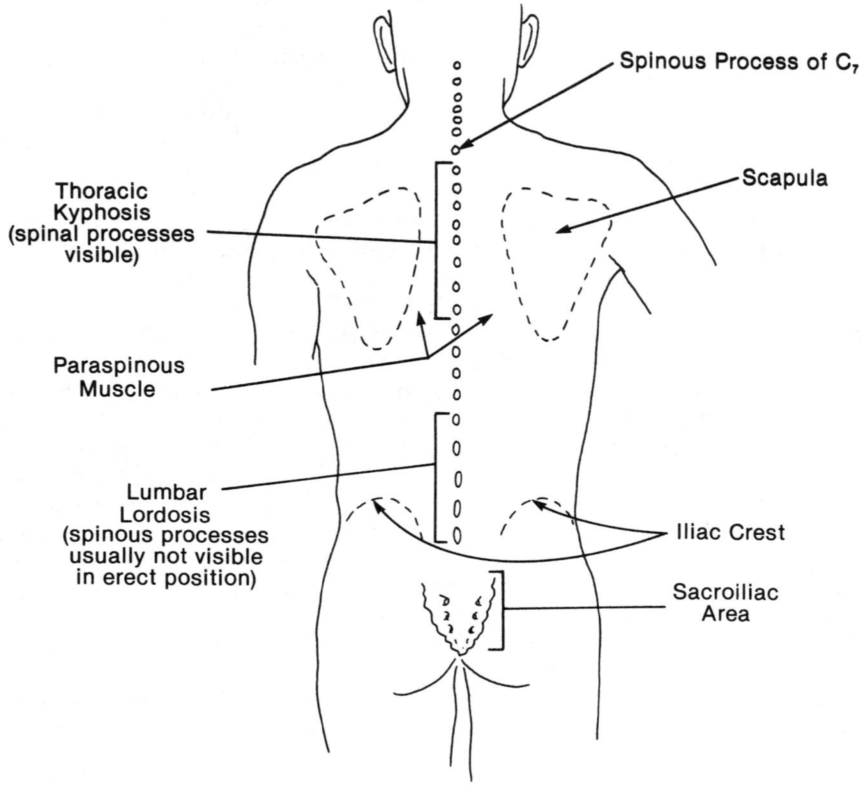

FIGURE 1.1 Posterior view of the thoracolumbar spine.

The lumbar vertebrae are more massive than the other vertebrae, the lumbar discs are relatively thick, and the articulating joints are placed in a sagittal plane. Because of this, the lumbar spine will move in flexion and extension but there is little rotation. After careful inspection and palpation, the patient should be asked to bend forward. This movement requires spinal and hip flexion and is often recorded by measuring the distance from the fingertips to the floor. Although this test is crude, it serves as a useful screening test for lumbar pathology. During forward flexion, normal lumbar lordosis is lost. Persistence of lordosis on forward flexion indicates either muscle spasm or a process within the spine itself. During forward flexion, the spinous processes should become more visible and the spinous processes should gradually separate. A means of measuring this more specifically is by the use of the Schober test (9). In this test, a perpendicular line is drawn from the midpoint between the posterior iliac crests and an arbitrary point 10 cm above and 5 cm below. Lengthening of the line joining these two points is measured on anterior flexion as shown in Figure 1.2. In a normal individual this 15-cm line should lengthen by 4–8 cm, although there is much variation with age. Lateral flexion can be measured in a similar way by using a 20-cm line in the midaxillary plane. A normal individual will distract this 20 cm to 25–32 cm. Extension is assessed with the patient standing with both feet on the floor and the support of the physician. Normally, the trunk will extend about 30° from the upright position.

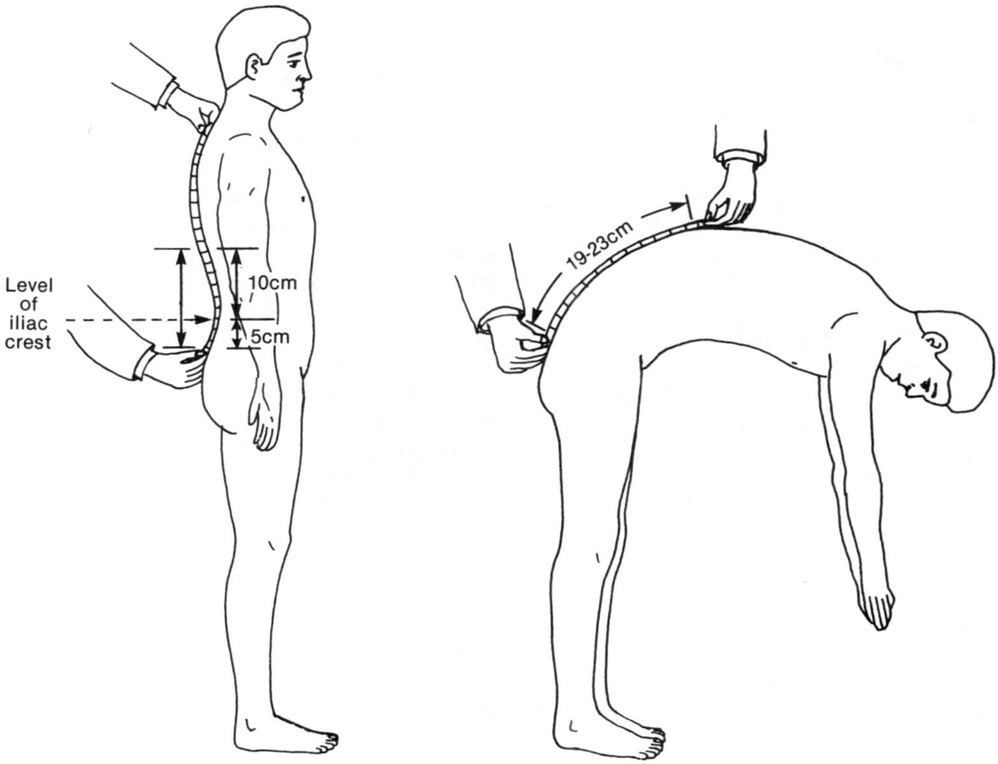

FIGURE 1.2 The Schober test, for measuring forward flexion of the lumbar spine (see text).

The sacrum articulates with the bony pelvis by means of the sacroiliac joints. These joints are narrow and stabilized by unusually strong dense ligaments and there is very little movement in these joints. Inflammatory disease of the sacroiliac (SI) joints is usually manifest by direct tenderness over the sacroiliac areas. This finding can be quite nonspecific, however, since there are several periarticular structures which may be tender, such as tendon-muscle attachments, muscle, bony prominences, and superficial fat pads. The SI joints can be more specifically compressed by having the patient lie on his side and using firm sustained downward pressure over the iliac crest. A positive response is obtained when pain is reproduced in the sacroiliac joint region.

Careful neurologic examination of the upper and lower extremities is an obviously necessary part of the evaluation of any condition involving neck or back pain. Careful attention to muscle strength, reflexes, and sensation is helpful in excluding significant nerve root irritation or spinal cord compression. Rectal and pelvic exam should be a routine part of the evaluation for low back pain.

The straight leg raising test is carried out with the patient flat on the examining table. The examiner gradually and passively flexes the thigh while holding the knee fully extended. The patient's other leg and thigh should be stabilized in extension while this test is being performed. This test will produce tension on the sciatic nerve and hamstring muscles, but normally each leg and thigh should be raised almost to a right angle without discomfort. This test is considered to be positive when pain is reproduced in the hip or low back region on the side being tested, and suggests nerve root irritation or muscle spasm.

The Shoulder

The shoulder is the most mobile joint of the body and is actually a composite of several joints which all contribute to the total motion; viewed anteriorly, the structures about the shoulder are demonstrated in Figure 1.3. The glenohumeral joint is a spheroidal or ball-in-socket joint formed by the articulation of the head of the humerus with the shallow glenoid cavity of the scapula. It is protected superiorly by an arch formed by the coracoid process, the acromion, and the coracoacromial ligament. Also contributing to shoulder movement are the joints on either end of the clavicle. Medially, the sternoclavicular joint is a simple spheroidal joint with a fibrous disc. This joint can become involved in a variety of articular processes and careful inspection and palpation here may reveal swelling, redness, or tenderness. Laterally, the acromioclavicular joint lies near the surface of the skin, and palpation here may reveal swelling and tenderness as well. The scapulothoracic articulation, although not really a joint, allows for most of the final 90° of vertical motion when the arm is raised above the head.

The glenohumeral joint is surrounded by a fibrous articular capsule which is very loose and allows considerable freedom of movement. The capsule has two openings. One is an aperture in the attachment of articular capsule to the humerus that allows the long tendon of the biceps to enter the bicipital groove and attach to the superior aspect of the glenohumeral fossa. Another opening permits a synovial reflection to function as a subscapular bursa. Above the joint capsule lies the broad flat tendons of the rotator cuff muscles: the supraspinatus, infraspinatus, subscapularis, and teres minor muscles. The tendons of these muscles merge together as they insert onto the lesser tubercle of the humerus and form a fibrous reinforcement to the articular capsule. The supraspinatus muscle lies mostly superiorly and functions primarily as an abductor. The subscapularis lies anteriorly and serves as an internal rotator. The infraspinatus and teres minor tendons lie mostly posteriorly and serve as external rotators. Overlying the

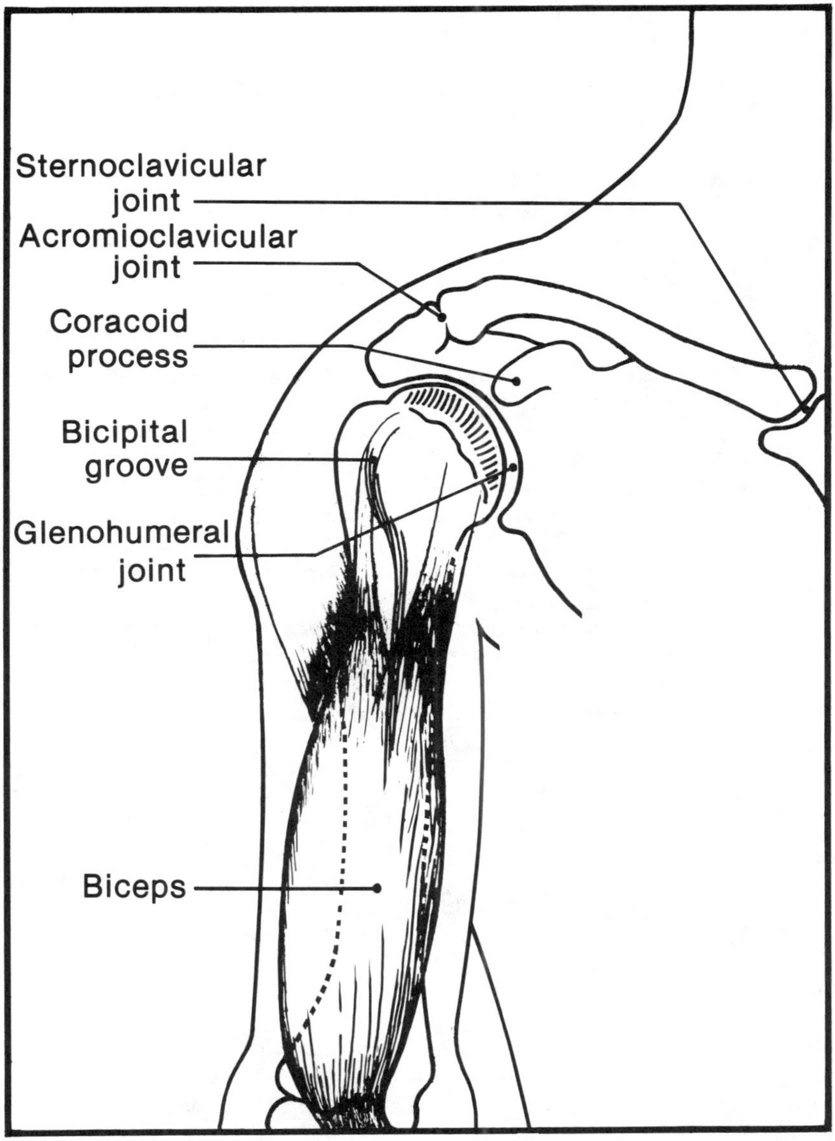

FIGURE 1.3 The shoulder: anterior view of external structures.

rotator cuff tendons is the subacromial bursa, which extends laterally as the subdeltoid bursa. This bursa communicates with the joint cavity in approximately 20-33% of individuals (6). Similarly, tears in the rotator cuff tendons are likely to result in a communication between the bursa and the joint cavity.

Inspection of the shoulder should begin with careful attention to symmetry. Glenohumeral swelling is usually not easily visible unless there has been extension into the subacromial bursa, although some distention may be detected over the anterior aspect of the joint. Palpation may reveal tenderness over the lateral aspect of the humeral head when there is pathology within the rotator cuff. The long head of the biceps tendon, as it travels in the bicipital groove anteriorly, is in a particularly good place for direct palpation. This tendon can be rolled under the fingertips while palpating along the anterior aspect of the humeral shaft. Severe pain can be elicited in this area by forced supination of the forearm against resistance (Yergason's sign).

Range of motion in the shoulder is very complex, but abnormalities here can be screened for by asking the patient to perform four simple maneuvers, as shown in Figure 1.4:

1. Each arm should be raised above the head in a wide sideways arc, finally attempting to touch the palmar surfaces of the hands together above the head.
2. With both elbows extended, the patient is asked to move both arms upward in a wide forward arch and touch the palms together above the head.
3. The patient should touch both hands on top of his head with elbows flexed and back as far as possible.
4. The patient should reach around to his back and place the back of his hand as high as possible between the scapulae.

If a patient can perform all of these movements smoothly, then glenohumeral pathology is essentially ruled out.

When abnormalities are found, careful assessment of internal rotation, external rotation, and abduction should be performed. During these maneuvers, the examiner should stabilize the scapula with one hand while he passively moves the arm with the other hand. Under these circumstances, about 90° of abduction should be possible as well as 90° of internal and external rotation.

Rotator cuff tears produce limitation of active abduction. Patients with a partial tear of the rotator cuff may be able to initiate abduction, but are unable to complete movement to a horizontal position. If the arm is passively abducted to a horizontal position, the patient may be able to raise the arm further by use of the deltoid muscle. Under these circumstances, if the arm is lowered slightly below the horizontal, it may fall suddenly to the patient's side. This test of the integrity of the rotator cuff is known as the "drop arm sign."

The Elbow

The elbow is a hinged joint formed by the articulation of the distal humerus with the olecranon fossa of the ulna and with the head of the radius. These articulations allow flexion and extension as well as some rotation of the forearm on the upper arm. All of these junctions are enclosed by an articular capsule with a common synovial cavity, making the synovial membrane relatively extensive. The synovial membrane itself is usually palpable only in the posterior aspect, as shown in Figure 1.5. Other important structures around the elbow include the large olecranon bursa and the epicondyles of the humerus. The lateral epicondyle serves as an attachment for the extensor muscles of the forearm, while the flexor muscles attach at the medial epicondyle.

The elbow joint itself is best assessed initially by screening range of motion. The normal elbow will extend to 0° (forearm directly in line with the upper arm). The joint should flex normally to 150–160°. About 90° of pronation and supination of the forearm should be possible. Full range of motion of the elbow joint without reproducing pain is very helpful in excluding an intrinsic articular problem as a cause for elbow pain.

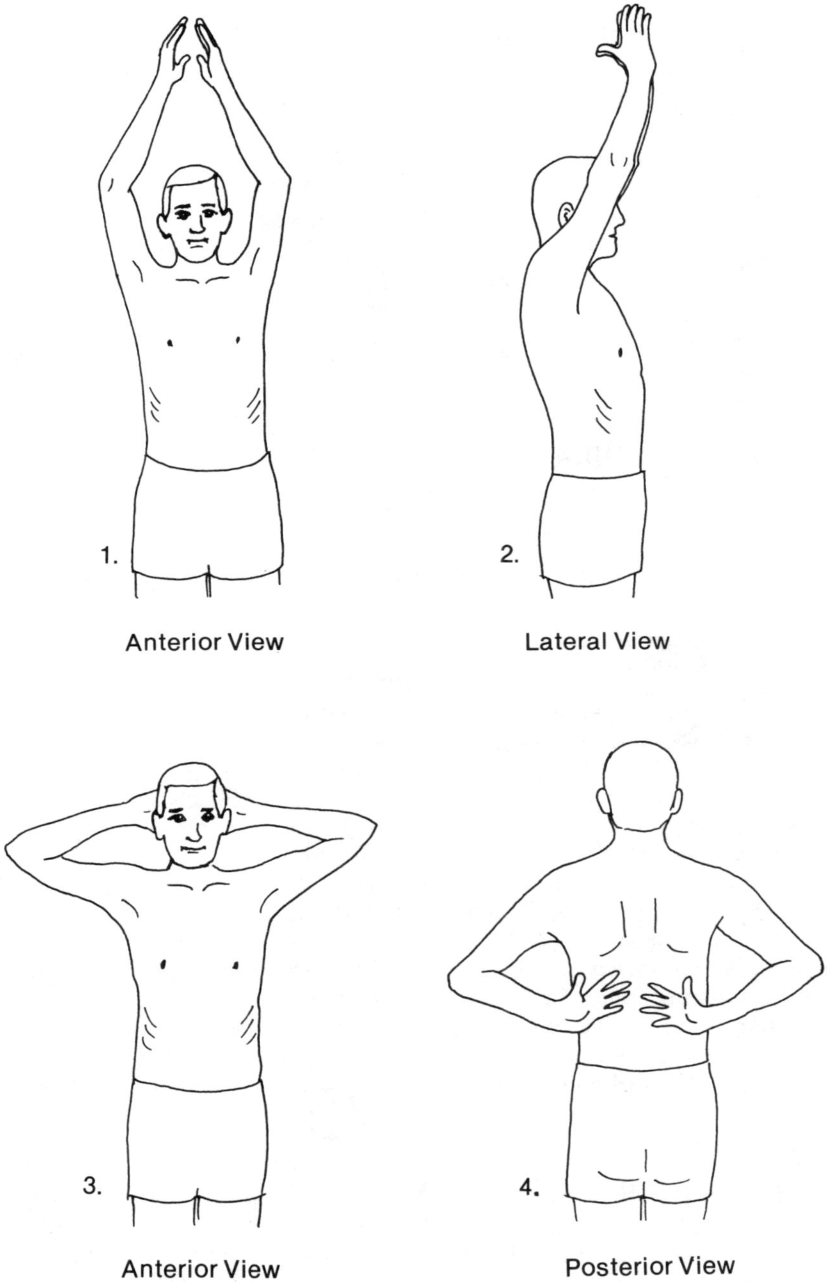

FIGURE 1.4 Exam for shoulder movement (see text).

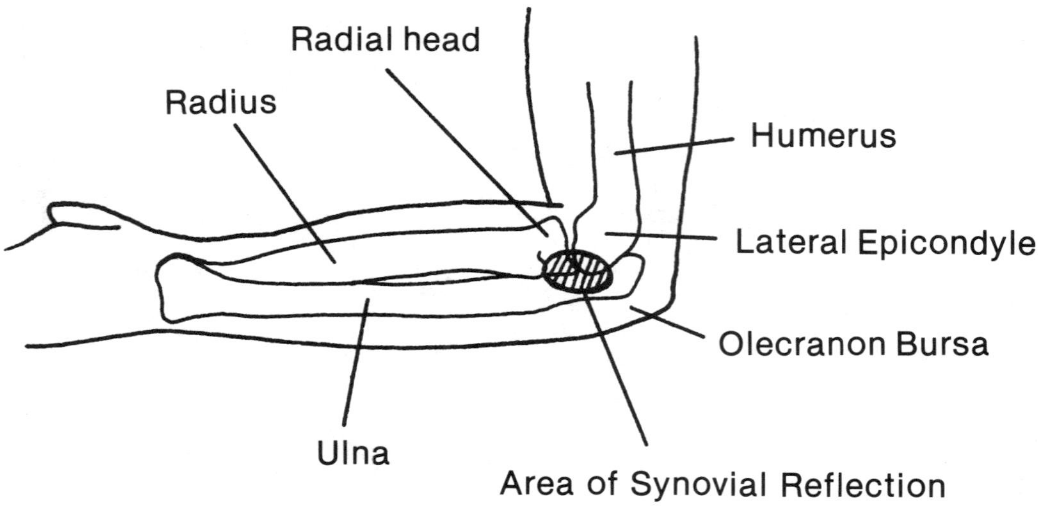

FIGURE 1.5 The landmarks of the elbow (lateral view).

Careful inspection and palpation of the elbow are necessary to evaluate the periarticular structures. The olecranon bursa, lying directly over the olecranon process, can be palpated easily for fluid, tenderness, or heat. This is a particularly common location for subcutaneous nodules which may be large enough to be seen, but sometimes are only palpable. These may occur in rheumatoid arthritis and gout and may also occur distal to the elbow along the ulnar shaft. Along the lateral aspect of the elbow is the lateral epicondyle. Tenderness here is commonly known as tennis elbow (lateral epicondylitis). The area between the olecranon process, the lateral epicondyle, and the radial head is the area where the joint capsule is closest to the skin and thus most easily palpable. This area should be carefully examined for synovial thickening, fluid, and tenderness and is the location at which arthrocentesis for synovial fluid is best accomplished. Synovial thickening may also be palpated in the groove medial to the olecranon process, where the ulnar nerve is also very close to the skin. The bony prominence of the medial epicondyle is also a site of irritation, and tenderness here is noted as golfer's elbow (medial epicondylitis).

The Wrist and Hand

No examination of the musculoskeletal system is complete without a thorough assessment of the physical findings and function of the wrists and hands. This functional unit is highly specialized in sensibility and complex movements that are important in the majority of activities of daily living. Thus, even the slightest compromise of function here will be quickly detected by the patient.

Hands and wrists are extremely important in the differential diagnosis of rheumatic diseases. Many disorders affect only the hands, and most involve them at one time or another (10). Probably more diagnostic information can be obtained by careful observation of the pattern of joint involvement in the hand and wrist than in any other part of the body.

The wrist is essentially three joints—the radiocarpal, the intercarpal, and the distal radioulnar joints—as demonstrated in Figure 1.6. Most of the movement of the wrist takes place at the radiocarpal joint. The small joint between the radius and ulna allows a small amount of pronation and supination, but generally allows very little movement unless diseased. The intercarpal articulation is a complex interconnecting joint that permits some degree of flexion and extension between the proximal and distal rows of the carpal bones. Swelling of the wrist is usually most evident on the dorsal aspect and may be localized or diffuse. Localized swelling may resemble cysts and result from synovial reflections from tendon sheaths or from the wrist joint itself. Ganglia are cystic enlargements that characteristically occur on the dorsal surface, but usually between the tendons or tendon sheaths. They do not communicate with the joints and rarely cause symptoms other than localized swelling or mild discomfort. Synovitis of the wrist is indicated by swelling or soft tissue fullness. This is usually characterized by tenderness and localized warmth and is best detected over the dorsal aspect as well. In the palmar aspect of the wrist, the long flexor tendons of the forearm muscles are enclosed in a common sheath that extends to the midpalm and lies within the relatively narrow carpal tunnel under the transverse carpal ligaments. The median nerve is contained within this area, and swelling or edema may cause compression, producing the carpal tunnel syndrome. Diagnostic signs for carpal tunnel syndrome include Tinel's sign and Phalen's sign. Tinel's sign is elicited by percussion of the

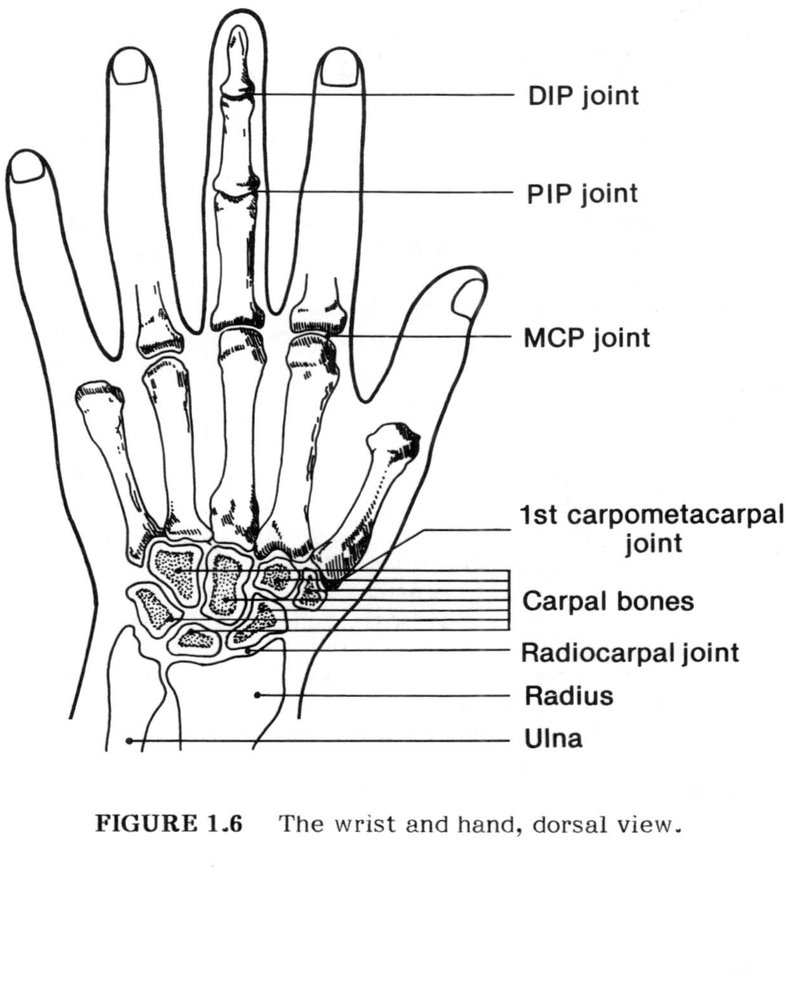

FIGURE 1.6 The wrist and hand, dorsal view.

volar aspect of the wrist over the median nerve and this will produce a tingling sensation over the distribution of the median nerve. Phalen's sign is positive when the wrist is maintained in palmar flexion for 60 seconds, producing numbness and paraesthesias over the same area. Subtle degrees of swelling can be detected in the palmar compartment as well, and the thenar eminence of the palm should be inspected carefully for atrophy and compared to that of the other hand.

The wrist should normally flex to about 90° from neutral position and extend to 70°. This can usually be done actively and passively and should not cause pain. Early synovitis of the wrist can be detected by the reproduction of pain with these maneuvers. The head of the ulna is usually prominent on the dorsal aspect of the wrist. Pressure over this area usually results in little or no movement. When the radioulnar joint is diseased, the distal ulna will become more movable, resulting in the characteristic "piano key sign" seen frequently in rheumatoid arthritis. Pain and tenderness localized to the radial aspect of the wrist can result from tendinitis of the abductor pollices longus and extensor pollices brevis as they pass near the radial styloid process. This is known as deQuervain's disease. This is confirmed by the Finklestein test performed by clenching the thumb tightly in the fist and placing the wrist in forced ulnar deviation, reproducing pain in this area. On the palmar surface of the hand, the tendons should be individually inspected for abnormalities. Idiopathic thickening and contracture of the palmar aponeurosis (Dupuytren's contracture) can be felt within individual tendons and is sometimes associated with bound-down skin in the involved area. More localized thickenings (tenosynovitis) can be palpated in the flexor tendons in the palm, usually at the level of the metacarpal head. Because of the relationship of the various flexor tendons here, such an enlargement may result in temporary or even persistent locking of the digit on flexion or extension. This can sometimes be released forcibly resulting in an audible or palpable click. This condition is known as a "trigger finger" and most commonly involves the first and fourth fingers (6).

As shown in Figure 1.6, the joints of the hand distal to the wrist consist of four parallel rows of articulations: the carpal-metacarpal (CMC), metacarpal-phalangeal (MCP), proximal interphalangeal (PIP), and distal interphalangeal (DIP). The first CMC is a relatively mobile joint and may characteristically be affected in osteoarthritis with resulting tenderness and bony enlargement. The rest of the CMC joints are relatively immobile except for some movement of the fifth CMC, and are rarely involved in arthritis except by extension from the wrist joint.

The MCP joints are hinged joints with dense palmar and collateral ligaments. These ligaments are loose in extension, permitting some ulnar and radial deviation here. The dorsal surface is protected by a thin capsule reinforced by extensor tendons across the joint. The PIP and DIP joints are hinged joints that permit flexion but little lateral movement.

An overview of hand function and involvement may be obtained by having the patient make a fist and then open and spread the fingers. Grip strength can be assessed by having the patient squeeze the examiner's second and third fingers as tightly as possible. This can be further quantitated by use of a folded blood pressure cuff as mentioned previously. Screening for synovitis in the MCP's can be accomplished by squeezing across the entire arch of MCP's. Tenderness elicited by this maneuver should be followed up with individual palpation of each MCP joint. The PIP's and DIP's should be similarly assessed for warmth, tenderness, and enlargement. Finally, the skin of the hand should be examined carefully for dorsal thickening and tightness as might be seen in scleroderma. Infarcts in the digital pulp and periungual areas can be visible in various types of vasculitis. Telangectasia may be noted in scleroderma, lupus, or overlap syndromes.

Characteristic abnormalities of the hands should be sought. Bony enlargement of the DIP's (Bouchard's nodes) and PIP's (Heberden's nodes) are characteristic of osteoarthritis. Diffuse symmetric swelling, particularly when it involves the MCP's and wrists, is more typical of rheumatoid arthritis. More active and long-standing rheumatoid disease may result in ulnar deviation at the MCP joints as well as characteristic subluxations of the IP joints (the swan-neck and boutonnière deformities discussed in Chapter 8). The fingernails should be inspected for irregularity or pitting as might be seen in the arthritis accompanying psoriasis or Reiter's syndrome.

The Hip and Pelvis

The hip is a ball-in-socket joint formed by the articulation of the rounded head of the femur with the cup-shaped cavity of the acetabulum. It is a weight-bearing joint with a wide range of motion and great stability. The hip has many similarities to the shoulder, being stronger and more stable but less mobile than the shoulder. The synovial membrane of the hip is not palpable or visible and must be examined indirectly. The hip joint is surrounded by powerful and well-balanced muscles that serve to move the extremity and maintain the upright position of the trunk. Extension is performed by the gluteus maximus and hamstring muscles as well as one head of the adductor muscle. Flexion is carried out by the psoas major, iliacus, tensor fascia lata, rectus femoris, sartorius, pectineus, and abductor longus. Abduction is achieved by the gluteus medius and minimus and adduction by a group of medial muscles (the adductor mechanism). Rotation involves a combination of these movements. There are several bursae located about the hip girdle, as shown in Figure 1.7. The iliopectineal bursa lies between the deep surface of the iliopsoas muscle and the anterior surface of the joint. The trochanteric bursa is situated between the gluteus maximus and the lateral surface of the greater trochanter. The ischiogluteal bursa overlies the ischial tuberosity posteriorly in close proximity to the sciatic nerve.

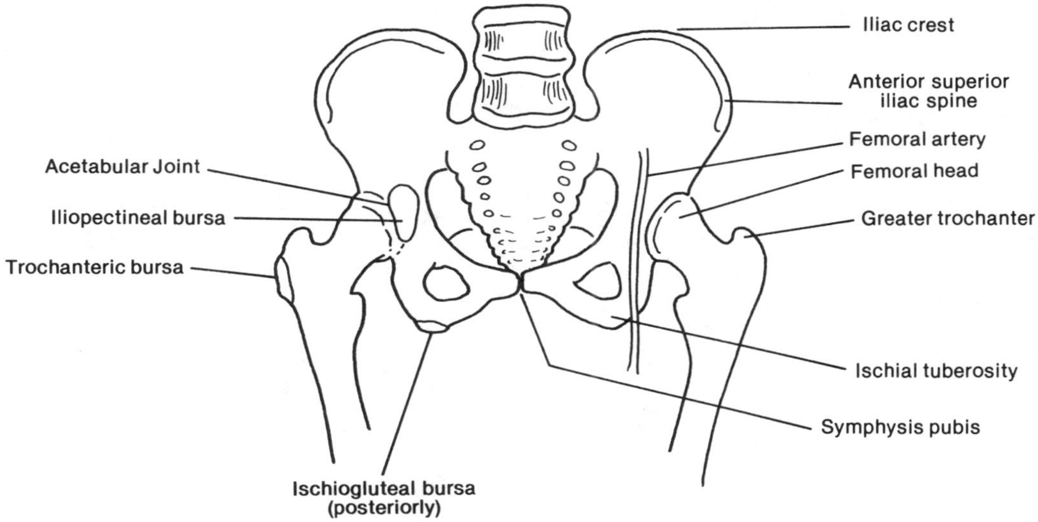

FIGURE 1.7 Structures around the hip.

Hip function is first assessed by observation of the patient's gait, body habitus, and pelvic tilt. Several types of limp or abnormalities of gait are associated with disease of the hip. In general, when a hip is painful or diseased, the body will tilt toward the involved side and become balanced in this position by leaning towards the affected side, thrusting the weight directly over the hip joint and decreasing the necessity for muscles to hold the pelvis level here. This is known as antalgic gait. With the patient standing, leg length discrepancy can be screened for by comparing the levels of the iliac crests. Some deformities may be apparent in a standing position, such as the placement of one hip in front of the other because of flexion contracture.

Palpation about the hip is best directed by the patient's symptoms. The area over the greater trochanter and over the ischiogluteal tuberosity should be palpated to detect bursitis in these locations. Pain originating from the hip joint itself is usually felt in the anterior thigh or groin. Sometimes the patient is unable to define the pain and can only locate the area as a deep general pain in the region of the hip.

Hip range of motion is best ascertained on the examining table. The normal hip has about 15° of extension, 120° of flexion (with knee flexed), 40° of abduction, and 40–45° of internal and external rotation. Extension is best tested in the prone position with the examiner pulling the straight leg back while stabilizing the pelvis. With the patient supine, a simple test for detecting most of the movements of the hip can be performed. This is known as the heel-to-knee test (Patrick test) shown in Figure 1.8. In this test the hip and knee are flexed so that the heel lies

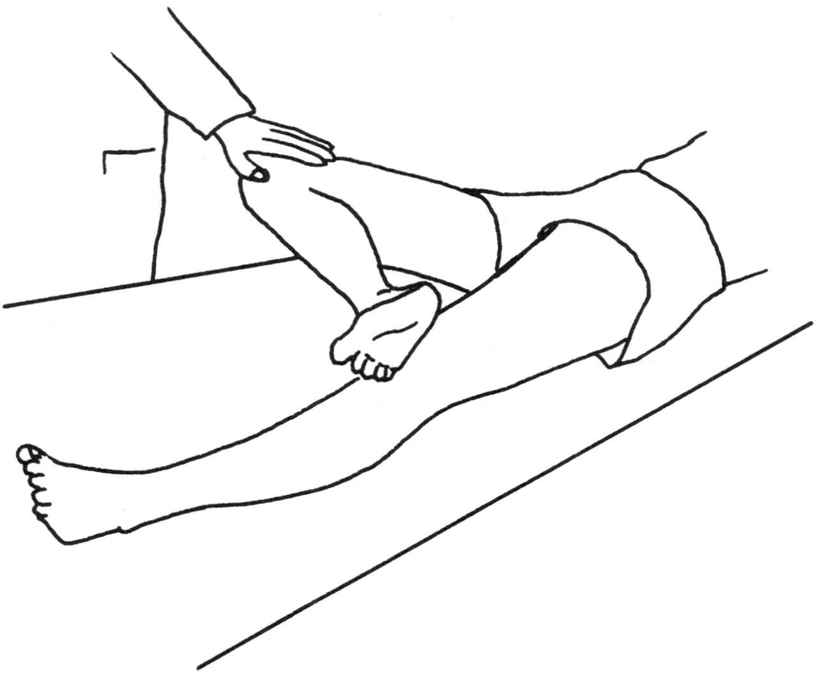

FIGURE 1.8 Fabere or Patrick test for assessing hip movement (see explanation in text).

beside or on top of the opposite extended knee. The hip is then abducted and externally rotated as far as possible. Pain, muscle spasm, or limitation of motion of the hip suggests an abnormality within the hip joint itself. In a normal hip, motion is normal and no pain or discomfort occurs. Motions of the hip tested in this maneuver are flexion, abduction, external rotation and, at the completion, extension. This test is sometimes designated as the "fabere sign," after the initial letters of these motions. Abnormality on this test should be followed up with more specific attempts to delineate exactly which motions are affected. It is important in assessing all hip movement to stabilize the pelvis with the opposite hand in order to avoid misinterpreting movement here.

The Knee

The knee is the largest and most complex joint in the body. It is functionally composed of three separate joints which share a common articular cavity. One articulation is located between the lateral femoral and tibial condyles and a similar articulation is formed medially. Each of these compartments contains a fibrocartilage meniscus in addition to hyaline cartilage over the articular surfaces. The third compartment lies anteriorly between the patella and the femur. The knee is stabilized by a combination of the articular capsule, the patellar ligament, the medial and lateral collateral ligaments, and the anterior and posterior cruciate ligaments.

As shown in Figure 1.9, the knee is complex both in its internal structure and surrounding landmarks. The synovial membrane is large and usually extends outside the actual joint and forms a pouch beneath the quadriceps muscle, normally extending as much as 6 cm above the superior pole of the patella. There are numerous bursae about the knee, many of which are inconsistent and variable from one patient to the next. A relatively large prepatellar bursa lies on the anterior aspect of the knee and separates the skin from the patella. There are other small

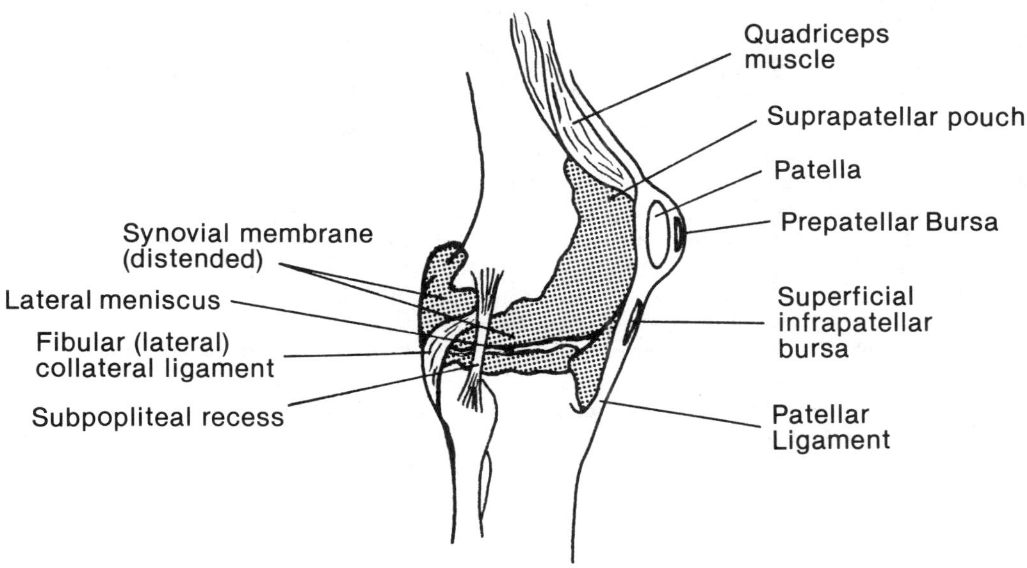

FIGURE 1.9 Structures around the knee (lateral view).

bursae located in the infrapatellar region anteriorly and the subpopliteal recess laterally. There are also small bursae in the area of the gastrocnemius muscle posteriorly and sometimes these communicate with the articular cavity. The anserine bursa is located on the medial aspect of the knee and is near the tendinous insertion of the sartorius muscle on the medial aspect of the tibia.

The knee should be examined in a standing position initially with careful attention paid to angular deformity, such as genu varus (bowlegs) and genu valgus (knock-knees) previously described. Backward bowing resulting from hyperextension of the joint is known as genu recurvatum. The knee should be carefully examined with the patient in a supine position so that all the muscles around the knee are fully relaxed and extended as fully as possible. Normal landmarks should be noted and both sides should be compared for swelling, changes in overlying skin color, and quadriceps tone and size. Significant synovial effusion is usually manifestested by swelling in the suprapatellar pouch. Swelling in the prepatellar bursa may be noted, and the popliteal space may be distended by herniation of the synovial membrane here (Baker's cyst). Palpation of the knee should begin with attention to temperature changes of the knee joint when compared to the opposite knee or surrounding skin. Effusions are probably better recognized in the knee than any other joint. The patella in a normal knee is easily compressed against the femoral condyles and produces a firm resistance. Fluid within the cavity of the knee joint will cause distension of the capsule on either side of the patella and a floating sensation when the patella is balloted. Smaller effusions may be identified by milking the fluid from the medial aspect of the knee into the suprapatellar pouch. Gentle pressure on the opposite side of the knee will result in the slow reaccumulation of fluid in the area milked and this is known as a "bulge sign." In obese patients, both of these signs can be very difficult to elicit and a large effusion may hide under large amounts of subcutaneous fat. It is often useful to place one hand over the suprapatellar area, while the other hand is placed with the thumb and index finger on opposite sides of the patella. Compression with one hand should result in the feeling of a fluid-filled sac pushing against the fingers of the other hand. Swelling and thickening from hypertrophic synovium will result in a doughy or boggy sensation rather than the feeling of fluid. Palpation of periarticular structures may reveal tenderness along the joint line without significant synovial thickening as is sometimes seen in meniscal injuries. Ligamentous stability should be tested by stressing the medial and lateral collateral ligaments. Cruciate ligaments may be tested by the "drawer test." With the knee in a flexed position, the examiner should be able to detect instability by pushing and pulling on the lower leg. Normal ligaments should allow very little movement with this maneuver.

The normal knee is a hinged joint that should extend to 0° and flex actively or passively to roughly 130-150°. Palpation of the knee during movement is useful for detecting crepitus, a common finding in osteoarthritis. To detect significant patellofemoral disease, the patella should be held distally and an isometric quadriceps contracture against resistance should be requested. Normally, a patient is able to produce a strong effective contraction. Patients with significant patellofemoral disease, such as chondromalacia, will have an initial contraction followed by reflex relaxation and discomfort (11). Other structures about the knee may be tender, particularly the prepatellar and anserine bursae.

The Ankle and Foot

As shown in Figure 1.10, the ankle articulation actually is composed of a true ankle joint (talocrural joint), subtalar joint, and intertarsal joints, between the talus and the other bones of the hind foot and midfoot. The true ankle joint is a

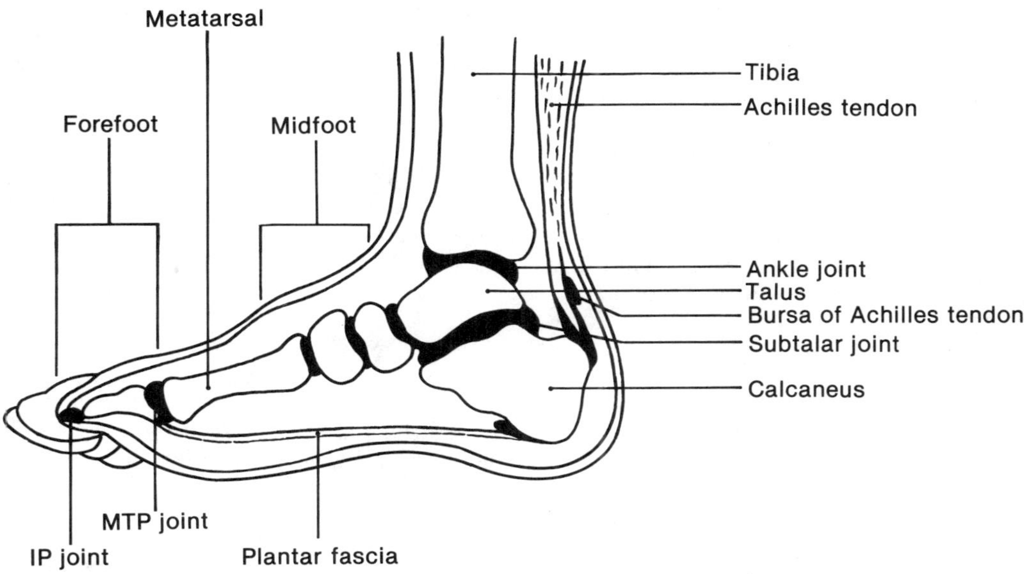

FIGURE 1.10 The foot and ankle.

hinged joint whose movement is limited almost entirely to plantar flexion and dorsal flexion. The subtalar and intertarsal joints allow the foot to invert and evert. The vast majority of the body weight is actually transmitted through the tibia to the talus, and the fibula produces lateral stability at the ankle. The metatarsophalangeal (MTP) joints and the proximal and distal interphalangeal joints of the foot are similar to the corresponding joints in the hand. Each has an articular capsule lined with a synovial membrane and various supporting ligaments. Several bursae are located about the foot. There are bursae located adjacent to the first and fifth MTP joints and several bursae are located about the heel, both posteriorly near the achilles tendon insertion and on the plantar surface near the attachment of the plantar fascia. Observation of the foot and ankle in a standing position will reveal subluxation of the ankle joint. Careful inspection of the feet for location of callus formation, subcutaneous nodules, bursal reactions, and also appearance of the nails can be helped in indicating areas of abnormal pressure or friction. Callus and bursal reactions in particular will indicate areas of unusual pressure related to underlying joint deformities. Examination of the patient's shoe will also help illustrate how the patient walks.

Palpation of the ankle should be performed with particular attention to the anterior aspect and the recesses under the malleoli on both sides. The synovial membrane is closest to the surface at these points, and thickening, warmth, and swelling may be detected. Swelling within the ankle joint should be differentiated from diffuse swelling seen in patients with peripheral edema of the extremity. From a neutral position perpendicular to the lower leg, the normal ankle joint should dorsiflex about 20° and plantar flex 45°. Inversion of 30° and eversion of 20° should be possible at the subtalar joint. The heel should be palpated for tenderness near the achilles tendon insertion and along the plantar aspect at the insertion of the plantar fascia. Swelling, tenderness, and warmth of the midfoot may be detected by careful palpation. Usually these signs are present on the dorsal rather than the plantar aspect. The MTP joints should be palpated for localized tenderness and the undersurface observed for abnormal callus formation and deformity.

Metatarsalgia, or pain and tenderness of the plantar surface, is a common complaint that may occur alone or in association with arthritis or overuse. Interdigital neuroma (Morton's toe) causes similar pain, but tenderness is usually between or distal to the heads of the metatarsals, most commonly between the third and fourth metatarsals. A tarsal tunnel syndrome, similar to the carpal tunnel syndrome in the hand, occurs when the posterior tibial nerve is irritated as it passes under the medial malleolus.

Hypermobile Joints

Although most arthritic processes result in loss of motion of joints, on occasion syndromes may be manifest by hypermobility of the joints. Heritable disorders of connective tissue such as Marfan's syndrome, Ehlers-Danlos syndrome, and osteogenesis imperfecta as well as the benign hypermobile joint syndrome may be characterized by generalized joint hypermobility. Criteria have been set forth for the diagnosis of generalized hypermobility, with three of the following five conditions being necessary: 1) the ability to hyperextend the elbows beyond 180°, 2) hyperextension of the knees beyond 180°, 3) ability to touch the thumb to the forearm on flexion at the wrist, 4) the ability to make the fingers parallel to the forearm on extension of the wrist and MCP joints, 5) the ability to dorsiflex the foot to greater than 45° (12). Patients with generalized joint hypermobility are probably predisposed to developing dislocation, subluxations, and possibly premature osteoarthritis.

In Marfan's syndrome, the feature of arachnodactyly results in elongation of the digits. One means of detecting this is by having the patient grip the wrist with the other hand about 4 cm proximal to the radial styloid. Appreciable overlapping of the thumb and fifth finger is abnormal. This is known as the "wrist sign of Walker and Murdoch." In another test of arachnodactyly and ligamentous laxity in the hands of patients with Marfan's, the patient makes a fist with the thumb inside the flexed fingers across the palm. In such patients, the distal portion of the thumb will extend well beyond the ulnar margin of the hand. This is known as the "thumb sign of Steinberg."

Fibrositis and Trigger Points

Many patients present with nonspecific musculoskeletal pains and few abnormalities can be found on specific examination of the joints. The fibrositis syndrome, or fibromyalgia, is an entity which has been described in which patients have such complaints and have various tender points throughout the body. Certain areas of the body appear to be more sensitive to pressure than other areas and these are particularly tender in patients with this syndrome. These include the trapezius skinfolds, the supraspinatus ligaments on the upper borders of the scapula, and the ligaments in the lower cervical intraspinous spaces. The anterior costochondral junctions and lateral and medial epicondyles at the elbows are areas in the upper extremity worth examining. In the low back, patients frequently have tenderness in the lower lumbar intraspinous ligaments and in the areas of the ligaments and bursae of the upper and outer quadrants of the buttocks. The greater trochanters and anserine bursa regions of the knee are also areas that seem to be particularly sensitive in patients with this syndrome. Attention to these areas is a worthwhile part of any physical exam in a patient with widespread pain and few specific findings on examination of the joints themselves. Further discussion of fibrositis can be found in Chapter 12.

The Differential Diagnosis of Musculoskeletal Complaints

Although the exact diagnosis is not always made on the basis of history and physical examination alone, several general questions should be answered before proceeding to laboratory examination, x-rays, or synovial fluid analysis:

1. Is this an articular or nonarticular process? Although the history will usually suggest the answer to this question, the physical examination is usually necessary. Not all musculoskeletal pain is related to pathology within the joint. A diseased joint will usually have findings localized to the joint, and range of motion is usually affected at the very least by pain on movement of the joint. The examiner should be able to elicit periarticular foci that may be responsible for the entire pain syndrome. Identification of periarticular causes of pain significantly alters the diagnostic and therapeutic approach to the patient.
2. Is this an acute or chronic problem? Problems lasting less than 4-6 weeks are usually considered acute or self-limited, while those lasting longer are considered chronic. Obviously, the distinction is artificial and several variations are seen. An additive pattern of arthritis is that in which the initial features persist while new features are added on over a period of time. A migratory pattern is one in which an initially painful joint will totally subside while other joints become symptomatic. Palindromic or intermittent patterns are those in which repetitive attacks occur and then completely remit between attacks.
3. Is this a monoarticular (localized) or polyarticular (diffuse) process? By definition, monoarticular means one joint or joint-related structure. In practice, involvement of as many as two or three separate joints, although actually oligoarticular, can still be approached as a more or less monoarticular problem. The distinction here again can be artificial, as many polyarticular diseases may have a monoarticular component, particularly at the onset of illness.
4. Is this an inflammatory or noninflammatory process? Probably the most important point in the history is the duration of morning stiffness. Noninflammatory processes may be associated with several minutes of morning stiffness, but inflammatory disorders are invariably associated with stiffness of at least 1 hour's duration. On physical examination, the detection of warmth is probably the most important feature in differentiating inflammatory from noninflammatory disease. Pain on movement and detection of synovial thickening and swelling are more compatible with an inflammatory process but are less specific.
5. Is this an axial or peripheral arthropathy? This feature of the pattern of joint involvement is very helpful in differentiating the various types of arthritis. The term axial refers not only to the spine but also to other centrally located joints, such as the temporomandibular, sternoclavicular, and shoulder joints as well as the hips and sacroiliac joints. The distinction here is particularly helpful in differentiating the seronegative spondyloarthropathies from those arthropathies which are more related to autoimmunity, such as rheumatoid arthritis or lupus.

6. Is this a symmetric or asymmetric process? This distinction is important in differentiating rheumatoid arthritis, the classic symmetric arthritis, from all sorts of other arthropathies and nonarticular problems.
7. Is the condition systemic or strictly limited to the joints? Several elements in the history should be helpful in suggesting this. Although many patients complain primarily of musculoskeletal symptoms, a careful review of systems will bring out symptoms of generalized systemic illness, such as fever, malaise, weight loss, or anorexia. Evidence of pulmonary, gastrointestinal, dermatologic, renal, or cardiovascular disease may provide important diagnostic information. Many systemic diseases present with musculoskeletal complaints while many rheumatic diseases have systemic manifestations which are either intrinsically part of the disease process (e.g., the rash of psoriatic arthritis, Raynaud's phenomenon, and pulmonary fibrosis in scleroderma or cutaneous ulceration in polyarteritis nodosa), or are recognized extraarticular complications of the disease (e.g., aortic sufficiency in ankylosing spondylitis, or pulmonary nodules in rheumatoid arthritis).

After answering these basic questions, the clinician should have at least a general idea of the nature of the illness being dealt with, if not a specific diagnosis. Only with more specific knowledge about the various disease entities can a reasonable differential diagnosis be considered.

Acute monoarthritis may be caused by several conditions, summarized in Table 1.3. Acute noninflammatory conditions often result from trauma, which may range from blunt trauma to subtle internal mechanical problems. In the proper racial and age setting, sickle cell arthropathy should also be considered. Gout and pseudogout should be top considerations in acute inflammatory arthritis, but the presence of fever or chills should suggest an infectious cause. The other conditions listed usually involve several joints, but may on occasion cause a monoarticular problem.

The differential diagnosis of chronic monoarthritis is listed in Table 1.4. Among noninflammatory causes, osteoarthritis is by far the most common, but the other entities should be suspected when the presentation is unusual or when radiographs show very few changes of osteoarthritis. Chronic, indolent infections, such

TABLE 1.3 Differential Diagnosis of Acute Monoarthritis

- Noninflammatory
    - Traumatic arthritis
    - Sickle cell arthropathy
- Inflammatory
    - Gout
    - Pseudogout
    - Infectious: gonococcal or other bacterial
    - Reiter's disease
    - Enteropathic arthritis
    - Palindromic rheumatism
    - Rheumatoid arthritis

TABLE 1.4 Differential Diagnosis of Chronic Monoarthritis

Noninflammatory
Osteoarthritis
Neuropathic arthropathy
Reflex sympathetic dystrophy
Traumatic arthritis
Tumor (bone)
Osteomyelitis
Bursitis and tendinitis
Nerve entrapment
Inflammatory
Tuberculous arthritis
Fungal arthritis
Rheumatoid arthritis
Reiter's syndrome
Psoriatic arthritis
Hemophilic arthropathy
Synovial neoplasm

as those seen with tuberculosis or fungi, should be considered first in any chronic inflammatory monoarticular condition, although many other conditions may cause this as well.

Acute polyarthritis may occur in a wide variety of conditions listed in Table 1.5. In a young, sexually active patient, gonococcal arthritis should be a first consideration and the physician should be alert to other possible signs of this, including tenosynovitis and characteristic pustular rash. Sarcoidosis, rheumatic fever, Reiter's syndrome and the prodromal stages of hepatitis B infection are all frequently associated with an acute polyarthritis, and should be suspected in the appropriate clinical setting. The other conditions listed may present in a variety of ways, but many are common enough to be suspected when other causes are not found. Rheumatoid arthritis, in particular, may present acutely in many joints with negative serologic tests, and may require careful follow-up before a diagnosis is established.

Chronic polyarthritis has many possible causes, listed in Table 1.6. Rheumatoid arthritis is probably the most common inflammatory type, while osteoarthritis is the most common noninflammatory type of chronic arthritis in multiple joints.

Arthritis localized to the axial skeleton should suggest the conditions listed in Table 1.7. Ankylosing spondylitis and the other spondyloarthropathies are characterized by sacroiliac disease and gradual loss of spinal mobility. Infectious sarcoiliitis or osteomyelitis should be considered when a relatively acute back syndrome is associated with fever. Osteoarthritis, osteoporosis with compression fractures, or herniated disc should be suspected in older patients or in those with a history of trauma, while referred pain syndromes should be considered where radiographic findings are minimal.

TABLE 1.5 Differential Diagnosis of Acute Polyarthritis

Gonococcal arthritis
Sarcoidosis
Rheumatic fever
Reiter's syndrome
Acute hepatitis B
Sickle cell arthropathy
Henoch-Schönlein purpura
Juvenile rheumatoid arthritis
Gout
Pseudogout
Enteropathic arthritis
Hypertrophic osteoarthropathy
Psoriatic arthritis
Leukemia
Polymyositis
Systemic lupus erythematosus
Rheumatoid arthritis

TABLE 1.6 Differential Diagnosis of Chronic Polyarthritis

Inflammatory
Rheumatoid arthritis
Systemic lupus erythematosus
Gout
Pseudogout
Juvenile rheumatoid arthritis
Psoriatic arthritis
Reiter's syndrome
Polymyositis
Polymyalgia rheumatica
Enteropathic arthritis
Hypertrophic osteoarthropathy
Noninflammatory
Osteoarthritis
Fibrositis
Metabolic bone disease
Hypothyroidism

TABLE 1.7 **Differential Diagnosis of Axial Arthropathy**

Ankylosing spondylitis
Reiter's syndrome
Psoriatic spondylitis
Enteropathic spondylitis
Infectious sacroiliitis
Osteomyelitis
Osteoarthritis (spondylosis)
Osteoporosis
Herniated disc
Referred pain

Arthrocentesis

The examination of synovial fluid is as important to the evaluation of joint disease as a urinalysis in renal disease (13). The synovial fluid provides direct information about the process occurring within the joint. Many common conditions may be diagnosed rapidly and definitively by synovial fluid examination even when only small amounts of fluid are available (see Chapter 2). Arthrocentesis should be performed as part of the diagnostic evaluation in any patient with joint disease. In patients with a known diagnosis, arthrocentesis should be performed whenever a superimposed secondary process, such as infection or crystal deposition, is suspected. Arthrocentesis may also be used to provide symptomatic relief in a painful swollen joint by removal of fluid, and is sometimes combined with local injection of an anesthetic or corticosteroid preparation for this purpose.

There are relatively few contraindications to arthrocentesis or local corticosteroid injection into joints (see Table 1.8) (14). The main risk of arthrocentesis is the introduction of infection into the joint. Although this is exceedingly rare, careful adherence to aseptic technique and avoidance of areas of cellulitis are absolute necessities.

The procedure may be performed on almost any synovial joint. Although sterile gloves and draping are unnecessary, strict asepsis should be observed. Most joints are most easily entered on the extensor surface where synovial fluid is palpable and closest to the skin. The area should be carefully palpated and the point of entry marked with a ballpoint pen with the writing portion retracted (this will leave an impression on the skin which will remain several minutes) (14). The skin should be carefully cleansed at least twice with an antiseptic-iodine solution. Local anesthetic is optional and may be achieved by topical ethylchloride spray or by intradermal-subcutaneous xylocaine. Using a 5-50-cc syringe with a 20-25-gauge needle, the joint should be entered through the previously made mark and fluid aspirated. Tubes for cell count, glucose determination, culture, and slides for wet preparation and gram stain should be available at the bedside (often a tray containing all the needed materials is convenient). If local corticosteroid is to be injected, the syringe may be removed, leaving the needle in place within the joint. As noted in Table 1.8, however, if infection is suggested by the initial appearance of the synovial fluid, corticosteroid injection should be deferred. When local corticosteroid is to be injected, the patient should be made aware of the small risk

TABLE 1.8 Contraindications to Arthrocentesis and Joint Injection

Contraindications to Arthrocentesis
- Periarticular infection
- Bacteremia (relative)
- Inaccessible joint (e.g., spine)
- Bleeding disorder (relative)

Contraindications to Local Corticosteroid Injection
- All of the above, plus:
  - Unstable joints
  - Articular infection
  - Intraarticular fracture
  - Frequent and multiple prior injections (relative)
  - Failure to respond to prior injection

of introducing infection, as well as the possibility of local skin atrophy or transient inflammation at the site of injection.

The knee is the easiest joint in the body to aspirate. The patient should be in a supine position, and the joint space is usually entered from the medial approach just under the midportion of the patella. The shoulder is best entered from an anterior approach with the patient seated or supine. The coracoid process should be palpated under the clavicle and a mark made 1-2 cm inferior and lateral from this point. With the arm held in external rotation, the needle should be directed slightly laterally to enter the joint. The ankle is best entered anteriorly at a point just above and lateral to the medial malleolus and medial to the extensor tendon of the great toe. The needle should be inserted about 1 in. to be within the joint. The subtalar joint may be entered laterally just beneath the lateral malleolus. The wrist is accessible from a dorsal approach just distal to the head of the radius. Although there is usually a depression here, fluid or synovial thickening may be felt here when the joint is affected. The elbow may be entered just below the lateral epicondyle and above the olecranon, at a point where thickened synovium or fluid may be palpated. The hip is a difficult joint to tap blindly, and fluoroscopic guidance is often necessary to ensure accuracy. With the patient supine, a needle may be inserted at a point 2-3 cm below the anterior superior iliac spine and 2-3 cm lateral to the femoral pulse. A $3\frac{1}{2}$-in. spinal needle may be needed for this approach. The small joints of the hands and feet are difficult to aspirate and inject. A small (22-25 gauge) needle should be inserted from a dorsal-lateral approach. Traction on distal part of the joint may allow the needle to enter the joint space more readily. As with any other joint with little fluid, care should be taken to express any small amount of fluid left in the bore of the needle (but not visible in the syringe), since even a single drop may be sufficient for some studies (such as crystal analysis).

References

1. Hollander JL: Introduction to arthritis and the rheumatic diseases. In DJ McCarty (ed.), *Arthritis and Allied Conditions,* 9th Ed. Philadelphia, Lea and Febiger, 1979, pp. 3-7.

2. Fries JF, Mitchell DM: Joint pain or arthritis. *JAMA* 235:199-204, 1976.

3. Arthritis Foundation, *Annual Report,* New York, 1976.

4. McCarty DJ: Differential diagnosis of arthritis; analysis of signs and symptoms. In DJ McCarty (ed.), *Arthritis and Allied Conditions,* 9th Ed. Philadelphia, Lea and Febiger, 1979, pp. 36-50.

5. Fries JF: General approach to the rheumatic disease patient. In WN Kelley, ED Harris, S Ruddy, CB Sledge (eds.), *Textbook of Rheumatology,* 1st Ed. Philadelphia, W. B. Saunders, 1981, pp. 353-358.

6. Polley HF, Hunder GG: *Rheumatologic Interviewing and Physical Examination of the Joints,* 2nd Ed. Philadelphia, W. B. Saunders, 1978.

7. McCarty, DJ, Gatter RA, Steele AD: A twenty-pound dolorimeter for quantification of articular tenderness. *Arthritis Rheum* 11:696-697, 1968.

8. Lee P, Baxter A, Dick WC, Webb J: Assessment of grip strength measurement in rheumatoid arthritis. *Scand J Rheumatol* 3:17-23, 1973.

9. Moll JMH, Wright V: Normal range of spinal mobility; An objective clinical study. *Ann Rheum Dis* 30:381-386, 1971.

10. Katz WA: The hands and wrists in the diagnosis of rheumatid diseases. In WA Katz (ed.), *Rheumatic Diseases: Diagnosis and Management,* 1st Ed. Philadelphia, J. B. Lippincott, 1977, pp. 27-70.

11. Convery FR, Convery MM: Examination of the joints. In WN Kelley, ED Harris, S Ruddy, CB Sledge (eds.), *Textbook of Rheumatology,* 1st Ed. Philadelphia, W. B. Saunders, 1981, pp. 359-383.

12. Wynne-Davies R: Acetabular dysplasia and familial joint laxity: Two etiological factors in congenital dislocation of the hip. J Bone Joint Surg 52B: 704-716, 1970.

13. Schumacher HR: Synovial fluid analysis. In WN Kelley, ED Harris, S Ruddy, CB Sledge (eds.), *Textbook of Rheumatology,* 1st Ed. Philadelphia, W. B. Saunders, 1981, pp. 568-579.

14. Owen DS: Aspiration and injection of joints and soft tissues. In WN Kelley, ED Harris, S Ruddy, CB Sledge (eds.), *Textbook of Rheumatology,* 1st Ed. Philadelphia, W. B. Saunders, 1981, pp. 553-567.

Chapter 2

LABORATORY TESTING IN RHEUMATOLOGY

Henry Rothberger, M.D., Tung-Kwang Lee, M.D., and Maria P. McGee, M.D.

In the practice of rheumatology, as in other medical specialties, laboratory testing is of importance for establishing diagnoses and monitoring disease activity. Tests described in this chapter are for the most part bioassays subject to considerable variation in performance from one laboratory to another. Although these tests are somewhat unique to rheumatology, it is surprising how often they are misunderstood or misinterpreted in view of the high prevalence of rheumatic disorders in the general population. As a supplement to information in this chapter, the reader is encouraged to inquire about details of quality assurance, specificity and sensitivity of tests offered by local laboratories. This knowledge is critical for interpretation of results.

Synovial Fluid Analysis

Synovial fluid is a plasma ultrafiltrate from subsynovial capillaries containing hyaluronic acid secreted by synovial cells. Hyaluronic-protein complexes account for the viscous nature of normal synovial fluid. The function of synovial fluid is to provide lubrication and nourishment for articular cartilage. Synovial fluid may be aspirated by arthrocentesis (see Chapter 1) or obtained during surgery. Normal synovial fluid is clear or pale-yellow, acellular, and highly viscous. Synovial fluid analysis is a simple method that permits immediate diagnosis of some diseases, particularly in establishing the diagnosis of infectious and crystal-induced arthritides (gout and pseudogout). All patients with synovial effusions and an undiagnosed arthritis should undergo arthrocentesis and synovial evaluation. Complete examination of the synovial fluid involves not only gross examination but also microscopic, biochemical, and bacteriologic evaluations.

Results of synovial analysis of normal and pathologic fluids are given in Table 2.1. Synovial fluids are typically grouped into one of three categories. Conditions

TABLE 2.1 General Grouping of Synovial Fluids Based on Synovial Analysis

	Normal	Group 1	Group 2	Group 3
Color	None	Yellow	Yellow	Varies
Clarity	Clear	Clear	Turbid	Purulent
Viscosity	High	Varies	Varies	Low
Mucin clot	Firm	Firm	Poor	Poor
WBC ($X10^3/mm^3$)	< 0.2	< 2	10-40	> 50
PMN's (%)	< 25	< 25	> 50	> 90
Glucose*	NL	NL	Low or NL	Very low
Complement	NL	Varies	Varies**	High
Culture	(-)	(-)	(-)	50% (+)
Crystal#	(-)	(+)	(+)	(-)

* Compared to blood
** Reduced in RA
\# Seen in crystal-induced arthropathies: monosodium urate crystals, seen in gout, are strongly negatively birefringent. Calcium pyrophosphate dihydrate (CPPD), seen in pseudogout, are weakly positively birefringent. (See further discussion in Chapter 11.)

associated with each type of fluid are as follows: 1) group 1 (noninflammatory): osteoarthritis, chronic crystal synovitis, neuropathic arthropathy, osteochondromatosis, sytemic lupus erythematosus (SLE), rheumatic fever, systemic sclerosis, aseptic necrosis; 2) group 2 (inflammatory): rheumatoid arthritis (RA), Reiter's syndrome, psoriatic arthritis, ankylosing spondylitis, acute crystal-induced synovitis, viral or fungal infection, SLE, rheumatic fever, psoriatic arthritis, systemic sclerosis, juvenile arthritis, Sjögren's syndrome, scleroderma, polymyositis; 3) group 3 (septic): bacterial infections.

The gross examination of synovial fluid includes inspection of volume, color, clarity, and viscosity. The existence of only a small amount of synovial fluid in the joint does not rule out the possibility of an important pathologic process. In rheumatoid arthritis, hundreds of ml of fluid may be present within the joint, but at other times there may be little appreciable increase of fluid. Clear fluids usually indicate a noninflammatory process, while opaque fluids usually indicate the presence of inflammation. Bloody synovial fluid is usually a result of trauma, tumor, or coagulopathy but may also be seen occasionally in RA, osteoarthritis, and pseudogout. Milky (chylous-like) fluid may occur in chronic RA, pancreatitis, SLE, or other miscellaneous conditions. Synovial fluid from patients with RA, acute crystal-induced synovitis and other chronic arthritides occasionally has a green color. In general, the viscosity of synovial fluid is decreased by inflammation, due to depolymerization of the hyaluronate-protein complexes (as seen in gout and RA patients).

At times it is preferable to add an anticoagulant to aspirated synovial fluid to prevent coagulation. Since citrate coagulants combine with calcium in synovial fluid to form crystals which confuse interpretation, the use of heparin is recommended.

The total white blood cell count (WBC) and differential counts of synovial fluid are very important in the diagnosis of arthritis. Under ordinary light microscopy, a direct smear of synovial fluid is helpful for estimating these counts. Since acid precipitates synovial fluid proteins, the use of 0.3% saline as a substitute for acetic acid to dilute the fluid and lyse red blood cells is important. The normal synovial fluid leukocyte count varies, but most authors accept 200 WBC/mm^3 as the upper limit. RA synovial fluid may have WBC counts from 2000 to 75,000 cells/mm^3 while the WBC count for bacterial arthritis is often greater than 100,000 cells/mm^3. In normal synovial fluids, the percentage of polymorphonuclear cells (PMN's) is less than 25%. The presence of only a few cells per high-power field suggests a noninflammatory disorder. In septic arthritis, smears usually reveal that more than 75% of cells are PMN's. Specimens from RA patients usually show numerous neutrophils containing phagocytized lipid and cell debris. The so-called RA cells or ragocytes which can be found among those patients with RA, gout, or septic arthritis are PMN's with small (0.5–2 μm), dark cytoplasmic granules primarily of immunoglobulins.

The purpose of polarizing microscopic examination of synovial fluid is primarily to detect crystals seen in gout (caused by monosodium urate crystals, MSU) and pseudogout (caused by calcium pyrophosphate dihydrate crystals, CPPD). This is a simple and rapid way to diagnose these diseases. Monosodium urate crystals of gout are usually needle-shaped (1–20 μm in length) and show strong negative birefringence. The property of birefringence results in changes of color (from yellow to blue) in visualizing the crystals as the microscope slide is rotated 90° in relation to a compensator. During an acute attack of gouty arthritis, the majority of MSU crystals are within neutrophils or macrophages. The CPPD crystals of pseudogout are usually rod-shaped or rectangular (1–20 μm in length and up to about 4 μm in width), and are positively birefringent. Cholesterol crystals can also be found in synovial fluid. These are found in RA and many other arthropathies and are irregular birefringent plates, often with notched margins. For further discussion of crystal-induced arthropathies, see Chapter 11.

The mucin clot test reflects polymerization of synovial fluid hyaluronates which will form a tight clot in contact with 2% acetic acid. The hyaluronate of synovial fluid in inflammation is degraded and diluted with exudates and does not form a normal mucin clot. The mucin clot becomes flocculent roughly in proportion to the degree of inflammation.

The normal concentration of glucose in synovial fluid is slightly lower than that of blood glucose. Infections often result in a very low level of glucose. Moderate decreases may occur in RA.

Bacteriologic culture is of prime importance in distinguishing group 2 from group 3 fluids, since overlap in the WBC count and other measures of inflammation occur between these groups. It is important to remember that septic arthritis and lupus, RA or crystal-induced arthritis can occasionally coexist. Further, in some types of infectious arthritis, such as that due to *Neisseria gonorrheae,* organisms are not readily cultured from joint fluids. This may be explained by the fact that joint inflammation in these processes may be mediated by immune complexes rather than by direct invasion of the synovial space by organisms. Synovial smears should also be examined for bacteria, using Gram stain, since information regarding the type of infecting organism will be available immediately, if the number of organisms is sufficient to give a positive stain. A further discussion of infectious arthritis may be found in Chapter 21.

Acute Phase Proteins (APP)

The acute phase proteins are a heterogeneous group of serum glycoproteins. Their concentration increases within the first few days following tissue damage or inflammation. This phenomenon is referred to as the acute phase response (APR), which may occur from a wide variety of stimuli. Protein changes during the APR may be classified into three groups (Table 2.2). The most widely used tests for APP in clinical medicine are measurements of the erythrocyte sedimentation rate and C-reactive protein.

Erythrocyte Sedimentation Rate (ESR)

After placing fresh homogenized and anticoagulated blood in a vertical standard glass tube, RBC's will tend to fall toward the bottom. The sedimentation rate of RBC in mm/hour is the ESR. This phenomenon is not totally understood but depends on rouleaux formation of RBC, which in turn likely depends on the negative surface charge (zeta potential) of the RBC. Increases in serum concentrations of asymmetrical molecules like fibrinogen or immunoglobulins will raise the dielectric constant of plasma, resulting in a reduction of the zeta potential. This promotes the aggregation of suspended RBC, leading to elevation of ESR. The concentration of any APP will affect the ESR, with fibrinogen having the greatest effect.

Among methods of determining the ESR, the Westergren technique remains the most useful. Two ml of homogenized venous blood (in 0.5 ml of a sodium citrate solution) are poured into a 30 cm x 2.5 mm (ID) tube and the sedimentation rate or ESR is measured as described above. The test should be set up within 2 hours after the blood is drawn since prolonged storage of blood or tilting of the calibrated tube will increase the ESR. Commonly accepted normal ESR values by this method for males and females are 0–15 mm and 0–20 mm, respectively. ESR values in the range of 20–30 mm are considered mildly elevated and those above 55 mm are considered markedly elevated. Aging and anemia with resultant changes in the erythrocyte-plasma ratio are commonly responsible for mild increases of the ESR.

The ESR has been employed in medicine for half a century; although it is nonspecific and is an indirect reflection of APP, it is still a useful diagnostic supplement to clinical evaluation of febrile and rheumatic diseases. It is largely of value

TABLE 2.2 Changes in Concentrations of Acute Phase Proteins in Inflammation

50% increase	2-4 fold increase	> 100 fold increase
Ceruloplasmin	α1-acid glycoprotein	CRP*
C3	α1-antitrypsin	SAA**
	α1-antichymotrypsin	
	Fibrinogen	
	Haptoglobin	

* C-reactive protein
**Serum amyloid A-protein

if it is normal, thus tending to exclude the presence of certain active diseases. Serial measurements of ESR can be used for follow-up of rheumatic fever and myocardial infarction, to confirm a diagnosis or a differential diagnosis, as with RA versus osteoarthritis, or to monitor the progress of an inflammatory disease like RA, polymyalgia rheumatica, or temporal arteritis (although it only roughly parallels disease activity in RA). High ESR values may be seen in a wide variety of conditions. In juvenile RA, an increased ESR often parallels the activity of the disease, but elevations may remain in spite of effective treatment. One-third of scleroderma patients have a normal ESR. The other two-thirds have mildly or markedly increased ESR measurements. The ESR is also usually increased in patients with SLE or Sjögren's syndrome but is often normal in polymyositis. Amos et al. (1) reported that the progression of RA, when judged by radiologic changes, was more likely to occur when serum CRP and ESR were consistently raised; when those levels were high, nearly all patients deteriorated. For those SLE patients with secondary infection, ESR also tends to rise.

C-Reactive Protein (CRP)

C-reactive protein is a serum component which appears in response to a variety of inflammatory stimuli. This plasma protein was named CRP because of its ability to yield precipitates with pneumococcal C-polysaccharides in the presence of calcium ion. The concentration of CRP can rise rapidly more than a thousandfold during inflammation.

The semiquantitative capillary precipitation test and the quantitative radial immunodiffusion assay are the most widely employed methods for detection of CRP. The most sensitive technique for CRP measurements is a recently developed radioimmunoassay. Using this technique, Claus et al. (2) studied 153 healthy blood donors and found that the serum CRP levels ranged from 0.0068 mg% to 0.82 mg% (mean = 0.13 mg%). Concentrations less than 0.5 mg% are normal but most apparently healthy individuals have serum CRP levels less than 0.2 mg%. Morley et al. (3) classified CRP concentrations lower than 1 mg% as normal.

The physiologic role of CRP in different states of inflammation and tissue damage is not yet clear, but it is known that CRP has the ability to activate the complement system and inhibit platelet function. This suggests that CRP participates in the modulation of the inflammatory process. CRP also probably stimulates the phagocytic activity of neutrophils as well as the motility of neutrophils. CRP may modify the immune response through binding to T cells and altering their functions, inhibiting the production of lymphokines and stimulating generation of suppressor T cells.

The uses of CRP measurements include the following, although none is specific: 1) as an indicator for inflammatory diseases or tissue damage; 2) to monitor the antiinflammatory effects of treatment; 3) for the detection of intercurrent infection.

High serum CRP levels are seen in bacterial infections, rheumatic fever, RA, juvenile arthritis, ankylosing spondylitis, polymyalgia rheumatica, systemic vasculitis, psoriatic arthritis, malignant tumors, myocardial infarction, and trauma (surgery, fracture). The measurement of serum CRP concentration in RA patients tends to correlate with radiographic changes. Conversely, in patients with other autoimmune diseases such as SLE, scleroderma, dermatomyositis, and Sjögren's syndrome, CRP levels rise only modestly regardless of the severity and activity of the disease. The significance of elevated CRP in SLE patients is uncertain. Morrow et al. (4) found that moderately high levels of CRP can be found in SLE patients without infection, and Zein et al. (5), using the same technique, found that elevations of serum CRP levels in SLE patients are associated with disease activity. Morley and Kushner found that marked elevations of serum CRP were almost exclusively seen in patients with bacterial infections (3). Moderate elevations were associated with a diagnosis of RA, SLE, scleroderma, dermatomyositis, or rheumatic fever. Thus, the monitoring of CRP levels may be useful in detecting bacterial infections in SLE patients, but discrepancies between studies limit usefulness of this test.

Rheumatoid Factor

Rheumatoid factors are antibodies which react with antigenic determinants in the Fc portion of immunoglobulin G. These factors react with autologous immunoglobulins and therefore are considered autoantibodies. Erick Waaler discovered rheumatoid factor (RF) in 1937 while working with a complement consumption test, using sheep erythrocytes (srbc) coated with anti-srbc rabbit antibodies. He noted that serum from rheumatoid arthritis patients contained a factor which could agglutinate the antibody-coated erythrocytes, and the antibodies were necessary to obtain agglutination (6). Later in 1948 Rose and associates, working with a complement fixation test for rickettsia, also noted agglutination induced by the serum of RA patients and pointed to the usefulness of this agglutination reaction for the diagnosis of RA (7).

Rheumatoid factors can be IgG, IgM or IgA antibodies and can be detected at very low concentration in the circulation of some healthy people. However in patients with rheumatic disease the presence of these factors is more prevalent and their concentration higher. Relatively high concentrations of rheumatoid factors are found not only in rheumatic disease but also in chronic inflammatory states, neoplastic disease, and other conditions associated with hyperglobulinemia. Table 2.3 lists some of the diseases more frequently associated with the presence of rheumatoid factor.

Rheumatoid factors of the IgM class are easily detected using routine techniques, but the detection of the more specific IgG and IgA rheumatoid factors requires more specialized techniques not available in routine hospital laboratories.

Rheumatoid factor found in rheumatoid arthritis is characteristically heterogeneous with respect to immunoglobulin class and specificity, i.e., these rheumatoid factors are a mixture of immunoglobulins of classes IgM, IgG, and IgA and can react with animal IgG determinants, species-specific human IgG determinants, and human IgG alloantigens (Gm).

Rheumatoid factors in the serum of rheumatoid arthritis patients have relatively low affinity for IgG determinants but can form labile complexes by self-aggregation (IgG rheumatoid factor) and by binding of aggregated IgG (IgM rheumatoid factor). In contrast, rheumatoid factors detected in synovial fluids are sometimes of greater avidity suggesting that high affinity blood rheumatoid factors forming stable and large complexes are removed from the circulation by the reticuloendothelial system (8).

Rheumatoid factor of the IgM class can be detected by immunoagglutination techniques similar to those originally described by Waaler and Rose. This factor is multivalent for IgG and can very efficiently agglutinate particles coated with human IgG. Particles commonly used are bentonite or latex beads which form a visible flocculus when the IgG in the particle is cross-linked by IgM rheumatoid factor. The amount of rheumatoid factor in the serum is expressed as the highest dilution given visible agglutination. Because the IgG used is human, the reaction may detect antibodies against alloantigens resulting from immunization by transfusion or pregnancy.

TABLE 2.3 Rheumatoid Factor in Various Clinical States

Clinical States	% Positive ≧ 1:160 dilution
Rheumatoid arthritis	80
Juvenile rheumatoid arthritis	20
Ankylosing spondylitis	<15
Infections	
S bacterial endocarditis	48
Nonspecific viral disease	15
Infectious hepatitis	24
Tuberculosis	11
Leprosy	24
Lung diseases	
Bronchitis	62
Asthma	17
Silicosis	15
Idiopathic pulmonary fibrosis	32
Miscellaneous disease	
Sarcoid	17
Cirrhosis of liver	36
Sjögren's syndrome	>90
Myocardial infarction	12

(Reprinted with permission from Zweiman, B, Lisar, RP. Autoimmunity and autoimmune disease. In JB Henry (ed.), *Clinical Diagnosis and Management by Laboratory Methods,* 16th Ed., vol. 2. Philadelphia, Saunders, 1979, p. 1271.)

The Waaler-Rose test, also called the sheep cell agglutination test (SCAT), is based on the same immunoagglutination principle, but for this test the particles are sheep red blood cells coated with rabbit antisheep red blood cell antibodies. This test is more specific for rheumatoid arthritis than the latex or bentonite agglutination techniques since rheumatoid arthritis RF reacts more frequently with animal IgG determinants than RF in other conditions. However, the titers are usually lower than those obtained by agglutination of particles coated with human IgG. A variation of these techniques utilizes bentonite or latex particles coated with animal IgG, thus avoiding possible agglutination of the red cells by antisheep antibodies.

Rheumatoid factor of the IgG class is more difficult to detect routinely because IgG is not a good agglutinator, has a tendency to self-associate, and is generally present in serum mixed with IgM rheumatoid factor. The IgG and IgA rheumatoid factors can be identified by their sedimentation rate or by agglutination techniques after removal of IgM rheumatoid factor.

Radioimmunoassay (RIA) and enzyme-linked immunoabsorbent assay (ELISA) are very useful techniques for the detection of any RF class. These tests are more sensitive than the latex or SCAT tests and larger number of samples can be tested at a time.

Antinuclear Antibody (ANA) Testing

ANA detection by immunofluorescence was described using sera from patients with SLE and other connective tissue diseases in 1957 (9). This was approximately a decade after initial descriptions of the LE cell phenomenon, which occurs in defibrinated blood due to ingestion of nuclei from damaged cells by blood phagocytes (e.g., PMN's) (10). The finding of LE cells is reasonably specific for SLE and is initiated in vitro using blood which is stirred and incubated to bring about the cell damage needed for release of free nuclei and the subsequent phagocytosis of nuclei by leukocytes. Serum antibodies that are reactive with deoxyribonucleoprotein (ANA's) opsonize the released nuclei and facilitate phagocytosis, giving rise to large homogeneous inclusions in phagocytes that can be identified as LE cells on Wright's stained smears. Disadvantages of the LE cell test are that it is relatively insensitive, tedious to perform, and has potential for misinterpretation due to the appearance of artefacts such as tart cells that occur in normal defibrinated blood. Therefore, this test has been large replaced by ANA assays using immunofluorescence and other methods capable of detecting antinuclear antibodies directed against not only deoxyribonucleoprotein, as in the LE cell test, but also many other classes of nuclear antigens.

The finding of ANA, when properly performed, indicates in the majority of cases an ongoing or latent inflammatory disorder within the broad classification of connective tissue disease (11, 12). However, other disorders, usually immunologic, are also characterized by this serologic abnormality. In addition, ANA is occasionally found in apparently normal subjects, but this is rare when the test is performed properly. ANA testing relies on use of biological reagents susceptible to great variability in performance and requiring careful standardization. To date, there are no universally accepted criteria for how the ANA test should be conducted, although current efforts are being made by the Center for Disease Control, which supplies a panel of reference sera with known specificities to clinical laboratories upon request. Regardless of the ANA test procedure chosen, quality control can only be assured by continual monitoring of disease prevalence in the patient populations studied. This goal is achievable when ANA laboratory results are reviewed periodically and correlated with additional diagnostic information. Whether there is reasonable monitoring of test results through feedback between the ANA laboratory and clinicians should be carefully evaluated when considering the validity of ANA test results. All too often, patients with vague protean complaints are referred to rheumatologists because of the finding of a positive ANA, which cannot be confirmed when retested by a well-standardized ANA assay. Despite potential shortcomings due to poor quality control and monitoring, ANA's are important markers of SLE and related syndromes, largely replacing the LE cell test, which is positive only in a small subset of SLE patients and negative in other rheumatic disorders for which the ANA now serves as a reliable marker.

To successfully interpret ANA results, the clinician should have some knowledge of the various laboratory techniques applied. Initial screening is usually with an indirect immunofluorescence assay. For performance of indirect immunofluorescence, a droplet of patient serum is pipetted onto a glass microscope slide coated with substrate cells fixed with acetone, methanol, or a combination of two fixatives. As many as 20 or 30 different sera can be examined on the same slide. The slide overlaid with test serum droplets is incubated for a brief period to allow tight binding of any serum ANA to target antigens in substrate cell nuclei. It is then washed to remove irrelevant immunoglobulin and all other serum components except bound ANA. The next step is to overlay the slide again, this time with antihuman immunoglobulin prepared in rabbits or other animals and chemically

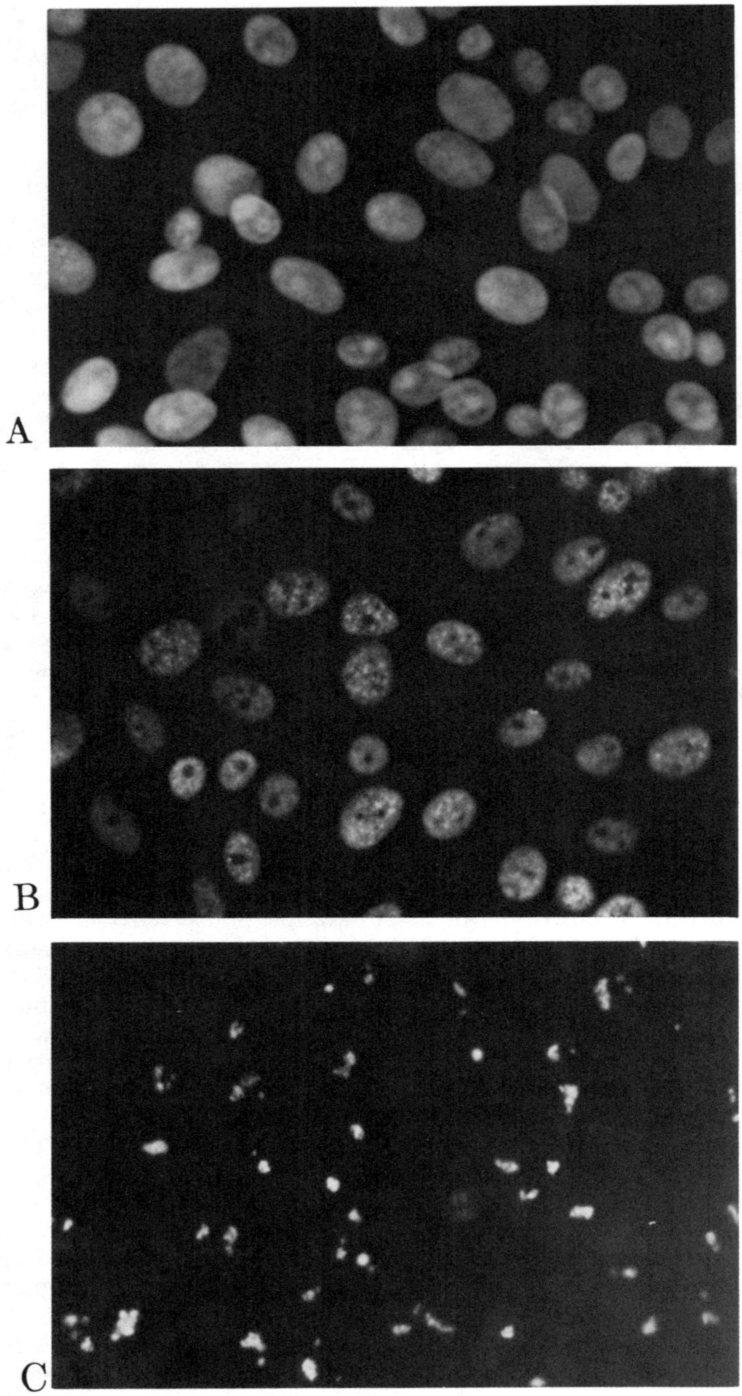

FIGURE 2.1 Typical staining patterns seen in flourescent antinuclear antibody (ANA testing; A: homogeneous, B: speckled, C: nucleolar.

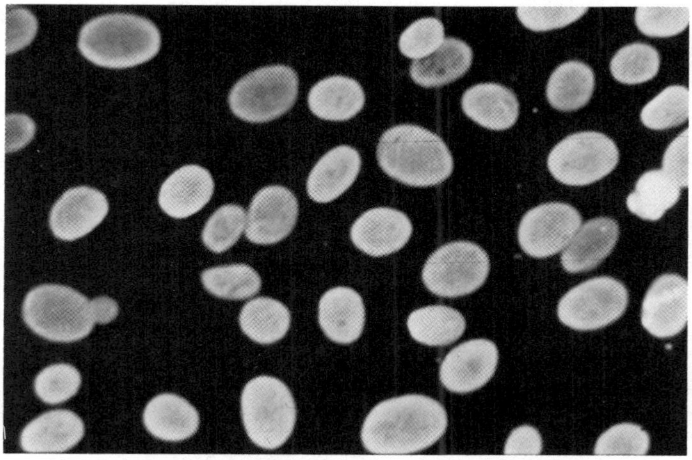

D

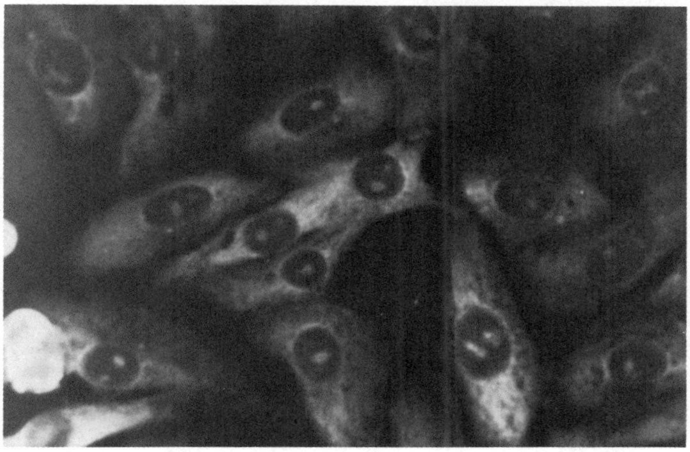

E

FIGURE 2.1 (Cont'd) Typical staining patterns seen in flourescent antinuclear antibody (ANA) testing; D: peripheral (rim), E: cytoplasmic. (Reproduced with the technical assistance of Mr. Phillip Heitman.) Magnification using Vero cell (cultured African green monkey kidney cell) substrate.

conjugated with fluorescein. This antiimmunoglobulin probe binds to any human ANA on the slide. The slide is washed again to remove unbound antiimmunoglobulin. The remaining antiimmunoglobulin, being bound to ANA and fluorescein conjugated, will emit visible fluorescence when exposed to the excitatory and filtered UV light system of a fluorescent microscope. By examining the substrate slide using such a microscope, ANA on cell nuclei can be visualized. The fluorescence patterns and titers observed are recorded and this information provides the clinician with diagnostic information. Typical staining patterns for fluorescent ANA testing are shown in Figure 2.1. Disease associations typically reported using monolayer ANA substrates prepared with "immortalized" cells such as the Vero cell line (available from the American Type and Culture collection and grown in tissue culture) are shown in Table 2.4.

TABLE 2.4 Correlations Between Diseases, Typical ANA Patterns, and Titers Determined by Immunofluorescence*

Disease	ANA Pattern	Titer
SLE	H, S, N, P	High
PSS	N, S	High
RA	H	Low
MCTD	S	High
Sjögren's syndrome	S	Low
CREST	C	High
ANA-negative SLE	Cyt	Low
Misc.	H	Low

* Abbreviations for patterns: H = homogeneous, S = speckled, N = nucleolar, P = peripheral, C = centromere, Cyt = cytoplasmic. Abbreviations for diseases: SLE = systemic lupus erythematous, PSS = progressive systemic sclerosis, RA = rheumatoid arthritis, MCTD = mixed connective tissue disease, CREST = variant PSS (see Chapter 14), Misc. = other nonspecific conditions and normals.

TABLE 2.5 Variables Important in the Outcome of ANA Testing*

Type of substrate (cell type)
Rigor of washing steps
Specificity of antiimmunoglobulin probe
Titer selected as positive

* ANA testing by the numerous immunofluorescent methods available yield results that are sometimes widely disparate. Some of the variables involved are listed. Results are only meaningful if the test is carefully standardized and monitored.

There are a number of important variables in performance of ANA testing that can lead to confusion in interpretation of results. These are listed in Table 2.5. ANA results may vary significantly on different substrate cells, yielding different staining patterns. This is shown, for example, by the transformation of the centromere (13) staining pattern seen using substrates containing rapidly dividing cells with metaphase plates to a discrete speckled appearance using substrates that predominantly contain cells in interphase. Moreover, certain substrates, such as mouse liver, have multiple rather than the two or three nucleoli present in other cell lines, so that nucleolar fluorescence on mouse liver yields a pattern that may be mistaken for speckled. Other patterns such as peripheral, cytoplasmic, and combinations of patterns may also vary significantly from one type of substrate to another.

An additional important variable is the source of substrate cells. Until recently, thin tissue slices obtained by cryostat sectioning were the preferred substrate. These are currently being replaced in many laboratories by monolayer cultures of human or animal cell lines which have the advantage of avoiding the problems encountered with relatively thick tissue sections in which subtle ANA patterns can be obscured due to overlap of individual cells on the slide. Cytocentrifuged cells from noncell line sources, such as human blood, can also be used, although this latter source is currently not convenient for adaptation to widespread clinical use. Another variable to consider is the specificity of the fluorescein conjugated antiimmunoglobulin, as some laboratories use conjugates reactive with human IgG and IgM, while others use conjugates reactive only with IgG. Some have preference for anti-IgG conjugates, as conjugates reactive with ANA of the IgM class have been reported to have less specificity for rheumatic diseases. The method of preparing substrate slides is another variable of importance, since certain cellular antigens (such as SSA/Ro and SSB/La) are soluble (14, 15) and can be washed off the slide, thus giving a falsely negative ANA result. Finally, the ANA titer selected as positive should yield appropriate sensitivity and specificity, and with new batches of substrate slides and fluorescein conjugates, results should be carefully standardized. Further, interobserver readings of pattern and titer should correlate highly. Titer is defined as the highest dilution of the test serum that gives a positive result with a discernible pattern such as nucleolar or homogeneous. It has been shown that many normal sera react with nuclear antigens. Therefore, careful test standardization and continuous monitoring of the disease categories identified are required for establishing and maintaining the correct cutoff titer distinguishing sera from patients with connective tissue disorders and other immunologic disease from normal sera containing ANA at lower titers.

Aside from using immunofluorescence, serum should be examined for ANA by double immunodiffusion and/or counterimmunoelectrophoresis. These methods are used to detect antibodies to soluble nuclear antigens which may not be observable by immunofluorescence. For clinical purposes, the utility of these tests is related not only to detection of antibodies missed by immunofluorescence, but because of correlations of the particular antibodies identified with SLE and other diseases. If a patient's serum reveals precipitin lines indicating the presence of ANA in these precipitin tests, the ANA responsible for forming these lines is classified as either identical or nonidentical with precipitin lines formed by prototype sera from patients known to have the antibodies of interest. Disease associations of ANA commonly detected as precipitin lines are shown (Table 2.6). Reactivities of anti-Sm and anti-nRNP (16) are directed against nonhistone nuclear antigens extractable with saline. Anti-SSA/Ro and anti-SSB/La are directed against protein antigens on cytoplasmic and/or nuclear RNA's (14). In the case of anti-SSB/La, the target antigens have been shown associated with products of Epstein Barr viral genomes present in mammalian cell nuclei. For detection of ANA to certain of these antigens, newer more quantitative tests such as gel electrophoresis Western blotting, and ELISA assays are now becoming available.

Another class of ANA of diagnostic importance is that directed against DNA. ANA reactive with DNA can be classified regarding specificity for double or single strandedness of the DNA molecule (anti-dsDNA or synonymously antinative DNA, and anti-ssDNA, respectively). For purposes of rheumatologic evaluation, it is desirable to be able to find anti-dsDNA specificity since this type of antibody

TABLE 2.6 ANA to Soluble Antigens*

Specificity	Disease Associations
Anti-SSA(Ro)	SLE, Sjögren's, neonatal SLE
Anti-SSB(La)	SLE, Sjögren's
Anti- Sm	SLE
Anti-RNP	MCTD, SLE, RA
Anti-Scl-1, Scl 70	Scleroderma

* ANA with the specificities shown are currently detected by counterimmunoelectrophoresis and immunodiffusion. Sera negative for ANA by immunofluorescence should be tested by these methods as well (see text).

has proven to be a reliable marker for SLE, especially when complicated by nephritis. In addition, DNA anti-dsDNA immune complexes have been shown to fix complement and have been isolated from sera and kidneys of patients with SLE nephritis, indicating that they may be pathogenic in production of nephritis. Measuring for the less specific anti-ssDNA, which is found in a number of rheumatic conditions such as RA, MCTD and SLE, may also be desirable in certain situations as a gauge of disease activity rather than for determination of particular diagnostic categories. (It is important to recognize a source of possible confusion in these tests: most anti-dsDNA antibodies cross-react with ssDNA thereby giving a positive test for ssDNA as well. By definition, anti-ssDNA antibodies, as commonly seen in RA, do not cross-react with dsDNA.) For practical purposes it is fortunate that sera containing anti-DNA of either specificity almost always show ANA by indirect immunofluorescence so that the routine ANA test can be used as an initial screen and the anti-DNA test can be performed as follow-up when needed. The staining pattern seen when sera positive for anti-DNA are tested by immunofluorescence for ANA may vary, although a number of reports have indicated that the peripheral pattern is common. To overcome the problem of DNA denaturation inherent in older methods of anti-DNA testing (e.g., the Farr assay using purified DNA) several newer assays have been devised. For example, one employs a synthetic DNA substrate, synthetic poly dAdT. Another utilizes the trypanosome *Crithidia luciliae* which contains an organelle rich in dsDNA and lacking significant amounts of ssDNA. This distinction allows rather convenient detection of anti-dsDNA using kinetoplasts in cultured *C. luciliae* as substrates and indirect immunofluorescence by methods analogous to the ANA test described above.

Complement

The complement cascade consists of a group of proteins with circulate in an inactive form. Once the first components are activated, the cascade proceeds rapidly, inducing an amplified effect which can mediate inflammation, and a sequence of defensive reactions including viral neutralization, chemotaxis, opsonization, and cell lysis. The circulating components of complement are designated by the letter

C followed by a number from 1 to 9. However the numbering of the first components (C1 to C4) does not correspond with the activation sequence which proceeds as follows: C1qrs, C4, C2, C3, C5, C6, C7, C8, C9.

The most abundant of the complement components is C3 and the activation of C3 is biologically the most important reaction of the complement cascade. There are two pathways for the activation of C3: the classical pathway which can be initiated by antigen-antibody reactions, and the alternate pathway which does not require antibodies and bypasses activation of factors C1qrs, C4, and C2.

The alternate pathway can be activated by a number of substances including yeast cell wall (zymosan), endotoxin, and cobra venom factor. The alternate pathway includes two additional proteins, factor B and factor D.

Once the first component of the complement sequence is activated each component is activated by its predecessor, which in turn activates the following component. The activation steps generally involve enzymatic cleavage of the components with the generation of biologically active fragments, i.e., C3a, C5a. Specific inhibitors such as C1 and C3b inactivators check the balance of the reaction at various points in the sequence, during physiologic conditions (17).

During complement activation in vivo, the levels of the various components in blood may be decreased and decay products may be detectable in various body fluids. The measurement of the levels of complement components and decay products may give a rough index of disease activity in conditions where complement activation is prominent.

Many of the complement components can be considered as acute phase proteins and their concentration changes during and following inflammatory reactions. Changes in the concentration of the proteins of the complement cascade are generally associated with activation of one or both pathways. In addition, proteolytic enzymes released during tissue damage can induce activation of some of the complement components. Therefore, pathologic activation of complement occurs not only in rheumatic diseases, but also during processes in which the pathogenic mechanism does not involve immune reactions directly, such as disseminated intravascular coagulation, endotoxemic and hemorrhagic shock, myocardial infarction, and some situations in which proteolytic enzymes are released as consequence of tissue damage. Furthermore, any inflammatory and infectious disorder involving antigen-antibody reactions can be associated with changes in the concentration and electrophoretic characteristics of complement components.

Assays for complement components are basically of two types: tests which determine functional or hemolytic activity and tests which detect the presence of protein components regardless of their functional state. This latter type of test can be either qualitative or quantitative. Functional tests detect either the activity of the complete complement cascade or the activity of single components. Functional tests of single components are for the most part relegated to research laboratories, because they require the use of highly purified expensive components and relatively complex procedures. These tests accurately quantitate functional individual components. In contrast, assays for the total activity of complement are not very sensitive to partial deficiencies in specific components. However, functional tests for total complement activity are reliable and sensitive for the assessment of the classical complement pathway as a whole. The most widely known and used of these tests is the total hemolytic complement, usually expressed as CH50. The CH50 represents the concentration of sample serum which lyses 50% of a standard cell suspension. The test is conducted by incubating dilutions of the sample to be measured with a standard suspension of sheep erythrocytes in the presence of rabbit antibodies against sheep erythrocyte Forssman antigen. The antibody solution is standardized precisely to a concentration that lyses half of the cells in a given time in the presence of 1 ml of standard guinea pig complement (a hemolytic or CH50 unit). The complement titer in a serum sample is obtained by determining the dilution of serum at which 50% lysis is obtained and expressing this dilution as a reciprocal. The complement titer represents the number of hemolytic units in 1 ml of undiluted sample.

Appropriate processing of samples is essential for correct analysis. Functional tests should be performed with serum because anticoagulants interfere with complement function. Samples which could possibly have cryoprecipitins (cold precipitating proteins) should be processed at 37°C because aggregated immunoglobulins may initiate complement activation. Serum samples should be aliquoted and stored at -40°C or -70°C and if transportation of samples is needed, dry ice should be used.

Immunochemical tests are easy to perform and the reagents are commercially available. However, since these assays measure the complement components using antibodies, detection of cross-reacting degradation products may affect the results. Components commonly measured by immunochemical techniques include C1q, C4, C3, C5, factor B (of the alternate pathway) and C1 inhibitor.

Activation of complement components alters their electrophoretic mobility and this can be detected by immunoelectrophoretic technique. This technique is useful to differentiate complement activation by the classical pathway, alternate pathway, or by endogenous proteolytic enzymes. Using antibodies against C3, C4, and factor B of the alternate pathway it is possible to detect by electrophoresis the presence of the intact components and their degradation products. Therefore, if the electrophoretic pattern shows degradation of C3 and C4, activation of the classical pathway is suspected. If the pattern shows degradation of factor B, then activation of the alternate pathway is suspected. If only degradation of C3 is detected, endogenous enzymes or other causes may be suspected.

All available techniques have shortcomings and require care in the interpretation of the results. Abnormal concentrations of complement components are not only due to activation, but can be caused by alterations in the rates of synthesis or catabolism. In addition, local synthesis of the components and/or deficient clearance mechanisms may result in a lack of correlation between complement levels in blood and other body fluids such as synovial fluid.

Immune Complex Testing

Immune complexes are found in the serum of patients with a variety of diseases (18). These molecules are currently of interest to rheumatologists because of the prospect that they may provide markers of specific immunologic illnesses, severity of manifestations, and clues about pathogenic processes. The possible importance of circulating immune complexes in human disease became emphasized by studies in animal models including "one shot" acute serum sickness in rabbits and spontaneous immune complex disease in murine (mouse) models such as the NZB-NZW hybrids. In such models, immune complexes are found as tissue deposits, and the appearance of soluble immune complexes in the circulation has been found to correlate with pathologic changes such as nephritis, vasculitis, myocarditis, and synovitis. Further, these changes in animal models, in certain instances, were accompanied by decreases of serum complement, as in human SLE. Circulating immune complexes also were found in a number of human infectious diseases due to many types of pathogens including bacterial, viral, fungal, and parasitic agents. The latter findings suggested that certain types of tissue damage during infection, such as the synovitis of *N. gonorrheae* infection and the vasculitis of bacterial endocarditis, are due to phlogistic effects of immune complex molecules rather than direct toxicity of infecting organisms. Examples of human diseases associated with circulating immune complexes are shown in Table 2.7.

An early expectation with development of assays for circulating immune complexes was that manifestations of SLE and other types of immune vasculitis would be predictable based on these tests. Although examples of patients whose clinical course parallels the rise and fall of circulating immune complex levels have been described, to date precise relationships between these measurements and disease activity in SLE and other connective tissue disorders of unknown etiology, such as RA and scleroderma, remain unclear. Certain associations have been established, such as that between vasculitis in RA and cryoglobulinemia, and that between myocardial involvement in scleroderma and the presence of circulating immune complexes detectable by the Raji cell assay. However, in general, the finding of persistently abnormal levels of circulating immune complexes can best be thought of as a marker of an immunopathologic process rather than as an indicator of disease exacerbation, a particular diagnosis, or disease manifestation.

In rheumatic illnesses that follow infection, more definite relationships between the occurrence of circulating immune complexes and disease activity are established. A prime example understood in considerable detail is in Lyme arthritis (19). In this disease, precipitated by tick bite and resultant infection with the *Ixodes dammini* spirochete, virtually all patients with the initial skin lesion, erythema chronicum migrans, show circulating immune complexes. These complexes persist only in those patients showing subsequent additional organ damage including nerve, heart, and joint involvement. In those patients with persistent joint involvement without other organ damage, the complexes become detectable in synovial fluids and diminish in the circulation. Other relationships between infection

TABLE 2.7 Immune Complexes: Disease Associations

Rheumatoid arthritis

Systemic lupus erythematosus

Systemic sclerosis

Sjögren's syndrome

Lyme arthritis

Miscellaneous connective tissue diseases (mixed connective tissue disease, polyarteritis nodosum)

Glomerulonephritis

Neoplasm (solid tumors and leukemia)

Infections
- Bacterial: endocarditis, meningococcemia, gonococcemia, leprosy, syphilis
- Viral: dengue, CMV, hepatitis B, mumps, varicella, infectious mononucleosis, Coxsackie B
- Parasitic: malaria, schistosomiasis, filariasis, toxoplasmosis

Miscellaneous immune diseases

and the appearance of circulating immune complexes have been described. Mixed cryoglobulinemia, polyarteritis nodosa, and glomerulonephritis are found in association with persistent infection with hepatitis B virus. Moreover, antigens from this virus can be identified in immune complexes isolated from the circulation of the infected patients. In acute bacterial endocarditis, circulating immune complexes are found, and often these can be identified before culture results become positive. Similarly, in many other infections, circulating immune complexes are found. However, in general, knowledge of precise mechanisms accounting for the specificity of organ involvement and relationships with disease activity and interactions with mediator systems such as the complement cascade and coagulation pathways are lacking.

Through animal models and in vitro testing, considerable information has accumulated regarding how physiochemical properties of antigen, antibody, and immine complexes may be related to pathogenicity. Certain properties determine immune complex size, such as the immunoglobulin class, antibody valence, and ratio of antigen/antibody molecules in the circulation (Table 2.8). Large immune complexes are rapidly cleared from the circulation by the mononuclear phagocytic system. Smaller complexes persist longer, enhancing potential for pathologic interactions, such as complement activation and build-up of high concentrations in the circulation. Certain antigens are considered to enhance pathogenicity due to properties of charge or other factors that influence clearance from the circulation and deposition in tissues. For example, DNA molecules are positively charged and are therefore capable of attaching to glomeruli which have a high negative charge. The attached DNA may then become complexed to anti-DNA antibody with intraglomerular formation of immune complexes containing these two components. On the other hand, preformed circulating immune complex molecules, especially those with high positive (cationic) charge, can become attached to glomeruli. Large molecular size can contribute to subendothelial localization and persistence of the cationic complexes. Other physiochemical properties can also greatly influence the behavior of immune complexes. Receptors on hepatocytes can account for clearance of immune complexes containing certain glycoprotein antigens, and small changes in the structure of these antigens can lead to persistent circulation of the complexes. However, Fc receptors on cells of the mononuclear phagocytic system, which remove complexes due to interaction with the antibody component, are the more classically recognized removal system. Saturation of this system

TABLE 2.8 Factors Influencing Pathogenicity of Circulating Immune Complexes

Properties of the antibody (Ig class, association constant for antigen)
Properties of the antigen (valence, size, chemical composition, tropism for specific tissues)
Properties of the immune complex (cryoprecipitability, attachment to tissue receptors)
Host's ability to remove immune complexes (solubilization, phagocytosis)

with excesses of circulating immune complexes or due to defects in the system, as described in primary biliary cirrhosis and SLE, can also account for persistence of immune complexes in the circulation. Other mechanisms of immune complex removal have been described, such as by attachment to C3 receptors on circulating red cells and removal from the circulation of immune complex laden erythrocytes after traversal through the liver. Mechanisms of immune complex solubilization by complement components have been described. The presence of defective solubilization of immune complexes by sera from patients with active but not inactive SLE raises the question of whether this defect contributes to high levels of immune complexes in SLE.

A large choice of methods exists for detecting immune complexes in the circulation and other body fluids, such as those collected from the pericardial, synovial, and pleural spaces. Available methods rely on different principles, and concordance is not always found when comparing results. The properties of immune complexes used for these measurements include: 1) adherence to cellular receptors or specific proteins, 2) inhibition or stimulation of cellular responses in vitro, 3) physiochemical characteristics such as size, 4) reaction with antibody directed against components of the complexes, and 5) other biologic effects such as fixation of complement. To date, there is no single preferred test for immune complexes, and some investigators have recommended use of a combination of tests to obtain definitive results. In almost all cases, immune complexes are quantitated relative to calibration curves prepared by measuring known amounts of an aggregated IgG standard rather than immune complexes known to be pathogenic in the particular disease studied. This type of standardization is less than optimal, since effects of biologically formed immune complexes in the test system may differ considerably from that of the standards, and the pathogenic complex may represent only a fraction of the total amounts of complexes measured. For clinical testing, specific immune complexes important in disease activity remain largely unidentified, and pathogenic complexes are not available for testing purposes at the present time. A list of the various methods now widely used for immune complex testing is shown in Table 2.9.

TABLE 2.9 Examples of the Tests Used for Measuring Immune Complexes

Relying on interactions with cellular receptors: (Raji cell assay, erythrocyte, antibody-complement rosettes) lymphocyte rosette inhibition, K-cell cytotoxicity inhibition, macrophage uptake inhibition)
Binding to complement components: C1q binding assays, conglutinin assay
Binding to antibodies: using monoclonal and polyclonal rheumatoid factors
Binding with staphylococcal protein A
Physiochemical techniques: polyethylene glycol precipitation, gel filtration, analytic ultracentrifugation, cryoprecipitation

Human Lymphocyte Antigen (HLA) Testing

Immunologic reactions involve recognition of antigen by lymphocytes and interaction between lymphocytes and other cells of the immune system. The recognition of antigen and the accompanying and subsequent cellular cooperation leading to immune reactions require interactions at the level of a specific group of surface molecules encoded by a chromosomal region designated MHC (major histocompatibility complex). Each individual within a population expresses a set of these molecules encoded by genes of the MHC. In the human, the MHC is located in the short arm of chromosome 6 and is designated HLA (human lymphocyte antigen) region (20). The genes of the HLA region are grouped in four loci, designated A, B, C, and D/DR, and code for three different classes of molecules or factors. Class 1 comprises proteins encoded by genes in the A, B, and C loci; class 2 comprises proteins coded by the D/DR locus; and class 3 includes certain components of complement coded by genes in a region close to the HLA-B locus. Class 1 and 2 factors are proteins expressed on the surface of cells and present considerable degree of polymorphism, that is, the amino acid composition of the proteins varies from individual to individual. These individual variations cause recognition of these proteins as foreign antigen. In addition, these differences are responsible for the MHC restriction phenomena which demonstrate that cell to cell interactions leading to immunologic responses require identity of the interacting cells at the level of the MHC antigens.

Class 1 molecules are expressed on the surface of all nucleated cells and can be detected by serologic methods using antisera induced by pregnancy, transfusions, and tissue grafts. A bank of antisera with known specificities is maintained by the National Institutes of Health and these antisera are available for research and histocompatibility testing for organ transplantation. Class 2 molecules can be detected by either cell culture techniques using mixed leukocyte cultures which detect D antigens, or by serological techniques which detect DR antigens on the surface of B lymphocytes. Another useful technique for the detection of D/DR coded antigens is the primed lymphocyte typing technique (PLT). This method is based on the specificity of the secondary response to D antigens of cells primed with known antigens. Only cells sharing antigen with the cells used for priming will stimulate a secondary response. Almost all (but not all) the D antigens correspond to DR antigens. This discrepancy could be due to the fact that although both methods detect the same group of molecules, the mixed leukocyte reaction technique detects a combination of antigens, whereas the serologic methods detect single molecules on the B lymphocyte. Individual HLA antigens or specificities are designated by a number preceded by a letter indicating the locus coding it, e.g., A2, B27, D/DR1. This nomenclature is established and revised in international histocompatibility workshops which take place regularly and where data are reviewed in order to designate new antigens. Recognized antigens that are not definitively accepted are designated by adding a "w" (for workshop) to the letter and the number, e.g., Bw39, Dw12.

The individual differences in HLA antigens are important in the determination of genetic predisposition to disease, and the incidence of many diseases has been found to be correlated with the presence of certain antigens or combination of antigens coded by the MHC. This correlation further emphasizes the importance of the MHC in the biology of the immune system. It is of interest that the majority of the diseases in which this association has been found are so-called autoimmune disorders, thus suggesting that inheritance of a certain set of surface molecules can give rise to an immunological dysfunction which in turn is the factor or one of the factors responsible for the development of disease. The typing of HLA antigens expressed by a particular individual and the discovery of disease association within populations are of interest not only for the understanding of genetic predisposition and mechanisms of immunologic disease but also for the prevention, diagnosis, and prognosis of certain diseases.

Association between HLA and disease is estimated by calculating the frequency with which a disease develops in individuals with a particular antigen and comparing it to the frequency with which the disease develops in individuals without the antigen. Comparisons must be done between individuals belonging to the same ethnic group, because antigen distribution among normal populations varies considerably depending on race. For example, A1 is found in more than 25% of European Caucasians but in only 1% of Japanese. The frequency of presentation of certain HLA antigens in patients with rheumatic diseases and in normals is depicted in Table 2.10 (20).

TABLE 2.10 HLA Disease Association in Caucasians

		Antigen Frequency %	
	Antigen	Disease	Control
Ankylosing spondylitis	B27	96	4
Reiter's syndrome	B27	76	6
Acute anterior uveitis	B27	55	4
Reactive arthritis			
Yersinia	B27	88	14
Salmonella	B27	94	14
Shigella	B27	85	14
Rheumatoid arthritis	Dw4	59	16
	DR4	70	28
Juvenile rheumatoid arthritis			
With iritis	DR5	71	19
Without iritis	DR5	52	19
Behcet's syndrome			
Ocular type	B5	50	12
Arthritis type	B27	27	3
Mucocutaneous type	B12	53	22
Sjögren's disease	B8	58	21
	Dw3	69	10
Psoriatic arthropathy	B27	24	7

(Reprinted with permission from Dewar PJ: *HLA Antigens, Clinics in Rheumatic Disease,* vol. 9. Philadelphia, W. B. Saunders, 1983, p. 1.)

Although HLA typing has proven to be an important research tool for the understanding of pathogenic mechanisms in several diseases, the clinical application of HLA typing to patient care remains uncertain. Even in the case of ankylosing spondylitis, where HLA-B27 is present in 96% of Caucasian patients, routine use of HLA testing is discouraged, and controversy remains as to whether the test should ever be obtained (see discussion in Chapter 10).

References

1. Amos RS, Constable TJ, Crockson RA et al.: Rheumatoid arthritis: Relations of serum C-reactive proteins and erythrocyte sedimentation rates to radiographic changes. *Brit Med J* 1:195-197, 1977.

2. Claus DR, Osmand AP, Gewurz H: Radioimmunoassay of human C-reactive protein and levels in normal sera. *J Lab Clin Med* 87:120-128, 1976.

3. Morley JI, Kushner I: Serum C-reactive protein levels in diseases. In I Kushner, JE Volanakis, and H Gewurz (eds.), *C-Reactive Protein and the Plasma Protein Responses to Tissue Injury.* London and New York, New York Academy of Sciences, 1982, pp. 39-47.

4. Morrow WJW, Isenberg DA, Parry HF et al.: C-rective protein in sera from patients with systemic lupus erythematosus. *J Rheumatol* 8:599-604, 1981.

5. Zein N, Ganuza C, Kushner I: Significance of serum C-reactive protein elevation in patients with systemic lupus erythematosus. *Arthritis and Rheumatism* 22:7-12, 1979.

6. Waaler E: On the occurrence of a factor in human serum activating the specific agglutination of sheep blood corpuscles. *Acta Pathologica et Microbiologica Scandinavica* 17:172-178, 1940.

7. Rose HM, Ragan C, Pearce E, Lipman MO: Differential agglutination of normal and sensitized sheep erythrocytes by sera of patients with rheumatoid arthritis. *Proc Soc Exp Biol Med* 68:1-6, 1949.

8. Allen C, Elson CJ, Scott DGI et al.: IgG antiglobulins in rheumatoid arthritis and other arthritides; relationship with clinical features and other parameters. *Ann Rheum Dis* 40:127-131, 1981.

9. Friou GJ: Clinical application of lupus serum-nucleoprotein reaction using flourescent antibody technique. *J Clin Invest* 36:890, 1957.

10. Hargraves MM, Richmond H, Morton R: Presentation of two bone marrow elements: The tart cell and the LE cell. *Proc Staf Meet Mayo Clin* 23:25-28, 1948.

11. Parker MD, Kerby GP: Combined titer and fluorescent pattern of IgG antinuclear antibodies using cultured cell monolayers in evaluating connective tissue diseases. *Ann Rheum Dis* 33:465-472, 1974.

12. Tesser JRP, Rothberger H, Agudelo C: The clinical significance of anticytoplasmic antibodies found on fluorescent antinuclear antibody testing. *J Rheum* 10:227-234, 1983.

13. Tromposch HD, Smith D, Sevecal J-L, Rothfield N: A long-term longitudinal study of anticentromere antibodies. *Arthritis Rheum* 27:121-131, 1984.

14. Lerner HA, Lerner MR, Hardin JA, Janeway CA, Jr., Steitz JA: Deciphering the mysteries of RNA-containing lupus antigens. *Arthritis Rheum* 25:761-766, 1982.

15. Scott JS, Maddison PJ, Taylor PV, Esscher E, Scott O, Skinner RP: Connective tissue disease, antibodies to ribonucleoprotein, and congenital heart block. *N Engl J Med* 309:209-212, 1983.

16. Munves EF, Schur PH: Antibodies to Sm and RNP. Prognosticators of disease involvement. *Arthritis Rheum* 26:848-853, 1983.

17. Atkinson JP, Frank MM: Complement. In CW Parker (ed.), *Clinical Immunology*. Philadelphia, W. B. Saunders, 1981, p. 219.

18. Theofilopoulos AN, Dixon FJ: Immune complexes in human diseases. *A J Path* 100:531-591, 1980.

19. Hardin JA, Steere AC, Malawista SE: Immune complexes and the evolution of Lyme arthritis. *N Eng J Med* 301:1358-1363, 1979.

20. Dewar PJ: HLA antigens. *Clin Rheum Dis* 9:93-116, 1983.

Chapter 3

DIAGNOSTIC RADIOLOGY IN THE RHEUMATIC DISEASES

Alan Klein, M.B., B. Ch. and Wells Martin III, M.D.

In the radiological investigation of joint diseases there are several signs which are helpful in making a diagnosis. Individually these signs will often suggest the presence of joint disease but may not be specific. However when present in combination or when considering the anatomic distribution, a definitive diagnosis is possible. Several of the signs of rheumatic disease can occur in other nonrheumatic conditions.

I. Soft Tissue Changes
   A. Soft Tissue Swelling. This may be diffuse or localized, unilateral or bilateral. If bilateral it may be either symmetrical or nonsymmetrical.
      1. Diffuse swelling: usually associated with nonrheumatic conditions.
         a) Soft tissue overgrowth, e.g., acromegaly
         b) Edema of any type
         c) Cellulitis
      2. Localized swelling
         a) Concentric: all the way around the joint and may involve one or many joints and be unilateral or bilateral. Can present as either increased soft tissue width or increased density about the joint.
            (1) Rheumatoid arthritis (periarticular soft tissue swelling is the earliest radiological change).
            (2) Systemic lupus erythematosus
            (3) Reiter's
            (4) Psoriasis (Figure 3.1)
            (5) Ankylosing spondylitis occasionally
            (6) Arthralgias associated with gastrointestinal abnormalities (ulcerative colitis, Crohn's disease, Whipple's disease, and small bowel bypass surgery).

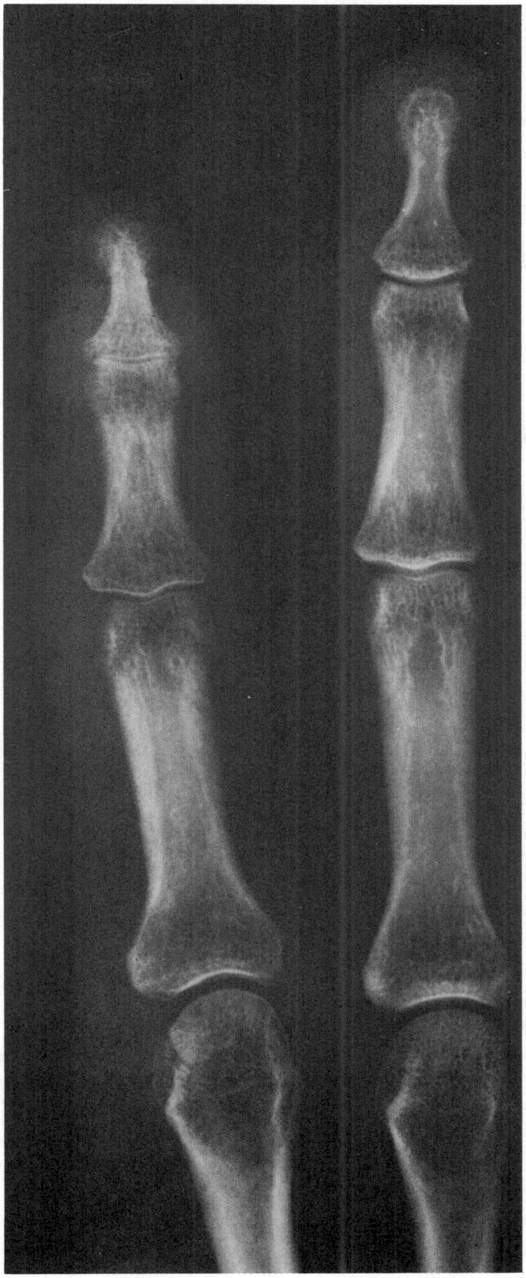

FIGURE 3.1 Soft tissue swelling of the index finger in psoriasis ("sausage finger").

(7) Gout
(8) Nonrheumatic conditions:
(a) Sarcoid in 25% of cases
(b) Hemarthrosis due to hemophilia or trauma
(c) Infections (Figure 3.2)
(d) Synovial and other soft tissue tumors

b) Eccentric
(1) Gout (Figure 3.3)
(2) Infective or foreign body granuloma
(3) Soft tissue infection (extraarticular)
(4) Tendon sheath xanthoma
(5) Subcutaneous nodules (in rheumatoid arthritis, rheumatic fever, systemic lupus erythematosus, and polyarteritis nodosa).

B. Decreased Soft Tissue
1. Diffuse: occurs with muscle atrophy.
a) Long-standing rheumatoid arthritis
b) Dermatomyositis
c) Systemic lupus erythematosus
d) Disuse from muscular or neurologic abnormalities
2. Localized: loss or atrophy mainly at the tip of the finger or fingers.
a) Trauma (most common)
b) Scleroderma (Figure 3.4)
c) Raynaud's
d) Rheumatoid arthritis
e) Psoriatic arthritis
f) Neuropathic disorders

II. Osteopenia. Loss of bone density (also known as osteoporosis). May be generalized or localized.

A. Generalized. In generalized osteopenia, especially if long-standing, the cortex of the bone is very thin and there is loss of trabeculation with a ground glass appearance. This type of osteopenia is seen in 1) long-standing rheumatoid arthritis; 2) juvenile rheumatoid arthritis [juvenile chronic polyarthritis (JRA)]; 3) dermatomyositis; and 4) systemic lupus erythematosus. The finding is often compounded by the long-term use of steroids in treatment of the underlying arthritis.

B. Localized
1. Juxtaarticular, polyarticular: the ends of the bones within the joint capsule are involved in the inflammatory process and become osteopenic. The diaphyses (the shaft portion of the bones) are spared.
a) Rheumatoid arthritis (early) (Figure 3.5)
b) Juvenile rheumatoid arthritis (Figure 3.6)
c) Reiter's
d) Scleroderma
e) Lupus erythematosus (late)
2. Juxtaarticular, monoarticular: isolated to one joint or group of joints (e.g., wrist)
a) Pyogenic arthritis
b) TB arthritis
c) Hemophilia

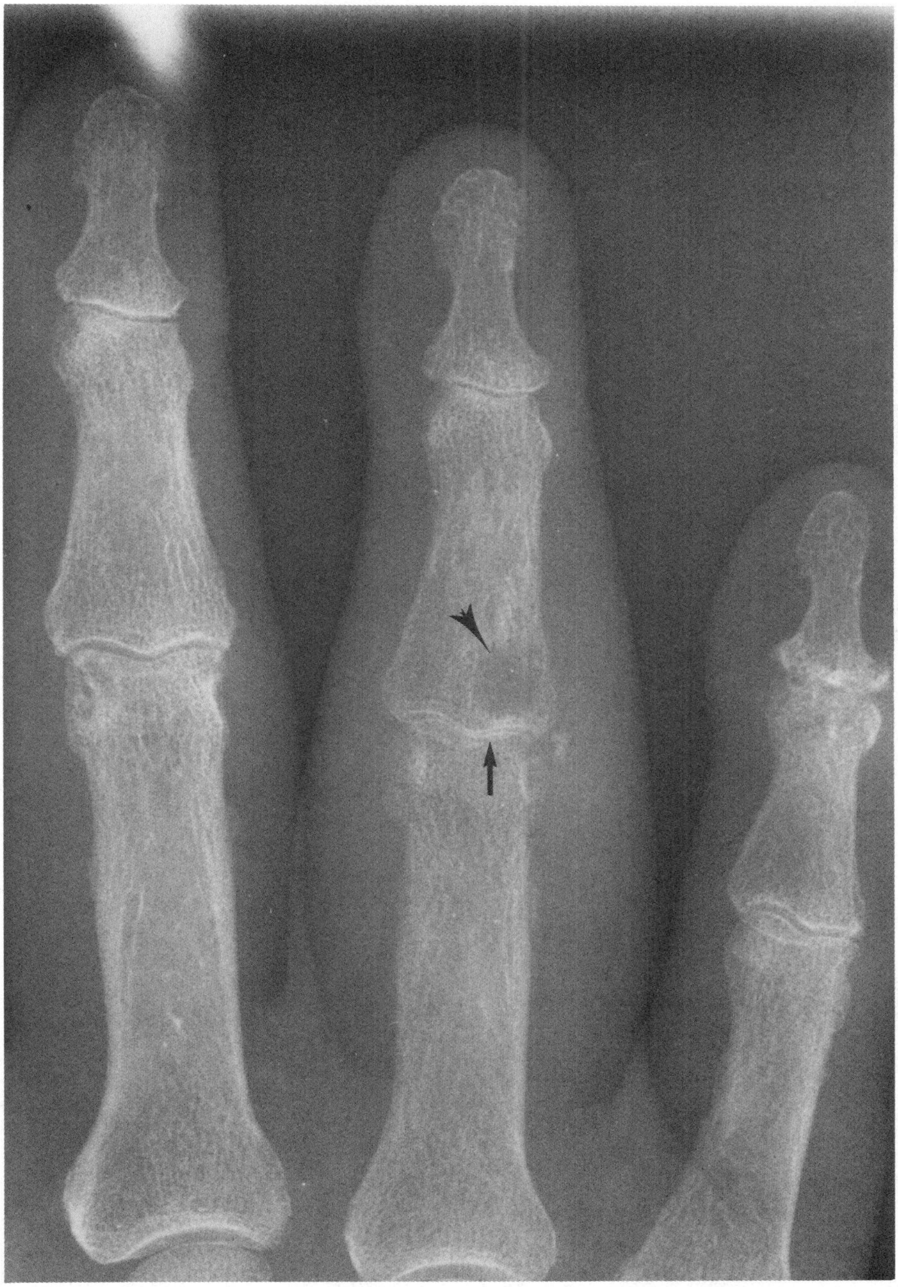

FIGURE 3.2 Localized soft tissue swelling in osteomyelitis and septic arthritis. In addition to the soft tissue swelling, note the bone destruction (arrow head) and narrowing of the proximal interphalangeal joint (arrow).

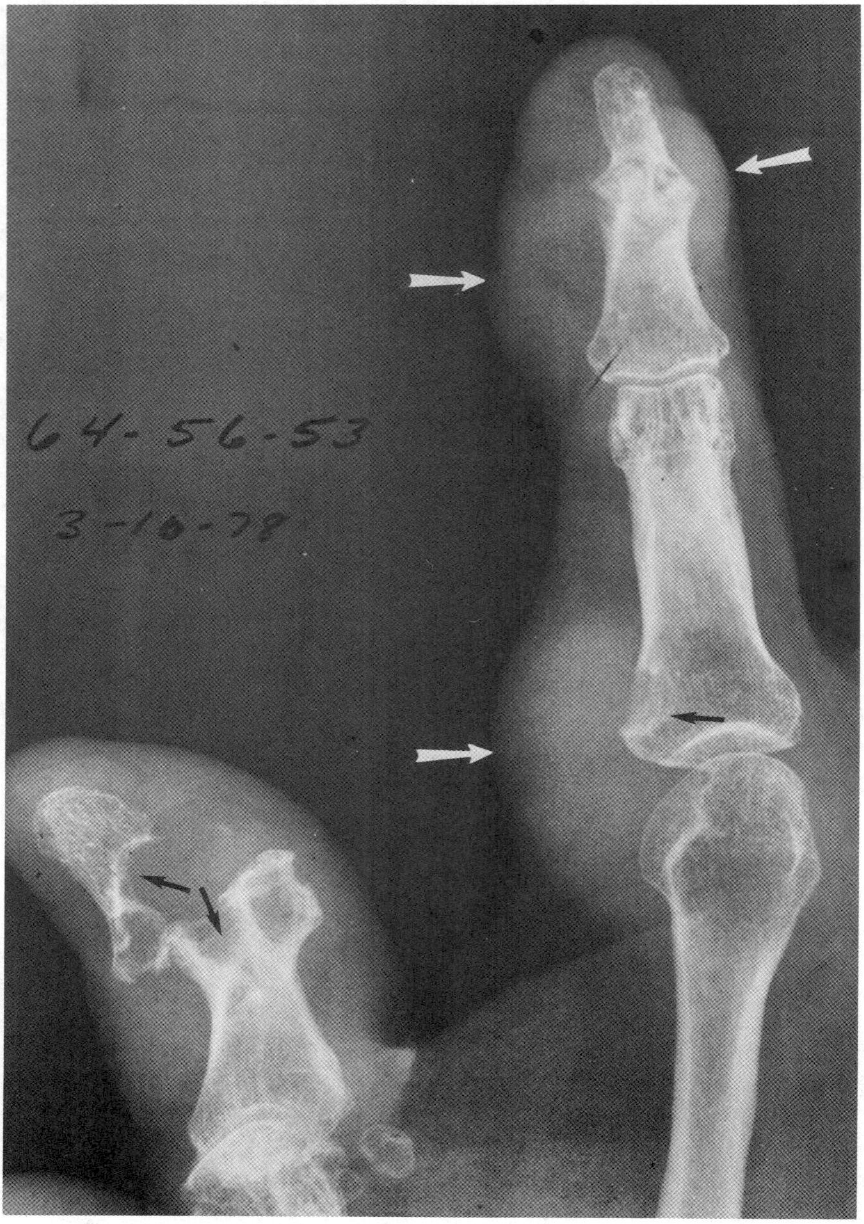

FIGURE 3.3 Gout with eccentric soft tissue masses due to tophi (white arrows). Note also well-demarcated erosions in the phalanges (black arrows).

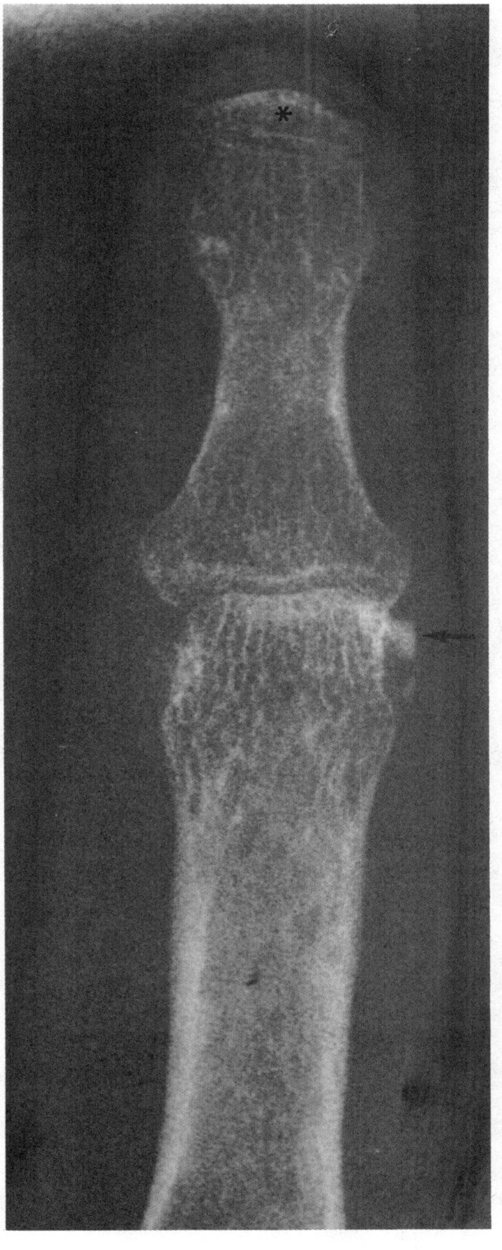

FIGURE 3.4 Scleroderma: Bone resorption of the terminal phalanx with a small residual fragment (*) and atrophy of the overlying soft tissues. Juxtaarticular calcification at the proximal interphalangeal joint (arrow).

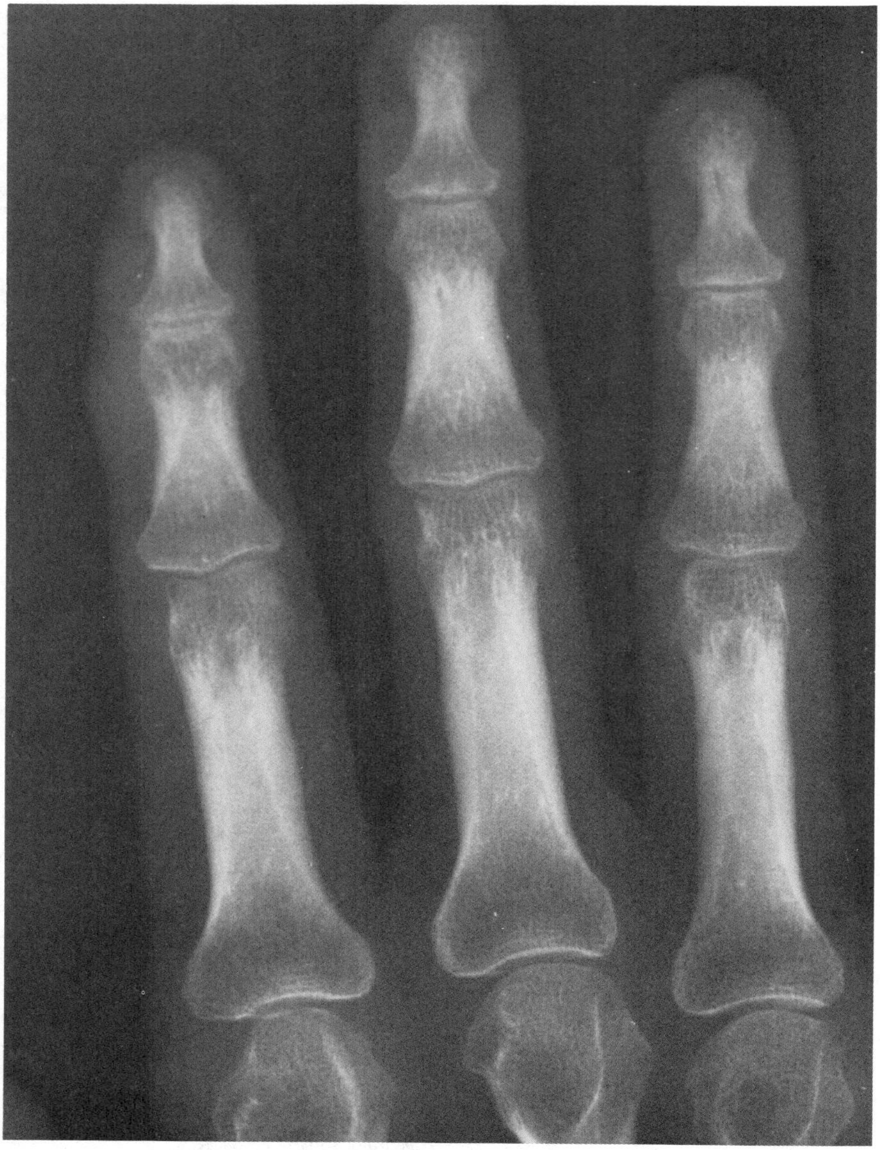

FIGURE 3.5 Juxtaarticular osteoporosis. Rheumatoid arthritis.

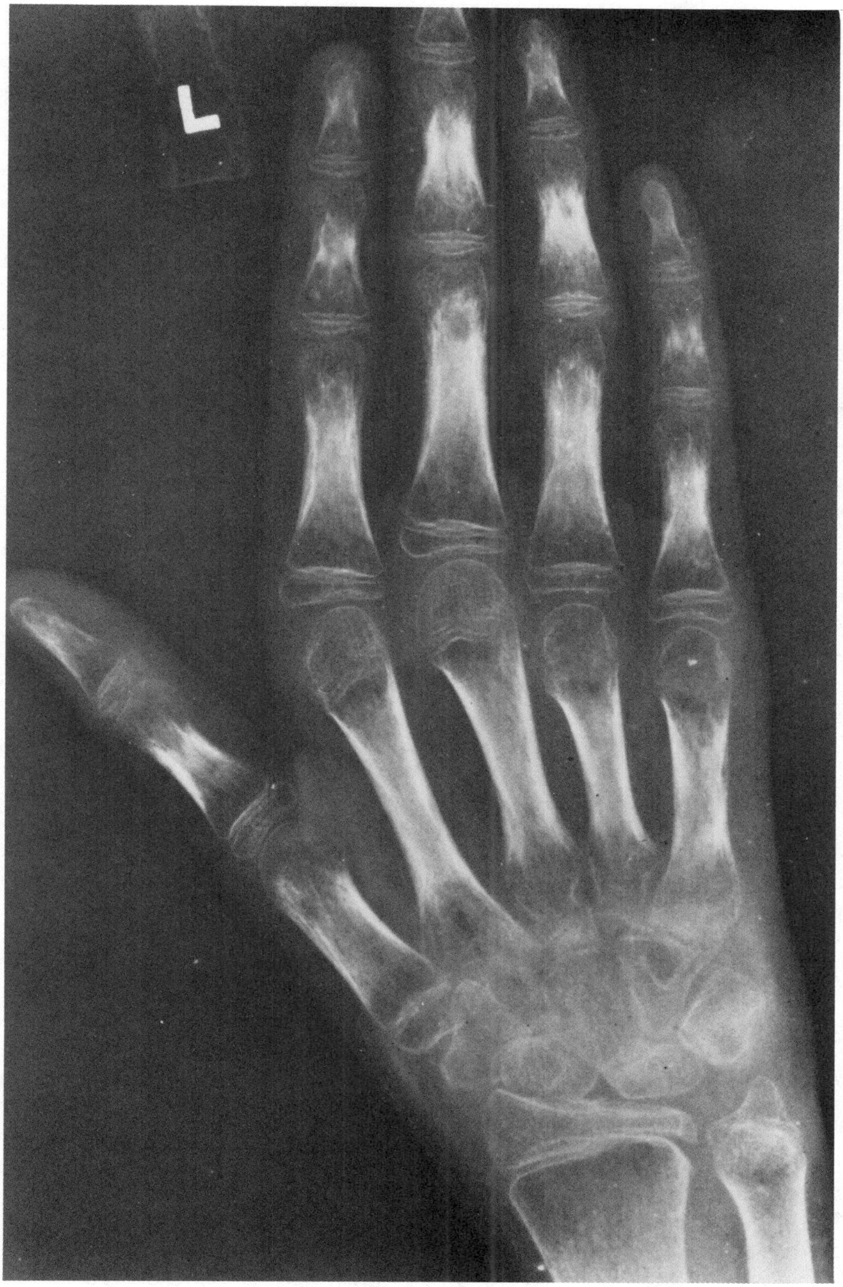

FIGURE 3.6 Marked juxtaarticular osteoporosis in juvenile rheumatoid arthritis. Note the unfused epiphyses indicating the patient age to be about 15 years.

III. Joint Space Changes. The joint space is not a true space but consists of radiolucent articular cartilage over the articular ends of each bone forming the joint with a small amount of interposed synovial fluid. Occasionally, ligaments are present within the joint such as the cruciate ligaments of the knee.

A. Joint Space Widening. Separation of the articular surfaces of a joint may occur in the presence of a large effusion of any type. This may occur in: 1) rheumatic diseases (in the early stages); 2) infection; and 3) hemorrhage (hemophilia or trauma).

B. Joint Space Narrowing. Results from the destruction of articular cartilages and may be:

1. Uniform narrowing
   a) Rheumatoid arthritis (Figures 3.7, 3.8)
   b) Lupus erythematosus
   c) Psoriasis
   d) Reiter's
   e) Ankylosing spondylitis
2. Nonuniform narrowing
   a) Hemachromatosis
   b) Calcium pyrophosphate deposition disease (Figure 3.9)
   c) Degenerative arthritis (Figure 3.10)
   d) Infectious arthritis (pyogenic or TB)
   e) Gout (as a late manifestation)

C. Joint Effusions. Easily seen as soft tissue prominence in the knee (suprapatellar bursa) (Figure 3.11), elbow, and ankle. Less easily seen in other joints. Occurs in:

1. Synovitis associated with any of the rheumatic diseases
2. Infection
3. Trauma
4. Degenerative arthritis

IV. Erosions. Bone erosions are commonly seen in or around joints in several of the arthritides and the cause and appearance of the erosions differ with each etiology.

A. Rheumatoid Arthritis and Juvenile Rheumatoid Arthritis. The erosions are poorly defined and are often referred to as "rat bite" because of the irregular margins. The erosions begin at the articular margins but enlarge to involve the articular surfaces. Any synovial joint may be involved but the hands (Figure 3.12) (mainly the metacarpophalangeal and proximal interphalangeal joints), wrists (Figure 3.13), and feet are most commonly involved. Erosions of the outer end of the clavicle (Figure 3.14) and superior surface of the upper ribs (Figure 3.15) may also occur.

B. Psoriasis (Figures 3.16, 3.17): The erosions are at the margins of the articulations in the early stages but spread to involve the central areas later. Initially, they may simulate the erosions of rheumatoid arthritis except that the distal interphalangeal joints of the hands and feet are most commonly involved. In the later stages bone destruction leads to "pencil in cup" deformity.

C. Reiter's. The erosions begin at the joint margins and often spread centrally. Erosions may occur in the appendicular and axial skeleton. Most frequently involved are the foot, hand, wrist, knee, and sacroiliac joints.

D. Systemic Lupus Erythematosus. Erosions are occasionally seen in the metacarpals, rarely in the metatarsals. These usually occur late in the disease and are classically hook-like.

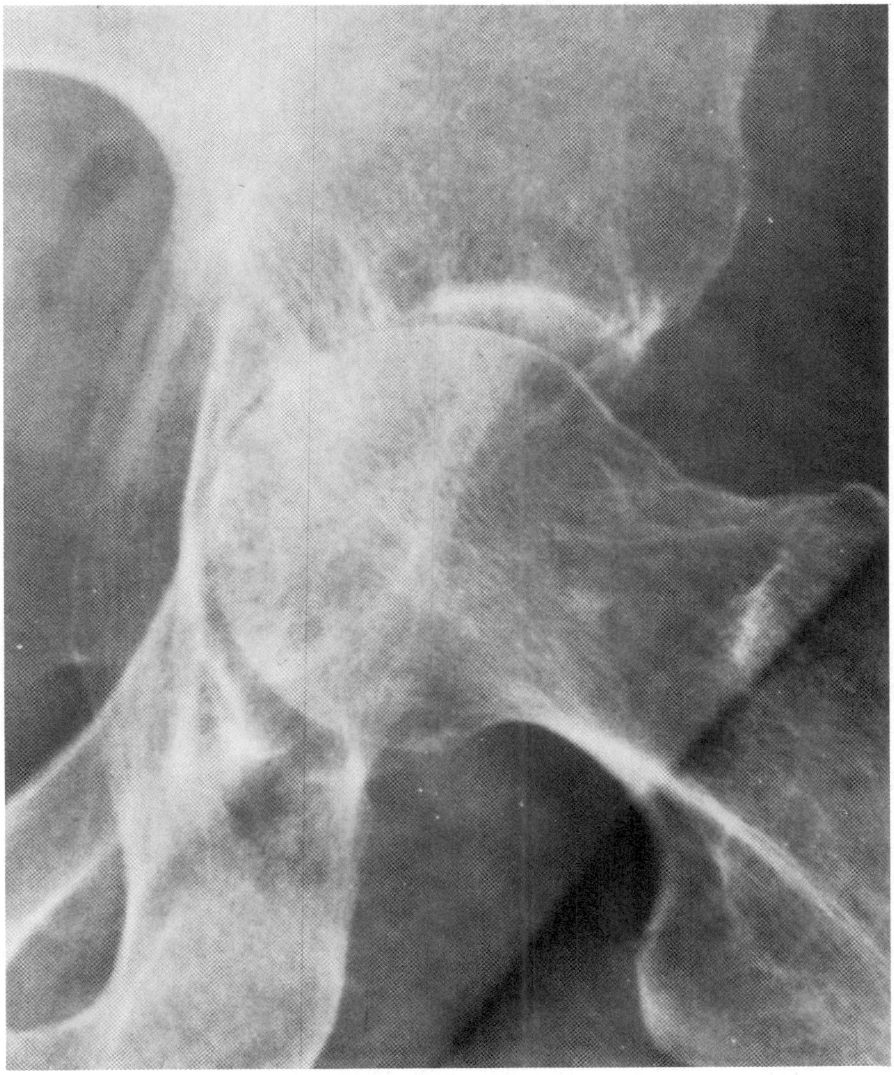

FIGURE 3.7 Rheumatoid arthritis of the hip with narrowing mainly medially and superomedially.

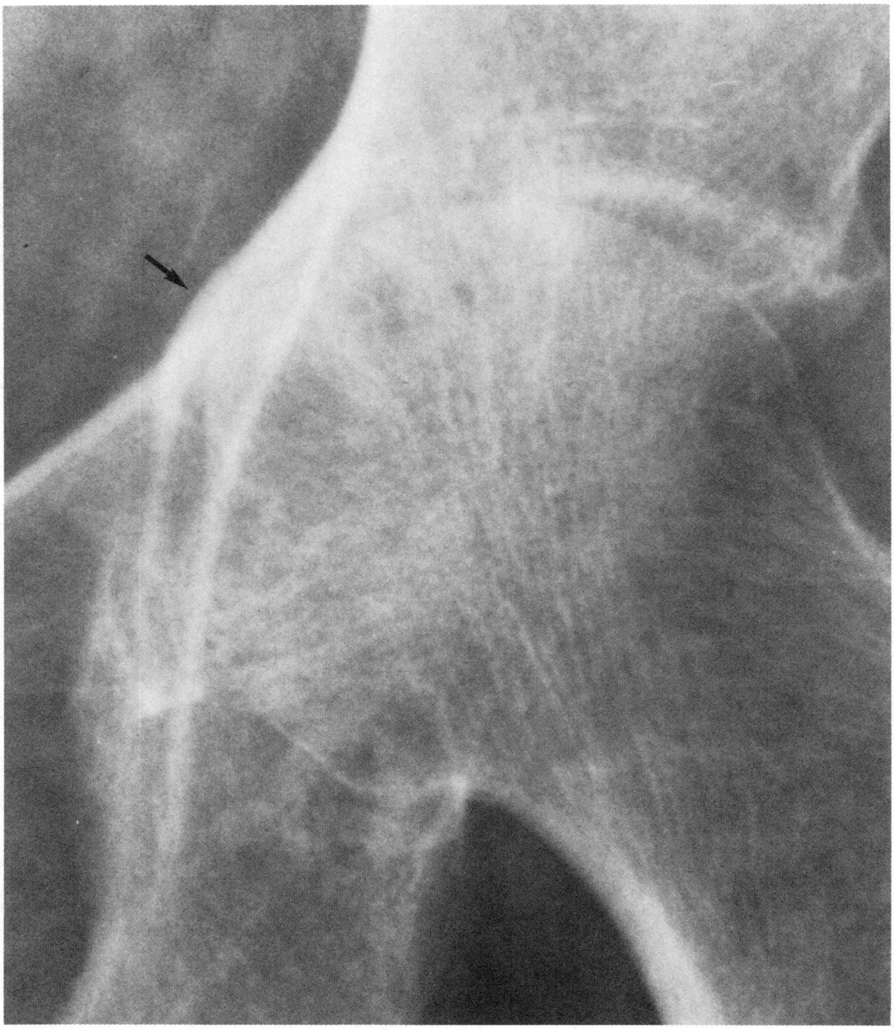

FIGURE 3.8 Medial and superomedial joint space narrowing with early protrusio acetabuli (arrow) in rheumatoid arthritis.

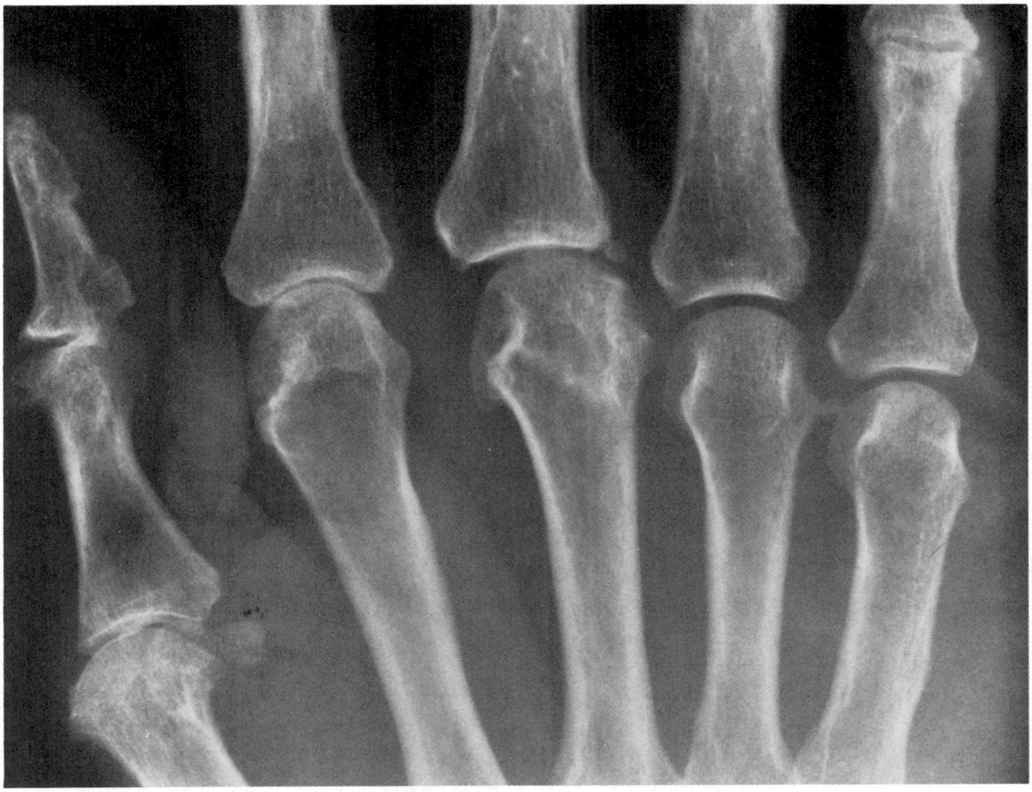

FIGURE 3.9 Nonuniform joint space narrowing of the second and third metacarpophalangeal joints in calcium pyrophosphate deposition disease

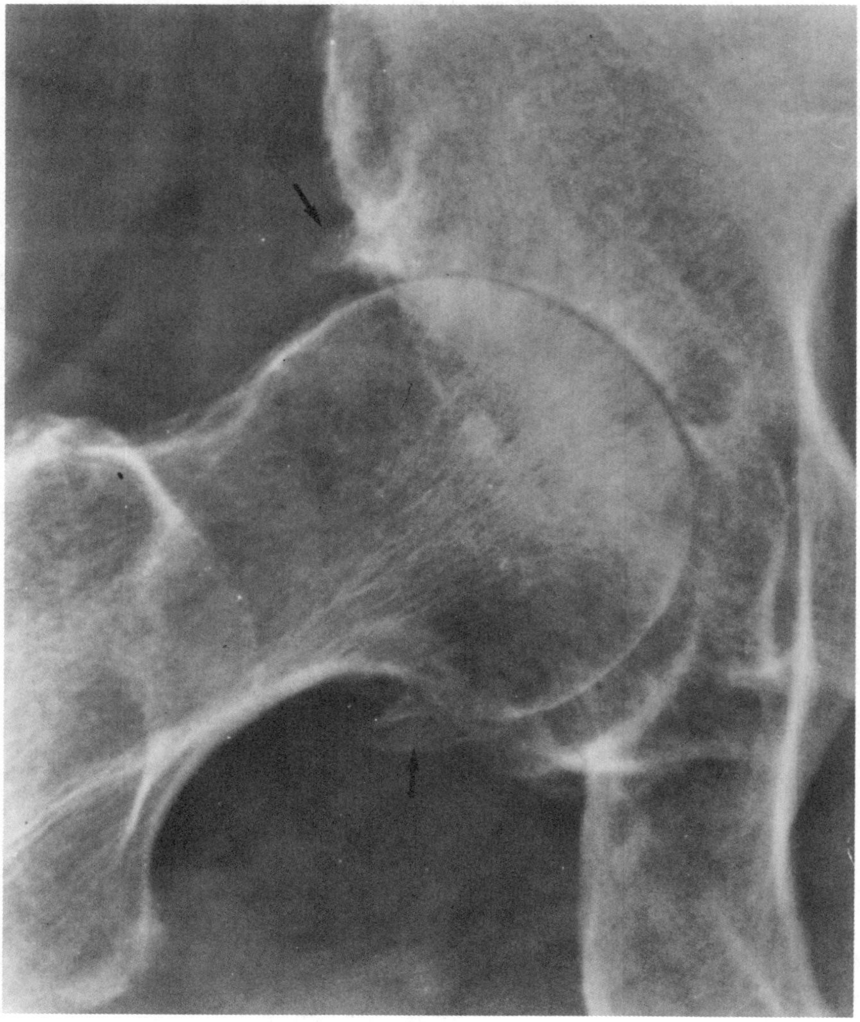

FIGURE 3.10 Degenerative joint disease (osteoarthritis) of the hip with joint space narrowing mainly superiorly and marginal osteophytes (arrow).

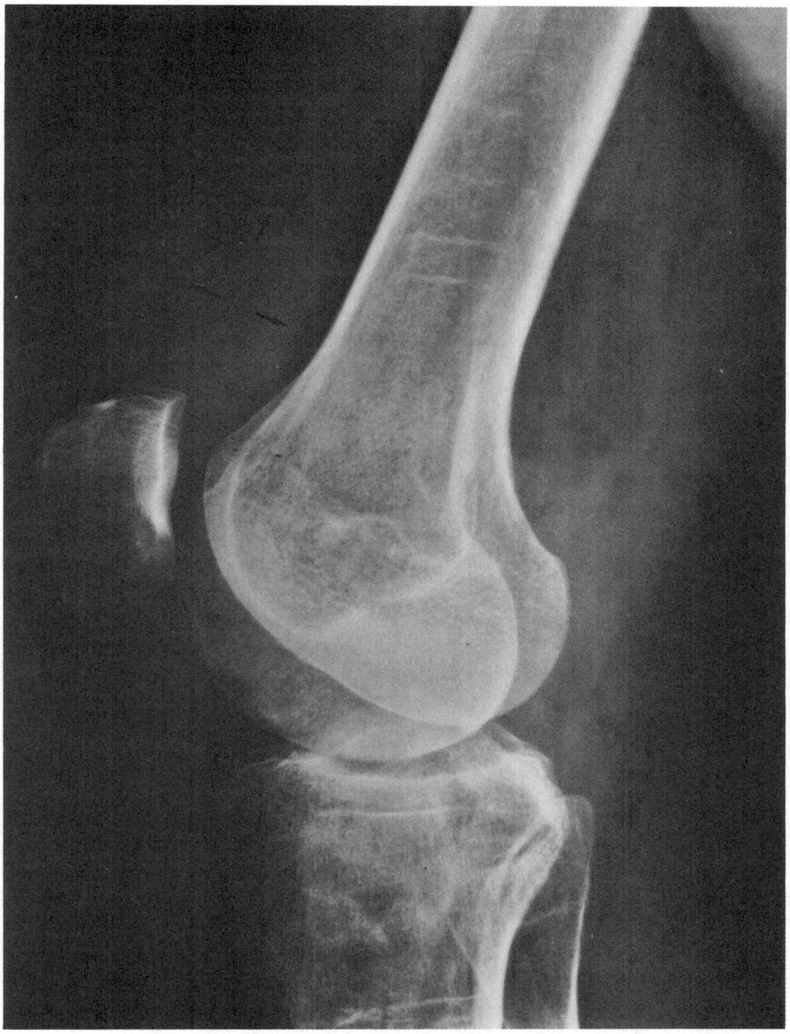

FIGURE 3.11 Knee joint effusion (arrows) posttraumatic.

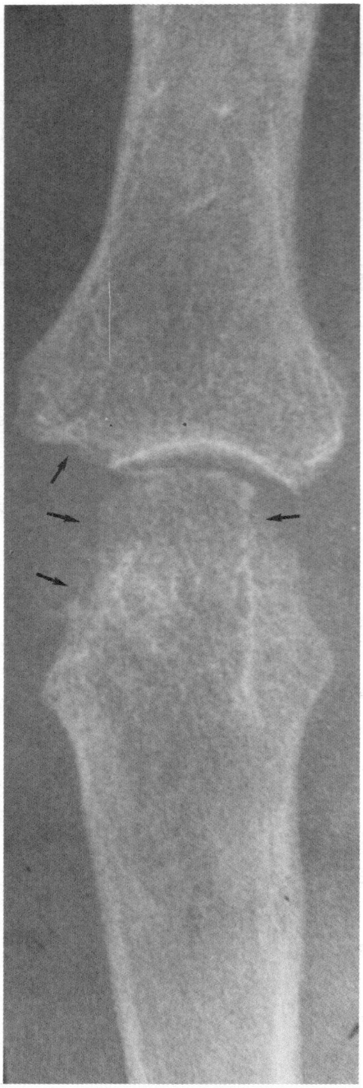

FIGURE 3.12 Rheumatoid arthritis. Early erosions about a metacarpophalangeal joint (arrows).

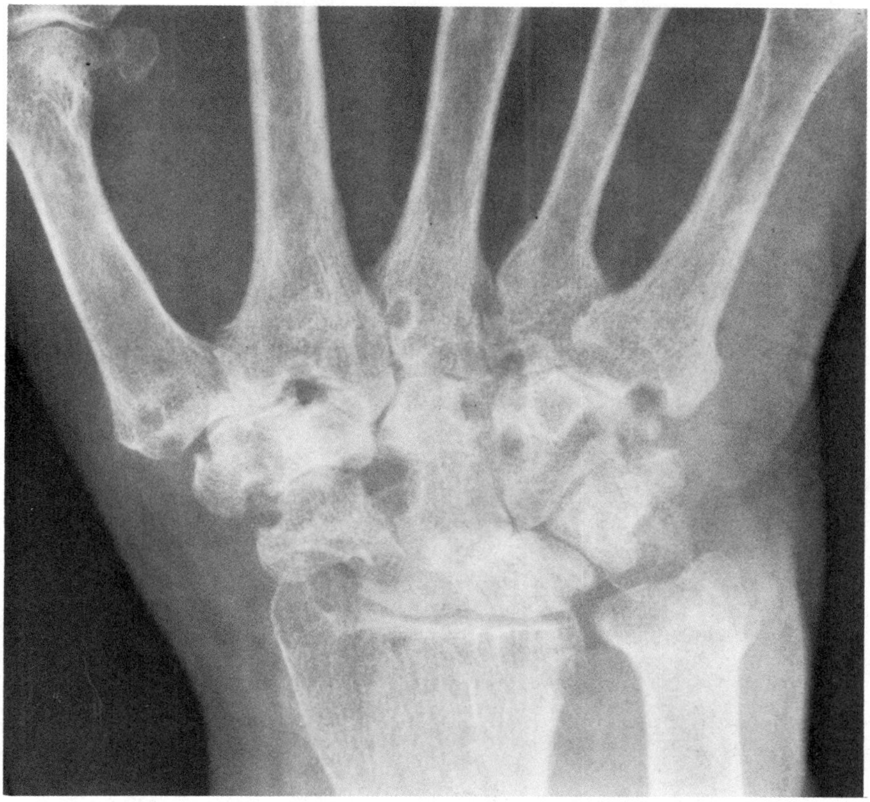

FIGURE 3.13 Extensive erosions of the distal radius and ulna, carpal bones and metacarpal bases in rheumatoid arthritis. There is also joint space narrowing.

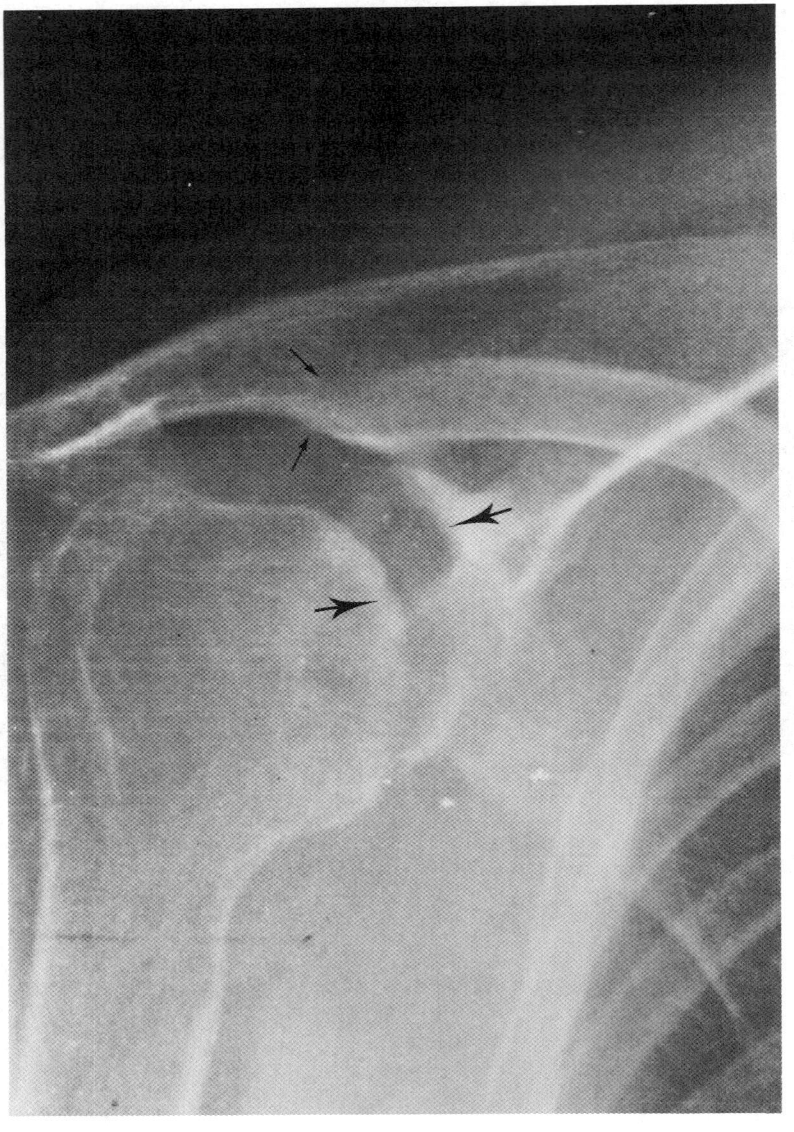

FIGURE 3.14 Erosion of the outer end of the clavicle (small arrows) in rheumatoid arthritis. Note also erosions in the glenohumeral joint (large arrows).

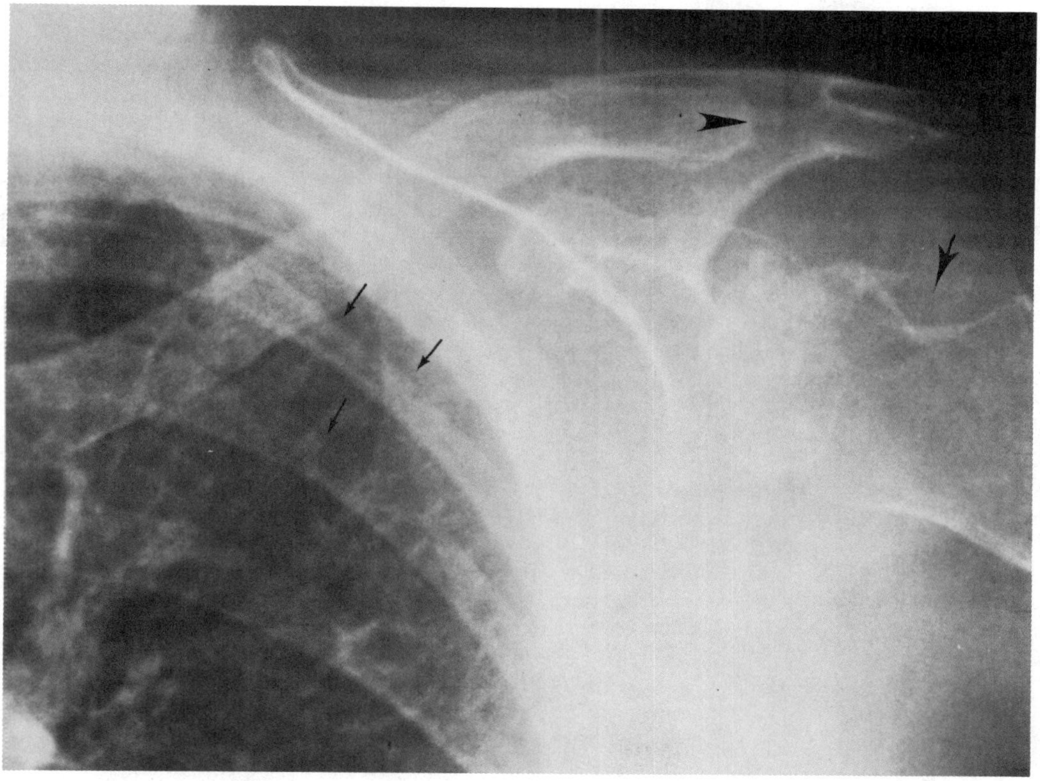

FIGURE 3.15 Rheumatoid arthritis with erosion of the superior surfaces of the fourth and fifth ribs (small arrows), outer end of the clavicle (arrow head) and humeral head (large arrow).

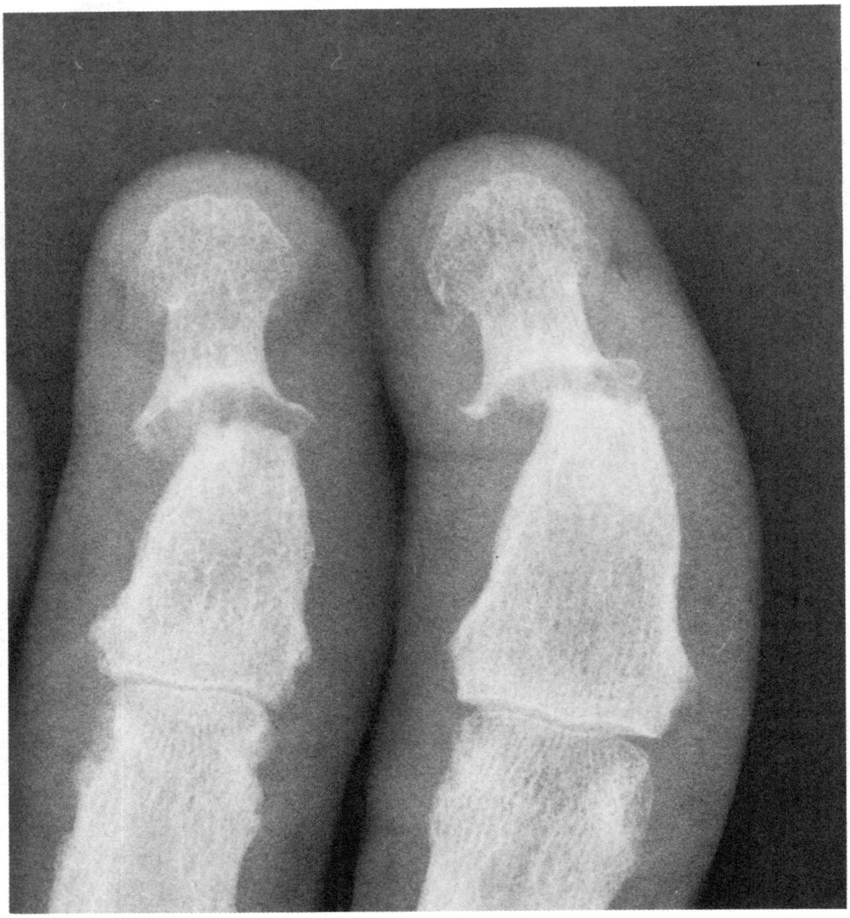

FIGURE 3.16 Psoriasis with erosions of the distal interphalangeal joints and "pencil in cup" deformity.

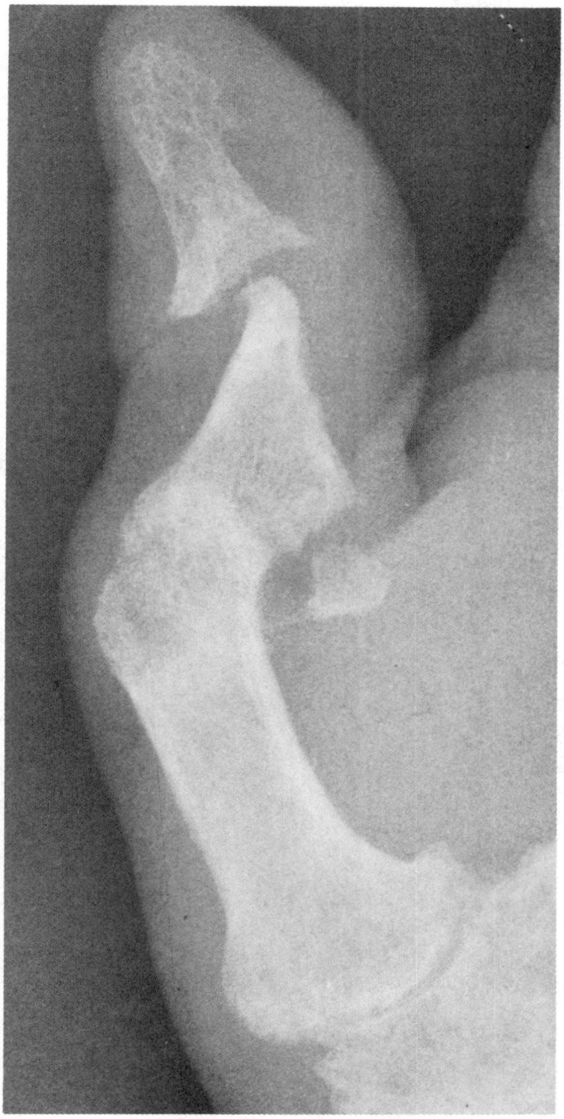

FIGURE 3.17 Psoriasis with erosions of the distal interphalangeal joints and "pencil in cup" deformity.

E. Gout. The erosions may occur centrally or adjacent to the joint (Figure 3.18). Those adjacent to joints are usually well defined with an overhanging or hook-like margin.

F. Degenerative Arthritis. In most cases of degenerative arthritis there are no true erosions. Subarticular cyst formation is common in the later stages and this may mimic en face erosions. Inflammatory or erosive osteoarthritis, an uncommon condition first described in 1961 by Crain, is characterized by true erosive changes involving the articular surfaces of the interphalangeal joints with associated proliferative new bone formation on the articular margins.

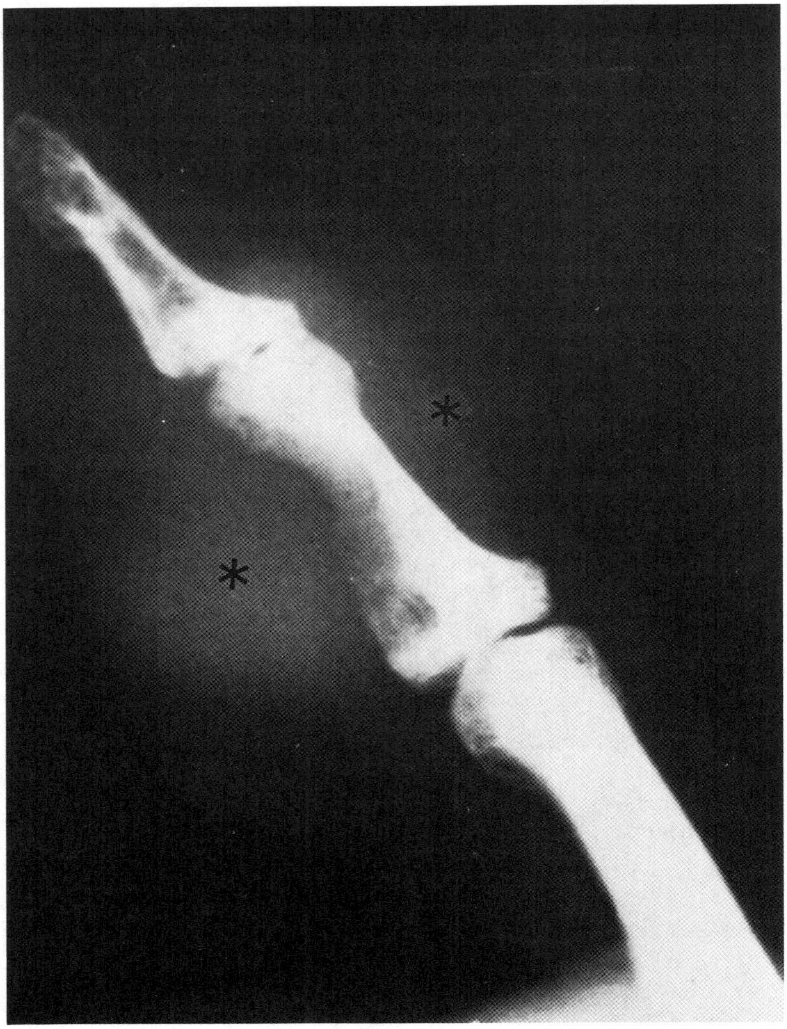

FIGURE 3.18 Erosion of a phalanx in gout. Note the adjacent soft tissue tophus (*).

G. Infection. Erosions usually begin at the articular margins similar to rheumatoid arthritis but progress to involve the subarticular bone with subchondral extension of pannus. This can occur with either pyogenic or tuberculous arthritis.

H. Erosions in Special Situations
   1. Atlantoaxial region. The atlantoodontoid articulation is a synovial joint and can be affected by any of the rheumatoid diseases. Erosions of the odontoid occur in rheumatoid arthritis (in up to 35% of cases) (Figure 3.19) and less commonly in JRA, ankylosing spondylitis, psoriasis, and Reiter's. It is frequently accompanied by atlantoaxial subluxation which may however occur without the presence of erosions.
   2. Sacroiliac joints. Erosions of sacroiliac joints may be bilateral (symmetrical or nonsymmetrical) or unilateral.

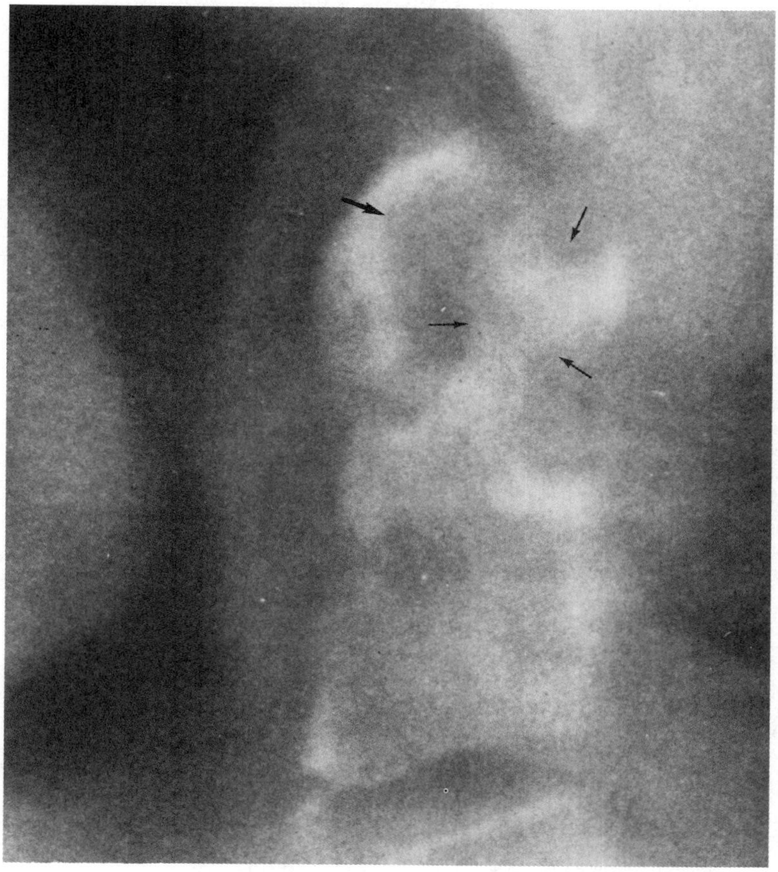

FIGURE 3.19 Erosions of the odontoid (small arrows) and anterior arch of the atlas (larger arrow) in rheumatoid arthritis.

a) Bilateral symmetrical
   (1) Ankylosing spondylitis (Figure 3.20)
   (2) Enteropathic sacroiliitis
   (3) Reiter's, uncommon
   (4) Psoriasis, uncommon
b) Bilateral nonsymmetrical
   (1) Reiter's
   (2) Psoriasis
   (3) Ankylosing spondylitis (early, occasionally)
   (4) Rheumatoid arthritis
   (5) Gout
c) Unilateral
   (1) Infection
   (2) Reiter's (occasionally)
   (3) Gout

3. Calcaneus. Erosions in the calcaneus may occur in:
   a) Psoriasis
   b) Reiter's
   c) Rheumatoid arthritis
   d) Gout
   e) Infection

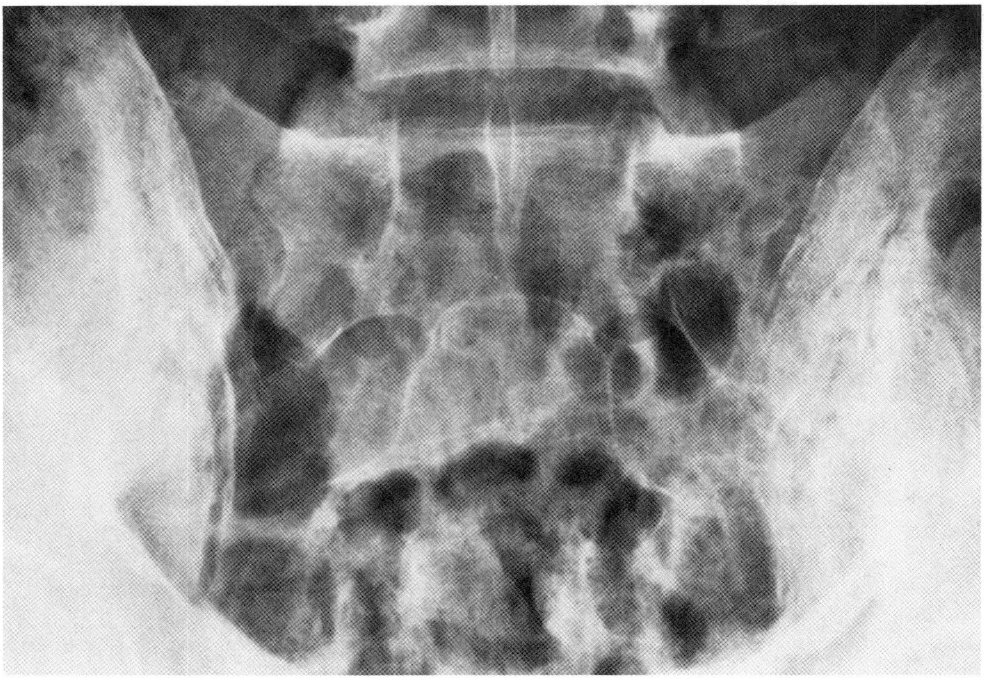

FIGURE 3.20 Ankylosing spondylitis. Erosions of both sacroiliac joints.

V. Alignment Changes. These occur as a result of changes in the articular cartilages or articular ends of bone, changes in the joint capsule and ligaments, or imbalance of muscular action around the joint. Any of the above causes, either singly or in combination, may contribute to the deformity. Alignment abnormalities may be classified as 1) flexion, 2) hyperextension, 3) deviation (the axis of the digits deviate from the normal), and 4) subluxation and dislocation.

A. Flexion Deformities
1. Psoriatic arthritis
2. Dupuytren's contracture of the palmar fascia
3. Posttrauma (Volkman's ischemic contracture, burns, and neurologic trauma)
4. Rheumatoid arthritis
5. Systemic lupus erythematosus

B. Hyperextension of the distal interphalangeal joints with flexion of the proximal interphalangeal joint (boutonnière deformity). Seen in 1) rheumatoid arthritis, 2) SLE, and 3) Jaccoud's arthropathy. Swan neck deformity (Figure 3.21) (opposite of boutonnière) and pure hyperextension deformity occurs in 1) SLE, 2) rheumatoid arthritis, and 3) psoriasis.

C. Deviation, Subluxation and Dislocation. In the hands the digits usually deviate towards the ulnar side (Figure 3.22). Likewise, subluxation (partial dislocation) is frequently but not invariably to the ulnar side. Atlantoaxial subluxation can also occur (Figure 3.23). Complete dislocation in the rheumatic diseases is not common but may occur. These findings may be seen in:
1. Rheumatoid arthritis
2. Jaccoud's arthropathy
3. Lupus erythematosus
4. Psoriasis
5. Gout (advanced)
6. Infectious arthritis (advanced)
7. Charcot's joints (neuropathic)
8. Trauma (subluxation and dislocation)

VI. Periosteal New Bone Formation. Also known as periosteal reaction or periostitis. New bone is laid down along the shafts of bone including the metacarpals, metatarsals, and phalanges. It may be fine (linear), coarse (thicker), or layered and may be parallel to the long axis of the shaft or may be radiating (sunburst) or perpendicular to the shaft. The layered, radiating, or perpendicular types are usually associated with bone tumors (Ewing's sarcoma and osteosarcoma), but may be seen in anemia (in the skull) or with stress fractures. The other types of periosteal reaction are seen in many different conditions including: 1) Reiter's disease (common, coarse) (Figure 3.24), 2) psoriatic arthritis (less common, coarse), 3) juvenile rheumatoid arthritis, 4) rheumatoid arthritis (occasionally, fine) 5) infectious (usually pyogenic, less commonly TB), 6) hypertrophic osteoarthropathy, and 7) trauma. The appearance produced by subperiosteal cortical bone resorption in hyperparathyroidism may mimic periostitis.

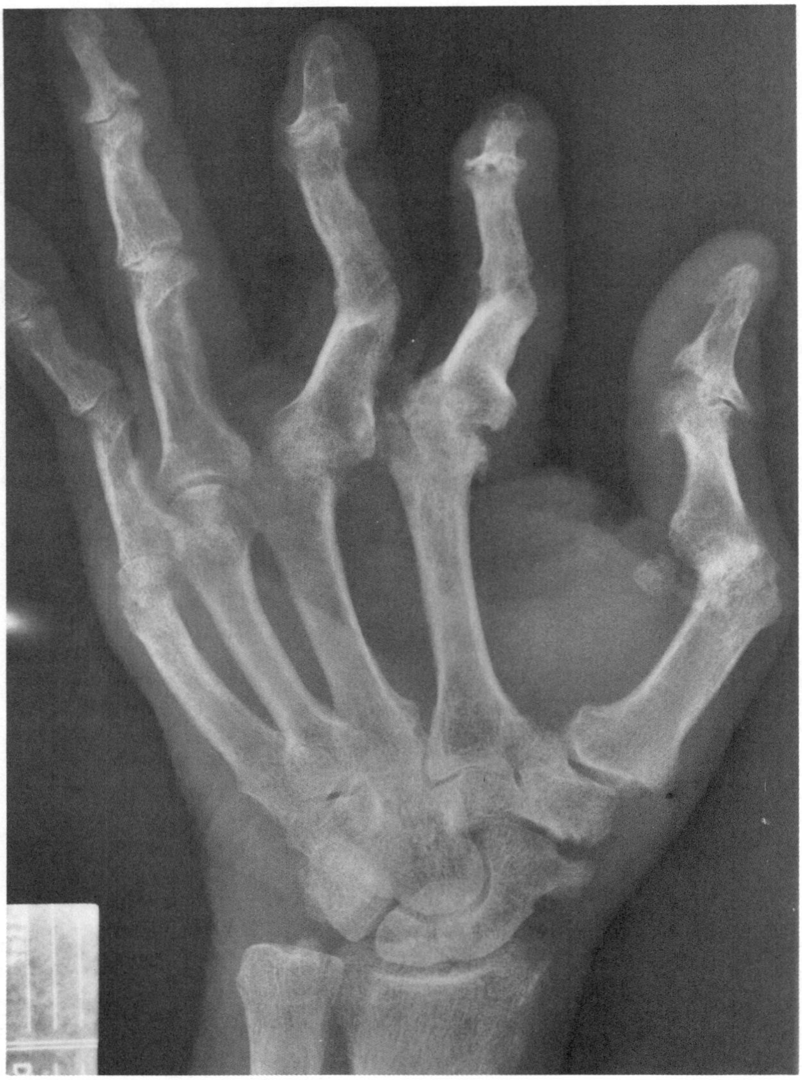

FIGURE 3.21 Swan neck deformity (hyperextension of the PIP joints and flexion of DIP joints) in psoriasis. Note the associated erosions.

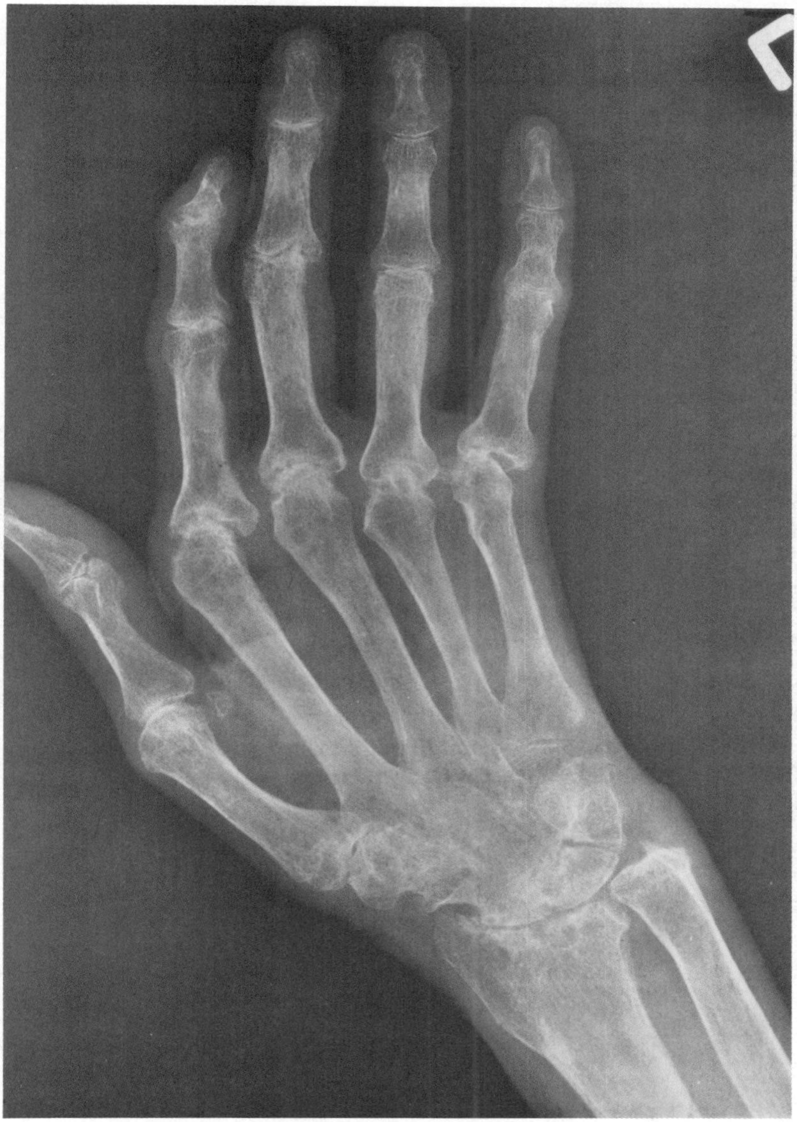

FIGURE 3.22 Rheumatoid arthritis with ulnar deviation at the MP joints. Joint space narrowing and erosions in the hand and wrist with ankylosis of several of the carpal joints.

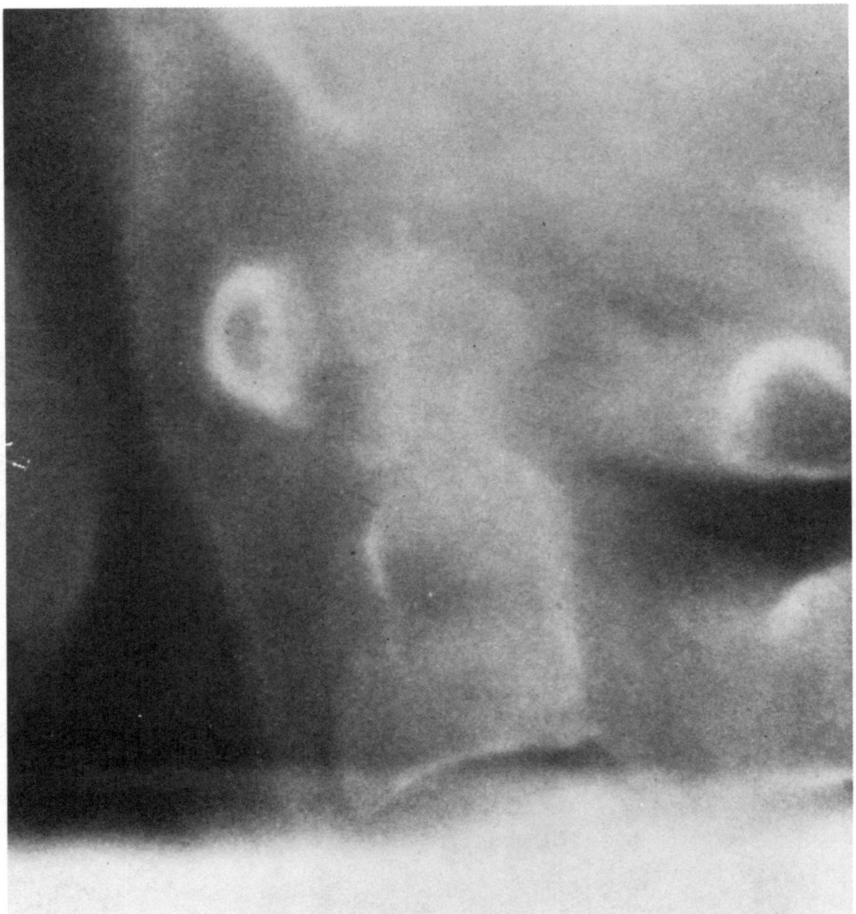

FIGURE 3.23 Atlantoaxial subluxation with odontoid erosions in rheumatoid arthritis (lateral tomogram of C1 and C2).

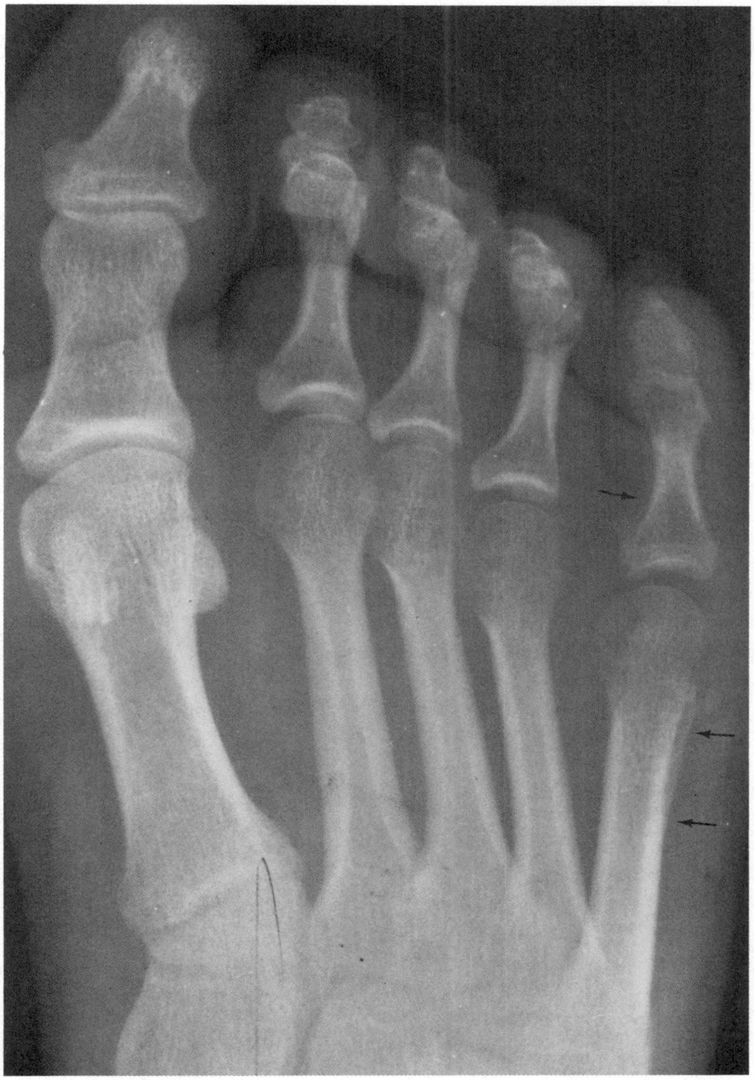

FIGURE 3.24 Periosteal reaction in Reiter's disease (arrows).

VII. Ankylosis. Following destruction of the articular cartilage there may be obliteration of the joint space by either fibrous tissue or bony fusion. Fibrous ankylosis is not usually visible radiologically but is a clinical diagnosis. Bony ankylosis is seen as bony trabeculae bridging the affected joint. Bony ankylosis may be seen in 1) rheumatoid arthritis (Figure 3.25) (carpal and tarsal bone ankylosis occurs late in the disease), 2) JRA (Figure 3.26 A and B), 3) psoriasis (interphalangeal joints), 4) ankylosing spondylitis, and 5) infectious arthritis: a) pyogenic, b) TB (common in the spine, uncommon elsewhere).

A. Ankylosis in Special Situations
   1. Sacroiliac joints
      a) Bilateral symmetrical
         (1) Ankylosing spondylitis
         (2) Enteropathic sacroilitis
         (3) Reiter's (uncommon)
         (4) Psoriasis (uncommon)
      b) Bilateral nonsymmetric
         (1) Reiter's (uncommon)
         (2) Psoriasis (uncommon)
      c) Unilateral: infection.

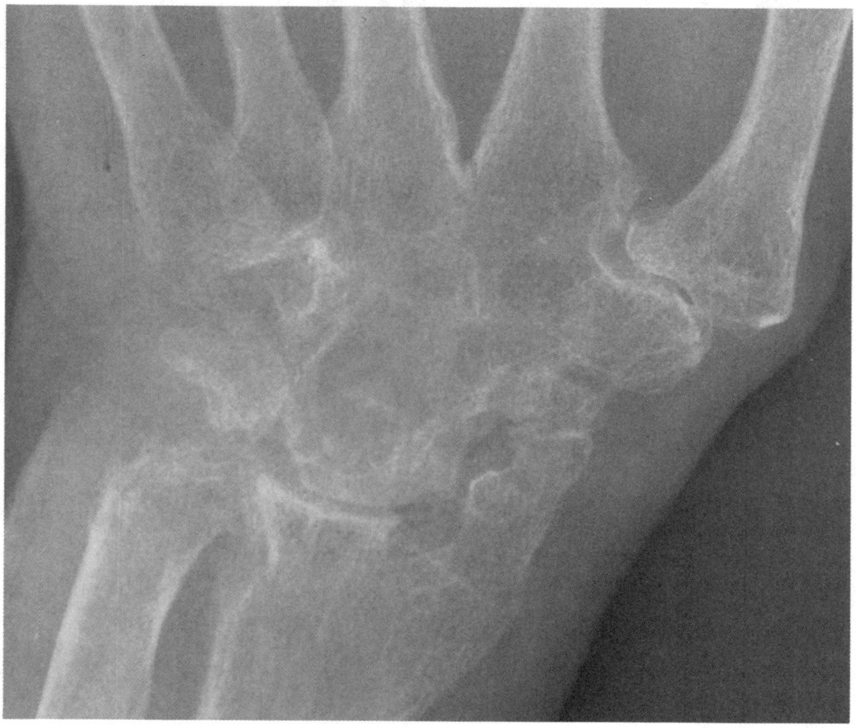

FIGURE 3.25 Ankylosis of carpal bones with erosions in long-standing rheumatoid arthritis.

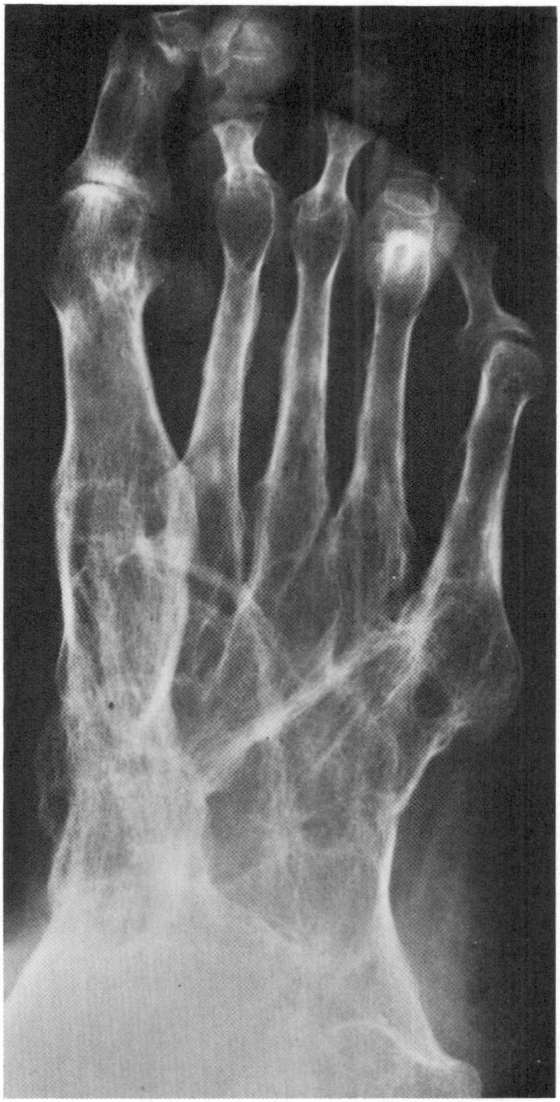

FIGURE 3.26 (A) Frontal view of the foot.

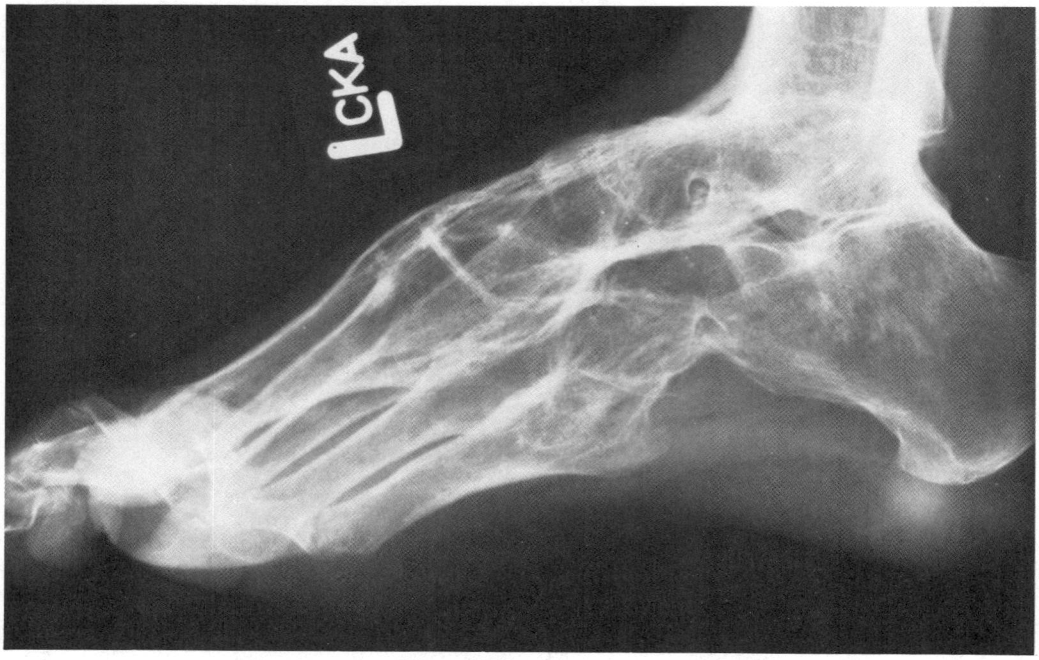

FIGURE 3.26 (B) Lateral view of the foot and ankle showing juvenile rheumatoid arthritis with ankylosis.

VIII. Phytes
   A. Osteophytes. This equals hypertrophic bone formation. It may occur at the articular margins of joints (degenerative joint disease) or arise from the vertebral bodies, several millimeters from the end plates (spondylosis or degenerative disease of the spine).
   B. Syndesmophytes. This is ossification of the annulus fibrosus. It is a fine linear calcific bridge extending vertically between the edges of the vertebral bodies and is usually symmetric. Seen in: 1) ankylosing spondylitis (Figure 3.27), 2) enteropathic arthropathy [e.g., ulcerative colitis (Figure 3.28 A and B)], and 3) alkaptonuria.
   C. Coarse Syndesmophytes. These are, in fact, ossification in the paravertebral connective tissues. They form coarse ill-defined or well-defined bridges between the vertebral bodies, separated from the edge of the vertebral body and the disc. They are usually asymmetric. These are seen in 1) psoriasis, and 2) Reiter's (Figure 3.29).

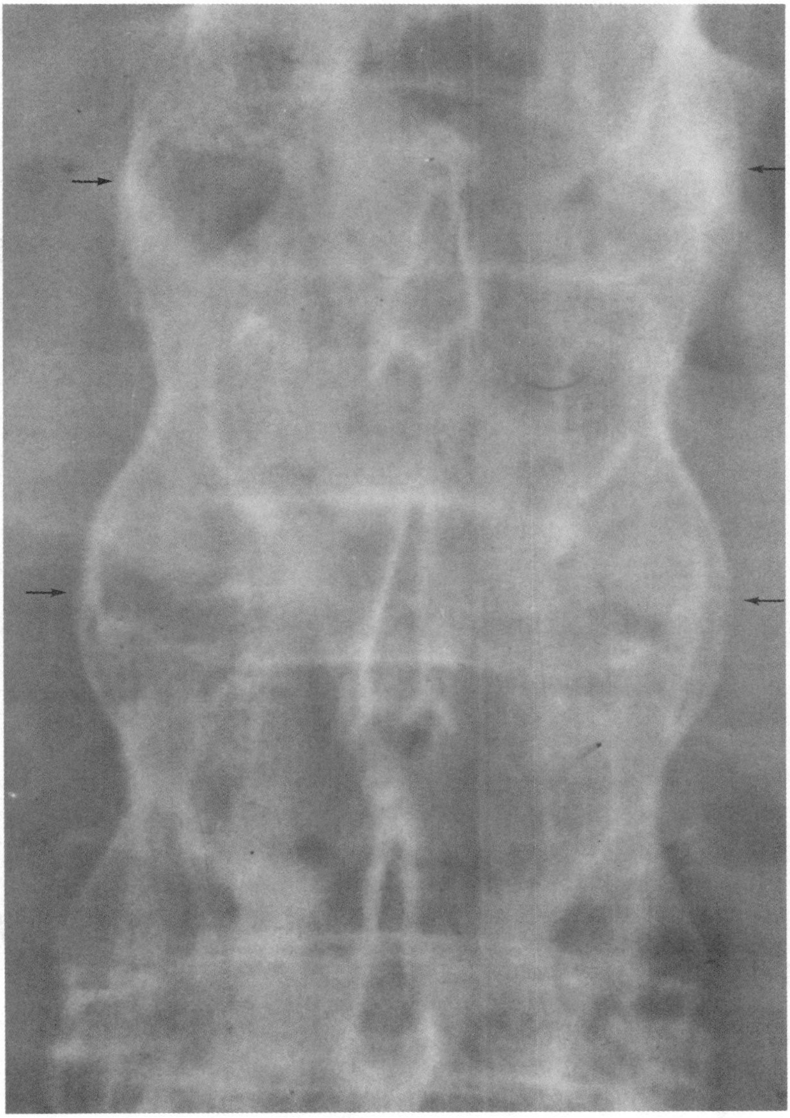

FIGURE 3.27 Fine symmetric syndesmophytes of ankylosing spondylitis in the lumbar spine (arrows).

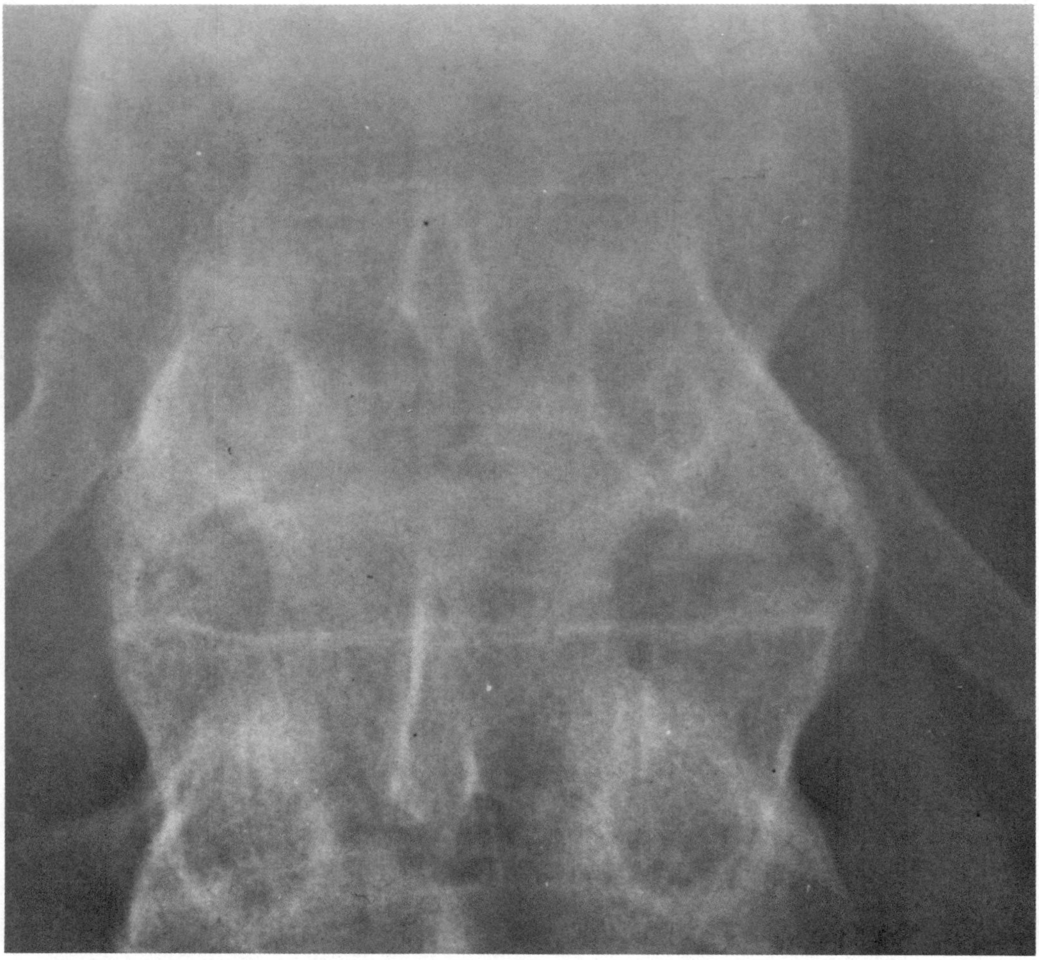

FIGURE 3.28 (A) Frontal views of the thoracolumbar junction showing fine syndesmophytes in a patient with ulcerative colitis.

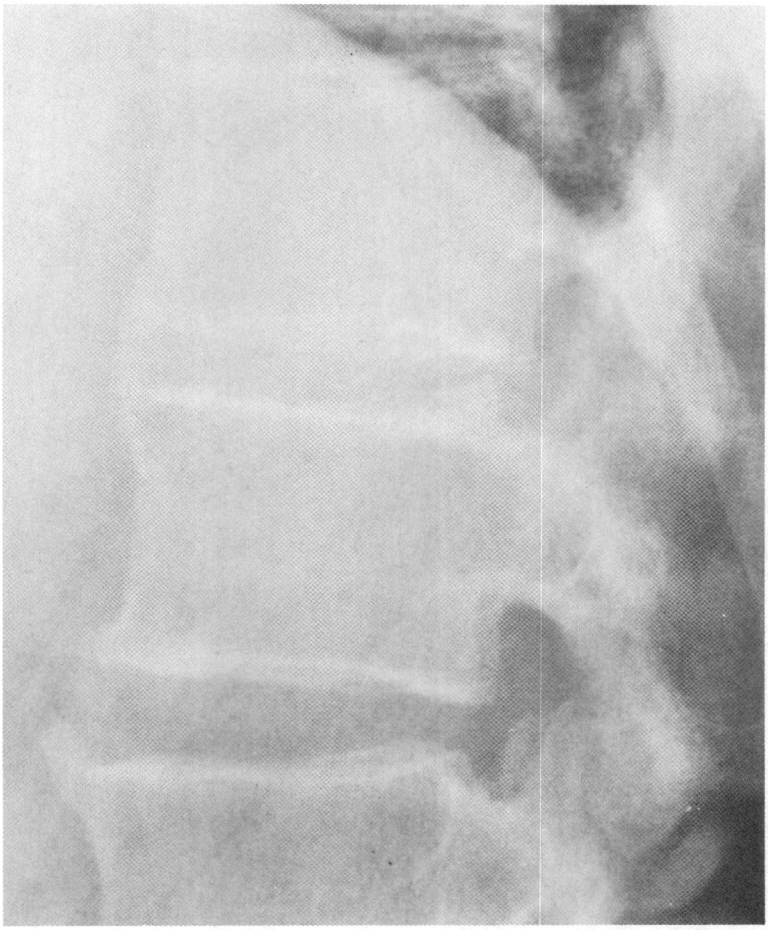

FIGURE 3.28 (B) Lateral views of the thoracolumbar junction showing fine syndesmophytes in a patient with ulcerative colitis.

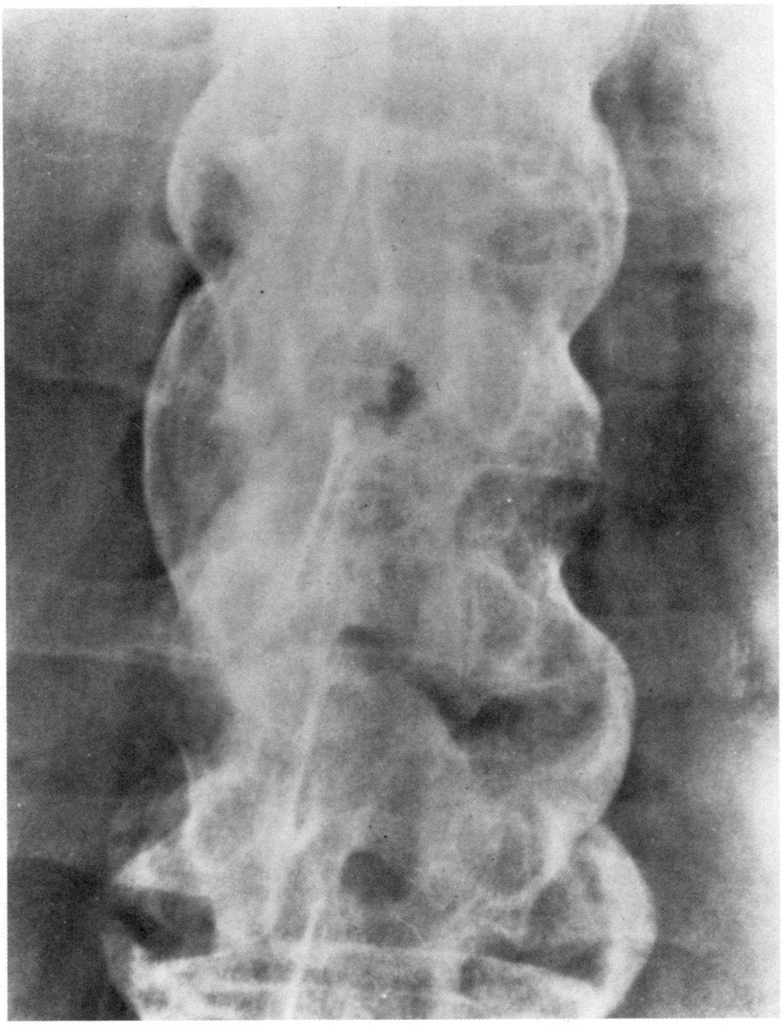

FIGURE 3.29 Reiter's disease with large coarse asymmetric syndesmophytes.

IX. Enthesopathy. This refers to bone erosion with proliferation at the site of ligament or tendon attachment to bone. It is seen mainly in the iliac crest, ischial tuberosities, femoral trochanters, humeral tuberosities, calcanei (plantar surface and Achilles' tendon insertion) and the patella. It occurs in 1) ankylosing spondylitis (Figure 3.30), 2) psoriasis, 3) Reiter's disease (Figure 3.31), and 4) rheumatoid arthritis (rarely).

X. Calcification

A. Calcification Within Joints

1. Chondrocalcinosis (calcification of articular cartilage or meniscus). Seen in:
    a) Calcium pyrophosphate deposition disease (Figure 3.32, 3.33, and 3.34)
    b) Gout
    c) Hemochromatosis
    d) Hyperparathyroidism
2. Calcified loose body
    a) Degenerative joint disease
    b) Trauma
    c) Osteochondritis dissecans (Figure 3.35)
    d) Neuropathic joints
    e) Synovial osteochondromatosis

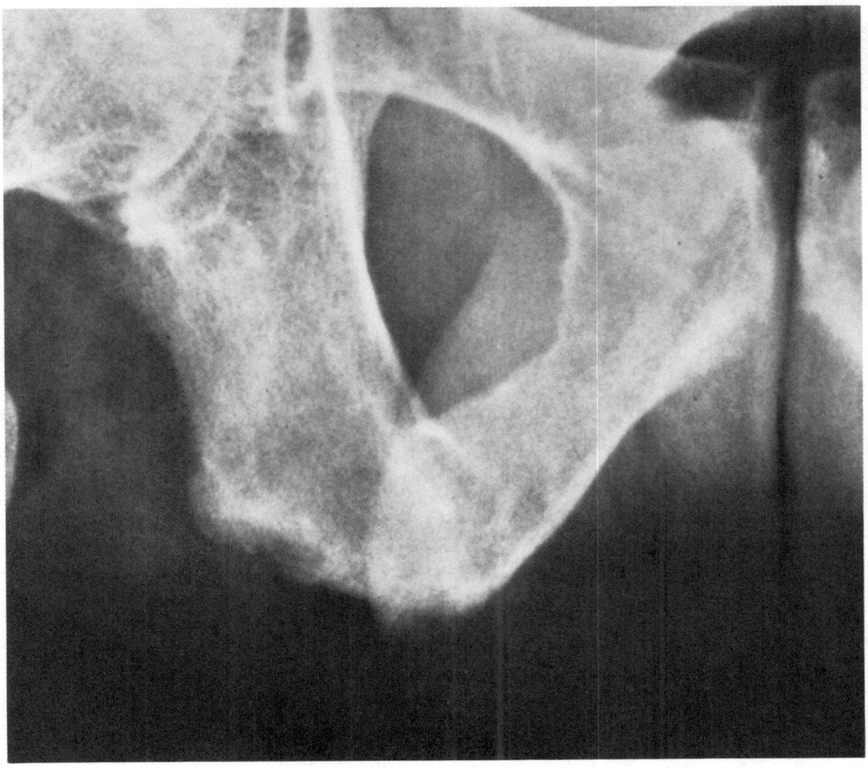

FIGURE 3.30 Erosions and new bone formation in the ischial tuberosity (enthesopathy) in ankylosing spondylitis.

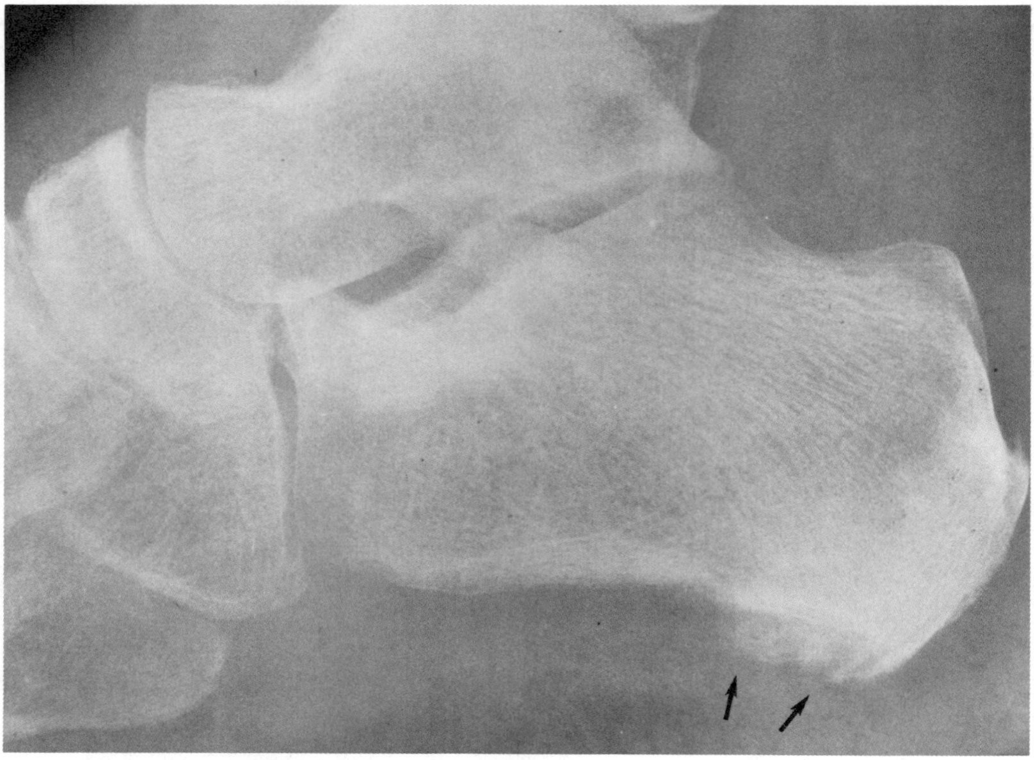

FIGURE 3.31 Enthesopathy of the calcaneus in Reiter's disease (arrows).

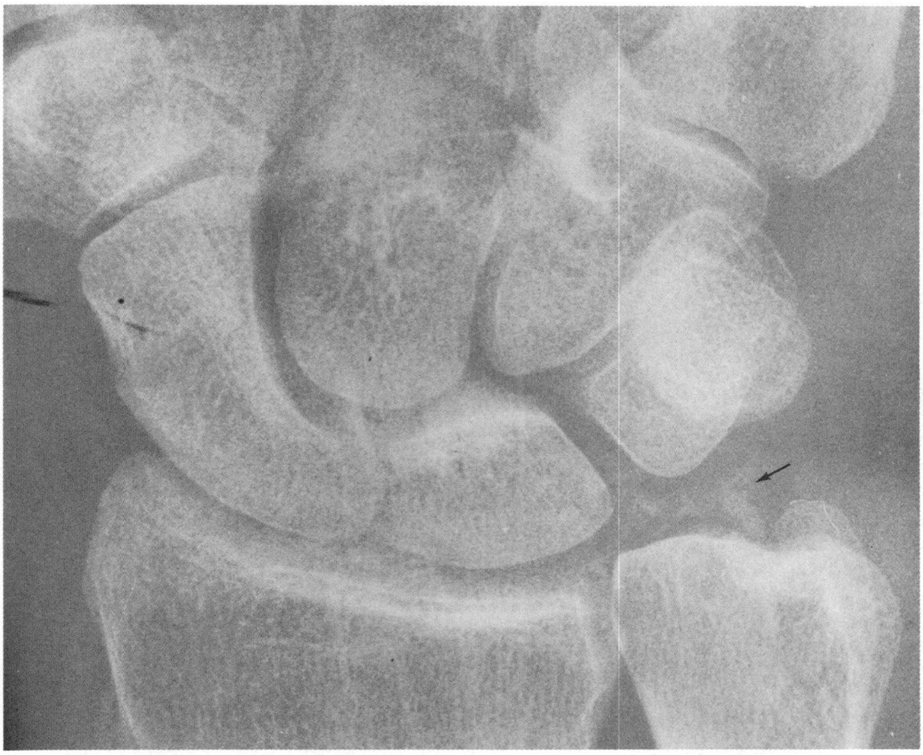

FIGURE 3.32 Calcium pyrophosphate deposition disease with calcification in the triangular cartilage of the wrist (arrow).

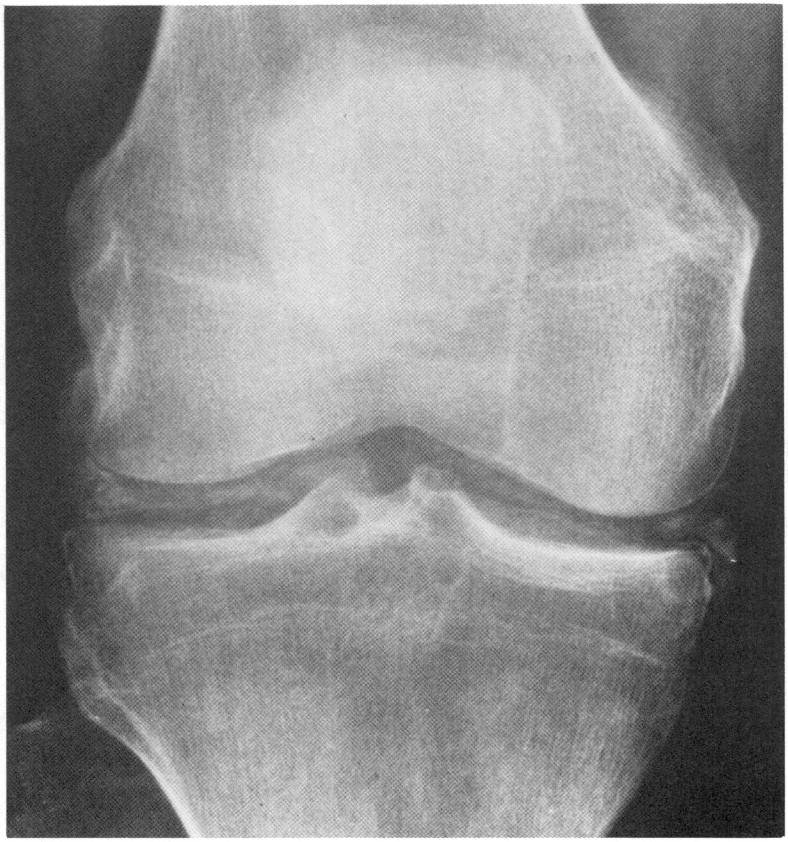

FIGURE 3.33 CPPD with meniscal calcification in the knee.

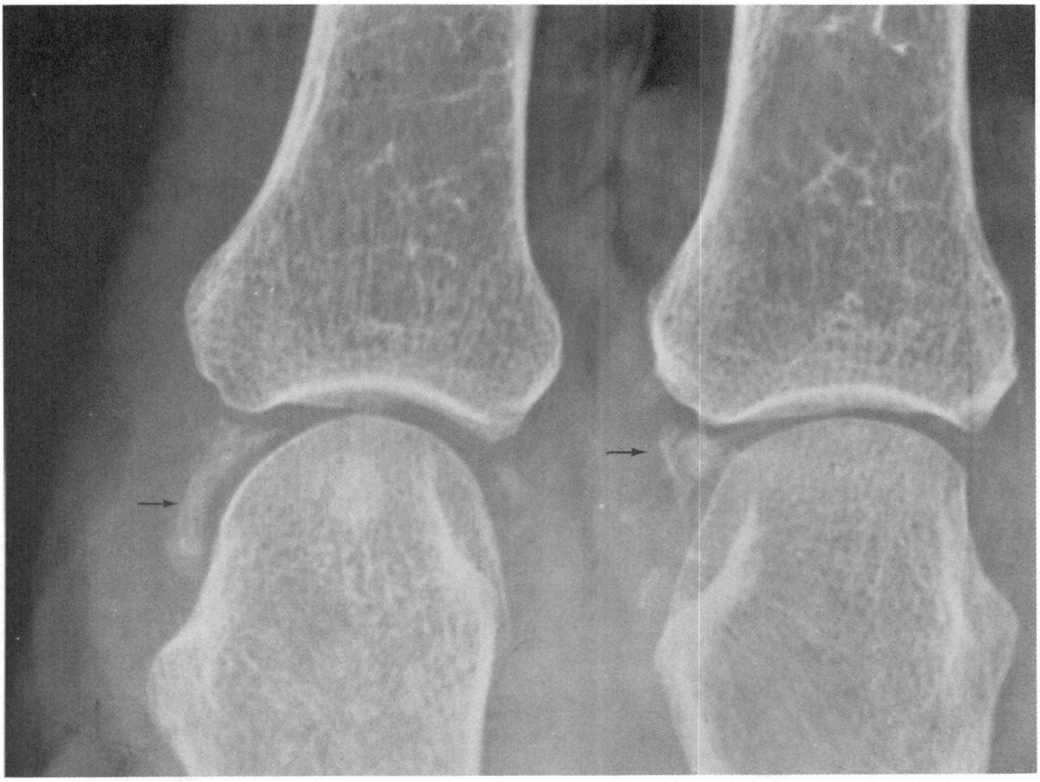

FIGURE 3.34 Articular cartilage calcification (arrow) in the metacarpophalangeal joints in CPPD.

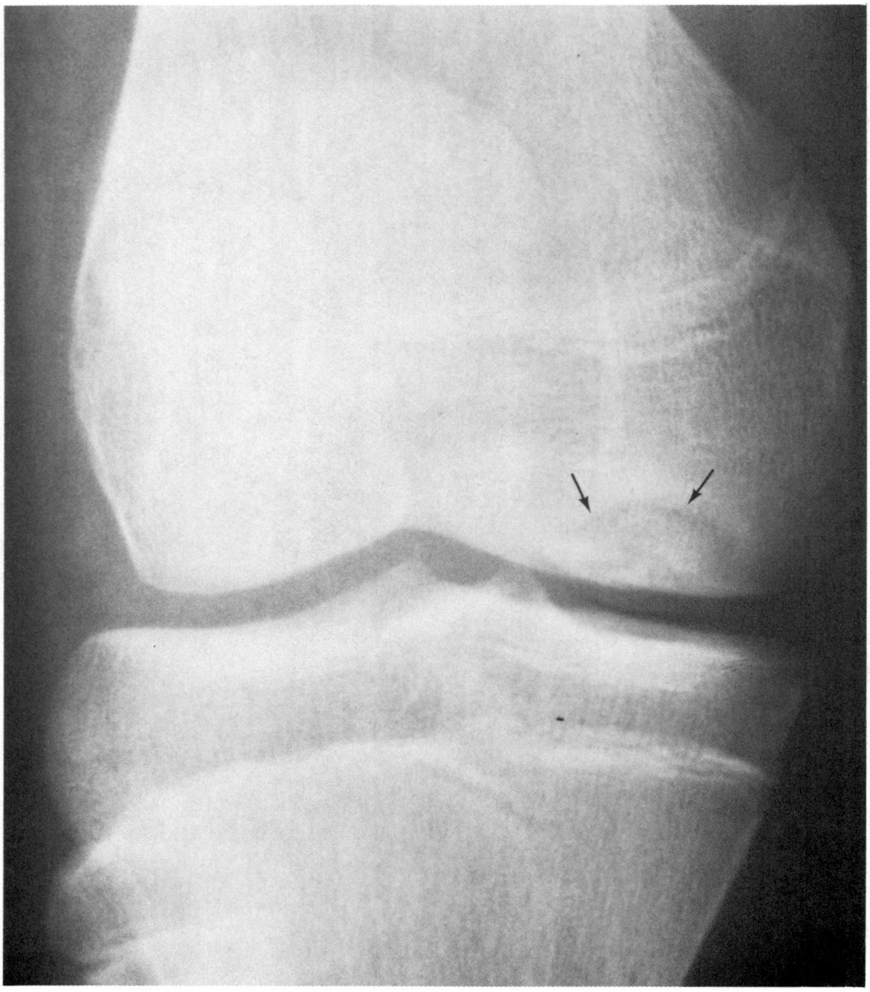

FIGURE 3.35 Osteochondritis dissecans of the knee with osteochondral fragment in the medial condyle (arrows).

B. Calcification in the Soft Tissues (Extraarticular)
   1. Scleroderma
   2. Rheumatoid arthritis
   3. Gout
   4. Neuropathic joints
   5. Trauma
   6. Dermatomyositis (Figure 3.36)

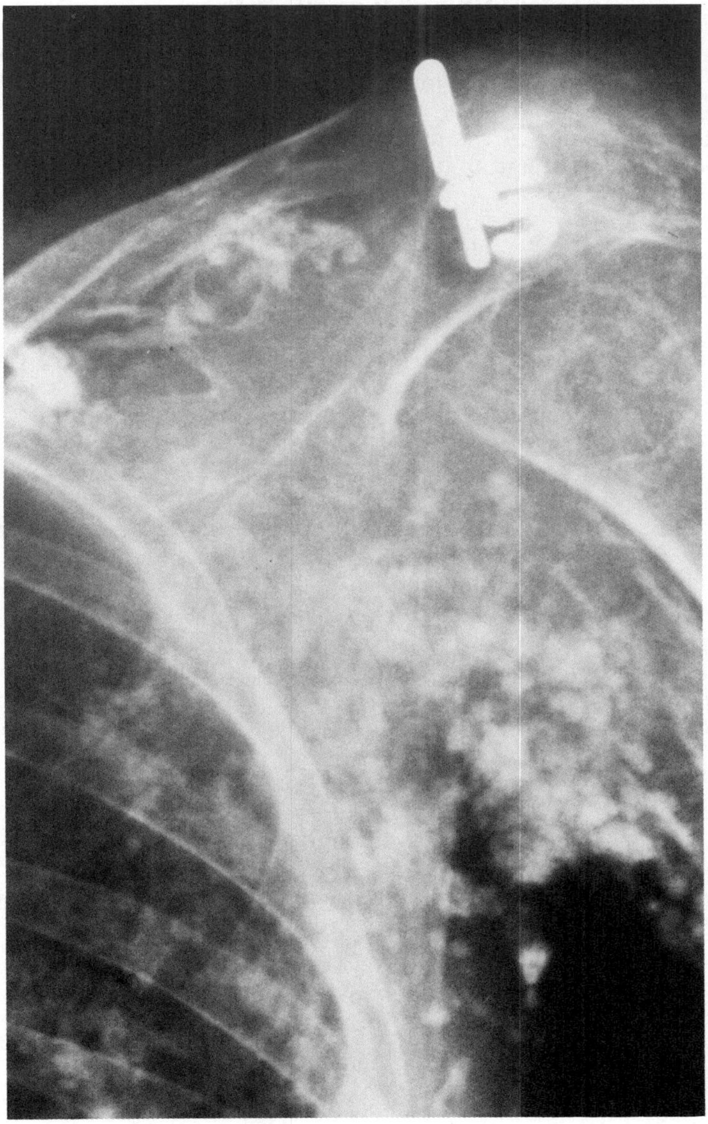

FIGURE 3.36 Extensive soft tissue calcification around the shoulder and upper chest in dermatomyositis.

Now that the radiographic features of joint disease have been outlined in a general manner, one can apply these particular radiographic features to specific arthritides. By systematically examining each radiograph with reference to the already described features of joint disease, one can formulate a differential diagnosis and often make a specific diagnosis from the radiographs. For the remainder of this chapter, the common radiographic changes seen in specific disease entities will be briefly listed.

Rheumatoid Arthritis

A description of the radiographic changes and their distribution in rheumatoid arthritis will be discussed first. This is a relatively common disease and thus is often portrayed as the gold standard in radiographic differential diagnosis of arthritis. For the remainder of the disease entities discussed, comparison will be made with rheumatoid arthritis.

Radiographic Changes

1. Osteoporosis (Figure 3.37).
2. Joint space narrowing. Within a particular joint itself, the narrowing is uniform throughout that joint. For example, in the knee, both the medial and lateral compartments are equally narrowed (Figure 3.40). In the hip, both the superior and medial portions of the joint space are narrowed.
3. Erosions. The location of the erosions is along the margins of the articular bone where the articular bone is directly in contact with synovium. These are termed marginal erosions (Figures 3.38, 3.39, 3.40).
4. Subchondral cysts.
5. Ankylosis. Ankylosis of the carpal bones is more common than ankylosis of the MCP joints or interphalangeal joints (Figure 3.41).
6. Subluxations and malalignment deformities. Subluxations at multiple joints can occur. Ulnar deviation of the phalanges with respect to the long axis of the metacarpals is often seen (Figure 3.42).
7. Several radiographic characteristics that are not part of the spectrum of rheumatoid arthritis include bony sclerosis, osteophytosis, and periosteal reaction.

Distribution

Symmetric. One of the hallmarks in rheumatoid arthritis is the marked symmetry in distribution of the radiographic changes listed above. Multiple joints are involved bilaterally and symmetrically and include those in the hand (MCP, PIP), wrist, foot (MTP, PIP), knee (all compartments), elbow, and C-spine.

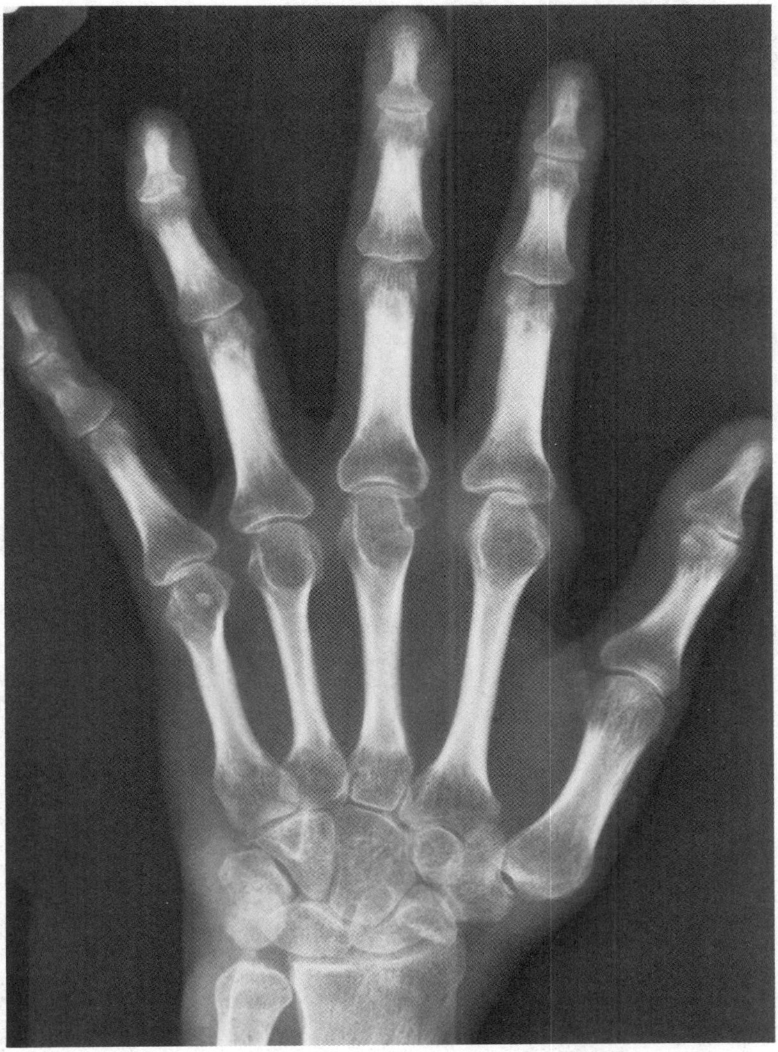

FIGURE 3.37 Hand in early rheumatoid arthritis. Marked juxtaarticular osteoporosis of the carpal, metacarpophalangeal, and interphalangeal joints with joint space narrowing in the metacarpophalangeal joints.

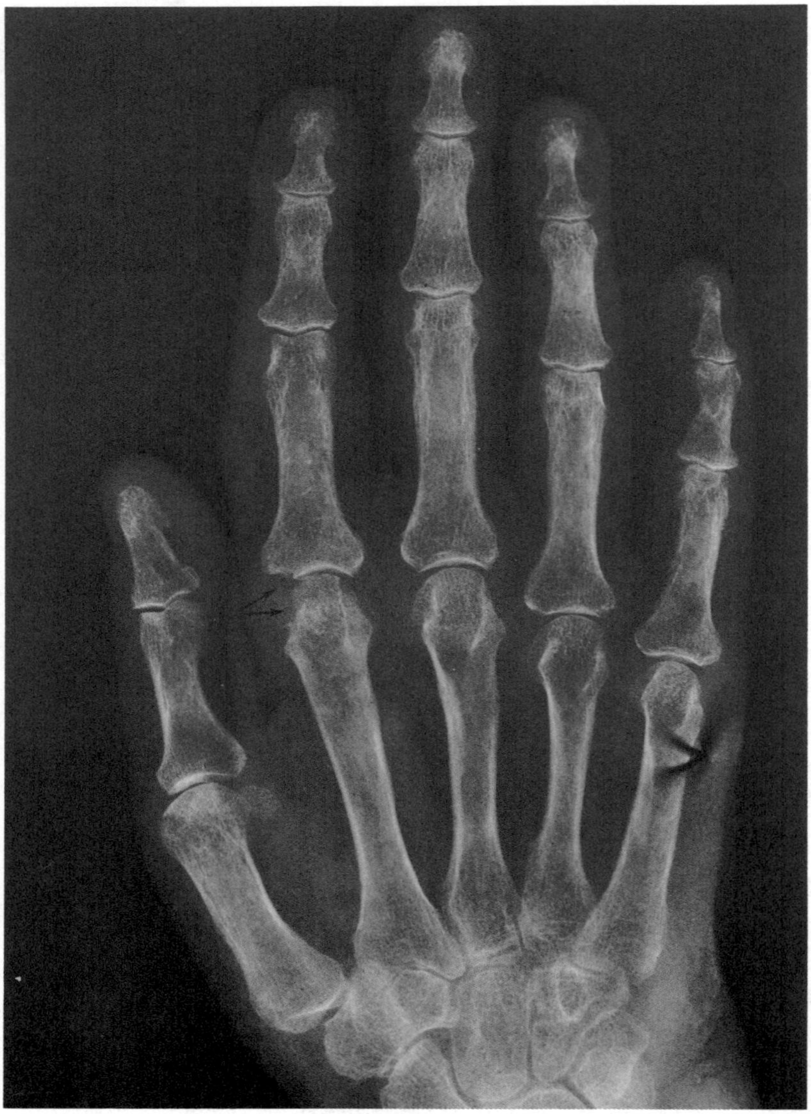

FIGURE 3.38 Rheumatoid arthritis. Erosions in the metacarpophalangeal joint of the index finger (arrow) and joint space narrowing in the metacarpophalangeal joints of the index and ring fingers.

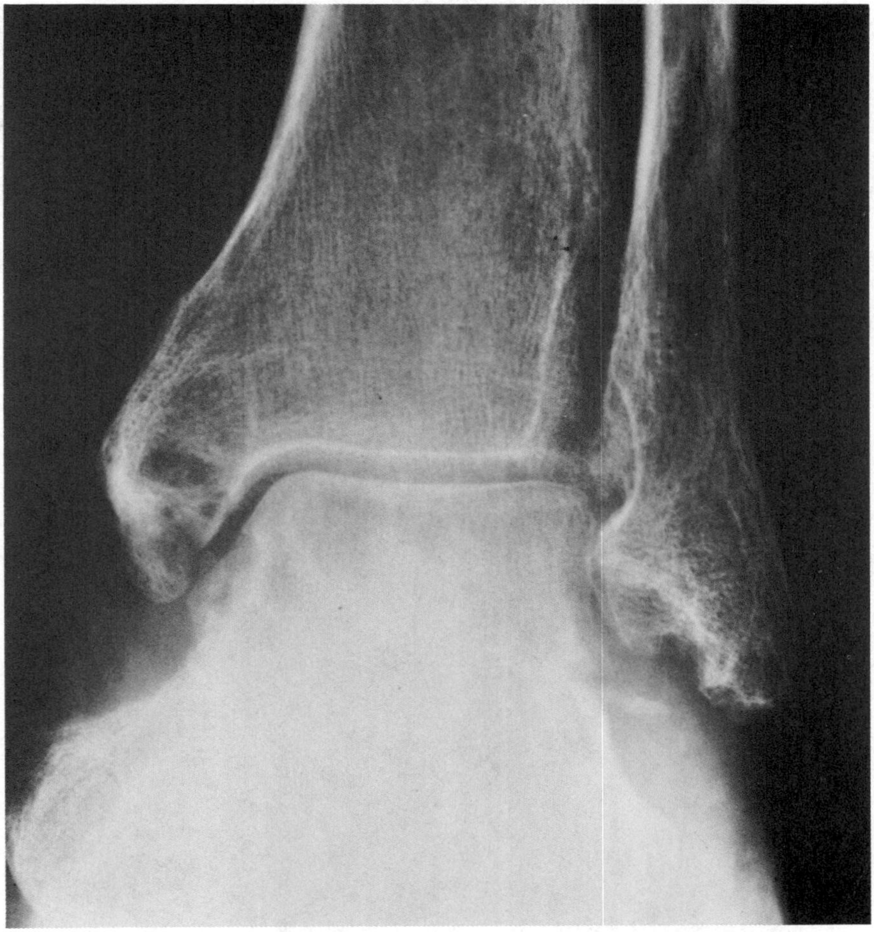

FIGURE 3.39 Large erosions around the ankle in rheumatoid arthritis. These erosions are similar to those seen in gout.

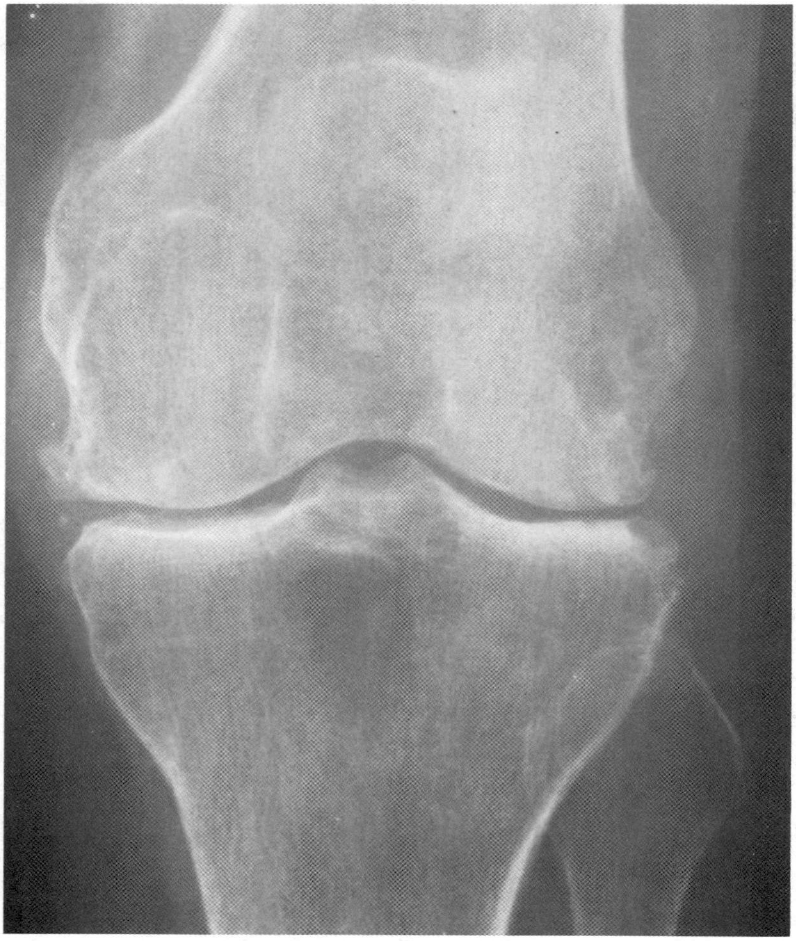

FIGURE 3.40 (A) Frontal view of the knee in rheumatoid arthritis.

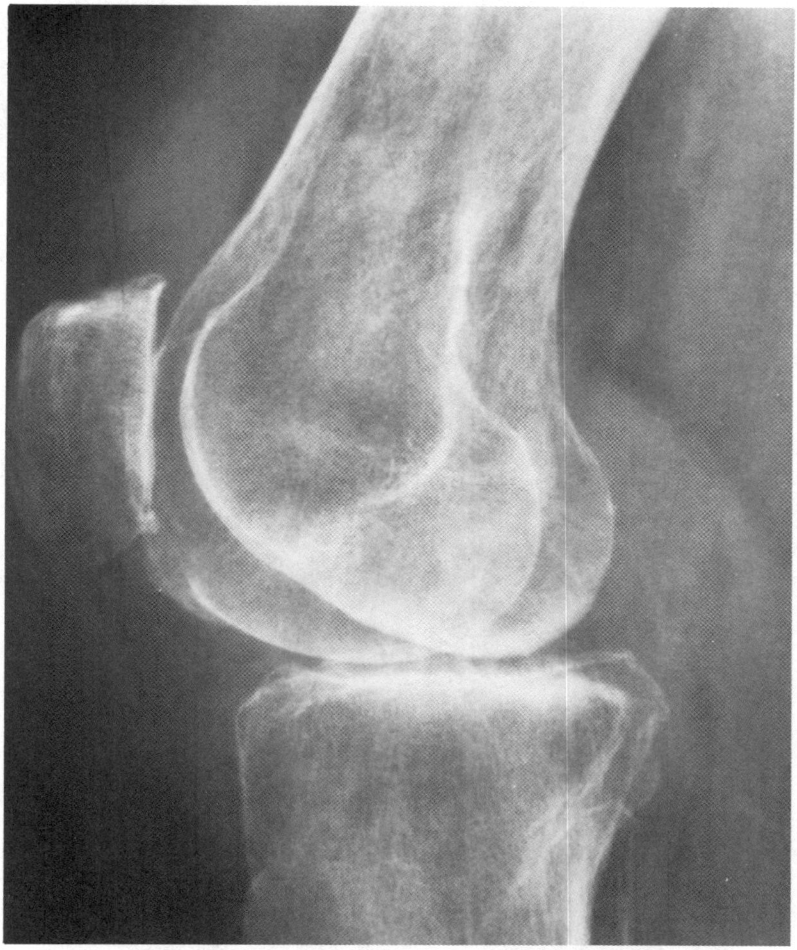

FIGURE 3.40 (B) Lateral view of the knee in rheumatoid arthritis. There is narrowing of the patellofemoral and the medial and lateral tibiofemoral compartments with marginal erosions. Note the relative absence of osteophytes. An effusion is present in the knee joint.

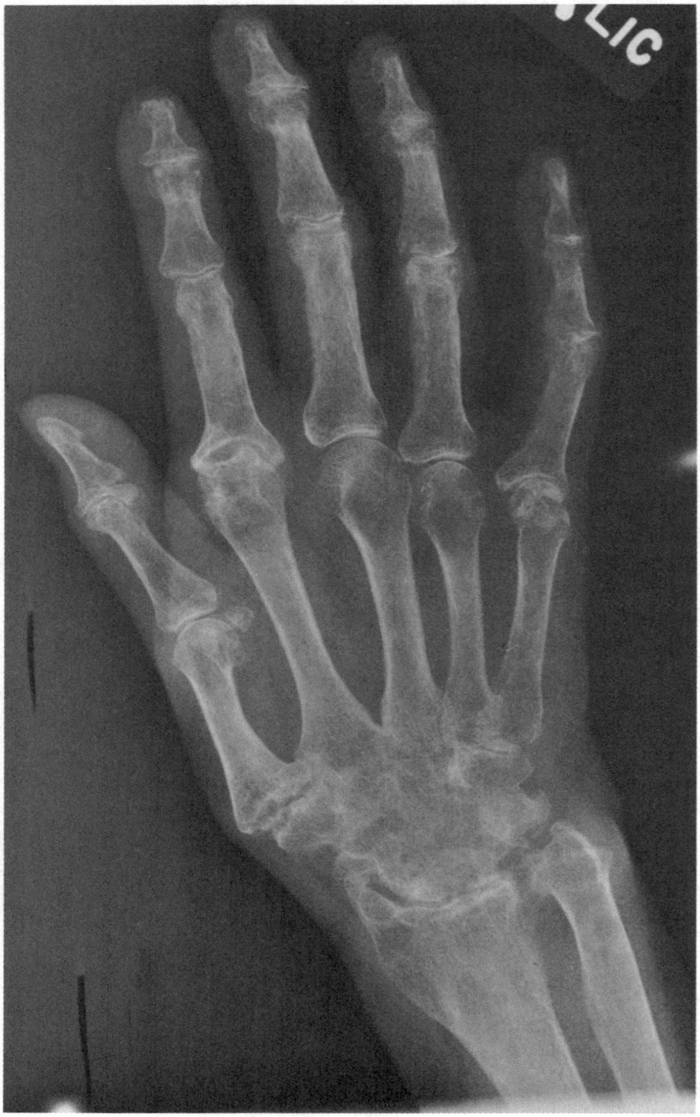

FIGURE 3.41 More advanced rheumatoid arthritis with ankylosis in the carpal and carpometacarpal joints. Erosions and joint space narrowing are present in the radiocarpal, metacarpophalangeal, and proximal interphalangeal joints.

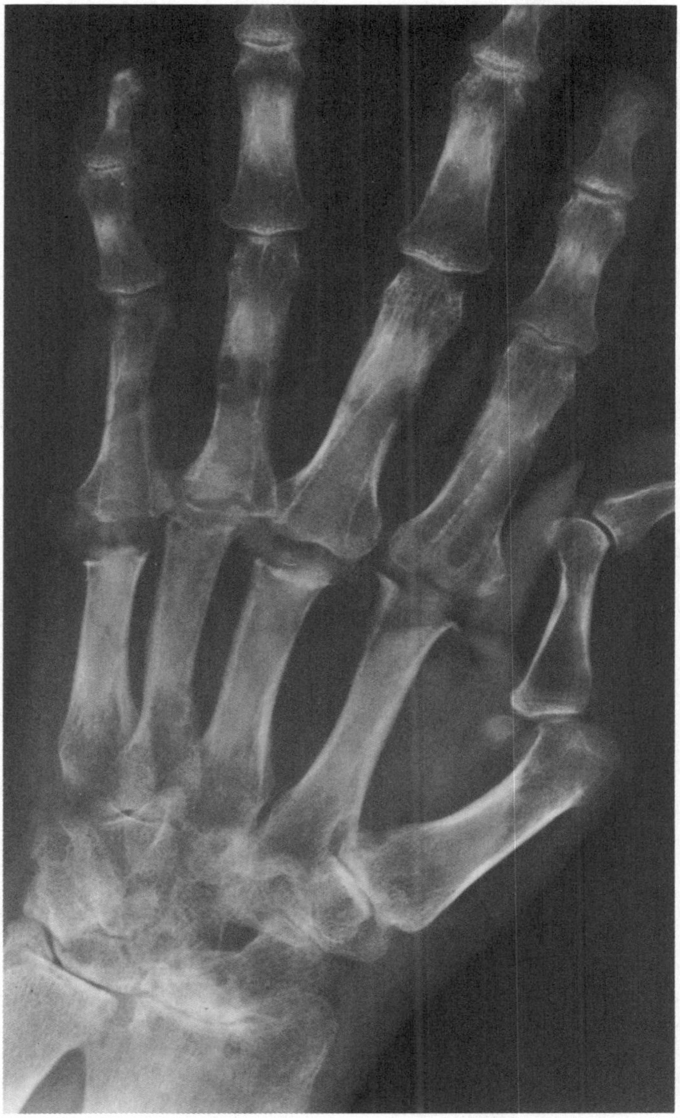

FIGURE 3.42 Late stage rheumatoid arthritis. Prosthetic joints have been placed in the second through fifth metacarpophalangeal joints.

Seronegative Spondyloarthropathies

The seronegative spondyloarthropathies are also referred to as rheumatoid variants. This implies that they have radiographic changes that are similar to those changes seen in rheumatoid arthritis. However, there are distinct differences as well. The seronegative spondyloarthropathies include ankylosing spondylitis, psoriasis, and Reiter's syndrome.

Ankylosing Spondylitis (Figures 3.43, 3.44)

Radiographic Changes

1. Syndesmophytes. These are very thin and delicate vertical bony bridges extending from one vertebral body to the next vertebral body and lying within the annulus fibrosis of the intervertebral disc.
2. Sacroiliitis. The stages of sacroiliitis include initial erosion with widening progressing to a bony repair response consisting of sclerosis. As this response continues, obliteration of the sacroiliac joint occurs with the result being complete bony fusion. The sacroiliitis is bilateral and symmetrical.
3. Vertebral body squaring. The anterior portion of a normal vertebral body is concave. Actual erosive changes occur at the anterior superior corner and anterior inferior corner of the vertebral bodies, thus causing loss of the normal concavity. The resultant appearance is that of a vertical or square anterior surface of the vertebral body.
4. Periosteal reaction, whisking. This is seen at sites of tendon insertion (entheses) and is referred to as an enthesopathy (Figure 3.30).
5. Joint fusion and joint narrowing.
6. Compared to rheumatoid arthritis, erosions, osteoporosis, and subchondral cysts are much less common.

Distribution

The major sites of abnormalities include the spine and sacroiliac joints. Often the sacroiliac joints will be initially involved with portions of the lumbar spine next becoming involved. The disease then gradually migrates up the spine to involve the thoracic and cervical spine. In long-standing ankylosing spondylitis, the hips are often involved as well.

Psoriatic Arthritis

Radiographic Changes

1. Erosions. Because this is also a disease of synovium, the locations of the erosions are at the margins of the joints just as occurs in rheumatoid arthritis.
2. Periosteal reaction.
3. Tuftal resorption.
4. Sacroiliitis and spondylitis with paravertebral ossification. In psoriatic arthritis, the sacroiliitis is bilateral but asymmetric. The spondylitis appears as large bulky bony bridges from one vertebral body to the next vertebral body. These bony bridges or paravertebral ossifications occur initially in the connective tissues outside of the intervertebral disc itself.

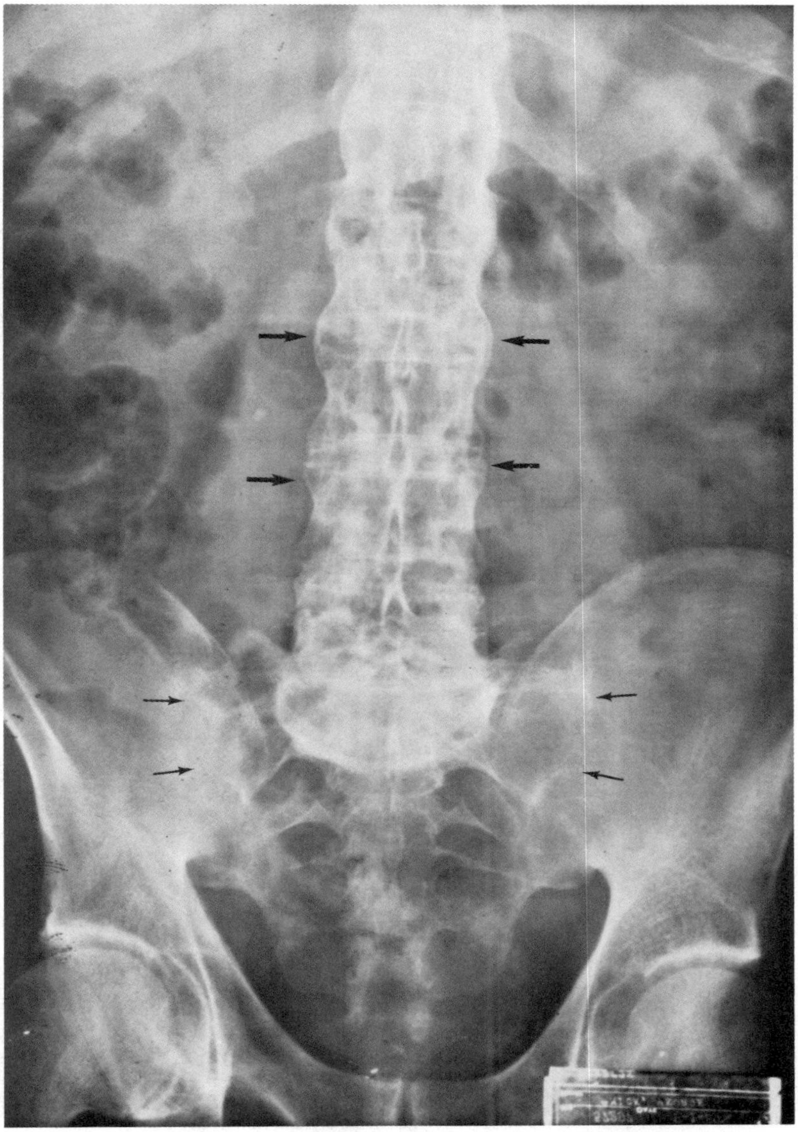

FIGURE 3.43 Ankylosing spondylitis with obliteration of the sacroiliac joints bilaterally (small arrows) and fine symmetric syndesmophytes in the lumbar spine (large arrows).

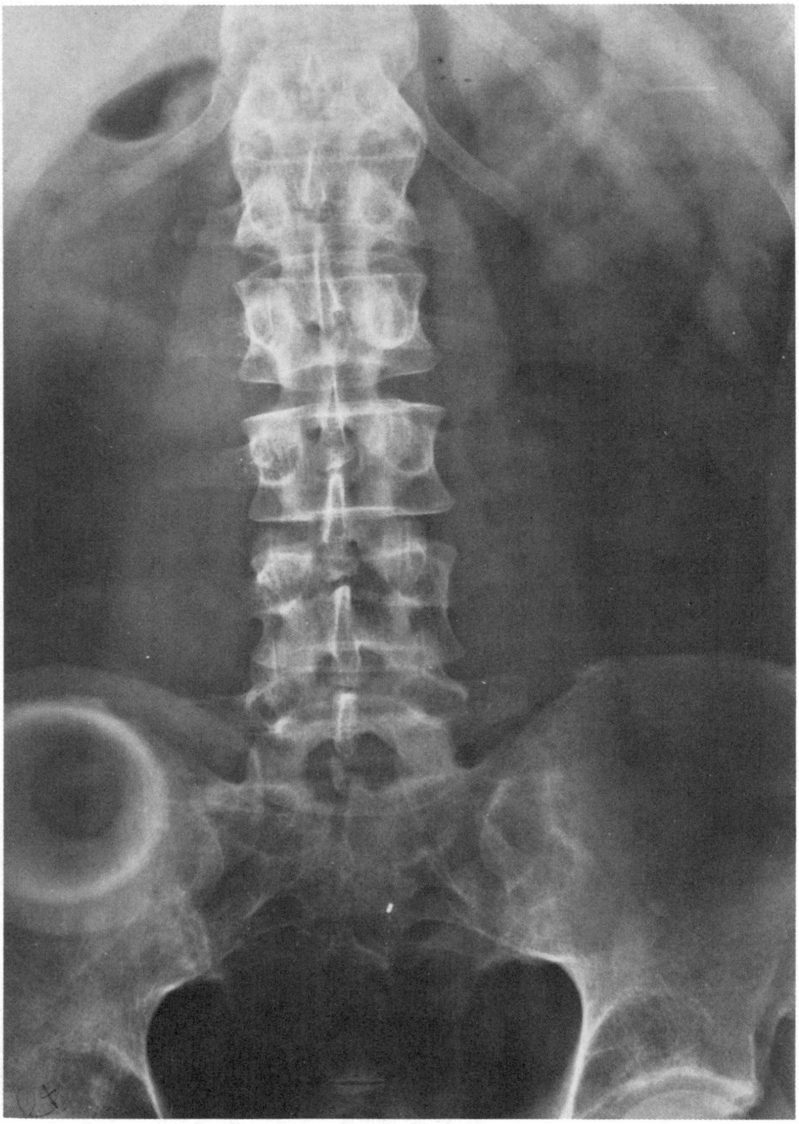

FIGURE 3.44 Ankylosing type spondylitis in ulcerative colitis (enteropathic arthropathy). Sacroiliitis and fine syndesmophytes in the thoracolumbar region. Note the ileostomy bag in the right lower quadrant; the patient had a colectomy for his bowel disease.

5. Ankylosis. In the hand and wrist, interphalangeal joint ankylosis is more common than carpal joint ankylosis.
6. Osteophytes and osteoporosis are relatively uncommon.

Distribution

The radiographic changes seen in psoriatic arthritis occur in an asymmetric distribution which is an important differentiating point with respect to rheumatoid arthritis. The joints asymmetrically involved include the hands and feet (DIP, PIP, classic), sacroiliac joints, and spine.

Reiter's Syndrome

Radiographic Changes

1. Erosions. The location of these erosions is also at the margins of the joint spaces just as in psoriatic arthritis and rheumatoid arthritis.
2. Periosteal reaction (Figure 3.24). This can occur along the long axis of the tubular bones of the feet as well as about the ankle. A commonly described location for periostitis or periosteal reaction includes the site of tendon insertion at the undersurface of the calcaneus.
3. Joint space narrowing. The joint space narrowing is uniform as in rheumatoid arthritis and psoriatic arthritis.
4. Osteoporosis. This is often juxtaarticular in location and occurs in the acute stage of the syndrome.
5. Sacroiliitis and spondylitis with paravertebral ossification (Figure 3.45). The appearance of these findings occurs as in psoriatic arthritis with the sacroiliitis being bilateral but asymmetric. The spondylitis consists of the large bulky bony bridges described in psoriatic arthritis.

Distribution

The distribution of the radiographic changes in Reiter's syndrome is often asymmetric. The most commonly involved joints are the small joints of the feet, the ankle, the knee, and the sacroiliac joints.

Connective Tissue Diseases

The connective tissue diseases represent another group of the arthritides and consist of systemic lupus erythematosus, scleroderma, dermatomyositis, and polymyositis, mixed connective tissue disease, and rheumatic fever.

Systemic Lupus Erythematosus

Radiographic Changes

1. Osteoporosis (45-55%)
2. Soft tissue swelling (25%)
3. Avascular necrosis (10-30%) (Figure 3.46)
4. Alignment abnormalities (5-40%).

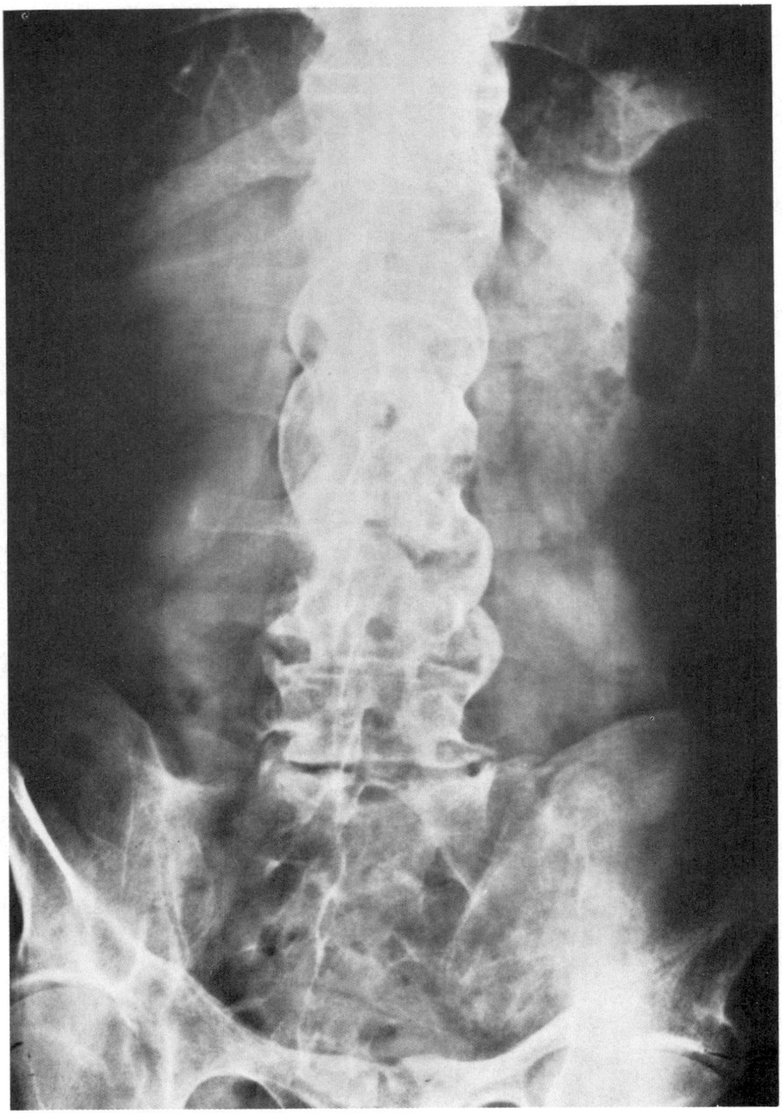

FIGURE 3.45 Reiter's disease. There is bilateral asymmetric sacroiliitis and coarse asymmetric paravertebral ossification (coarse syndesmophytes).

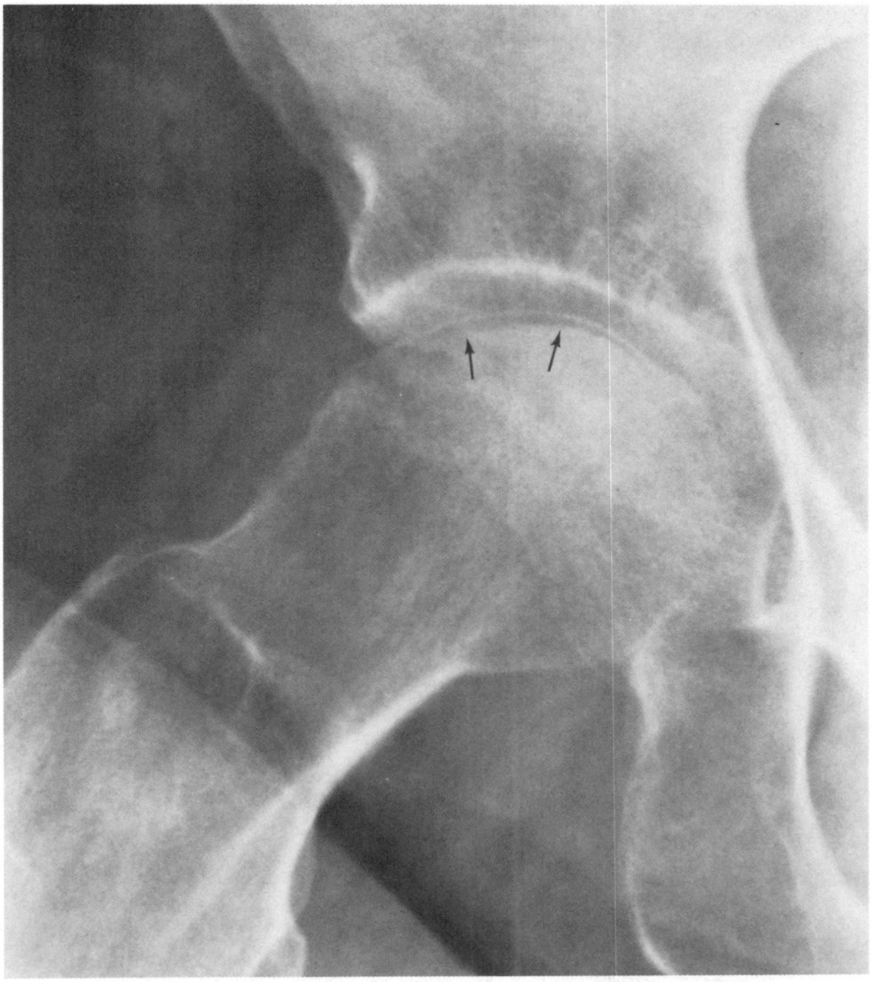

FIGURE 3.46 Aseptic necrosis of the femoral head with patchy sclerosis and crescentic subarticular lucent line (arrow). The patient had systemic lupus erythematosus and was on steroid therapy.

Deforming nonerosive arthropathy is the classically described characteristic abnormality seen in systemic lupus erythematosus. The other radiographic changes described are relatively less characteristic for this disease.

Distribution

Deforming nonerosive arthropathy occurs in the hand and usually consists of ulnar deviation of the phalanges at the MCP joints. Avascular necrosis most often invades the hip and shoulder joints.

Scleroderma (Figure 3.47)

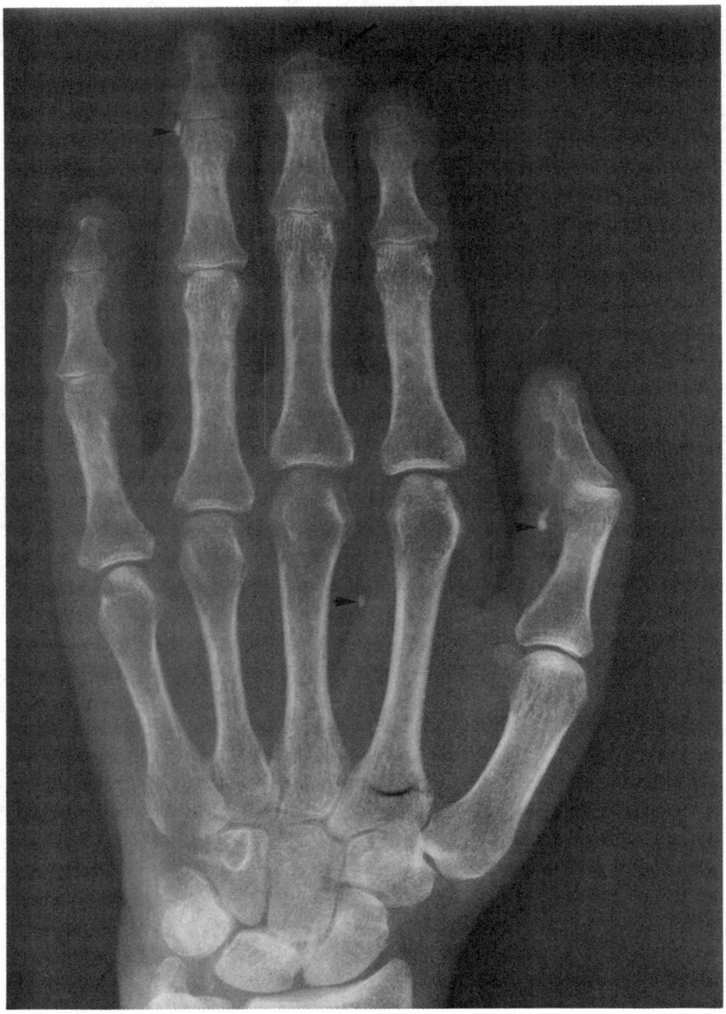

FIGURE 3.47 Hand in scleroderma with bony and soft tissue resorption of the ends of the fingers (arrows) and soft tissue calcification (arrowheads).

Radiographic Changes

1. Soft tissue resorption and bony resorption (80%). This phenomenon is described as a characteristic radiographic change for scleroderma and is secondary to Raynaud's phenomenon.
2. Soft tissue calcification.
3. Articular involvement is relatively uncommon in scleroderma.

Distribution

The classic site of distribution is within the small joints of the hands and wrists. Other sites including the elbow are less commonly involved.

Dermatomyositis and Polymyositis

Radiographic Changes

1. Soft tissue edema
2. Soft tissue calcification.

Distribution

The radiographic changes most often occur about the knees and elbows but can occur about multiple joints.

Jaccoud's Arthropathy (Rheumatic Fever)

Radiographic Changes

1. Malalignment abnormalities. Flexion and ulnar deviation occurs at the MCP joints as in systemic lupus erythematosus. Radiographically, these two malalignment deformities are identical. In the foot, flexion and fibular deviation occurs at the MTP joints.
2. Osteoporosis, joint space narrowing, and erosions are uncommon.

Mixed Connective Tissue Disease

The radiographic changes of this disorder include those seen in scleroderma, systemic lupus erythematosus, polymyositis, and rheumatoid arthritis.

Radiographic Changes

1. Osteoporosis.
2. Soft tissue swelling or atrophy.
3. Joint space narrowing. This is most often uniform.
4. Subluxations and malalignment deformities.
5. Tuftal resorption.
6. Soft tissue calcification.

Extraspinal Degenerative Joint Disease Figures 3.48, 3.49)

Radiographic Changes

1. Joint space narrowing. As opposed to the uniform joint space narrowing seen in the arthritides already described, in degenerative joint disease the joint space narrowing is nonuniform. For example, in the knee, the medial compartment is often narrowed with preservation of the joint space of the lateral compartment.
2. Sclerosis. Bony sclerosis or eburnation is characteristic of degenerative joint disease.
3. Subchondral cysts.
4. Osteophytes. The formation of bony exostoses or osteophytes is also characteristic of degenerative joint disease.
5. Erosions and ankylosis are uncommon.

Distribution

The distribution of radiographic changes is markedly different from those seen in rheumatoid arthritis and some of the other inflammatory diseases. Asymmetry is characteristic in degenerative joint disease. The areas involved include the hand (DIP, PIP, MCP joints), wrist (first carpometacarpal joint, trapezioscaphoid joint), foot (first MTP and tarsometatarsal joint), knee (as noted above, the medial compartment) is narrowed more often than the lateral compartment (Figure 3.50), hip (again the distribution of joint space loss involves the superior portion of the joint space relatively greater than the medial portion).

Extraspinal Erosive (Inflammatory) Osteoarthritis

This is a special form of extraspinal degenerative joint disease and represents an acute inflammatory process.

Radiographic Changes

All of the findings described in extraspinal degenerative joint disease can be seen in inflammatory osteoarthritis. In addition, the following radiographic changes are seen:

1. Erosions. The hallmark of erosive osteoarthritis is erosions occurring in the midportion of the joint space and not at the margins of the joint space. This is in marked contrast to the inflammatory arthritides such as rheumatoid arthritis.
2. Ankylosis.

Distribution

The DIP and PIP joints of the hand and the first carpometacarpal joints are most often involved.

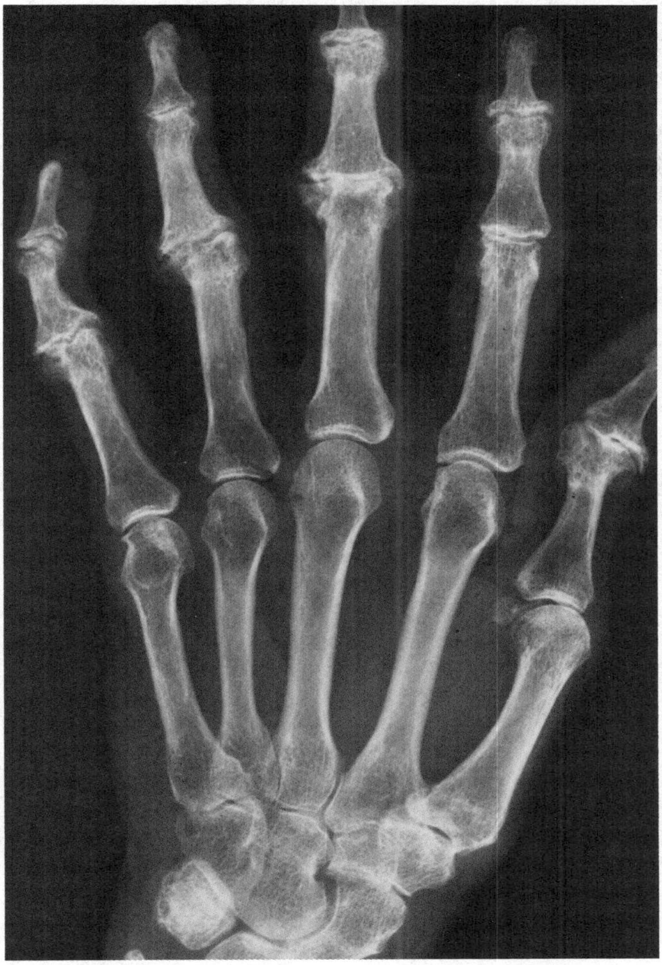

FIGURE 3.48 Osteoarthritis (degenerative joint disease) in the hand with involvement of the interphalangeal joints and first carpometacarpal joint. Note the joint space narrowing and osteophytes.

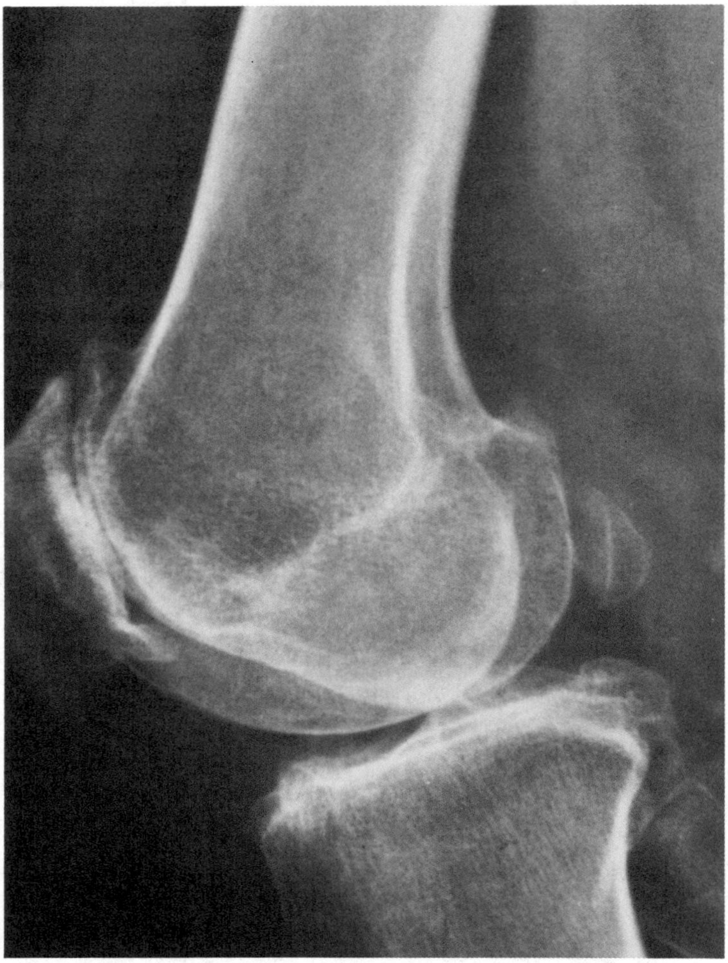

FIGURE 3.49 (A) Lateral view. Knee in osteoarthritis with joint space narrowing and osteophytes.

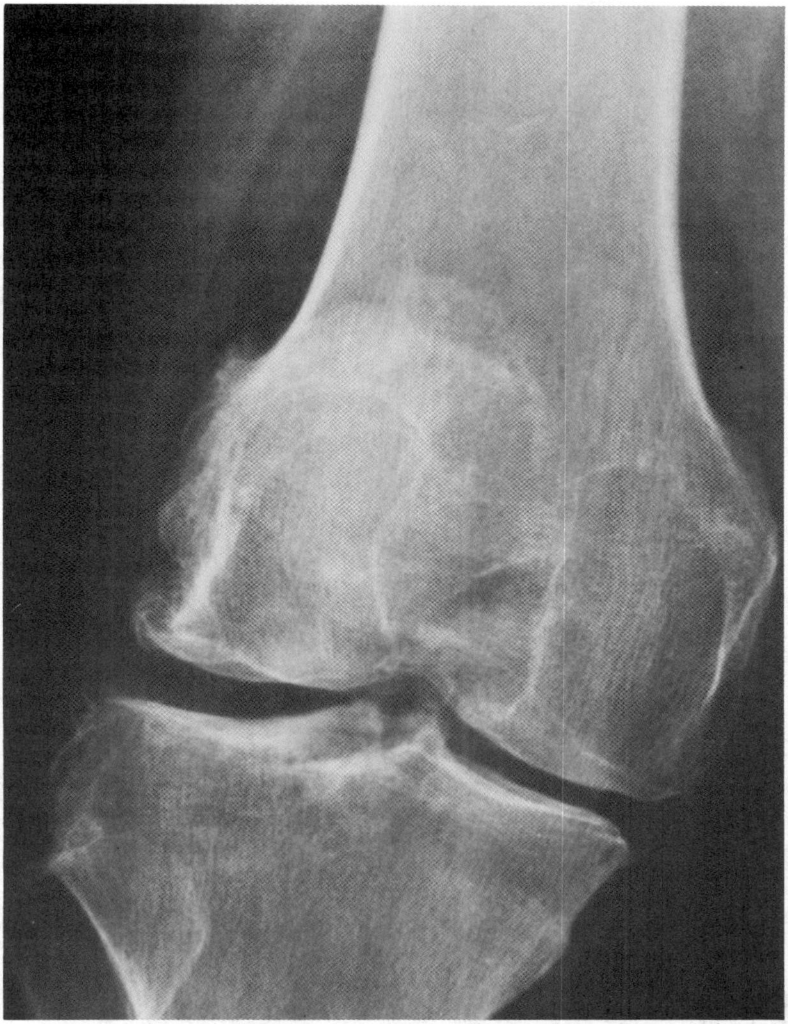

FIGURE 3.49 (B) AP view. Knee in osteoarthritis with joint space narrowing and osteophytes.

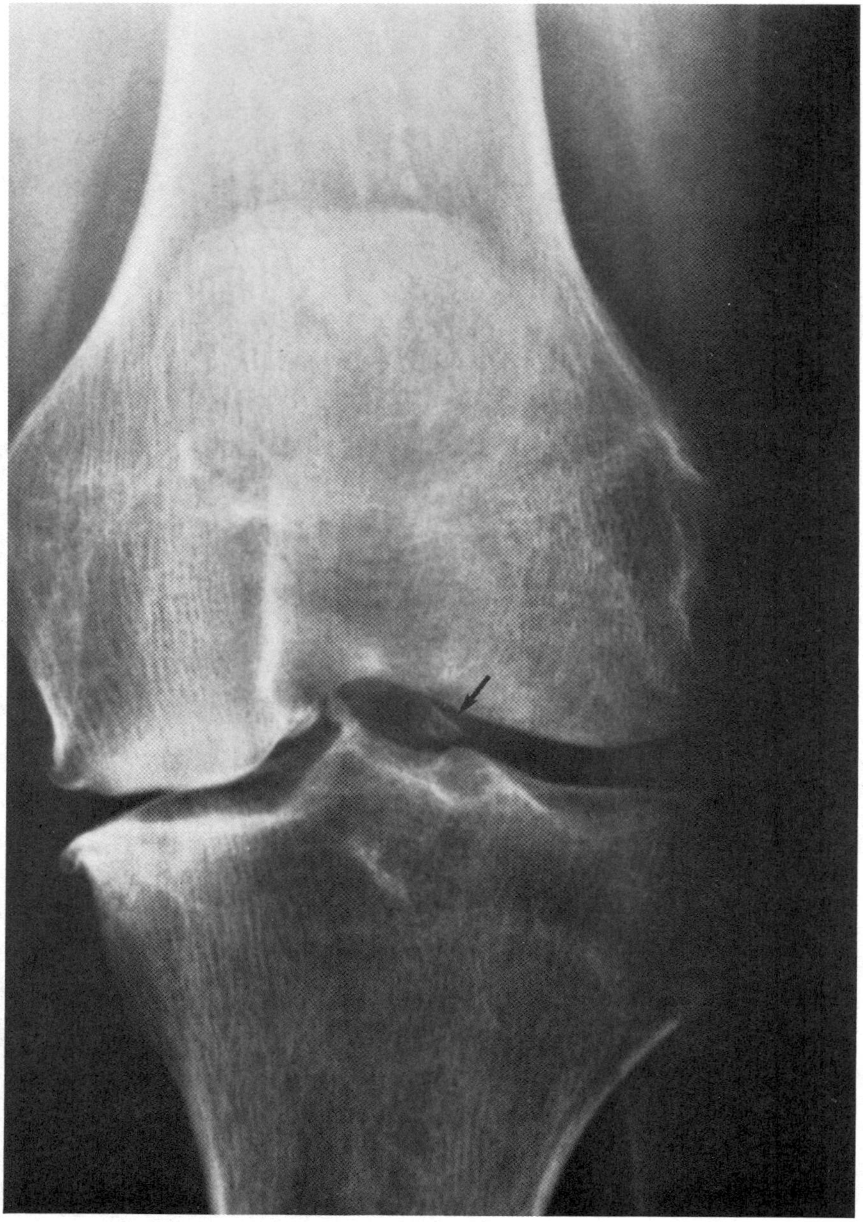

FIGURE 3.50 Knee in osteoarthritis with joint space narrowing and osteophytes. Note the predominantly medial compartment involvement and loose body (arrow).

Crystal Deposition Arthritides

The crystal deposition arthritides form another subcategory in the radiographic spectrum of arthritis and include gout and calcium pyrophosphate dihydrate crystal deposition disease.

Gout (Figures 3.51, 3.52)

Radiographic Changes

1. Soft tissue prominence (tophus). This represents a soft tissue collection of urate crystals.
2. Erosions. Erosions occur centrally within the joint. They also can occur near the peripheral portions of the joints and classically have a "hook" appearance.

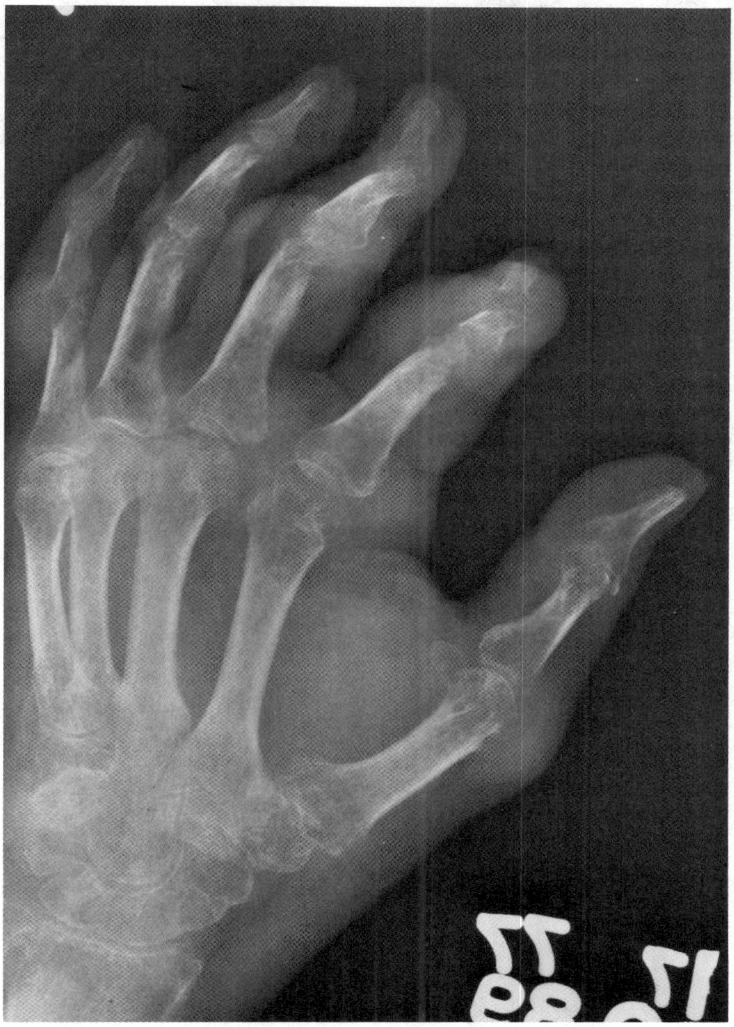

FIGURE 3.51 Hand in gout. Soft tissue tophi and bony erosions.

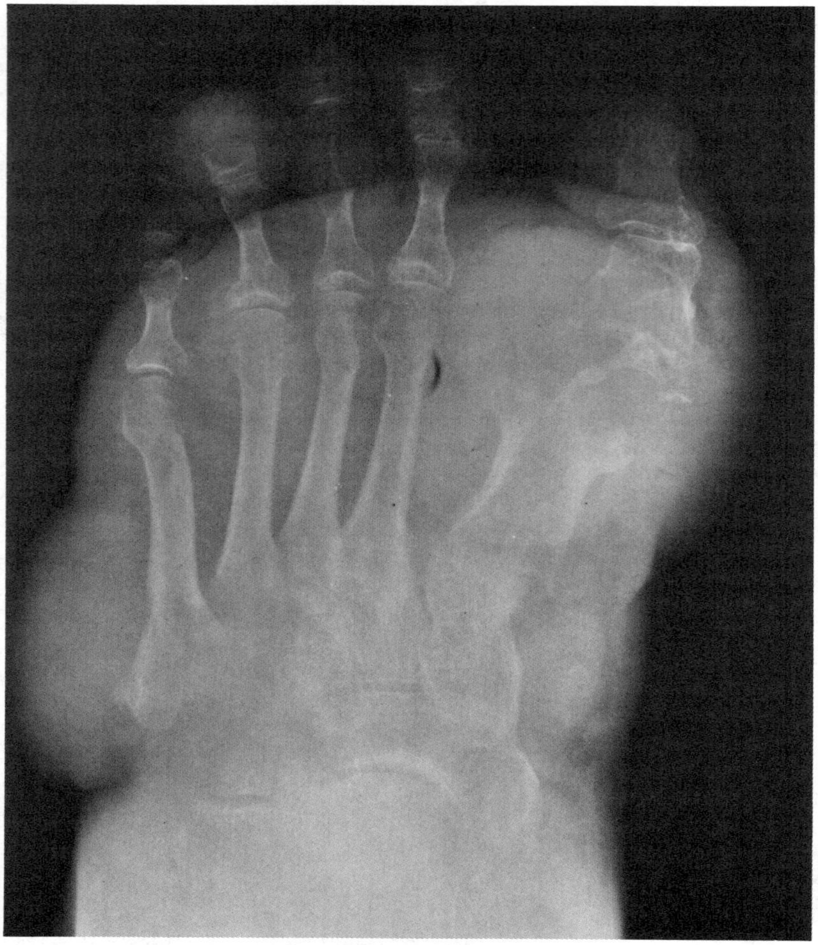

FIGURE 3.52 Foot in gout. Large tophi and extensive erosions.

3. Joint space preservation until late. In the presence of erosions, the joint space remains intact because a normal thickness of cartilage and bone between erosions is present. It is only until the entire articular cartilage has been destroyed that joint space narrowing occurs. In the inflammatory arthritides such as rheumatoid arthritis, this occurs much earlier because of the diffuse destruction caused by the synovial proliferation.
4. Subchondral cyst.

Distribution

The radiographic changes are most often distributed in an asymmetric manner and classically involve the first MTP joint. However, multiple other joints of the hands, wrists, and elbow often are involved.

Calcium Pyrophosphate Dihydrate
Crystal Deposition Disease (CPPD)
(Figures 3.9, 3.32, 3.33, 3.34)

Radiographic Changes

1. Chondrocalcinosis.
2. Arthropathy. Many features of degenerative joint disease are present in the pyrophosphate arthropathy. However, the distribution of these features as described below helps differentiate this disease from degenerative joint disease.
   a) Joint space narrowing
   b) Sclerosis
   c) Subchondral cysts
   d) Bone destruction and fragmentation

Distribution: Arthropathy

Multiple joints are involved including the knee (the patellofemoral compartment is initially narrowed with later narrowing occurring in the medial and lateral compartments), the wrists, the hands (MCP joints), and the hip (uniform joint space narrowing occurs).

Distribution: Chondrocalcinosis

The cartilage of the knees, wrists, and symphysis pubis are the most common sites of chondrocalcinosis.

References

1. Forrester DM, Brown JR, Nesson, JW: *The Radiology of Joint Disease,* 2nd Ed. Philadelphia, W. B. Saunders, 1978.

2. Resnick D, Niwayama G: *Diagnosis of Bone and Joint Disorders.* Philadelphia, W. B. Saunders, 1981.

Chapter 4

CLINICAL PHARMACOLOGY OF ANTIRHEUMATIC DRUGS

Jack W. Strandhoy, M.D.

This chapter will consider the clinical pharmacology of antirheumatic drugs through a discussion of the pharmacotherapeutic management of the major arthritides: rheumatoid arthritis, osteoarthritis (degenerative joint disease), and gouty arthritis. Although some of the drugs are useful in all three diseases, others have specific applications. The principles involved in the pharmacotherapy of these diseases, with differing immunopathogenic and management problems, can be extrapolated to aid in developing rational therapy programs for the over 70 types of arthritis which may be encountered in clinical practice.

Pharmacotherapy of Rheumatoid Arthritis (RA)

General management of the RA patient should include consideration of all of the modalities available for therapy, along with counseling of the patient and his family concerning the variable and remittive nature of rheumatoid disease (1). Not all patients require drugs. Adequate rest is important, and physical and occupational therapy may decrease pain while increasing mobility and function. Surgical therapy of chronic deformities including joint replacement has been rewarding. A goal of drug therapy is to relieve pain and inflammation and to potentially slow or reverse the damage to joints. The damage that occurs is related to the intensity of the inflammatory process and, therefore, reduction of inflammation during periods of disease activity should retard the rate at which tissues such as articular cartilage are damaged (2). Unfortunately, since the course of RA is unpredictable, it is difficult to prove that drugs arrest or retard joint damage. Nevertheless, new and existing antiinflammatory and immunomodulating agents relieve pain and stiffness and continue to be useful in the management of RA.

Nonsteroidal Antiinflammatoary Drugs (NSAID's)

These agents should be the first line of medical treatment for patients with RA. This class includes derivatives of salicylic acid and a wide structural diversity of compounds that inhibit prostaglandin synthesis.

Salicylates

Of the salicylates, aspirin is the most used since it is still the cheapest and most effective of the available preparations. It is the most extensively used analgesic, antipyretic, and antiinflammatory agent worldwide and is the standard for comparison and evaluation of the others.

Salicylates are present in the barks of trees belonging to the willow family and in certain other plants and derive their name from the botanical name for the willow family, *Salicaceae*. Extracts of barks were used medicinally by ancient civilizations and rediscovered in the eighteenth century by Reverend Edward Stone in an attempt to find a cheap substitute for quinine (3). Willow bark contains a bitter glycoside called salicin which was first extracted in 1827. From it, salicylic acid was prepared and later synthesized directly from phenol. Sodium salicylate was first used therapeutically in 1875. Later, acetylsalicylic acid was synthesized by Hoffman of the Bayer Company and introduced into medicine under the name aspirin in 1899. Although it has enjoyed widespread use for over 80 years, its mechanism of action and complex pharmacokinetics have only recently been elucidated.

Salicylates are absorbed rapidly from the stomach and upper intestine by passive diffusion (4). The pK_a of aspirin is low (3.5) and it therefore exists predominantly in the nonionized, more lipid-soluble form in the low pH (1.0) of the stomach. The pH of the intestine is considerably more alkaline, and salicylates are predominantly ionized. However, the rate of absorption actually exceeds that of the stomach because of the much greater surface area. Procedures that hasten gastric emptying time therefore hasten absorption. In order for tablets of aspirin to be absorbed, they must first undergo disintegration into granules or particles. These particles must then undergo the rate limiting step of dissolution in order to form a solution of drug molecules for absorption. Dissolution depends on the intrinsic solubility of the drug crystals, the pH of the environment, and the physicochemical properties of the dosage form (4). Soluble and buffered aspirins are more rapidly, but not necessarily more completely, absorbed than plain aspirin. Whereas this may be a slight clinical advantage for acute pain relief such as headache, it is not important in chronic dosing of aspirin in RA.

After absorption, salicylate is distributed throughout most body tissues and most transcellular fluids, primarily by pH-dependent diffusion (5). The volume of distribution of aspirin in normal subjects averages about 150 ml/kg body weight, a value equivalent to extracellular space; since salicylate is present within cells in some tissues, this suggests an uneven distribution of salicylate in the body. Salicylate crosses the blood-brain barrier slowly and is actively transported out of the CSF across the choroid plexus. The drug readily crosses the placental barrier. The distribution reflects the extent to which the drug is bound to plasma albumin and equilibrates with the tissues. Protein-bound drug molecules are pharmacologically inactive and as such cannot gain access to sites of action, biotransformation, or excretion since only the free drug leaves the circulation and diffuses into the tissues. However, protein binding is reversible and serves as a reservoir which is gradually depleted as the unbound drug is metabolized or excreted.

At concentrations encountered clinically, from 80 to 90% of the salicylate is bound to plasma albumin. In conditions associated with decreased plasma albumin, such as RA, the total blood concentration may be relatively low but more exists in the free state and more is concentrated in the tissues. The plasma albumin of young children is relatively low and consequently toxicity may result from ingestion of even comparatively low doses. Recent studies have additionally emphasized the potential importance of factors in addition to plasma albumin in determining the serum free fraction of salicylate (6) and the importance of erythrocyte-linked metabolic enzymes in determining the pharmacokinetics of aspirin in blood (7).

Ingested aspirin is mainly absorbed as such, but some enters the circulation as salicylic acid after hydrolysis by esterases in the gastrointestinal mucosa and liver. Aspirin is pharmacologically active itself but is rapidly hydrolyzed to salicylic acid which is also active. The plasma half-life for aspirin is 22 minutes (7). Consequently, plasma concentrations of aspirin are low and rarely exceed 20 μg/ml whereas salicylate levels of RA patients may approximate 200–300 μg/ml. Salicylate is eliminated by renal excretion, by glycine conjugation, and by microsomal oxidation. The metabolic pathways follow both first-order and zero-order kinetics (8, 9). At low doses, increments result in proportional increases in serum levels, since most of the drug is converted to salicylurate by conjugation with glycine and subsequent urinary excretion. Eighty percent of a low dose is metabolized by this major pathway. Therefore, when this pathway is saturated at higher doses, a small increase in dose will result in a relatively large increase in the serum level. The dose-dependent rate of elimination also explains why the plasma half-life of salicylate is 2–3 hours with low doses and 15–30 hours at high doses.

Renal excretion of salicylate and metabolites is the sum of glomerular filtration, active and passive proximal tubular secretion, and passive tubular reabsorption. Excretion of salicylate is extremely variable. In alkaline urine up to 85% of the ingested drug is eliminated as free salicylate, whereas in acidic urine this may be as low as 5% (5).

The discovery by Vane in 1971 (10) that aspirin and other NSAID's inhibit the biosynthesis of prostaglandins, along with the observation that prostaglandins are important mediators of inflammatory reactions, has shed new light on the mechanisms by which these drugs act. As shown in Figure 4.1, prostanoids are products of several enzyme reactions beginning with the liberation of arachidonic acid from phospholipids through the action of a phospholipase. The rapid formation of oxygenated products including a cyclic endoperoxide intermediate is catalyzed by a cyclooxygenase. Products of this intermediate include prostaglandins, prostacyclin, and thromboxanes. In the generation of at least some of the endoperoxides by cyclooxygenase, the free radical, superoxide, is formed and converted in turn into the hydroxyl free radical. Both of these strong oxidizing agents appear to have a role in the tissue damage accompanying inflammation. These free radicals are also produced by neutrophils and macrophages during phagocytosis (11). Superoxide generation is inhibited by a number of NSAID's, including aspirin, at therapeutic concentrations.

Aspirin inhibits cyclooxygenase by means of an irreversible covalent acetylation of the enzyme, in contrast to the action of other NSAID's which are reversible inhibitors. Although most cells can synthesize new cyclooxygenase, platelets cannot. Therefore, acetylation of their cyclooxygenase lasts for the approximate 7-day life of the platelet and explains why very low doses of aspirin are effective in reducing prostanoid-mediated platelet aggregation. Aspirin, as well as other NSAID's, probably inhibits inflammation by other pathways in addition to interrupting prostaglandin biosynthesis. For example, salicylate has been shown to be

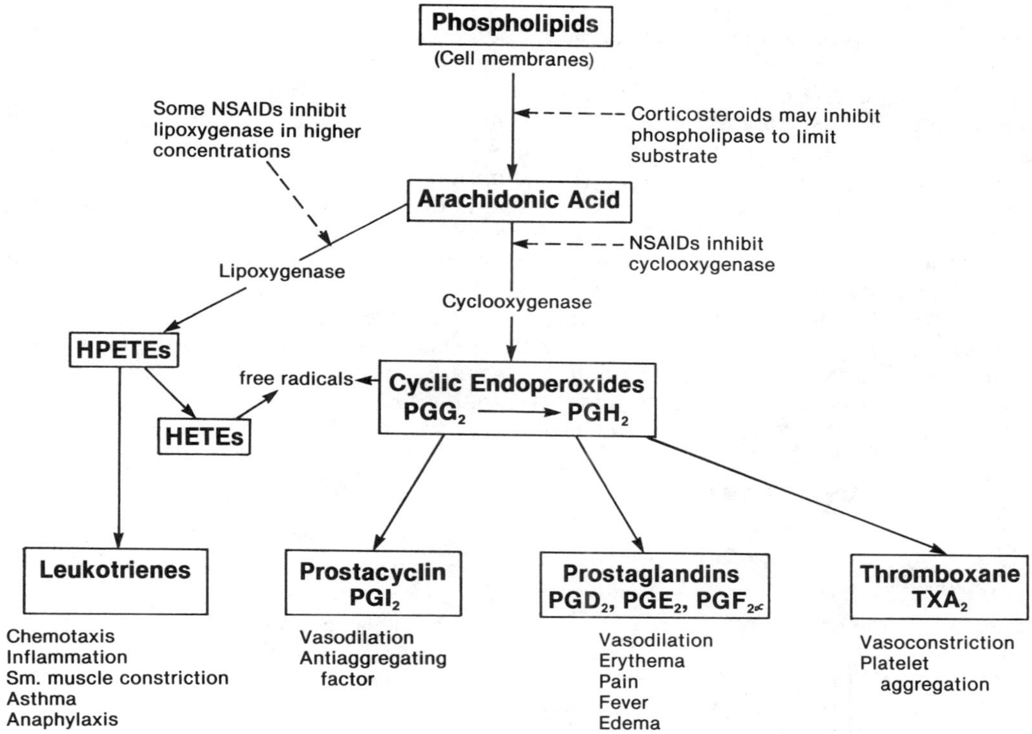

FIGURE 4.1 Inhibition of the production of prostanoids from phospholipids by antiinflammatory drugs.

a scavenger of free radicals and suppresses mononuclear leukocyte migration into the site of inflammation (12–14). Since the doses of NSAID's necessary to produce significant antiinflammatory responses are usually much larger than those necessary to achieve effective analgesia, antipyresis, and inhibition of cyclooxygenase (15), the exact mechanisms by which these drugs reduce inflammation is still an open question.

Therapy of RA and osteoarthritis (OA) requires relatively large doses of aspirin; adults usually require 4–6 g/day (about 12–20 regular tablets) in at least four divided doses in order to maintain a plasma salicylate concentration of 150–300 μg/ml. Compliance with such a demanding regimen becomes a problem. Children with juvenile chronic RA, as discussed in Chapter 19, tolerate aspirin better than adults but also require higher doses (80–100 mg/kg/day) in order to keep plasma salicylate levels up to about 300 μg/ml (2 mM) (16).

Aspirin toxicity is expressed in two general ways, both of which may be related to inhibition of prostaglandin synthesis. Aspirin may induce a hypersensitivity response in about 1 in 500 people. The reaction, which may be produced by small doses, includes rashes, urticaria, angioneurotic edema, nasal polyps, and severe asthma. The syndrome appears to be less a classical drug allergy and more an exquisite sensitivity to inhibition of prostaglandin synthesis in that patients hypersensitive to aspirin also react to many other chemically unrelated NSAID's (17). Several possible mechanisms have been hypothesized to contribute to the hypersensitivity reaction: inhibition of cyclooxygenase may favor production of more lipoxygenase prostanoids from arachidonate such as leukotrienes. They have been identified as the slow-reacting substances of anaphylaxis. Secondly, prostaglandins E_2 stabilizes mast cell membranes. Its inhibition may make these cells more liable to release histamine. A third possible contributing factor may involve the prior sensitization of patients to aspirin contained in over-the-counter medications prior to a prescribed regimen with an NSAID. All these factors, and undoubtedly others, may contribute. Additionally, about 15% of aspirin-sensitive asthmatics are also sensitive to the food and drug coloring agent, tartrazine, which may be incorporated into other drug formulations. Interestingly, sodium salicylate is a weak inhibitor of prostaglandin biosynthesis and does not precipitate the hypersensitivity reaction (18). Other nonacetylated salicylates such as salsalate and choline magnesium trisalicylate (discussed below) may be used in hypersensitive patients. Direct toxic reactions of aspirin (Figure 4.2) include ringing of the ear

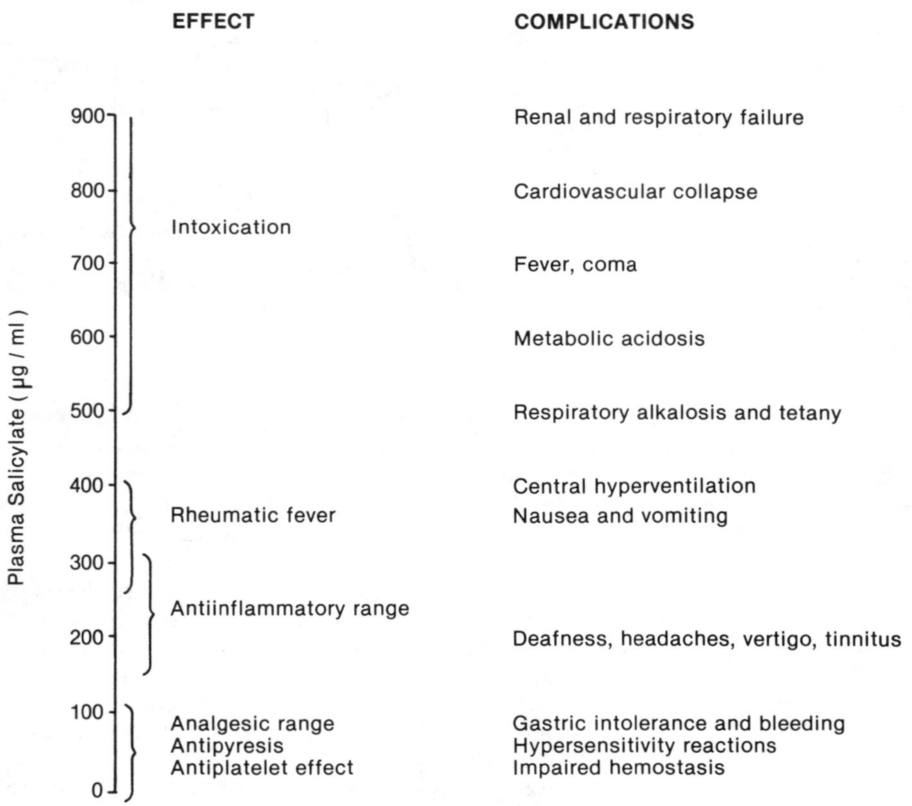

FIGURE 4.2 Relationships between plasma salicylate levels, effects, and complications. (Reprinted with permission of Applied Therapeutics, Inc., Spokane, Washington, from the chapter "Salicylates" in WE Evans, JJ Schentag, and WJ Jusko (eds.), *Applied Pharmacokinetics: Principles of Therapeutic Drug Monitoring.*)

(tinnitus) as an early sign which may progress to reversible hearing loss. Since this toxic effect is expressed in the therapeutic range for treating RA, the onset of tinnitus has been used to titrate the dose of aspirin. This indicator has proved to be unreliable in older patients with preexisting hearing loss (4) and in children who complain less of tinnitus. Larger toxic doses of aspirin lead to metabolic imbalances expressed as hyperventilation, metabolic acidosis, and cardiovascular collapse.

As is widely recognized, the most consistently troublesome major side effect produced by aspirin is gastrointestinal irritation. A serious, but infrequent, consequence of this has been the development of peptic ulcer disease. The cause of gastrointestinal irritation relates not only to the acidic, irritating chemical nature of the drug but also to its pharmacological inhibition of protective prostaglandins which normally inhibit gastrointestinal acid production and maintain blood flow to the gastric mucosa. Aspirin is therefore given in divided doses after meals and at bedtime with milk to minimize gastrointestinal irritation. Antacids may also be administered.

As with all medications, the prescribing physician should remain alert to renal side effects produced by aspirin. It should be used cautiously in sodium-restricted patients since the drug has been shown to depress renal blood flow and glomerular filtration rate in these circumstances (19). This occurs because the reduction of vasodilator prostaglandins in the kidney leaves unopposed an enhanced renin-angiotensin and sympathetic neural renal vasoconstriction heightened by sodium restriction. Renal failure may occur in some patients, associated with drug-induced acute interstitial nephritis possibly due to a delayed hypersensitivity reaction (20). Aspirin in high doses may also produce elevated levels of liver enzymes; however, serious liver damage with aspirin therapy in RA has not been a major problem in adults although hepatic necrosis has been reported in children treated for juvenile RA.

Use of NSAID's during the third trimester of pregnancy should be avoided since they may delay parturition and cause premature closure of the ductus arteriosus. Salicylates distribute throughout the body, cross the placenta easily, and appear in the milk of nursing mothers. They have not been proven to be teratogens (21, 22); however, babies born to habitual aspirin users were smaller, bruised easily, and were born late. The use of aspirin in children with influenza or chickenpox should be avoided during these acute illnesses. An epidemiological association between aspirin use in these conditions and an increased incidence of Reye's syndrome has been noted by the Center for Disease Control. Reye's syndrome may be very serious with 20-30% mortality.

Several drug interactions occur with aspirin. It decreases platelet aggregation to increase bleeding time and antagonizes vitamin K to prolong prothombin time. Since it may also displace oral anticoagulants from albumin binding sites, it should be used with caution in patients receiving anticoagulant therapy. Ingestion of alcohol also potentiates aspirin-induced prolongation of bleeding time and patients should be advised against concomitant use. The risk of gastrointestinal ulceration is increased when salicylates are given with steroids, phenylbutazone, or alcohol. Patients receiving high doses of salicylates along with a loop diuretic such as furosemide may experience salicylate toxicity at lower dose because of competition for renal excretion, exacerbated ototoxicity, and decreased effectiveness of the diuretic. This results because parts of the excretory and renal vasodilatory effects of furosemide depend upon increased renal prostaglandin synthesis. Aspirin also antagonizes the diuretic effects of spironolactone by inhibiting its binding to the tubule membrane. Aspirin partly antagonizes the effects of many of the other NSAID's by reducing their blood levels. This probably is due to a displacement from protein binding sites and greater metabolism of the free drug. Therefore, aspirin or one of the other NSAID's should usually be used alone.

Although aspirin is relatively safe and inexpensive, its frequent administration and gastrointestinal intolerance have simulated a continuing search for new agents and have produced numerous alternatives which should be considered.

One therapeutic alternative is enteric coated aspirin, which seems to have less gastrointestinal toxicity than regular aspirin preparations. It has been known for some time, however, that enteric coated aspirin preparations in some patients may be erratically absorbed (and occasionally not absorbed at all). Careful monitoring of clinical effects, careful questioning of patients for evidence of tinnitus, which would suggest adequate absorption, and/or monitoring of blood salicylate levels are therefore recommended when employing enteric-coated aspirin preparations. These drugs should be used carefully in patients with poor gastric emptying, as salicylate intoxication has recently been reported in patients with gastric outlet obstruction (23).

Nonacetylated salicylates have been utilized in an attempt to decrease especially the gastrointestinal side effects produced by acetylsalicylic acid (Figure 4.3). Many of these compounds have not been tested in careful trials against aspirin and, in the existing trials, they seem to produce less or at best equal antiinflammatory activity compared to aspirin. These agents are less potent inhibitors of the cyclooxygenase enzymes and some, such as choline magnesium trisalicylate,

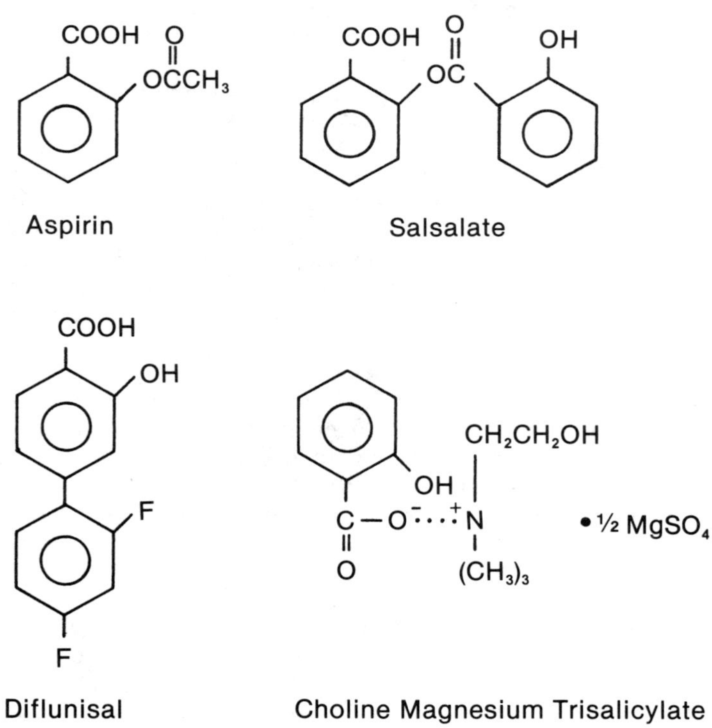

FIGURE 4.3 Aspirin and nonacetylated salicylates.

have been shown not to impair platelet aggregation when utilized in the doses employed in the usual therapeutic situations (24). Salsalate (salicylsalicylic acid) is an ester that is slowly hydrolyzed to two molecules of salicylic acid. It is insoluble in gastric juice and not absorbed until it reaches the small intestine.

A new addition to the nonacetylated salicylates is the difluorophenyl derivative of salicylic acid, diflunisal. This agent is available in 500 mg tablets, and may be given in the dose of 500 mg 3 times a day. Since food and antacids have been shown to affect peak blood levels of this agent, a reduction in dosage to 500 mg twice daily perhaps given between meals can be attempted if the agent is well tolerated and adequate antiinflammatory activity has been produced (25). This agent is approved for pain relief and treatment of osteoarthritis as well as for the treatment of RA, where double-blind trails with aspirin have suggested equal or better antiinflammatory activity in RA patients utilizing diflunisal (26). This agent is not metabolized to salicylic acid, but is a potent prostaglandin inhibitor, and has other activities much like other new NSAID's. It is therefore contraindicated in patients hypersensitive to aspirin or other NSAID's. It probably should not be used as an additive analgesic agent in patients who are under treatment with other nonsteroidal antiinflammatory agents. Since many of these agents are good analgesic agents in their own right, such additional therapy is rarely required. When such therapy is indicated, acetaminophen, which has good analgesic but no antiinflammatory or ulcerogenic activity, may be the drug of choice.

Diflunisal, like aspirin, displays concentration-dependent pharmacokinetics so that a doubling of the dose produces a greater than doubling of drug accumulation. The effect becomes more apparent with repeated doses. Since it is highly protein bound, it may displace oral anticoagulants and prolong prothrombin time. Interactions with renal function and diuretic drugs are similar to those with aspirin. Although diflunisal causes frequent (3-9%) gastrointestinal upset, it is better tolerated than aspirin in antirheumatic doses. Additional careful studies of both efficacy and side effects will be necessary to determine the value of the many available nonacetylated salicylate compounds in the therapy of RA. Diflunisal increases the renal excretion of uric acid and this modest uricosuric effect may lower plasma urate. It is not known whether diflunisal interferes with the activity of other uricosuric agents, and it is not yet approved as a primary agent in the treatment of gout.

Propionic Acid Derivatives

One of the largest classes of new drugs available for inflammation control in RA and OA are derivatives of propionic acid. Three are currently available clinically: ibuprofen, fenoprofen, and naproxen (Figure 4.4). A fourth agent, benoxaprofen (Oraflex) has been withdrawn from the market. At least five others are available in other countries and many more are undergoing clinical tarials. These agents also inhibit cyclooxygenase and are good analgesics but generally are weaker antiinflammatory drugs than aspirin (27). Even so, they are often first choice drugs in the treatment of joint disease because they have the lowest incidence of side effects. All of these drugs are potential anaphylaxis-producing agents in patients with aspirin allergy.

Ibuprofen was the first of this class to be marketed in the United States and derives its name from the isobutyl moiety. It is approved for use in acute episodes and chronic treatment of RA and OA. It is well absorbed and achieves peak plasma levels in 1-2 hours after a single dose. Since the half-life is only about 2

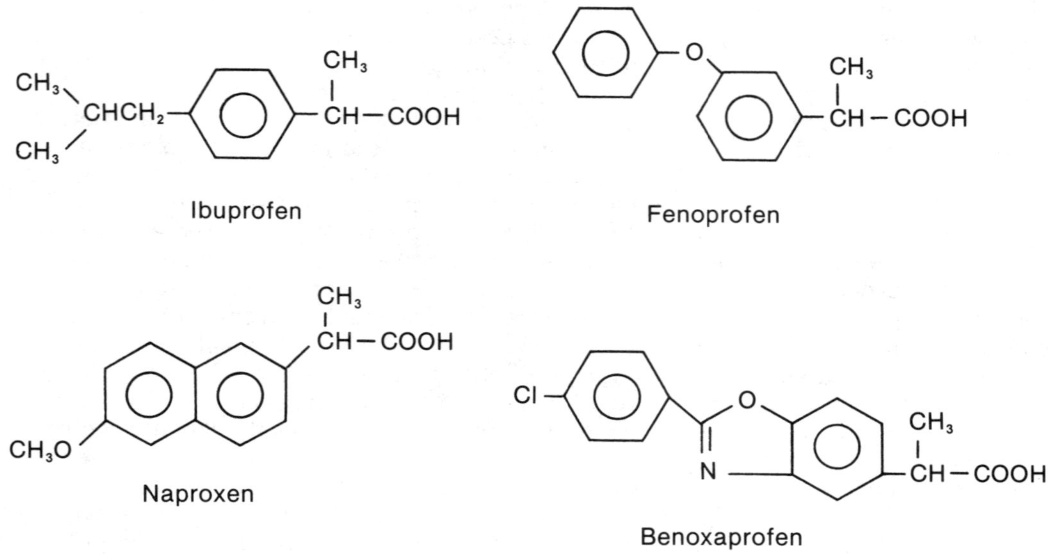

FIGURE 4.4 Propionic acid derivatives.

hours, 3-4 doses per day are necessary. Ibuprofen has been shown to readily penetrate the synovial fluid, with synovial fluid levels being about half those in serum (28). Moderate doses of ibuprofen are primarily analgesic, and indeed its most current use is as an over-the-counter analgesic. Doses of 2400 mg/day do show antiinflammatory activity (29). It is also especially effective for treatment of dysmenorrhea (30).

Although ibuprofen is well tolerated, there are some potentially serious toxicities. Liver function abnormalities may present as reversible increases in enenzymes such as alanine aminotransferase, LDH, and alkaline phosphatase. Hepatitis, sometimes cholestatic, has been reported in patients taking ibuprofen as well as with sulindac, indomethacin, and naproxen (31-33). These drugs should be used cautiously in patients with impaired hepatic function and liver function tests should be monitored. All NSAID's may cause fluid retention and diminished renal sodium excretion. Agranulocytosis and aplastic anemia have been reported with ibuprofen, fenoprofen, and naproxen as well as other NSAID's such as indomethacin, tolemetin, piroxicam, and sulindac (33). Toxic ambliopia has been reported with ibuprofen and patients who develop ocular disturbances should discontinue the drug. Ibuprofen can inhibit platelet aggregation since it inhibits prostaglandin biosynthesis but has been reported not to interfere with the protein binding of warfarin-like anticoagulant drugs (34).

Although all the NSAID's are generally safe, potential hepatic, renal, gastrointestinal, and hematological toxicities suggest that patients should have periodic white cell counts and determinations of serum creatinine concentrations and hepatic enzyme activities.

Fenoprofen is used as its calcium salt in RA and OA patients and is also well absorbed after oral administration. It achieves a peak plasma level about 2 hours after a single dose and has a half-life of approximately 3 hours. This, like ibuprofen, requires dosing 3-4 times per day. Fenoprofen, as well as other agents in this class, has been shown to be as effective as aspirin in the treatment of RA in trials using these drugs alone and in the presence of gold induction therapy. Its analgesic efficacy is comparable to codeine and low dose capsules have been marketed for analgesic use.

Fenoprofen is relatively well tolerated as compared with aspirin and causes less occult gastrointestinal bleeding. It shares in the potential hepatic, renal, and hematological toxicities outlined above. Paradoxically, headache can be a common side effect with some NSAID's that are effective analgesics. Headache and somnulence have been reported in 15% of patients taking fenoprofen. In addition, acute interstitial nephritis, sometimes presenting as nephrotic syndrome, has been described in patients taking NSAID's, particularly fenoprofen. This effect, which appears to be idiosyncratic and not related to prostaglandins, generally takes weeks or months to develop (35).

Naproxen has the longest half-life (16 hr) of the propionic acid derivatives currently available in the United States. This gives it an advantage clinically since it requires only twice daily dosage. It is approved for use in RA and OA as well as in the relief of acute gouty arthritis. Comparative trials between naproxen and other propionic acid derivates have shown naproxen to be marginally superior, but individual and unpredictable patient preference for one or another drug is more apparent than consistent pharmacological differences between the drugs (16). One study has suggested that combination therapy with aspirin was more efficacious than aspirin therapy alone, and it was suggested that side effects might be no greater in the combination therapy group (36). This is unusual in that combinations of aspirin and other NSAID's usually provide less than additive antiinflammatory activity. The short duration of this study (8 wks) and the relatively low dose of naproxen utilized (500 mg/day) do not answer the question of whether higher doses of this agent, which have recently been shown to be more efficacious (37), might produce equivalent antiinflammatory activity and less side effects than long-term combination therapy with this agent plus aspirin. Naproxen is effective in reducing the bone lesions in adjuvant arthritis which is a somewhat unsatisfactory but often used animal model for RA. Long-term studies underway with high doses of this agent should determine whether it has unique disease modifying properties among this class of antiinflammatory agents.

Naproxen is also available as its sodium salt which is more rapidly absorbed than the parent drug. This makes it more useful as a primary analgesic and antipyretic. This drug form is rapidly and completely absorbed from the gastrointestinal tract and achieves peak plasma levels and analgesia in 1-2 hours. The analgesic effect lasts for up to 7 hours. It is useful for mild to moderate pain relief and for the treatment of primary dysmenorrhea.

A fourth derivative of propionic acid, benoxaprofen, was marketed briefly under the trademark, Oraflex. It was voluntarily withdrawn from the market because it was associated with fatal cholestatic jaundice, especially in the elderly (15). Since it is a relatively weak cyclooxygenase inhibitor, its antiinflammatory effectiveness was suggested to be related more to its ability to inhibit 5-lipoxygenase and subsequent production of chemotactic leukotriene products. This reduces the migration of mononuclear leukocyte migration into sites of joint inflammation. Dahl and Ward (15) argue that this effect on other pathways of the arachidonic acid cascade may not be unique to benoxaprofen and that other "cyclooxygenase" inhibitors may have broader effects on prostanoid production.

It should be kept in mind that the daily cost to the patient of maximum dose therapy with these new agents ranges from 5 to 10 times that of aspirin. However, the greater potential safety and ease of administration make these new agents first choice with some physicians and patients for the treatment of RA and OA.

Acetic Acid Derivatives

This group consists of indoleacetic acid derivatives (indomethacin and sulindac) and pyrrolacetic acid derivatives (tolmetin and zomepirac) (Figure 4.5). The indole, indomethacin, is the oldest and best known of this group. Its acute antiinflammatory activity has been useful in the relief of acute gouty arthritis in addition to the therapy of RA and OA. Although it is a more potent inhibitor than aspirin of cyclooxygenase, doses that are tolerated by patients usually do not produce effects that are superior to salicylates. This is because of the potential of this drug for producing gastrointestinal irritation and severe frontal headache in a substantial percentage of patients (38). The untoward side effects of indomethacin cause about 20% of patients to discontinue it. Dyspepsia is the most common complaint with this drug, which probably is as ulcerogenic as aspirin and more ulcerogenic than the newer medications. The headache and light-headedness appears to be associated with plasma concentrations in excess of 5 μg/ml, and such concentrations may be seen as peak levels after doses in excess of 25 mg (39). Perhaps because indomethacin is related to serotonin, the central nervous system effects are greater than with unrelated NSAID. It should be used with caution, therefore, in patients in whom neurologic or psychiatric problems are already present (38). It may aggravate depression, epilepsy, and parkinsonism. It may also increase plasma levels of lithium to toxic levels in some individuals, presumably because of decreased renal clearance of lithium.

Indomethacin is absorbed well from the gastrointestinal tract and achieves a peak plasma concentration from a single dose in 2 hours. Its half-life of 4.5 hours dictates three or four times a day dosage. In order to increase compliance and reduce dose-related side effects, a sustained release (SR) capsule is now available which allows once or twice daily administration.

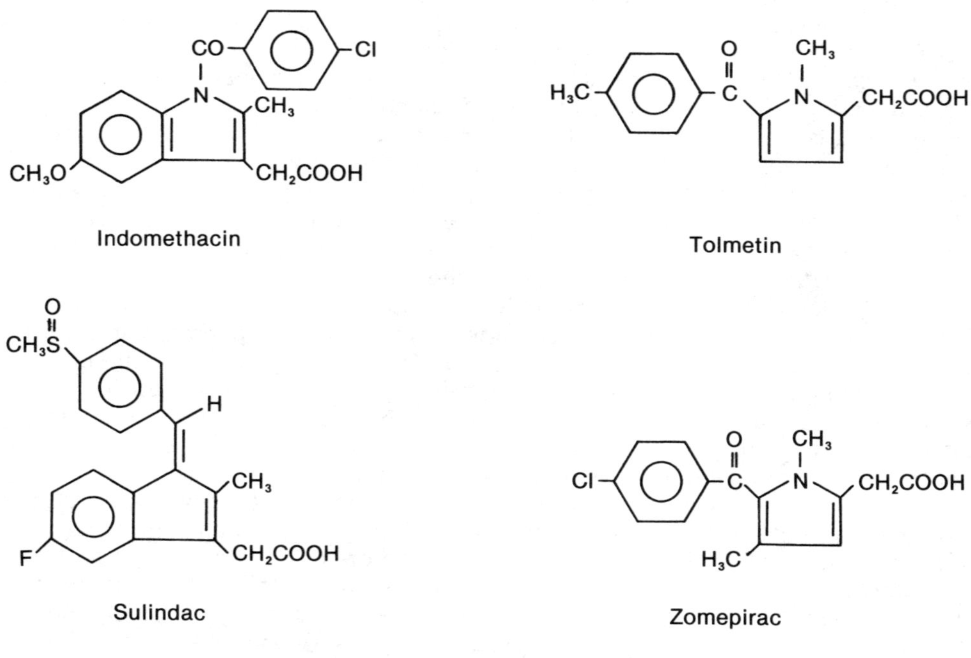

FIGURE 4.5 Acetic acid derivatives.

Although the drug is largely metabolized by the liver, acute renal failure and hepatotoxicity have been reported. The renal toxicity is thought to be an extension of its inhibition of cyclooxygenase, which results in decreased renal blood flow especially in patients who are already compromised with regard to renal blood flow status. It also antagonizes the natriuretic effect of furosemide. Coronary vasoconstriction may result, again as a consequence of decreased vasodilatory prostaglandins. Indomethacin is said not to modify the effect of oral anticoagulant agents. However, concurrent administration could be hazardous because of increased risk of gastrointestinal bleeding.

While indomethacin has not been proven teratogenic, safety for use during pregnancy has not been established and is not recommended. All NSAID's have the potential to delay parturition and cause constriction of the ductus arteriosus and should therefore be especially avoided during the third trimester. Most NSAID's are excreted in breast milk, and therefore nursing should not be undertaken while on therapy with these drugs.

Sulindac is useful in RA, osteoarthritis, and episodes of acute gouty arthritis. It has the advantage of a long half-life, requiring only twice daily dosage. Upper gastrointestinal complaints of dyspepsia and nausea are fewer than with aspirin, but problems with constipation are frequent (38). Aplastic anemia, severe hepatotoxicity, azotemia, and the Stevens-Johnson syndrome are associated with the use of this drug as well. This necessitates close follow-up of patients treated with this potentially useful NSAID.

The reason for sulindac's longer duration of action and relatively less gastrointestinal irritation lies in its structure. This newest of the indole derivatives has the nitrogen removed from the indole nucleus. It is given as an inactive prodrug, the sulfoxide, which is metabolized in the body to an active sulfide and an inactive sulfone. Whereas the half-life of the parent drug is about 8 hours, the half-life of the active sulfide is 16 hours. There seems to be little or no placental transfer of the drug, but it appears in breast milk.

Tolmetin is a pyrrolacetic acid derivative with a structure resembling indomethacin but an action and toxicity more like those of the propionic acid derivatives. It is used in the management of RA in adults and children and in OA. Although earlier studies suggested a short half-life of only 1 hour, more recent data show a longer half-life of 4.5-6 hr, so that three or four times a day dosage can be recommended (40). This drug appears to have an ulcerogenic potential as low as many of the other new NSAID's and does not appear to produce the central nervous system problems that may occur with indomethacin. It, however, shares other side effects of NSAID including peptic ulcer, hypersensitivity reactions, prolonged bleeding time, edema due to sodium retention, abnormal results of liver function tests, and a reversible rise in blood urea nitrogen.

At present, tolmetin and naproxen are the only NSAID's, other than aspirin, approved for the treatment of juvenile RA in children under 14 years of age and good studies exist concerning effectiveness (41). Theoretically, there is little reason not to believe that some of the other NSAID's will prove equally as safe for the treatment of juvenile RA.

Zomepirac is a pyrrole derivative which is a better analgesic than tolmetin but a weaker antiinflammatory agent. For this reason, it has been marketed soley as an analgesic for mild to moderate pain. A 100-mg dose compares in analgesic effect with 8 mg morphine intramuscularly. In patients taking zomepirac, especially in repeated, short courses of therapy, a higher incidence of anaphylactoid reactions than with other NSAID's was observed (33). For this reason, it has been withdrawn from the market although it may be reintroduced in the future with greater restrictions on its use.

Pyrazolon Derivates

Phenylbutazone and oxyphenbutazone, which is one of its major active metabolites, are two of the oldest and most potent NSAID's, but also two of the potentially most toxic (Figure 4.6). Both are used primarily for relief of acute exacerbations of RA, OA, and gouty arthritis. They are chemically and pharmacologically related to amidopyrine and antipyrine, which are analgesics no longer used because of bone marrow suppression. In fact, phenylbutazone was originally incorporated with amidopyrine as its solubilizing agent but was recognized to have activity of its own. It was introduced in 1949 for the treatment of RA and allied disorders.

These drugs have significantly more toxicity than newer agents. In addition to dyspepsia, gastric ulceration and hemorrhage, renal and hepatic damage have been reported and mouth ulcers and skin reactions are not uncommon (16). Salt and water retention may be pronounced and should preclude the use of these drugs in the elderly or those with heart disease. These drugs may be useful in short-term therapy, but are infrequently used for longer periods because of the potentially devastating side effects of marrow aplasia, which occurs with a frequency of 0.001-1% depending on reporting sources utilized. Half of all cases are fatal and these drugs are responsible for more than a third of all drug-induced blood dyscrasias in the United Kingdom and from 25 to 50 deaths a year (16). Agranulocytosis is more common in younger people in the early stages of treatment while aplastic anemia is more likely to occur in the elderly after a prolonged period of treatment. Although many rheumatologists are reluctant to use these agents in the treatment of RA, they certainly are potent antiinflammatory drugs, and may be used for up to 3-4 months if other drugs cannot control symptoms, if the physicians and patients understand the potential risk and if careful monitoring of the patients is performed (42). Oxyphenbutazone is being withdrawn from the market and phenylbutazone is now restricted to acute use only after other therapy has failed.

Oxyphenbutazone, the active metabolite of phenylbutazone, appears to have no clinical advantage over the parent agent either in efficacy or side effects, and may be more expensive. A European analog, azapropazone, is free from the risk of marrow suppression. Like phenylbutazone it is uricosuric, potentiates anticoagulants, and causes salt and water retention. In other respects, its profile of moderate efficacy and mild gastrointestinal irritation resembles more the propionic acid derivatives (16).

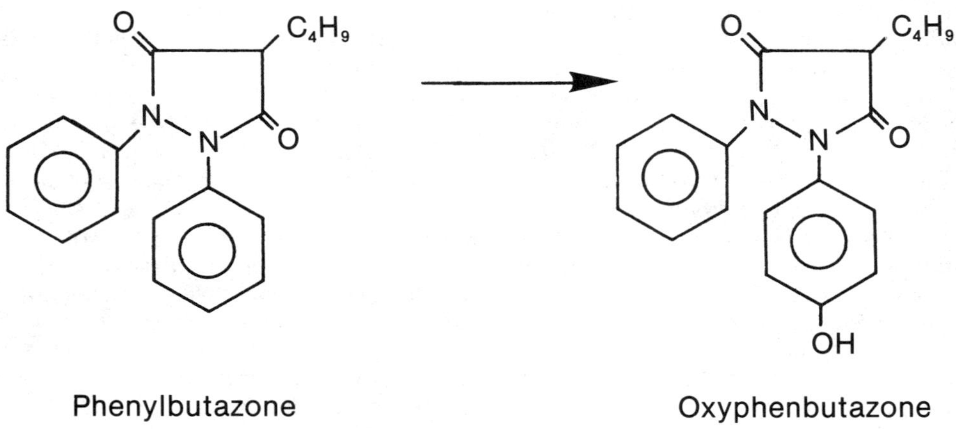

FIGURE 4.6 Pyrazolon derivatives.

Fenamic Acid And Oxicam Derivatives

These two chemical categories include some newer agents (Figure 4.7). The fenamates are anthranilic acid derivatives that are well absorbed after an oral dose. Meclofenamate sodium reaches peak concentration in 1 hour and has a half-life of 2–3 hours. Although it is moderately effective in RA and osteoarthritis, it is not recommended as the initial treatment choice because of gastrointestinal side effects. Diarrhea is a special problem with the fenamates probably due to enterohepatic recirculation of the drug, and renal insufficiency has been reported in elderly patients who have become dehydrated because of the diarrhea. Mefenamic acid also inhibits prostaglandin synthesis and may additionally block its cellular receptors (43). It is approved for use as an analgesic for moderate pain when therapy will not exceed 1 week because of the possibility of more serious side effects than with some of the other agents. It appears also to be an effective agent in the relief of dysmenorrhea.

Piroxicam is the only member so far of a new class of NSAID's, the oxicams. It has now become the most widely used NSAID worldwide (16) and is gaining popularity in the United States for both RA and OA treatment. It is a potent antiinflammatory agent with a plasma half-life of 40 hours, permitting the convenience of once a day dosing. The long half-life also makes rapid swings in blood levels unlikely even if the patient misses occasional doses.

Corticosteroids

Steroids reduce inflammatory reactions by preventing the formation of prostanoids. Rather than inhibiting the cyclooxygenase as do NSAID's, corticosteroids inhibit the phospholipases that release arachidonic acid from cell membrane phospholipids (see Figure 4.1). They therefore prevent the formation of products of the

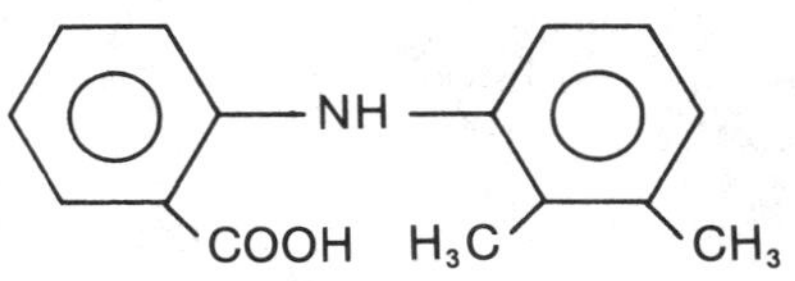

Mefenamic Acid

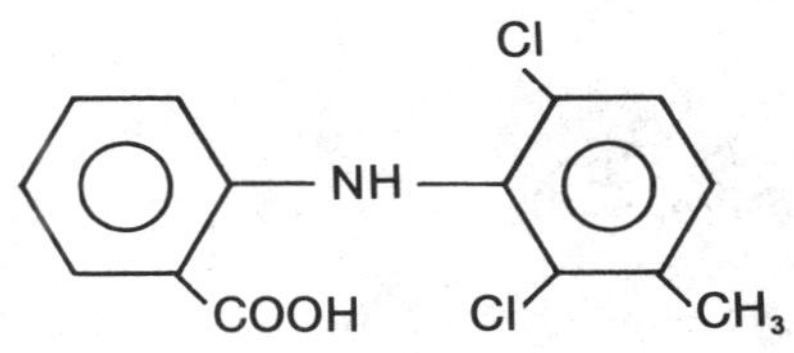

Meclofenamic Acid (Meclofenamate)

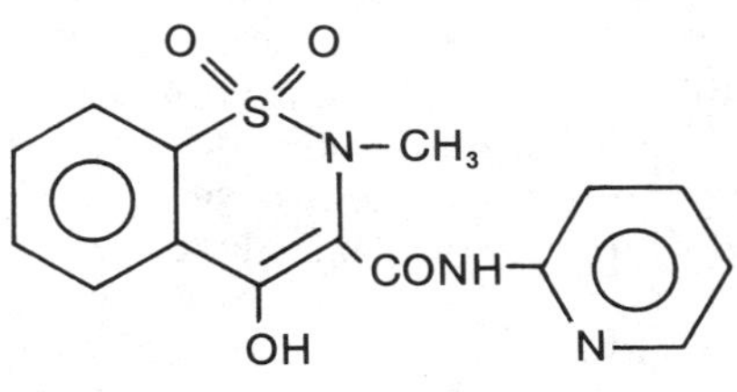

Piroxicam

FIGURE 4.7 Fenamic acid and oxicam derivatives.

lipoxygenase pathway as well as cyclooxygenase products. They also interfere with cell membrane fluidity. The antiphospholipase activity appears to be due to induced proteins, one of which is called macrocortin. It is released and generated by macrophages and probaby other cells and acts as the second messenger for some of the acute antiinflammatory actions of steroids (44).

Corticosteroids have been used both by local intraarticular injection and systemically to control RA inflammation. Systemic steroids are warranted in patients who develop severe extraarticular manifestations of RA, with life-threatening complications such as pleuritis with respiratory compromise or pericarditis with tamponade. Smaller doses of steroids are sometimes used systemically while awaiting for some of the slow-acting immunomodulating drugs to work. In virtually no instances should systemic steroids be used as sole therapy for several reasons. Neither steroids nor NSAID's have been shown to retard the radiographic progression of RA. Their potent antiinflammatory effect, however, may dissuade patients from taking other drugs thought to arrest or retard RA progression. Secondly, induction of a pharmacologic dependency may require increasing dosages to control symptoms and requires gradual tapering of doses when discontinuing therapy to allow adrenal recovery and to avoid rebound flares of disease. Thirdly, late side effects of steroids such as poor wound healing, impaired host defense mechanisms, osteoporosis, and other problems associated with Cushing's syndrome occur with prolonged therapy. In juvenile RA, corticosteroids may also interfere with growth and development. Since OA is a localized joint disease, systemic steroids are not appropriate therapy.

In contrast to systemic steroid therapy, intraarticular steroid injection has been a fairly well accepted treatment when used infrequently to attempt to control the inflammatory process in a single joint in a patient who is responding to the usual medical methods of RA therapy. Depot, long-acting suspensions of poorly soluble corticosteroids give most prolonged effects. These include prednisolone tebutate, methylprednisolone acetate, triamcinolone acetonide, and triamcinolone hexacetonide. Judicious use of this type of therapy is warranted inasmuch as systemic absorption of steroids may occur, septic arthritis of the injected joint is more likely, and increasing cartilage and bone breakdown may occur with repeated injections. Nevertheless, intraarticular steroid injections may be quite effective in alleviating for weeks to months the inflammation occurring in the injected joint.

Neither corticosteroids in normal therapeutic doses nor NSAID's have been shown to alter the course or rate of progressive joint damage in rheumatoid arthritis.

Immunomodulating Agents

The drugs in this category for the treatment of RA include antimalarials, thiol derivatives, and immunosuppressives (Figure 4.8). They are similar in that they may decrease both inflammation and progress of the disease. Improvement due to these so-called remission-inducing drugs has a striking latency period, occurring weeks or months after the initiation of therapy; the improvement often persists, usually for months or years, while therapy is continued, and it may last for weeks or months after therapy has ceased (45).

Claims of remission of RA are based on biochemical and radiological evidence. Several biochemical laboratory measurements appear to parallel the severity of the clinical disease. A family of proteins, possibly unrelated to the underlying cause of the disease, nevertheless increases in concentration in the plasma during an acute inflammation episode. These acute-phase proteins include the

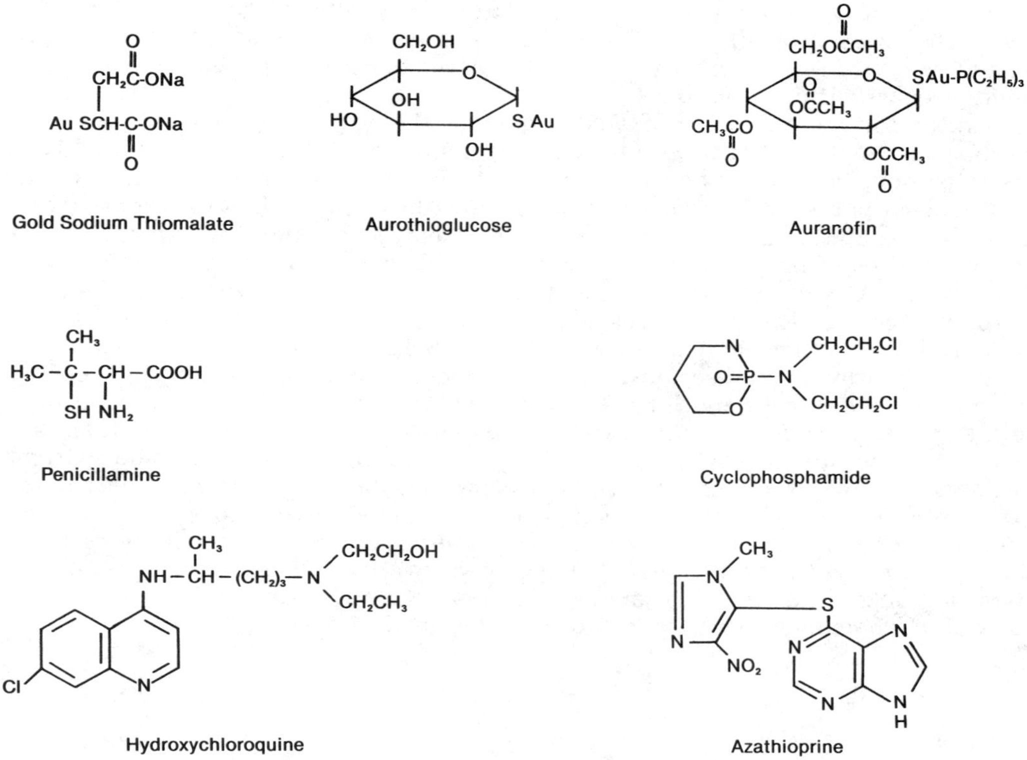

FIGURE 4.8 Immunomodulating agents used in treatment of rheumatoid arthritis.

C-reactive protein. Changes in similar proteins are reflected physiologically in an increased erythrocyte sedimentation rate (ESR). Rheumatoid factor, usually measured as an IgM anti-IgG, also rises with RA severity. All these biochemical markers may be decreased by immunomodulating agents more so than by NSAID's or steroids (46). Furthermore, the progression of radiologically-assessed joint destruction may be slowed, but probably is not reversed, by immunomodulating agents. The price paid for potentially improved disease management and slowed progression is increased toxicity and side effects with these agents.

Antimalarials

In 1951, Page (47) reported that the antimalarial, mepacrine, improved RA. Subsequently, chloroquine and later hydroxycloroquine, other antimalarials, gained wide use in RA treatment (48). The mechanism by which chloroquine or hydroxychloroquine ameliorates this disease is not completely understood. It concentrates in nuclei and lysosomes and stabilizes lysosomal membranes. It can reduce superoxide production since it traps free radicals. In vitro, chloroquine and hydroxychloroquine suppress lymphocyte responsiveness and impair chemotaxis (44, 48).

Mepacrine, another antimalarial, inhibits phospholipase and hence arachidonic acid liberation, but it is not clear if this contributes to hydroxychloroquine's effectiveness. The onset of beneficial effects of these drugs is subtle, occurring between 3 and 6 months after beginning of therapy. After cessation of therapy, arthritis usually recurs within 3 months.

In the United States, hydroxychloroquine is the only antimalarial regularly in use because of the belief of greater ocular toxicity with chloroquine. In reality, the later-developed hydroxychloroquine has been used in smaller, safer doses now that ocular toxicity is recognized. The retinopathy occurs because of selective ocular accumulation of drug in the retinal pigment, and toxicity may progress even after cessation of drug therapy. Corneal deposits visible by slit-lamp biomicroscopy usually do not affect visual function and they disappear if the drug is stopped or the dosage is reduced (49). There is no correlation between corneal deposits and retinal toxicity. Corneal deposits do not require discontinuation of the drug.

Retinopathy is more serious. Since chloroquines bind to melanin, they concentrate in the uveal tract and retinal pigment and may be retained for years in the retina and other tissues. Blurred vision or eventually a dense central scotoma may result. The problem occurs most with long therapy, high doses, or in older patients. Patients with RA receiving hydroxychloroquine should have a baseline ophthalmologic examination and reexamination every 6 months. Current doses of less than 3.5 mg/kg/day of hydroxychloroquine seem safe and seldom require stopping the drug. Other significant side effects have been exfoliative dermatitis and psoriasis flare-up, leukopenia, and neuromyopathy. Although undoubtedly effective in RA, newer immunomodulating agents may supplant antimalarials in the future.

Thiols

Gold Salts

Sulfur-containing compounds in the immunomodulating agent category include gold salts and penicillamine. Gold compounds were first used for RA in Europe over 50 years ago. Because of toxicity, their use declined, but in the past 20 years the use of gold compounds has risen again (48), in part because of successful controlled studies. These studies have shown a reduction in the number of inflammed joints, a lowered erythrocyte sedimentation rate, and retarded progression of radiologic evidence of RA in joints.

Intramuscular injectable gold compounds in current use are gold sodium thiomalate (GST) and gold thioglucose (Figure 4.8). Gold in these chelates is bound to a thiol ligand. In practice, gold salts are injected weekly for about the first 6 months, and then monthly maintenance is continued for up to many years. On such regimens, up to 80% of patients may respond (50). It is thought that the best candidates for chrysotherapy are patients with active disease of less than 1 year's duration.

Since these gold compounds are concentrated in synovial membranes and lysosomes, they are thought to suppress the activity of lysosomal enzymes in macrophages and lower the phagocytic activity of macrophages in RA. Gold also decreases the concentration of rheumatoid factor immunoglobulins and impairs proliferation of lymphocytes, but the correlation between these changes and clinical response is not always clear. As with other immunomodulators, there is a 3-month delay before benefits are observed. Withdrawal of gold therapy because of toxicity may be 15-20% of patients in the first year. About 10% of patients develop rashes, while potentially serious side effects such as bone marrow suppression and development of the nephrotic syndrome occur less frequently. These more serious reactions require close monitoring of white blood cells and renal function.

Recently, an oral gold preparation, auranofin, has been developed. It is a trialkylphosphine gold complex and, in contrast to parenteral gold agents that exist as polymers of simple subunits, auranofin is a monomeric, lipid soluble, stable compound. Some differences appear to exist between the ways GST and auranofin reduce inflammation. Unlike GST, auranofin primarily affects T rather than B lymphocyte function. Auranofin is more potent at inhibiting inflammation and lysosomal enzyme release. In contrast, both gold compounds equally suppress phagocytosis and macrophage function (51).

Auranofin produces significantly less mucocutaneous and renal toxicity but significantly more gastrointestinal problems (especially diarrhea) than parenteral gold (51, 52). This is because oral auranofin undergoes enterohepatic circulation without reabsorption from bile so that 95% of it is excreted in the feces and only 5% in the urine. By contrast, 70% of gold from GST is found in the urine (51).

D-Penicillamine

Penicillamine is a potent agent in the treatment of RA whose structure resembles the amino acid cysteine. The D-isomer shows less toxicity and is used clinically. The rationale for use in RA came from a demonstration of its ability to dissociate macroglobulins and rheumatoid factor. Even though the exact mode of action of penicillamine in RA therapy remains unknown, suggested mechanisms may include some known actions of the drug to decrease immune complexes and immune responses, suppress T and B cells, interfere with complement activity, and chelate calcium and zinc (48).

As with gold, the onset of clinical response is slow, and side effects requiring withdrawal of the drug may occur in up to 30% of patients. Since many are dose-related, the "go low, go slow" approach is recommended. Loss of taste (dysgeusia) is common and is reversed in 1-2 months even with continued drug use. Gastrointestinal symptoms may range from mild anorexia to intractable vomiting which may require discontinuing drug. Skin rashes may occur and vary in severity. Thrombocytopenia occurs in about 10-15% of patients and can be severe and develop suddenly (48). Renal toxicity is usually expressed as proteinuria. It may be mild but is significant ($>$ 2 g/24 hr) in about 10% of cases. Kidney biopsies may show basement membrane abnormalities and dense deposits. Proteinuria may persist for long periods when the drug is discontinued in spite of normal renal function and should warrant long-term follow-up. Other thiol drugs such as the gold salts and the antihypertensive agent, captopril, also produce proteinuria. Aggravation of autoimmune disease may occur with penicillamine and a lupus-like syndrome produced by uncertain immunologic mechanisms may be accompanied by antinuclear antibodies. One should keep in mind then that a patient with RA who experiences joint pain might actually need less penicillamine rather than more, because of the development of a lupus-like syndrome.

Immunosuppressives

Several immunosuppressive, or cytotoxic agents, used primarily in cancer patients and renal transplant recipients have been used in RA. The rationale for their use centers around a decrease in IgM and IgG rheumatoid factors and lymphocytes found in RA synovial fluid. Principal drugs used have been cyclophosphamide and azathioprine, although methotrexate has received more attention in recent studies. These agents should be reserved for severe progressive RA that is unresponsive to more conservative measures.

Cyclophosphamide is a bivalent substituted nitrogen mustard and the most potent alkylating agent known. The drug is activated by the liver and excreted by the kidneys. It is a powerful immunosuppressive and has clearly been shown in double-blind clinical trials to prevent progressive joint destruction and improve RA. This too is a slow-acting form of therapy. The side effects of cyclophosphamide can be considerable and include increased infections, sterility due to azospermia or ovarian fibrosis, leukopenia, alopecia which is usually reversible, gastrointestinal intolerance, cystitis or bladder hemorrhage which can be severe, and an increased incidence of cancer.

Azathioprine is often used to control transplant rejection and is also approved for treatment of RA. It was originally developed as an agent that was less toxic but as effective as 6-mercaptopurine (6-MP). Azathioprine is quickly converted to 6-MP in man and most, but not all, of its actions are due 6-MP. The exact connection between purine antagonism, immunosuppression and amelioration of RA is not at all well understood. Since xanthine oxidase is responsible for the breakdown of 6-MP, the dose of azathioprine should be reduced by two-thirds if allopurinol, a xanthine oxidase inhibitor, is used concurrently.

Azathioprine can also clearly improve the clinical course of RA. The most characteristic toxicity is a dose-related leukopenia which usually resolves on lowering the dose of the drug. Gastrointestinal intolerance, superimposed infections, and rashes may also occur. Azathioprine does not cause the genital or bladder toxicity seen with cyclophosphamide. Transplant patients receiving this agent are known to have a higher incidence of neoplasia but careful trials to verify this risk in RA treatment have not been done. Nevertheless, an assumed risk of neoplasia suggests that immunosuppressive drugs be reserved for RA patients who have not responded to or who have developed intolerable side effects on conventional NSAID and immunomodulating agent therapy. In order to minimize the individual toxicities of the drugs, a combination of cyclophosphamide, azathioprine, and hydroxychloroquine in moderate doses has been used in intractable RA (53).

Other Drugs; Special Considerations

Levamisole is an antihelmintic drug that has been shown to be an immunostimulant and to be effective in the management of RA (54). It stimulates some of the cellular elements of the immune response, but its mechanism of action in RA is not known. Early studies showed an unacceptably high incidence of agranulocytosis, but newer low dose regimens with weekly doses show better clinical results (55). Newer agents in this category with fewer side effects continue in various stages of development.

Dimethyl sulfoxide (DMSO) is a colorless oily liquid that readily penetrates the skin and mucous membranes. It localizes within the interstitium of tissues but is not found to any extent intracellularly. As a penetrant carrier solvent, it increases the dermal absorption of many other chemicals. Some of its pharmacologic effects have made it fashionable to consider as an antirheumatic agent (56). DMSO has local anesthetic activity and decreases nerve conduction. It enhances the action of other anesthetics. The acute antiinflammatory activity may result from its ability to scavenge free radicals generated by phagocytes. It also appears to have some ability to stabilize lysosomal membranes. Enthusiasm for DMSO was tempered by reports of increased lens opacity in animals studies; although these changes have not been documented so far in humans, they warrant caution. DMSO, when used topically for short periods, may be relatively nontoxic. It may have acute analgesic and acute antiinflammatory effects (56). It does not appear as if it will be of benefit in a chronic inflammatory disease such as RA.

Juvenile rheumatoid arthritis (JRA), discussed in Chapter 19, is a chronic inflammatory disease of childhood with onset before age 16. It may occur even in very young children accompanied by fevers and rashes and may affect only a few or many joints. Regardless of onset pattern, the long-term prognosis for life is excellent. Greater than 75% of treated patients have good function after 10 years of disease (57). For this reason, drug therapy may differ in JRA from adult RA. As with adult RA, aspirin is a first choice therapy. If hypersensitivity is present, a nonacetylated salicylate may be substituted. Since salicylism may be more serious in children, special attention to doses and over-the-counter medications is recommended. At present, the only NSAID's approved for children under 14 are tolmetin sodium and naproxen and some JRA patients respond better to them than to salicylates. These drugs suppress inflammation but do not prevent progressive joint damage. Gold, antimalarials, and D-penicillamine induce remission but, since JRA has generally a better prognosis than adult RA, are less frequently required. Corticosteroids cause the characteristic Cushing's syndrome but additionally interfere with growth and development in children so they should be reserved for temporary use with severe needs. Intraarticular steroids are effective when used infrequently and selectively in affected joints. Cytotoxic agents are used experimentally in JRA. Because of potentially life-threatening complications from the drugs, as well as the risks of infertility and cancer, the use of these drugs should be relegated to a few seriously ill children.

Pharmacotherapy of Degenerative Joint Disease (Osteoarthritis)

Degenerative joint disease, or osteoarthritis, is characterized by loss of articular cartilage which secondarily can affect the synovial membrane and underlying bone. As is discussed in Chapter 9, this disease is relatively uncommon in patients less than 40 years old, and is seen in 85% of patients over 70. Although osteoarthritis (OA) is not considered a systemic inflammatory arthropathy, there is often evidence of local inflammation and mildly inflammatory polyarthritis. It may constitute a group of diseases with different pathogeneses. One form of OA is generalized, has an unknown origin, and a genetic predisposition. A second form involves local trauma or overwork of a specific joint and often has an occupational cause. In any case, relief from pain and local inflammation is a therapeutic goal. Modifiers of the immune system are not a component of OA therapy as they are with RA.

Aspirin and other NSAID's are used both for analgesic and antiinflammatory effects. Since elderly patients are often treated, the decrease in renal function that NSAID's can produce needs consideration. Toxic effects of aspirin of hearing loss and tinnitus and of mental confusion may be interpreted as senility instead of salicylate intoxication. Individual response and preference of one NSAID over another varies as it does with RA treatment. There is no evidence that any NSAID alters the course of osteoarthritis once articular cartilage has been lost. Some evidence suggests that early antiinflammatory therapy decreases cartilage damage in minimally affected joints.

Intraarticular corticosteroids reduce arachidonic acid metabolism and membrane fluidity. They also depress chondrocyte metabolism and cartilage matrix production that is increased in OA to compensate for the degredative process. Consequently, although intraarticular steroids are effective over the short term (weeks), the long-term effects may be harmful. They should be used sparingly in a single joint along with oral NSAID's. Systemic corticosteroids have no role in the treatment of OA.

The nonsteroidal antiinflammatory drugs have analgesic efficacy as well, but some patients require additional pain control. To their regimen, analgesics such as acetaminophen, propoxyphene, or pentazocine may be added. Muscle spasm adjacent to inflamed joints may be relieved with muscle relaxants. Clinical priorities for the treatment of degenerative joint disease or osteoarthritis are summarized in Figure 4.9.

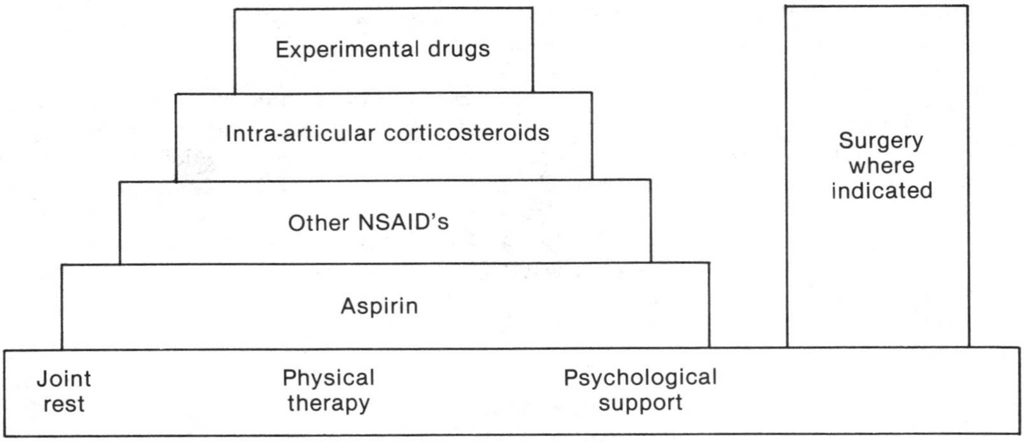

FIGURE 4.9 Pyramid of care in the treatment of osteoarthritis (degenerative joint disease).

Pharmacotherapy of Gout

As will be discussed in Chapter 11, gout is a consequence of the deposition of crystals of monosodium urate monohydrate in tissues. We live on the brink of urate crystallization (about 7 mg/dl). Small deposits of crystals are called tophi and these may eventually elicit an inflammatory response. Uric acid (mainly urate at body pH) is the end product of purine metabolism derived from two general sources: dietary purines and purines resulting from the normal metabolic turnover of cells. The biochemical scheme for urate production is shown in Chapter 11. Most other species possess uricase which further metabolizes urate to the much more soluble compound, allantoin. In an adult man on a purine-free diet, the total body urate averages 1200 mg. About 50% of the urate pool is turned over each day, resulting in an excretion of about 600 mg/day. Two-thirds is excreted in the urine and one-third in the feces.

The renal handling of urate is quite complex. Its final excretion is the result of filtration, active secretion, and active reabsorption in at least two sites (Figure 4.10). The balance between net secretion and net reabsorption varies among species. Both processes appear to occur in all species studied, but the ratio varies. Man undergoes net reabsorption of urate. Nearly all the urate in plasma is filterable at the glomerulus, and most of it is reabsorbed early in the proximal tubule. Approximately 50% of the original filtered load is then actively secreted back into the proximal tubule. Postsecretory reabsorption also occurs in the late proximal

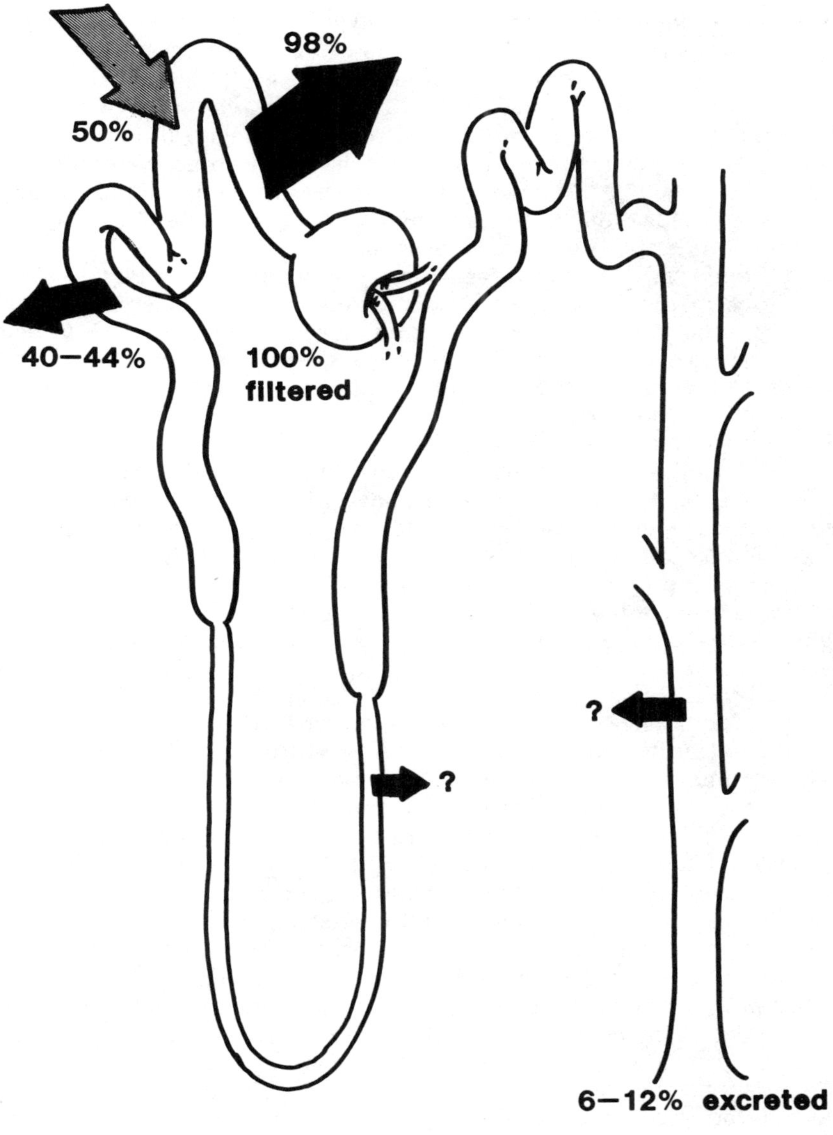

FIGURE 4.10 Renal handling of uric acid. Arrows denote active reabsorption and secretion while percentages refer to the fraction of the filtered load that is reabsorbed, secreted, and excreted.

tubule, pars recta, and possibly to a small degree in other nephron segments. An average of 6-12% of the original filtered load of urate is excreted.

Since plasma urate concentrations average 7-8 mg/dl in normal man, elevated values may be considered hyperuricemic. Even though chemical supersaturation of urate in the plasma should occur at concentrations of 7 mg/dl, crystallization does not always occur. Whereas about 13% of men have serum urate levels consistently over 7 mg/dl, only about 0.3% develop gout. Hyperuricemia incidence increases in postmenopausal women. Asymptomatic hyperuricemia in the absence of arthritis, tophi, or renal stones does not require drug therapy.

Hyperuricemia may have several primary or secondary causes. Overproduction of uric acid, in which > 600 mg/day is excreted in the urine, accounts for about 25% of the cases. These patients may be at an increased risk of urolithiasis (stones). Underexcretion of urate (< 600 mg/day) accounts for 75% of the patients. Several drugs or disease states may also influence plasma urate concentration as discussed in Chapter 11.

Hyperuricemia may result in acute gouty arthritis which usually occurs to men in their 40's and 50's. Without treatment, attacks tend to resolve in 3-10 days. Intercritical, or quiescent periods of gout, separate acute episodes of increasing frequency. Untreated gout results in tophaceous urate deposits around joints and extremities such as the helix of the ear and may also result in uric acid nephrolithiasis. The goal of therapy then is to relieve and prevent acute attacks, resolve tophi, and prevent sequelae of chronic tophaceous gout.

Colchicine is a unique antiinflammatory agent effective almost exclusively against gouty arthritis and a few less common forms of crystal-induced arthritis (Figure 4.11). Until recent years, it was unchallenged in treating acute attacks and preventing recurrence, but currently several NSAID's, especially indomethacin, offer alternative therapy. Colchicine is a cytotoxic alkaloid extracted from bulbs of the autumn crocus (*Colchicum autumnale)* and contains two unusual seven-membered rings. It disrupts microtubule formation and probably relieves the inflammation by breaking the cycle through which phagocytes digest urate crystals and recruit more phagocytes. Mobility of white cells depends upon intact microtubules so that colchicine reduces neutrophil migration.

The incidence of successful treatment of acute gout is as high as 75-95% when colchicine is begun within 12 hours after the onset of articular symptoms (58). However, many physicians prefer a NSAID for the treatment of recurrent attacks once the patient has demonstrated responsiveness to colchicine. Oral colchicine is given at 0.5 mg every hour until either relief of the attack or unacceptable toxicity occurs. The total dose should not exceed 8 mg. Diarrhea usually occurs with effective doses, and this is distressing for patients with severe pain in weight-bearing joints who have to run to the bathroom. Intravenous colchicine may be useful in patients who cannot take NSAID's or are unable to take oral medications. Diarrhea is less frequent, but this route of colchicine is very irritating to tissues so it must be diluted and given carefully to avoid extravasation. The usual dose is 2 mg colchicine diluted in 20 ml of saline infused slowly. A second dose of 1 mg may be given 6 hours later, up to a total dose of not more than 4 mg. Long-term oral colchicine in lower doses reduces recurrence of acute gout and can be used with urate-lowering drugs which hasten urate excretion or inhibit its synthesis.

Urate-reducing drugs should not be started during an acute attack. The patient should be asymptomatic for 2-4 weeks and may receive chronic colchicine to prevent precipitation of an attack when urate levels are altered by other drugs. If urate-lowering agents are advised, either enhanced renal excretion with uricosuric drugs or decreased synthesis of uric acid is an option. Allopurinol is an inhibitor of xanthine oxidase, the enzyme responsible for the formation of xanthine

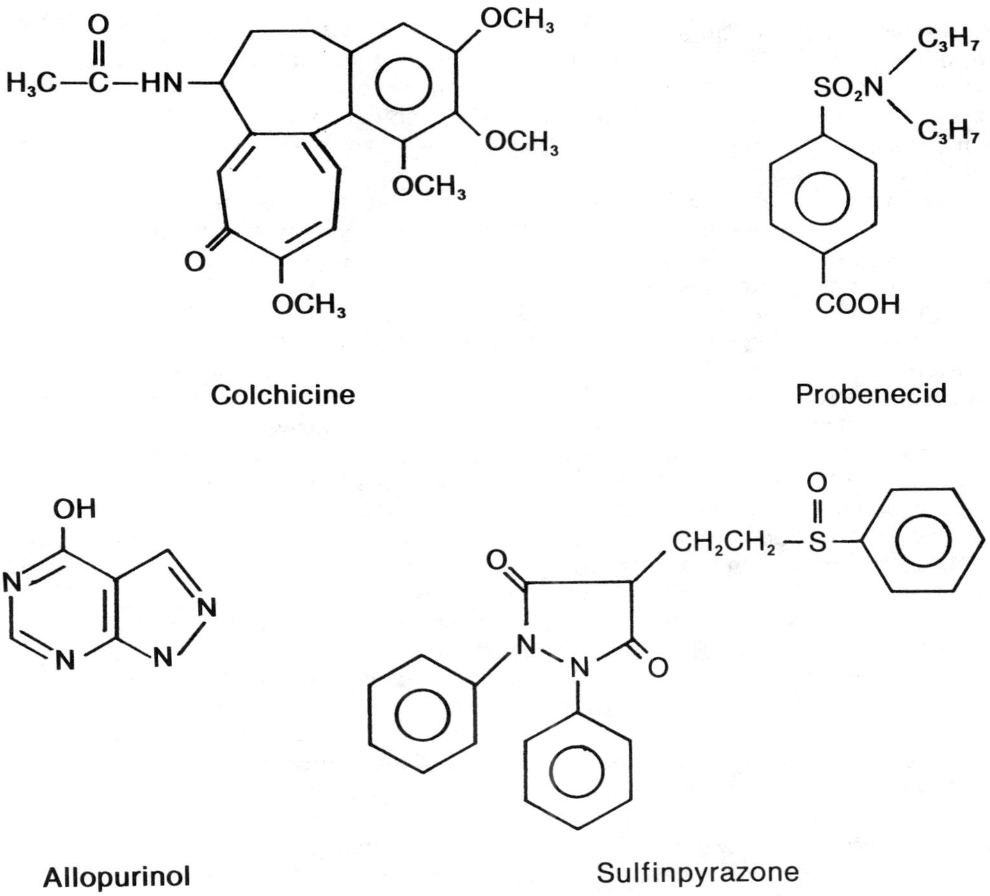

FIGURE 4.11 Drugs used in the treatment and prevention of gouty arthritis.

and uric acid from hypoxanthine. Allopurinol is a structural isomer of hypoxanthine and has a much greater affinity for xanthine oxidase than does xanthine. It decreases the rate of formation and the blood levels of urate considerably but does not appreciably affect that of the more water soluble xanthine. Since the metabolite of allopurinol, oxypurinol, is also active, it can usually be given only once a day. It is especially indicated in patients who develop untoward reactions to the uricosuric drugs, in overproducers, in patients with renal insufficiency, or in persistent stone formers. Patients may require 200–300 mg/day with mild gout or as much as 600–800 mg/day with more severe tophaceous gout to reduce serum levels of uric acid to below 7 mg/dl. In order to avoid precipitating an acute attack, allopurinol may be started as low as 100 mg/day and increased gradually. An adequate urine output of at least 2 L/day will help prevent urate precipitation or calculi formation. In patients with severely impaired renal function or decreased urate clearance, the half-life of oxypurinol in the plasma is greatly prolonged. A dose of only 100 mg/day or 300 mg twice a week may be adequate to maintain xanthine oxidase inhibition. Since it inhibits purine metabolism, the metabolism of azathioprine and 6-mercaptopurine is greatly reduced and these chemotherapeutic agents should be given in a reduced dose. Allopurinol has an incidence of about 20% side effects including gastrointestinal intolerance, rashes, blood dyscrasias, and vasculitis. An interaction of unknown mechanism occurs between allopurinol and ampicillin. The incidence of rashes due to ampicillin is increased approximately threefold by the concurrent administration of allopurinol (58).

Uricosuric agents are organic acids that reduce the net reabsorption of uric acid in the proximal tubule. In small doses, secretion is preferentially inhibited and uric acid retention is actually increased, but in larger doses used clinically both secretion and the quantitatively greater reabsorption processes are inhibited so that urate excretion is increased. Uricosuric drugs should not be given to patients with declining renal function or stones since the tubular load of urate will be increased. Overproducers should not be treated with these agents alone unless there is an allergy to allopurinol. Like allopurinol, these drugs are for the treatment of intercritical gout and should not be started during an acute attack. However, patients who are already receiving urate-lowering drugs and who have an acute attack can continue their therapy while the attack is being treated.

Probenecid was developed to inhibit the tubular secretion of penicillin and has been used since the early 1950's to inhibit the net tubular reabsorption of uric acid. It should be started gradually and often in combination with colchicine to avoid precipitating an acute attack. The usual starting dose is 250 mg twice a day. This is gradually increased to an average maintenance dose of 1.0–1.5 g/day. Serum urate levels decline gradually over several weeks. The biological half-life of probenecid is 6–12 hr so that it should be spaced throughout the day. The most common adverse reactions to probenecid are gastrointestinal upset and rashes. Rarely, there are more serious hypersensitive reactions.

Sulfinpyrazone is a congener of phenylbutazone with much less toxicity. It does not cause the severe blood dyscrasias seen with phenylbutazone. It is about 3–6 times more uricosuric than probenecid and additionally appears to inhibit platelet aggregation and has been used in the prevention of cardiovascular occlusive disease. However, since it is related to phenylbutazone, it is contraindicated in persons with allergy to other pyrazoles, in persons with blood dyscrasias or in the presence of gastrointestinal ulcer disease (59). Gastrointestinal upset or rash is the most common adverse reaction. Sulfinpyrazone decreases the metabolism of warfarin and tolbutamide (58), and since it alters platelet aggregation by itself, the concomitant use of warfarin and sulfinpyrazone must be monitored carefully. In contrast to these drugs, sulfinpyrazone may slightly enhance the metabolism of theophylline. Sulfinpyrazone is usually started at 50 mg twice a day. This is gradually increased to a maintenance dose that averages 200–800 mg/day in 3 or 4 divided doses.

The uricosuric activities of both probenecid (60) and sulfinpyrazone (61) are decreased by salicylate levels greater than 50 μg/ml which is an analgesic level obtained after only a few tablets of aspirin. Therefore, aspirin substitutes or at most only occasional doses of aspirin or other salicylates should be given to patients taking uricosurics. Since many over-the-counter preparations contain aspirin, this caution needs to be communicated to the patient.

References

1. Ehrlich GE: Treatment of rheumatoid arthritis. In J Yetiv (ed.), *Recent Advances in Clinical Therapeutics.* New York, Academic Press, 1981, pp. 223-234.

2. Simon LS, Mills JA: Nonsteroidal antiinflammatory drugs. *New Eng J Med* 302:1179-1185 and 1237-1243, 1980.

3. Bowman WC, Rand MJ: *Textbook of Pharmacology,* 2nd Ed. Oxford, Blackwell Scientific Publications, 1980.

4. Dromgoole SH, Furst DE: Salicylates. In WE Evans, JJ Schentag, WJ Jusko (eds.), *Applied Pharmacokinetics.* San Francisco, Applied Therapeutics Inc., 1980, pp. 486-517.

5. Flower RJ, Moncada S, Vane JR: Analgesic-antipyretics and antiinflammatory agents; drugs employed in the treatment of gout. In AG Gilman, LS Goodman, A Gilman (eds.), *The Pharmacological Basis of Therapeutics.* New York, Macmillan, 1980, pp. 682-728.

6. Costello PB, Green FA, Jung CY: Free versus bound salicylate concentration in adults and children with chronic inflammatory joint disease. *Arthritis Rheum* 25:32-37, 1982.

7. Costello PB, Green FA: Aspirin survival in human blood modulated by the concentration of erythrocytes. *Arthritis Rheum* 25:550-555, 1982.

8. Levy G: Clinical pharmacokinetics of aspirin. *Pediatrics* 62:867-872, 1978.

9. Graham GG, Champion GD, Ray RO, Paull PD: Patterns of plasma concentrations and urinary excretion of salicylate in rheumatoid arthritis. *Clin Pharmacol Ther* 22:410-420, 1977.

10. Vane JR: Inhibition of prostaglandin synthesis as a mechanism of action of aspirin-like drugs. *Nature* 231:232-237, 1971.

11. McCord JM, Fridovich I: The biology and pathology of oxygen radicals. *Ann Intern Med* 89:122-127, 1978.

12. DiRosa M, Papadimitriou JM, Willoughby DA: A histopathological and pharmacological analysis of the mode of action of nonsteroidal antiinflammatory drugs. *J Pathol* 105:239-256, 1971.

13. DiRosa M, Sorrentino L, Parente L: Nonsteroidal antiinflammatory drugs and leukocyte migration. *J Pharm Pharmacol* 24:575-576, 1972.

14. Meacock SCR, Kitchen EA: Some effects of nonsteroidal antiinflammatory drugs on leukocyte migration. *Agents Actions* 6:320-325, 1976.

15. Dahl SL, Ward JR: Pharmacology, clinical efficacy, and adverse effects of the nonsteroidal antiinflammatory agent benoxaprofen. *Pharmacotherapy* 2:354-366, 1982.

16. Nuki G: Nonsteroidal analgesic and antiinflammatory agents. *Brit Med J* 287:39-43, 1983.

17. Szceklik A, Gryglewski RJ, Czerniawska-Mysik G: Clinical patterns of hypersensitivity to nonsteroidal antiinflammatory drugs and their pathogenesis. *J Allergy Clin Immunol* 60:276-284, 1977.

18. Weinberger M: Analgesic sensitivity in children with asthma. *Pediatrics* 62: 910-915, 1978.

19. Muther RS, Potter DM, Bennett WM: Aspirin-induced depression of glomerular filtration rate in normal humans: Role of sodium balance. *Ann Intern Med* 94:317-321, 1981.

20. Linton AL, Clark WF, Driedger AA, et al: Acute interstitial nephritis due to drugs. *Ann Intern Med* 93:735-741, 1980.

21. Turner G, Collins E: Fetal effects of regular salicylate ingestion in pregnancy. *Lancet* 2:338-339, 1975.

22. Wilson JG: Factors determining the teratogenicity of drugs. *Ann Rev Toxicol* 14:205-217, 1974.

23. Halla JT, Fallahi S, Hardin JR: Acute and chronic salicylate intoxication in a patient with gastric outlet obstruction. *Arthritis Rheum* 24:1205-1207, 1981.

24. Stuart JJ, Pisko EJ: Choline magnesium trisalicylate does not impair platelet aggregation. *Pharmatherapeutica* 2:547-551, 1981.

25. Tobert JA, DeSchepper P, Tjandramaga TB et al.: Effect of antacids on the bioavailability of diflunisal in the fasting and postprandial states. *Clin Pharmacol Ther* 30:385-389, 1981.

26. Fishel B, Weiss S, Yaron M: Diflunisal in rheumatoid arthritis. *Inflammation* 5:253-261, 1981.

27. Kantor TG: Ibuprofen. *Ann Intern Med* 91:877-882, 1979.

28. Whitlam JB, Brown KF, Crooks MJ et al.: Transsynovial distribution of ibuprofen in arthritic patients. *Clin Pharmacol Ther* 29:487-492, 1981.

29. Godfrey RG, de la Cruz S: Effect of ibuprofen dosage on patient response in rheumatoid arthritis. *Arthritis Rheum* 18:135-137, 1975.

30. Chan WY, Dawood MY, Fuchs F: Relief of dysmenorrhea with the prostaglandin synthesis inhibitor ibuprofen: Effect on prostaglandin levels in menstrual fluid. *Am J Obstet Gynecol* 135:102-108, 1979.

31. Dhand AK, La Brecque DR, Metzger J: Sulindac (Clinoril) hepatitis. *Gastroenterology* 80:585-586, 1980.

32. Fenech FF, Bannister WH, Grech JL: Hepatitis with biliverdinaemia in association with indomethacin therapy. *Brit Med J* 3:155-166, 1967.

33. Anonymous: Toxicity of nonsteroidal antiinflammatory drugs. *Med Letter* 25:15-16, 1983.

34. Penner JA, Abbrecht PH: Lack of interaction between ibuprofen and warfarin. *Curr Ther Res* 18:862-871, 1975.

35. Finkelstein A, Fraley DS, Stachura I, Feldman HA, Gandy DR, Bourke E: Fenoprofen nephropathy: Lipoid nephrosis and interstitial nephritis. *Am J Med* 72:81-87, 1982.

36. Willkens RF, Segre EJ: Combination therapy with naproxen and aspirin in rheumatoid arthritis. *Arthritis Rheum* 19:677-682, 1976.

37. Day RO, Furst DE, Dromgoole SH et al.: Relationship of serum naproxen concentration to efficacy in rheumatoid arthritis. *Clin Pharm Ther* 31:733-740, 1982.

38. Moore ME: A rheumatologist's view of nonsteroidal antiinflammatory drugs. *Clin Ther* 4:137-149, 1981.

39. Orme ML'E: Plasma concentrations and therapeutic effect of antiinflammatory and antirheumatic drugs. *Pharmac Ther* 16:167-180, 1982.

40. Ayres JW, Weidler DJ, Sakmar E et al.: Linear and nonlinear assessment of tolmetin pharmacokinetics. *Res Commun Chem Pathol Pharmacol* 17:583-593, 1977.

41. Gewanter HL, Baum J: The use of tolmetin sodium in systemic onset juvenile rheumatoid arthritis. *Arthritis Rheum* 24:1316-1319, 1981.

42. Box J, Box P, Turner P, Pisko E: Piroxicam in rheumatoid arthritis: A double-blind 16-week study comparing piroxicam and phenylbutazone. *International Congress and Symposium Series of the Royal Society of Medicine* 1:41-46, 1978.

43. Tolman EL, Partridge R: Multiple sites of interaction between prostaglandins and nonsteroidal antiinflammatory agents. *Prostaglandins* 9:349-359, 1975.

44. Flower RJ, Wood JN, Parente L: Macrocortin and the mechanism of action of glucocorticoids. In I Otterness, R Capetola, S Wong (eds.), *Advances in Inflammation Research,* vol. 7. New York, Raven Press, 1984, pp. 61-70.

45. Anastassiades TP: Remission-inducing drugs in rheumatoid arthritis. *Canad Med Assn J* 23:405-412, 1980.

46. Laurent MR, Panayi GS: Biochemical parameters in the assessment of anti-inflammatory drugs - A review. *Agents Actions Suppl* 7:310-317, 1980.

47. Page F: Treatment of lupus erythematosus with mepacrine. *Lancet* 2:755-758, 1951.

48. Bunch TW, O'Duffy JD: Disease-modifying drugs for progressive rheumatoid arthritis. *Mayo Clinic Proc* 55:161-179, 1980.

49. Nylander U: Ocular damage in chloroquine therapy. *Acta Ophthalmol* (suppl)92:5-71, 1967.

50. Sharp JT, Lidsky MD, Duffy J: Clinical responses during gold therapy for rheumatoid arthritis. *Arthritis Rheum* 25:540-549, 1982.

51. Bernhard GC: Auranofin therapy in rheumatoid arthritis. *J Lab Clin Med* 100:167-177, 1982.

52. Lawrence JS: Comparative toxicity of gold preparations in treatment of rheumatoid arthritis. *Ann Rheum Dis* 35:171-173, 1976.

53. McCarty DJ, Carrera GF: Intractable rheumatoid arthritis: Treatment with combined cyclophosphamide, azathioprine, and hydroxychloroquine. *JAMA* 248:1718-1723, 1982.

54. Schnieden H: Levamisole - A general pharmacological perspective. *Int J Immunopharmacol* 3:9-13, 1981.

55. Multicentre Study Group: Levamisole in rheumatoid arthritis. *Ann Intern Med* 41:159-163, 1982.

56. Jiminez RAH, Willkens RF: Dimethyl sulfoxide: A perspective of its use in rheumatic disease. *J Lab Clin Med* 100:489-500, 1982.

57. Bernhard GC: Juvenile rheumatoid arthritis. In HF Conn (ed.), *Conn's Current Therapy*. Philadelphia, W. B. Saunders, 1983, pp. 787-790.

58. Talbott JH: Drug treatment of gout. In EC Huskisson (ed.), *Antirheumatic Drugs*. New York, Praeger, 1983, pp. 693-708.

59. Hasselbacher P: Hyperuricemia and gout. In HF Conn (ed.), *Conn's Current Therapy*. Philadelphia, W. B. Saunders, 1983, pp. 432-436.

60. Paschale LR, Dubin A, Bronsky D, Hoffman WS: Inhibition of the uricosuric action of Benemid by salicylate. *J Lab Clin Med* 45:771-777, 1955.

61. Yu TF, Dayton PG, Gutman AB: Mutual suppression of the uricosuric effect of sulfinpyrazone and salicylate. *J Clin Invest* 42:1330-1339, 1963.

Chapter 5

ARTHRITIS NURSING AND THE TEAM APPROACH IN THE MANAGEMENT OF RHEUMATIC DISEASE

Nirma Perricone, B.S.N., R.N. and
Jo Ann Fahey, B.S.N., R.N.

Until very recently the medical community has concerned itself primarily with the acute illnesses which once killed large numbers of the population in rather short periods of time. People are now living longer and our attention must now shift from the acute disorders to an older population that will suffer from chronic aging diseases. Physicians have not been adequately prepared to deal with these problems and research has not kept pace. Studies indicate that American health scientists may soon be facing a potential health crisis unless major scientific breakthroughs occur (1, 2).

Though chronic illnesses are not by any means limited to the elderly, the rapidly growing numbers of this age group will certainly have an impact. Consider that 11% of our population or 21 million people are now over 65. Within 35 years predictions are that percentage will double and in 60 years the percentage of people 85 and over will triple! (2) The rheumatic diseases will be a significant part of the chronic disease explosion. Rheumatology is a relatively new subspecialty and few physicians, or other health professionals for that matter, receive a focused experience in their basic programs. As a result, many lack experience with the spectrum of therapeutic and diagnostic strategies, yet 85% of arthritis patients will continue to be managed by primary care physicians.

Despite the progress which has been made in the treatment and pathogenesis of arthritis and connective tissue disease, the complex and chronic nature of these disorders can be frustrating and sometimes overwhelming to the primary care physician (3). The difficulty is that of managing the multiplicity of problems which confront these patients and their families, and which frequently run the full gamut from physical to psychosocial. A good therapeutic outcome often requires a variety of strategies and resources which may not be available or within the realm of the physician's training. Lack of time and limited resources tend to sometimes generate a "bandaid approach," rather than the well-coordinated comprehensive therapeutic program these patients require and deserve (4).

Developing a comprehensive management program for the rheumatic disease patient can be accomplished. Today, there are a variety of medical specialists available who are helpful in dealing with the myriad of problems that patients with a chronic disease must face. Rheumatologists, surgeons, nurses, physical therapists, occupational therapists, vocational counselors, sexual counselors, and educational consultants are just a few of the specialists who may be part of the treatment team. Although nursing specialists have been recognized for many years in the areas of maternal and child health, rehabilitation, critical care, and oncology, the rheumatology nurse specialist is a relative newcomer to the field.

At this time, a nurse who wants to specialize in rheumatology does not have a wide variety of programs available to choose from. A study done by Jette and Becker (5) in 1980 demonstrated that even at the undergraduate level the amount of clinical rheumatology exposure made available to nursing, physical therapy (PT), and occupational therapy (OT) students was extremely limited. Recognition of this situation by the Allied Health Professionals Section of the Arthritis Foundation and others has resulted in the development of professional education programs in arthritis for the various allied health professions as well as for the medical profession itself.

Multipurpose Arthritis Centers (MAC's) are also available in various parts of the country and are contributing significantly to the educational process. These are usually hospital-based and contain full diagnostic and therapeutic services by qualified professionals. They are referral organizations who emphasize and organize a team approach for the rheumatic disease patient, and are dedicated to complete assessment, diagnosis, and total management of such patients (6). In addition, the Arthritis Foundation offers fellowships to promote further study and research projects for qualified arthritis health professionals (AHP's).

White et al. (7) have identified the following three reasons why more nurses are specializing in rheumatology: 1) as the field of rheumatology expands, more rheumatology patient units are established with a subsequent need for specially trained nursing staff, 2) in general, there is an increased interest in the quality of life for chronically ill patients, and 3) with current statistics showing an increasing life span for patients with rheumatic illness, there is a general need for nurses educated in this area.

Nurses trained in the management of rheumatic illnesses can be found in a variety of settings including hospitals, outpatient clinics, and physician offices. They are also holding positions as nurse practitioners and nursing consultants. Regardless of the place of practice, the basic definition of rheumatology nursing is that "nursing is the diagnosis and treatment of human responses to actual or potential health problems." (7).

The Rheumatology Team

Philosophy

Successful treatment of the more severe rheumatic disorders necessitates a team approach with patient/family participation and long-range planning as well as frequent reassessment and modification (6). It requires not only the diversified skills of various health professionals, but health professionals with specific training and skills in the management of rheumatological disorders who are willing to communicate with each other and to organize and coordinate the patient's program.

Figley (9) states that "Multidisciplinary care evolves from the concept that the patient is a 'whole person' whose life may be disrupted in many ways by a medical disorder. It assumes that isolated medical treatment may not be adequate to address the total scope of problem areas caused by the illness or disability."

Team Structure

The structure of the rheumatology team may vary from place to place and setting to setting. Some facilities may be fully equipped and staffed with numerous disciplines of allied health professionals and physician specialists, while others with fewer personnel and resources may require their staff to wear many hats and extend their range of duties more liberally. For example a smaller facility may have a nurse and a physical therapist (PT), but no occupational therapist (OT). The nurse and PT may then have to "fill in" for the OT with the PT doing the splinting, and the nurse teaching the principles of joint protection and energy conservation. Such overlapping of roles is required to a lesser degree in the more specialized facilities, but remains important in that consistent reinforcement by various personnel is often essential to patient learning and compliance to therapeutic regimens. Bearing in mind there is much overlap in the roles of the various health disciplines, an attempt will be made to describe the basic roles of the various health professionals who are most frequently called upon to participate as members of the rheumatology team. The patient and his family of course are the most important members of the team and should be given every opportunity to take an active part in the decision-making process. They in turn should, to the best of their ability, attempt to participate in all aspects of the program. It is to their advantage to be familiar with the nature of the disease and treatment and to relate symptoms, problems, and untoward effects of the treatment to the appropriate physician and/ or health professional.

Team Management of the Patient with Rheumatic Disease

Role of Physician

Arthritis rehabilitation is a process which frequently is started late in the disease process and sometimes only after severe problems have developed. Swezey emphasizes the need for early preventive and comprehensive intervention when dealing with catastrophic disorders,* as the key to healthy adjustment and satisfactory therapeutic outcome (4).

The primary care physician is in a position to make the initial diagnosis and provide primary therapy early on. This is the setting in which the rehabilitative process should and frequently does begin. It is therefore important that he have a basic knowledge of the rheumatic diseases and their treatment as well as the roles of other team members so that he can initiate and implement appropriate treatment and move rapidly to consultative referrals by rheumatologists, orthopedist, vocational rehabilitation, psychiatry, etc. when appropriate. His role may be viewed as somewhat of a liaison role between the patient and the various other medical specialties. Continued maximal involvement and participation in all aspects of the program may be desirable and necessary as he is frequently called upon to implement, monitor, or reinforce the therapies initiated by other team members.

---

*Any disorder necessitating a meaningful change in lifestyle.

Many patients with rheumatic diseases can be managed by primary care physicians with the proper interest and training. Some family physicians, however, do not feel comfortable taking care of these patients and refer them on to the rheumatologist. Others who elect to manage these patients themselves often find a rheumatology consult indicated at some point in their care.

The rheumatologist's expertise and experience in the diagnosis and management of rheumatic diseases is especially helpful when: 1) the diagnosis is unclear or requires confirmation; 2) when the disease is severe and/or rapidly progressive; 3) when recommendations for a total management program are needed; 4) for specialized diagnostic studies such as synovial fluid analysis or joint aspiration; 5) for follow-up care of complicated cases; 6) when a systemic illness presents puzzling rheumatic manifestations; or 7) for expertise and administration of certain drugs and therapeutic modalities such as gold, immunosuppressive agents, corticosteroids, etc. (6). The rheumatologist may coordinate the activities of the total team and cooperates and communicates with the referring physician. He makes both long- and short-term medical management recommendations, and informs the patient of his illness and the use of therapeutic modalities. He may also consult with other specialists in regard to the patient, and provides reassurance and psychological support to the patient and his family. If he is connected to an academic setting he may also participate in the training of other physicians and in basic and/or clinical research in arthritis.

The physiatrist precisely evaluates the patient in regard to his functional capacity, and prescribes a comprehensive program. He may prescribe physical and occupational modalities, and assesses the need for braces, splints, and assistive devices. He may also make recommendations for transportation training and monitors the progression of ambulation training as well as the work of the physical and occupational therapists.

The orthopedic surgeon may also recommend manipulative or orthopedic devices such as braces or splints. His expertise, however, is in reconstructive joint surgery, and other arthritis-related surgery such as synovectomy, arthrodesis, osteotomy, and joint biopsy. He explains both long- and short-term goals to the patient and other rheumatology team members, and provides close postop follow-up as indicated.

The radiologist, of course, helps with the interpretation of bone and joint x-rays. The psychiatrist may help assess and care for the patients that have great difficulty adjusting and coping with problems inflicted on them by a chronic illness.

Role of the Nurse

The role and skills of the professional nurse in 1984 are significantly different from those envisioned by Florence Nightingale in the late 1800's. Ms. Nightingale and her staff had little more to work with than a sense of dedication and caring, plus their own ingenuity, while attempting to meet the needs of their wounded soldiers.

Today's professionals still have the same sense of dedication and caring; however, in addition the nurse now has a plethora of highly technical skills and resources available to assist in the nursing practice. Influenced in part by increasing consumer awareness and the pressures of accountability, today's nurse is educated, and expected to possess an expertise that will help assure that the patient receives safe and therapeutic care.

In general, a nursing department will include nurses with a variety of educational backgrounds and qualifications. Basic educational programs are from 1 to 4 years in length, providing both theoretical and practical experiences for the student. Associate and baccalaureate degree programs introduce management and leadership skills in their curriculum along with the practical skills. Nurses who choose to expand their qualifications delve into clinical specialty areas, administration, and education.

As a member of the rheumatology team, the nurse has a unique position relative to the total amount of actual contact time spent with the patient. As a result of this contact, the nurse can evaluate and communicate the effects of the total rehabilitation program on the patient's day-to-day functioning. For example, the nurse can determine how the patient incorporates newly learned OT and PT skills; what are the effects of medication and rest on disease activity; what is the quantity and quality of the patient's knowledge about his disease and its prognosis; and how do family interactions and understanding effect the course of the disease.

Within this general framework, the nursing plan of care is established. Together, the nurse and patient identify those problem areas which must be addressed. The nurse then assumes responsibility for assessing, planning, coordinating, and evaluating the patient's care as stated (10).

To facilitate discussion of the nurse's role, we have identified nine problem areas which are frequently experienced by patients with a rheumatic disease. The list includes problems associated with pain, stiffness, fatigue, medications, the need for education, nutrition, psychosocial concerns including the area of sexuality, discharge planning, and the need for referrals. Fortunately, not many patients experience all of these problems at the same time or to the same degree, but at some point in the patient's management each of these areas will need to be considered.

Pain

Considerable research has been done in the past to study the various causes, perceptions, and the mangement of pain. For example in one text of approximately 300 pages, 400 references were listed (11). Despite the vast amount of study, the understanding and management of a patient's pain eventually depends on two basic concepts. The first concept deals with the definition of pain. McCaffery defines pain as "whatever the experiencing person says it is, existing whenever he says it does" (12). The professional must assure the patient that he believes the patient experiences pain, and that he will help the patient develop methods for managing and coping with this pain. The second concept deals with the circuitous quality of pain. The perception of pain is a combination of physical stimuli and mental events regardless of the initiating cause of the pain (12). Once pain is perceived the patient becomes more anxious and tense. His anxiety and tension cause the perception of pain to be sharpened. This pattern continues to occur, thus becoming circuitous. If a person's pain is to be relieved he must be believed and the circuitous pattern interrupted.

With respect to the rheumatic illnesses, pain is frequently the reason the patient seeks medical evaluation. The pain is caused by active inflammation, joint damage, and anxiety. If the professional is going to develop a trusting rapport, one of the first actions he must take in managing the patient is to begin to treat the patient's pain. Although medications such as the nonsteroidal antiinflammatory drugs (NSAID's) are quite helpful, thought should also be given to referring the patient for such treatments as rest, splinting, the application of heat or cold, whirlpool baths, and exercise. In some instances, instruction in relaxation or biofeedback techniques may be useful.

In addition to the previously mentioned physical modalities, educating the patient as to his disease process and allowing him to discuss his psychological concerns will also help to decrease the pain perception, as these areas deal with the mental events affecting his pain.

Another aspect of pain management relates to dealing with the patient who experiences chronic pain and is depressed. Depression may be a significant problem for patients with rheumatoid arthritis (13). Treating the patient's depression may markedly decrease his perception of pain.

Narcotic analgesics are used infrequently in managing the rheumatic illnesses. Due to the chronic nature of these diseases, early use of narcotics may develop into a dependency problem. Secondly, as the narcotic removes the body's own warning signal, that is, pain, the patient is at risk of actually causing joint damage by overusing the joint.

In summary, when dealing with the patient's pain experience, the professional must remember that the pain is real and a warning signal. Pain must be aggressively addressed, medication such as the NSAID's used, other resources actively employed, and the use of narcotics avoided whenever possible.

Stiffness

Patients with rheumatic illnesses will usually complain of two types of stiffness. The first they will describe as a generalized morning stiffness which they experience upon awakening. The duration of this stiffness is often associated with the degree of disease activity (14). The second type of stiffness is described as rest-induced gelling. This stiffness occurs after a period of inactivity. Stiffness must be taken into account when organizing the patient's day. Early morning commitments to PT or OT should be avoided when possible. X-rays and tests should be arranged in the afternoon. An early morning shower will help the patient limber up as will taking the first dose of an antiinflammatory medicine approximately one-half hour before arising. If the patient experiences gelling, a balance between activity and rest must be determined in an attempt to keep gelling to a minimum.

Fatigue

Ongoing fatigue and decreased endurance are common problems associated with rheumatic diseases. Daily activity should be spaced to allow for adequate rest. It is often difficult to impress on patients the value of pacing and prioritizing their activities to accommodate the need to rest. The patient should be taught to rest before he becomes overly fatigued, and if he is working, encouraged to take a short rest period during the day. The patient may need a note from the physician outlining this need. Fatigue is not an easy symptom for the patient to handle; like pain, it is completely subjective and difficult for the employer, friends, and family alike to comprehend. The patient will need the support of the professionals caring for him in helping others recognize the significance of the problem and its management.

Medications

The administration of medication is considered to be a traditional nursing role. The nurse must be aware of the possible benefits and side effects of each medication, as well as have knowledge as to whether the medication is given with or without food, its duration of action, and the need for laboratory follow-up if necessary.

The nurse usually expands the role of administration to include time for instructing the patient about his medications, including the discussion of the previously mentioned considerations. In some institutions, the patients may be given permission by the physician to keep their arthritis medication at the bedside and follow through with self-administration. The benefits of this approach are threefold for the patient: 1) he will be able to take his medication at the proper time, for example, with his meal; 2) he will recognize that the physician expects and encourages him to be responsible for certain aspects of his disease management; and 3) if questions arise about the medication, there are resource people easily available to respond to the situation.

As part of the educational process, the patient should be provided with written information about his medications. This information should include the name of the medication, its mode of action, times when taken, possible side effects, how long it will take before the patient will realize the benefit from the medication, and the name and telephone number of the person he should contact if he has a question or suspects a side effect.

Time should be provided to allow the patient to restate the information provided him about his medications. This will give the practitioner an opportunity to clarify any misunderstandings.

It is important to complete this process prior to the day of discharge. Last minute instructions are frequently misinterpreted or forgotten. It is equally important to remember that while the nurse is most frequently the educator, the physician should reinforce the information provided. The more frequently an individual hears the same information, the greater the degree of understanding and, hopefully, compliance.

Patient Education

Patient education is one of the cornerstones of a rheumatic disease management program as illustrated in Figure 5.1. Both the patient and his family must be actively involved in the educational process. Effective long-term care requires that team members assist the patient in identifying his learning needs. From the earliest stages the patient should be encouraged to be an active partner in the struggle against disease rather than a passive recipient of care (15). For example, see Table 5.1 which illustrates what guidelines a patient could be taught with respect to contacting the physician.

There is evidence to support patient education as essential. Intelligent compliance leads to a more successful management program, as it encourages patient decision-making within certain parameters (15).

Traditionally, patient education has been a nursing role. However, it is important to remember that any team member can be a teacher and should take advantage of opportune moments to introduce, demonstrate, or reexplain information.

Learning or a change in behavior is influenced by many factors. Stress, body knowledge, previous experiences, physical and mental capabilities, cultural influences, language, and family relationships can all affect the patient's ability to learn. When presenting material, proceed in an organized fashion going from the

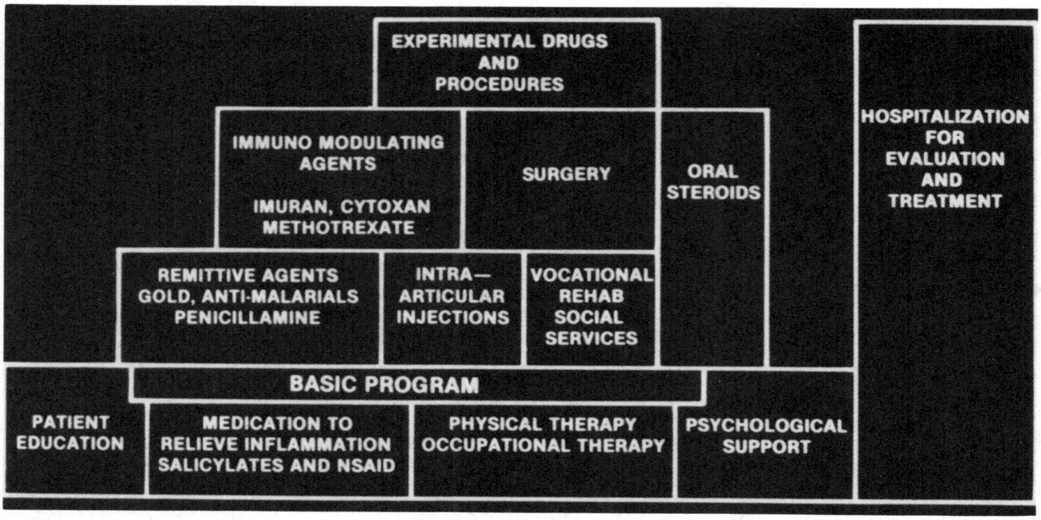

FIGURE 5.1 Rheumatic disease management program.

simple to the more complex. Remember to use terms and descriptions that the patient will understand. Allow time for questions, and always provide positive reinforcement for a job well done. In areas where it is possible, such as medication or exercising, provide the patient with flexible guidelines so that he may "juggle" his program. For example, if he is on aspirin and is taking 16 tablets a day, give him permission to decrease that dose to 12 tablets a day if he feels his arthritis is improved. This allows the patient to have a degree of self-control, and will increase compliance not only with medication, but in other areas as well.

Twelve topics (Table 5.2) which frequently need to be discussed with the rheumatic disease patient are disease process, short- and long-term goals, medications, pain control, the role of physical and occupational therapist, pacing and joint protection, range of motion exercises, sexual concerns, surgical options, nutrition, quackery, and the availability of community resources.

Printed materials and audiovisual aids to reinforce learning are readily available through the Arthritis Foundation, the Arthritis Information Clearing House, and many other manufacturers of audiovisual aids. These materials should be made available to all patients who are dealing with a rheumatic disease.

Nutrition

At this point in time, there has not been any scientific proof that one type of diet or the addition or elimination of any certain food can alter the course of a rheumatic disease (6). However, this is an area in which the public is frequently deluged with reports of new causes and cures for all forms of arthritis. The nurse and physician are frequently questioned about these reports.

TABLE 5.1 Patient Guidelines for Physician Contact

Is severe pain, swelling and/or heat present in one or two joints only Is numbness or tingling related to pain present Is fever present Is patient unable to use joint Is pain due to recent injury Does pain/stiffness keep patient from getting out of bed at all.	→ YES →	Call Physician Today
↓ NO ↓		
Has condition persisted more than 6 weeks Has condition progressed rapidly and/or seems alarmingly severe Are systemic symptoms present	→ YES →	Make Appointment With Physician
↓ NO ↓ Apply Home Treatment		

The Arthritis Foundation has a pamphlet available that answers more commonly asked questions about diets and attempts to help the patient identify those diets which might be harmful (16). Fries and Lorig in *The Arthritis Health Book,* also have a relevant chapter on nutrition (17). Included in this chapter is a description of the value of clinical trials in determining the efficacy of scientific treatment.

TABLE 5.2 Topics for Patient Education

Disease process
Establishing short- and long-term goals
Medication
Pain control
Physical and occupational therapy
Pacing and joint protection
Range of motion (ROM) exercises
Sexual concerns
Surgical options
Nutrition
Quackery
Community resources

Most rheumatologists now recommend a well-balanced diet for their arthritis patients with foods from all four food groups (6). Patients who are taking corticosteroids should limit their salt intake as the corticosteroids encourage fluid retention. Patients who are overweight are encouraged not only to decrease their caloric intake but also to increase their activity level. Decreased endurance and restriction of motion limit the choice of exercise programs available to the patient with arthritis. However, swimming as an exercise is frequently recommended, as it affords a therapeutic form of exercise.

Many forms of arthritis are characterized by the anemia of chronic disease. The patient demonstrates low serum iron, but usually total iron stores are adequate. Therefore, supplementation is not beneficial. Should the anemia be produced by gastrointestinal irritation from medication, supplementation may then be useful (6).

As food has so many individual and social implications, it will probably remain an active topic of discussion with respect to arthritis. For now, we should assure the patient that we will keep abreast of all the latest developments in this area and make new information available to him.

Psychosocial and Sexual Concerns

The identification of psychosocial and sexual concerns is a major part of managing a rheumatic illness. Patients and families who are learning to live with a chronic illness are under a significant amount of stress. The unpredictability of the symptoms and disease progression greatly adds to the burden the patient and his family must bear. Even when the disease has been quiescent for a period of time, the patient can never feel assured that it will stay that way.

Coping strategies vary from patient to patient and family to family. It is presumed that this variance is derived from earlier experiences with illness, family attitudes toward health and sickness, different biological sensitivities, varying social definitions, etc. (13). The physician as well as the other team members must reassure the patient that these concerns are normal and acceptable. Patients and family should be given the opportunity to voice their concerns in quiet, unrushed settings. When appropriate, referrals to social service, psychology, psychiatry, vocational rehabilitation, sexual counselors, or the chaplain should be arranged. As Baker states, it is important that interactions and plans convey a positive attitude towards self-help (13).

Patients suffering from rheumatic diseases, particularly the systemic forms such as rheumatoid arthritis, lupus, scleroderma, and ankylosing spondylitis, have many strategies they incorporate into their everyday life to help them appear normal. Among the strategies commonly used are covering up, keeping up, and pacing (18). In covering up, patients attempt to conceal their disability or pain. In keeping up, they follow through with activities they consider normal despite the risk of increased pain or fatigue. Pacing is one of the healthier strategies for appearing normal because this behavior allows for rest periods between covering up and keeping up. Pacing helps restore the patient's energy and interest for what he considers to be normal activities.

Arthritis patients fear becoming dependent. They are slow to elicit help from family and friends (18). Support groups are often helpful in that they provide the patient with contacts who truly understand his problems, and help is often more easily accepted within the group.

Depression is a common and important complication of rheumatoid arthritis (13). Physicians should be aware of the signs and symptoms of depression and treat with antidepressants as indicated. Baker recommends using an adequate dose of an antidepressant for at least 3 weeks before deciding that the drug is not working. It is also essential to stop the drug if no benefit has been received after that time (13).

In addition to recognizing the more obvious psychological concerns, sexual concerns should also be addressed. Despite the sexual revolution in recent years, sexuality is a difficult topic for most men and women to discuss. Sexual functioning has finally been recognized as worthy of medical inquiry and assistance. A disorder such as arthritis that causes pain and interferes with motion must have consequences in sexual functioning (19). Fortunately, there is increasing recognition of sexuality as a birthright of all people whether young or old, man or woman, healthy or ill (20).

All patients with any degree of disability should be asked about the effect of their illness on their sexual functioning. Inquiries should be straightforward, such as "How does your illness affect your sexual relationship?" or "Many people with your type of disability have sexual concerns, how has your illness affected your sexual relationship?" rather than "Is everything allright with your husband or wife?" (13). Direct questioning makes it easier for the patient to provide a legitimate response, and he feels you are willing to listen to his concerns.

Sexuality is an integral part of living. Self-esteem, self-worth, and reassurance of the strength of a loving relationship depend a great deal on sharing intimacy. The disabilities which result from arthritis do not mean there is no chance for a successful intimate relationship. Sexual fulfillment does not need to depend entirely on penile-vaginal penetration. Caressing, fondling, bathing together, use of a vibrator, or oral sex may be very stimulating and satisfying alternatives to the more traditional forms of intercourse. The Arthritis Foundation has a well-written publication for the patient entitled *Living and Loving* (21). Included in the pamphlet are suggestions for alternate positions for intercourse when pain limits the use of the face to face position. It also discusses accepting change in body image, communication skills, and planning for sexual interaction. If the patient is a young woman, you will need to discuss family planning with her and her partner. Referral to a gynecologist may be indicated if birth control is recommended.

Psychological and sexual concerns must be discussed openly and with a positive attitude. The physician must acknowledge that these problems require his attention and they are as important as prescribing a medication. Referrals to supporting disciplines are frequently helpful. Patients should be encouraged to maintain as much normalcy as is possible in their life patterns.

Referrals

There are many dimensions to the referral system. Referrals are not just limited to the in-hospital experience. For example, the primary care physician may need to refer the patient to a rheumatologist. The rheumatologist may need to refer to a specific discipline such as the physical therapist or occupational therapist for evaluation and treatment. Referral to a nurse may be indicated for patient education or to assist in monitoring medication administration and side effects. Social workers and vocational rehabilitation counselors may be needed to help the patient adjust to the limitations of his illness. An orthopedic surgeon may be consulted for surgical replacement of a joint. See Table 5.3 for frequently identified problems and appropriate referrals.

There are many reasons which may necessitate a referral. The important point is that the referral is timely, appropriate, and well planned. This helps to emphasize to the patient that consideration is being given to his individual needs when they occur.

Discharge Planning

Planning for the patient's discharge should be incorporated into the patient's plan of care from the onset of his hospital stay. It should be assumed that everyone to a greater or lesser degree will need discharge planning. This may be as simple as arranging a follow-up appointment with the physician or as complicated as organizing a multidisciplinary home care program. Far too often, this process is not addressed until the day the patient is leaving the hospital.

In general, patients who are dealing with a chronic illness will need more assistance with follow-up than those dealing with an acute illness. The ultimate goals of the plan should be to assist the patient and his family in maintaining optimum health and functioning by appropriately utilizing the health care system. The nursing staff or a specially designated home care coordinator will assist the team in identifying and organizing the discharge plan. In metropolitan areas, there are a large variety of resources available. Certified health care agencies can often provide some or all of the following services: skilled nursing care, physical therapy, occupational therapy, social services, home health aids, meals, transportation, supplies, and equipment. Unfortunately, the patient who lives in a rural area may not have as much available in the way of formal services, but often there are local community support groups such as churches, schools, and fellowship organizations which may help meet the need.

It is important to the patient and his family to know that they will continue to receive support and guidance once they have left the umbrella of the hospital setting. The professional's interest in the discharge plan reassures the patient that the professional cares about the patient's well-being. In addition, the patient senses that you understand he must continue to deal with his arthritis on a day-to day basis.

TABLE 5.3 Problem Oriented Team Referrals

Patient Problem	Who to Refer to	Modalities and Expected Outcomes
Unclear diagnosis or severe and rapid progressive symptoms	Rheumatologist	Performs physical exam and specialized diagnostic studies including laboratory evaluations and synovial fluid analysis Provides expertise in administration and follow-up of certain drugs such as gold, immunosuppressive agents, and/or corticosteroids Assists in coordination of a total team approach Assists patient and primary care physician in establishing and revising both short- and long-term goals
Incapacitating joint pain and deformity	Orthopedic Surgeon	Evaluates for possible benefit and complications associated with such procedures as synovectomy, arthroscopy, and reconstructive joint surgery Arranges for appropriate follow-up with PT and OT Refers for braces and/or splints when indicated
Educational needs	Nurse	Evaluates both quantity and quality of patient's knowledge in such areas as disease process, medications, pain control, sexual concerns, quackery, and community resources Recommends referral to other team members as needed Assists with coordination of information between patient and family members
	OT	Instructs patient in such areas as joint protection, pacing, and activities of daily living (ADL's), thus promoting patient independence and decreased joint stress
	PT	Instructs in use of ambulation aids such as canes, walker or wheelchair, paraffin dips and application of heat and cold as part of total treatment program
	Dietician	Instructs patients in need for well-balanced diet, with emphasis on maintaining a desirable weight and the effects of exercise

TABLE 5.3 (Continued)

Patient Problem	Who to Refer to	Modalities and Expected Outcomes
Difficulty performing ADL's	OT	Assesses patient's ability to function physically, emotionally, and socially Instructs patient in techniques such as joint protection, pacing, and work simplification to decrease joint stress Provides patient with adaptive equipment to allow for more independent functioning Fabricates splints for upper extremity joints to decrease joint pain and improve function
Limitation in joint motion	PT	Assesses joint range of motion (ROM), muscle strength endurance and functional ability Instructs patient in ROM exercises to either maintain or improve ROM Instructs in importance of good body mechanics to decrease stress placed on joints and soft tissues Along with other team members, encourages the patient's family to participate in the therapy program
Depression	Social Worker	Assists in evaluation of the psychosocial impact of a chronic illness on the patient and family Counseling will be provided as needed
	Psychologist	Performs psychological testing if indicated to evaluate functional components to an illness Instructs patients experiencing chronic pain in relaxation techniques and biofeedback, thus promoting decreased pain perception and an increased sense of control by the patient
	Psychiatrist	Evaluates patients experiencing significant difficulties coping with their illness and recommends appropriate treatment

Financial and employment concerns	Social Worker	Investigates availability of insurance and community support to aid the patient and family Assists with discharge planning and arranges for referrals as indicated
	Vocational Rehabilitation Counselor	Evaluates patient in terms of educational resources, abilities, and interests with respect to employment If indicated assists with job retraining May assist financially (i.e., drug treatment program or hospitalization to prevent or slow disability)

Role of the Occupational Therapist

Another essential member of the team treating the patient with a rheumatic illness is the occupational therapist (OT). There appears to be much confusion and lack of knowledge by other health professionals as well as patients as to the role of this team member (22). The title itself may be misleading in that many assume OT's concern themselves primarily with occupations or job training or with keeping patients occupied with crafts or recreational activities. In actuality, the OT's primary concern is to encourage the physical, emotional, and social independence of the rheumatic disease patient. He assesses the ability of the individual to function physically, socially, and emotionally and participates in the organization and implementation of an appropriate program to achieve these goals.

The therapeutic program for the arthritis patient usually emphasizes joint protection, energy conservation, and work simplification techniques to enable the patient to function with a minimum of fatigue and stress to the joints (4). The OT has specialized training in these areas of management, and is also qualified to provide and fit the patient with adaptive equipment. A brief discussion of some of the basic principles of joint protection, assistive devices and energy conservation follows. More in-depth information is readily available from other resources (17, 23, 24).

Joint Protection

Inflamed or unstable joints can be further damaged by the stresses of ordinary daily activities. Factors such as time and force can contribute to joint damage. Strong forces over a short period of time or mild forces over long periods of time may result in increased levels of pain as well as damage to the joint. Stressful forces often occur during activities involving squeezing, pushing, pulling, twisting, and lifting, or activities that place an extra load on joints such as excessive body weight, climbing stairs, or carrying groceries (17).

Joint protection techniques are a major part of the therapeutic program and are most valuable in their effectiveness for reducing pain, stress to the joints, and inflammation. It is also thought by many that diligent application of joint protection principles prevent deformities by preserving joint integrity, but this has not yet been adequately demonstrated, primarily due to the difficulty of achieving long-term steadfast compliance by patients (24).

Some principles of joint protection are offered to serve as guidelines for the appropriate type and amount of activity for optimum joint function (see Table 5.4).

Assistance Devices

Assistive devices or tools suitable to the task allow us to help the arthritis patient to a) simplify the task, b) increase his independence, and c) utilize available function in a pain-free and nontraumatic manner. There are available a wide variety of assistive devices which can be purchased, see Figures 5.2 and 5.3, but with a little effort and ingenuity many can be made inexpensively. For example, handles can be extended for easier reach by attaching dowels to items patients already have, or foam may be added to pens, pencils, forks, etc., in order to reduce stress to the joints as well as making them easier to grasp. Some guidelines to keep in mind when recommending assistive devices or equipment are suggested in Table 5.5.

TABLE 5.4 Principles of Joint Protection

PRINCIPLE 1

Use the strongest or largest joint possible to accomplish a task. The larger the area the more pressure, weight, and/or force the joint can tolerate. Example: use the palm of the hand rather than the fingers for opening doors and jar lids.

PRINCIPLE 2

Distribute the load over several joints. This minimizes the stress on individual joints. Example: use both hands or arms to accomplish a task one normally would do with one.

PRINCIPLE 3

Use each joint in its most stable and functional position. The most stable and functional position is usually the position in which the joint is in straight alignment, not bent or rotated to the side. Using this principle avoids excessive stretching of joint ligaments.

PRINCIPLE 4

Use good body mechanics. This principle is especially important for patients with back and neck problems.

PRINCIPLE 5

Avoid positions and activities leading to possible joint deformities. Patients tend to keep painful joints in the position which is most comfortable. This is frequently a flexed position which may lead to flexion contractures or other deformities. Patients should be encouraged to stretch out arms and legs when lying or sitting and to avoid using pillows under the knees.

PRINCIPLE 6

Avoid keeping joints in one position for prolonged periods of time. This is important for two reasons: 1) joints affected by arthritis tend to become stiff (gel phenomenon), 2) muscles become fatigued when fixed or tensed and such stress can cause pressure on damaged articular surfaces.

PRINCIPLE 7

Avoid activities that cannot be stopped. Activities which cause sudden or severe pain can cause joint damage if not stopped immediately.

PRINCIPLE 8

Reduce the effort required to do the job. Reduction of effort results in less stress and pain to involved joints and also improves total endurance allowing the patient more energy for other activities.

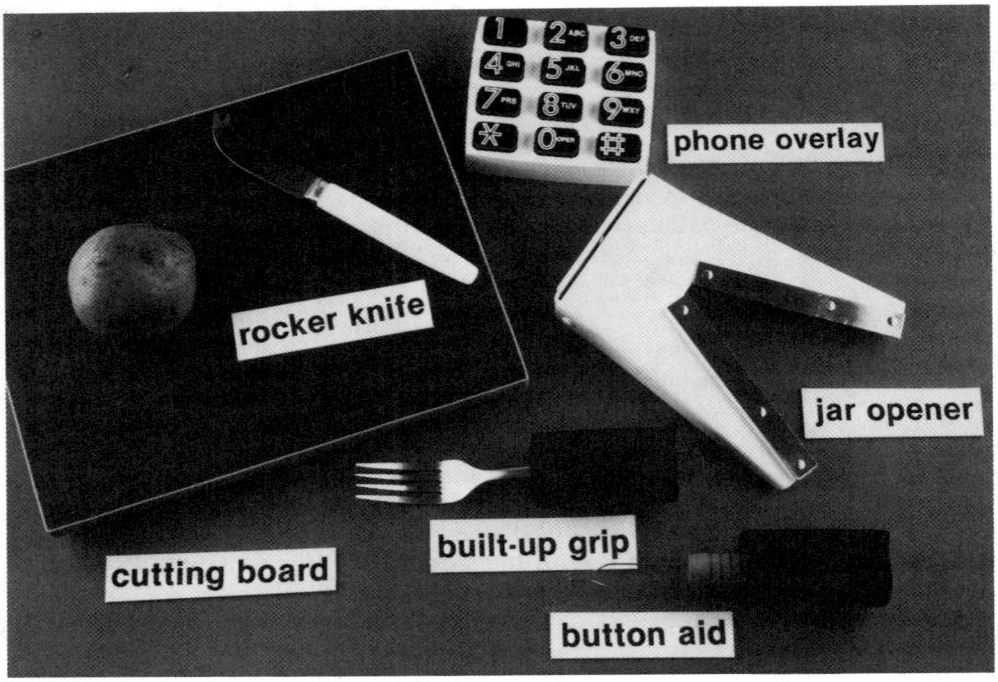

FIGURE 5.2 Assistive devices.

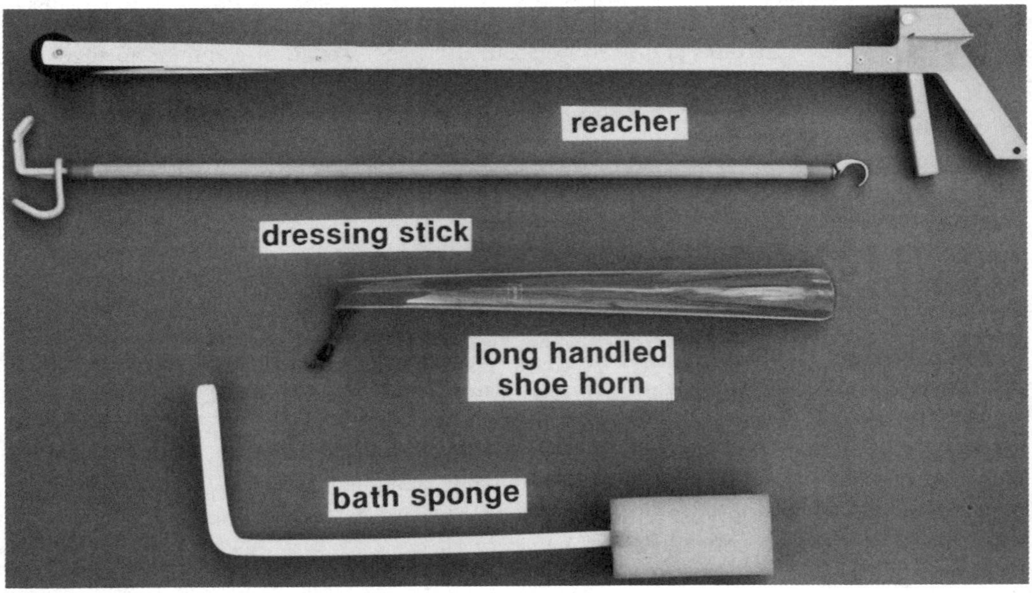

FIGURE 5.3 Assistive devices.

TABLE 5.5 Guidelines for Assistive Devices

Patients' needs for assistive devices may vary from morning to afternoon as well as during periods of exacerbations and remissions.

The equipment may affect other joints of the body. For example, canes, crutches, and walkers protect the lower extremities, but may place additional stresses on other involved joints such as the wrist, hand, or shoulder.

Activities involving tight grasps are contraindicated for patients with metacarpophalangeal involvement.

Be familiar with the devices you recommend. Convenience appliances may be too heavy or have buttons which are difficult to operate.

Teach patients to use their assistive aides correctly in order to derive full benefit (24).

Energy Conservation/Work Simplification

The supply of energy available to patients with systemic disease is often limited by pain, anemia, fever, or depression (26). It is therefore useful to incorporate the principles of energy conservation listed in Table 5.6 into the management program, and to help the patient recognize that it may take him longer and require more effort to perform a task. The OT can assist the patient to simplify and organize his environment and activities by helping to 1) identify and eliminate unnecessary tasks, 2) organize his work, 3) use efficient storage, and 4) pace his activities properly throughout the day. Simple suggestions or modifications in the home or work place (Figure 5.4) can be the difference between an independent, functioning member of society and a dependent, disabled one.

Splinting

The OT is also involved in upper extremity interventions such as the fabrication of supportive or corrective splinting (Figure 5.5), and in assisting the surgeon in the postoperative management of surgery of the upper extremities. Splints are utilized for arthritis patients primarily for the purpose of reducing inflammation by immobilizing the joint and to support the joint in optimal position of function in order to prevent deformities resulting from chronic improper positioning (23, 24). Splinting can help relieve muscle spasms, decrease pain on motion and decrease stress on inadequately supported structures.

TABLE 5.6 Principles of Energy Conservation

Alternate work with rest
Plan ahead
Set priorities and eliminate unneccessary tasks
Alternate heavy and light tasks
Learn activity tolerance

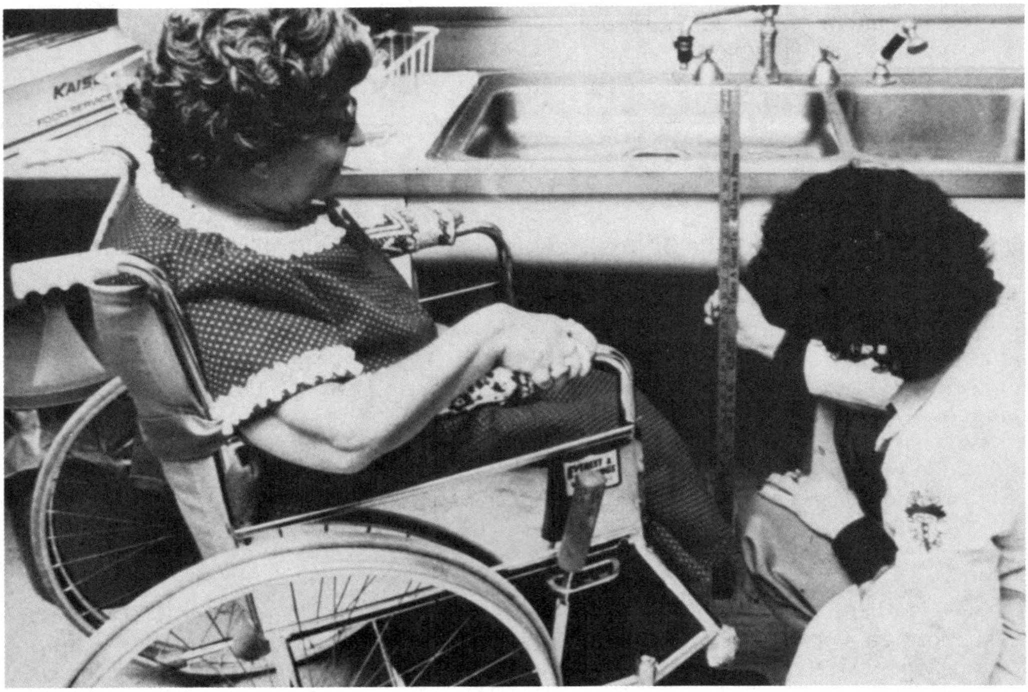

FIGURE 5.4 Minor adjustments in the home or work place can increase patient independence. (From the Arthritis Teaching Slide Collection, copyright 1980. Used with permission of the Arthritis Foundation.)

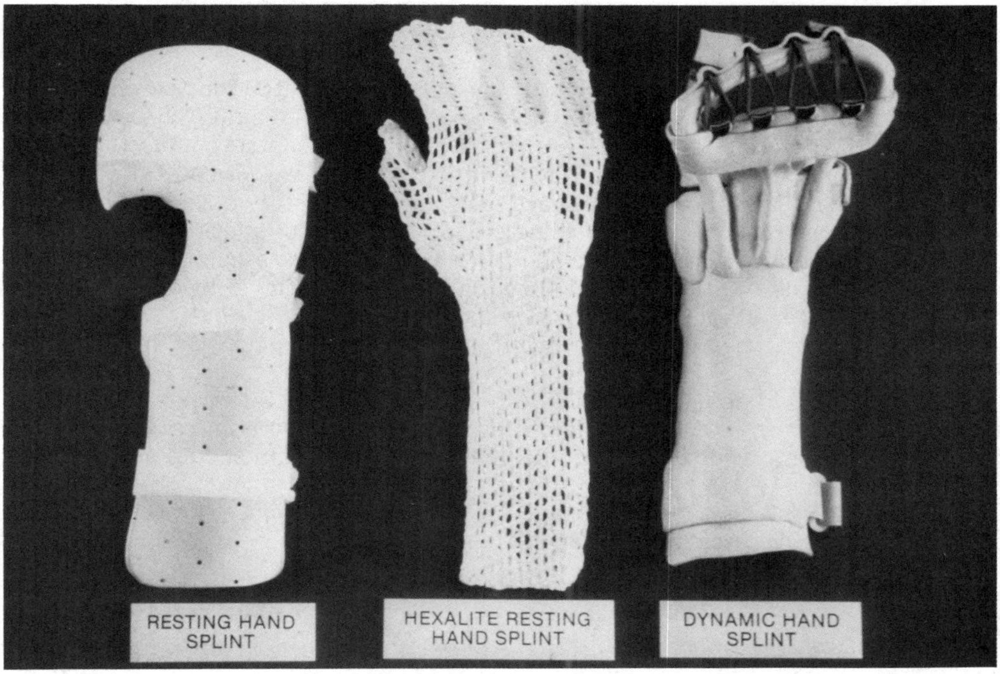

FIGURE 5.5 Examples of supportive and corrective hand splints.

Role of the Physical Therapist

The physical therapist (PT) is trained to evaluate the musculoskeletal system in terms of assessing joint range of motion, muscle strength, endurance, sensation, and functional ability. He is concerned with restoring function, pain relief, and the prevention of deformities through the use of treatment modalities such as exercises to maintain or increase range of motion or improve muscle strength, ambulation, and transportation techniques, body mechanics and positioning, use of ambulation assistive devices, heat, cold, traction, diathermy, and water.

It is beyond the scope of this text to delve into a discussion of each of these modalities. However, the role of exercise, heat, ice, and rest will be described as these modalities are frequently used by physicians and other health professionals apart from the PT.

Exercise

The role of exercise in the therapeutic regime of the patient with a rheumatic disease is a source of much confusion to most patients. The key to a successful exercise program is to maintain a proper balance between rest and exercise and to exercise properly (17). Exercise is a way of preventing loss of function by maintaining range of motion (ROM) and muscle strength. There are basically three types of ROM exercise: active, active assistive, and passive.

Active ROM exercises are those in which the patient moves body parts through full ROM without assistance. Active assistive ROM exercises are those in which the patient actively puts the body part through partial ROM then to full

ROM with assistance from an external force such as a pulley or the use of other body parts. Finally, in passive ROM, the body part is moved through complete ROM by another person or other external force.

Gentle stretch at the end of ROM is used to increase ROM in the chronic active or chronic inactive phases, but should be avoided in the acute phase as this places additional stress on structures already on maximum stretch due to swelling (24). How much and how often a patient should exercise to maintain or improve ROM varies, and there are no hard and fast rules. Melvin recommends that with stable chronic disease each joint be put through its complete ROM up to a maximum of 10 repetitions once a day; with active disease, a maximum of 2-5 repetitions twice daily. If exercises appear to increase inflammation, and pain is present 1 hour after exercise, repetitions should be reduced by half then increased by one repetition per day until maximum repetitions are reached or inflammation recurs.

Exercises should be done at a time of day when the patient feels the most limber, perhaps after or during the morning shower or 30-60 minutes after taking regular medication. Additional pain medication to mask pain should not be taken prior to exercise.

Exercises for strengthening require further consideration. The OT or PT can help develop specific programs for specific problems.

Heat/Ice/Rest

Frequently, the best relief for acute joint pain is to rest the affected joints and allow inflammation to subside. Total relaxation allows stress relief which allows the muscles to become less tense, making it easier and less painful to move the joints. Relaxation exercises are therefore frequently helpful in relieving pain and promoting sleep.

Heat and ice are secondary additives to rest in promoting pain relief and to reducing muscle spasms and stiffness. Ice compresses in the form of ice packs are sometimes beneficial for acute inflammation and tenosynovitis. Generally, the ice is most effective for very hot joints and is effective in reducing swelling as well as pain.

As swelling decreases, heat may become more effective. Moist heat in the form of hot packs or compresses, hot paraffin dips, hot showers as well as moist or dry heating pads are some of the more common forms of home heat therapy. The personal preference of the therapist and/or the patient may determine the particular modality used (25). Diathermy or deep heating by electromagnetic or ultrasound instrumentation may also be used but thus far the advantages of these modalities over superficial heating modalities have not been demonstrated (23).

A variety of methods of hydrotherapy ranging from arm or leg basins to whirlpools, Hubbard tanks, and conventional swimming pools may be utilized for providing both heat and buoyance of water for relief of articular pain. Many communities offer pool exercise programs for arthritis patients which are conducted by PT's and OT's and frequently supported by the local Arthritis Foundation. These programs are relatively inexpensive and have thus far had good community response. Patients must have their doctor's recommendation in order to participate.

Generally, the duration of treatment with heat or cooling modalities is 20-30 minutes except for ultrasound which is usually given for 5-15 minutes. Precautions should always be taken to avoid excessive elevation of either local or general body temperature. Local burns, or in the case of total immersion in warm water, weakness, collapse and/or injury may result if temperatures are too high, especially in patients with compromised circulatory resources (23).

After assessing the individual patient program, based on patient needs, the PT gives instruction to the patient and his family so that the program may be carried out at home.

Role of the Vocational Rehabilitation Counselor

The vocational rehabilitation counselor (VRC) who is knowledgeable in the rheumatic diseases can be a valuable resource. Many of these patients are afflicted in their most productive years, and may not be able to do their present jobs during periods of disease flares or when disabled by disease progression. Patients whose jobs involved physical labor or repetitive motions often find it difficult to continue these jobs, and early intervention by a vocational counselor can prepare them for more appropriate jobs and prevent them from going on disability. The VRC is trained to vocationally evaluate the patient in terms of the individual resources such as education, mental capacities, abilities, interests, work history, physical factors, etc. They have resources which can provide the training or education necessary for a patient to obtain a more appropriate job.

Role of the Social Worker

The role of the social worker in the rehabililtation of the rheumatic disease patient involves six major areas: evaluation, education, counseling, communication, discharge planning, and community referral (19). The training of the social worker prepares him to assist in the evaluation of the psychosocial impact of arthritis on the patient and his family. The social worker helps identify the problems and helps the patient deal with them. Social workers have skills in individual, family, and marital counseling. They also are concerned with promoting understanding between patient and staff members. They participate in discharge planning for inpatients and make community referrals as indicated, often times providing resources that help the patient maintain economic stability.

Role of the Psychologist

The psychologist is often needed to assist the patient to deal with the stresses inflicted on him by chronic illness, drug-induced psychological disturbances (19, 22), and the problems associated with chronic pain syndromes. He should be familiar with the psychosocial problems associated with the rheumatic diseases, and often times has expertise in biofeedback and other pain relief measures such as relaxation techniques. He can often provide useful psychological testing to identify specific psychosocial problems or to help differentiate between the symptoms of organic disease and those of emotional problems. For example, is loss of appetite, weight loss, and fatigue due to rheumatoid arthritis or to depression?

Numerous other health professionals make important contributions to the team but cannot be described in detail in this chapter due to space constraints. We will mention briefly that patient educators, podiatrists, and rehabilitation counselors as well as pharmacists often play key roles in the management of such patients as well as numerous others such as nutritionists, volunteers, and clerical personnel.

Summary

Throughout this chapter, we have emphasized the need for utilizing a team approach in managing the patient who has a rheumatic illness. The descriptions that have been provided about each discipline are by necessity brief. However, we believe these descriptions are in depth enough to assist you in developing a working knowledge of what expertise is available to you and the patient. Patients who must learn to adapt to a condition that can affect almost every aspect of their lives are entitled to the benefits of a multidisciplinary management program. Each member of the team supports and reinforces the information and guidance provided by the other team members. The reinforcement encourages patient understanding and compliance with the medical program. The core team should include the physician, nurse, physical and occupational therapists and, of course, the patient. Referrals to other professionals such as the rheumatologist, orthopedic surgeon, social worker, rehabilitation counselor, psychologist, sexual counselor, nutritionist, and podiatrist should be timely and organized. We expect that by carefully guiding the patient through the wealth of expertise that is available to him, we can help the patient decrease the amount of disability he experiences, and assist him in maintaining his self-esteem and independence.

References

1. Schneider E: Teaching nursing homes. *New Engl J Med* 308(6):336-337, 1983.

2. Freeland M et al.: Projections of national health expenditures 1980, 1985, and 1990. *Health Care Financ Rev 1980,* pp. 1-27.

3. Plotz CM: Introduction. *Postgraduate Medicine* 58(5):5, 1975.

4. Swezey RL: Arthritis rehabilitation: Staff facilities and evaluation. In GE Erlich (ed.), *Rehabilitation Management of Rheumatic Conditions.* Baltimore, Williams and Wilkins, 1980, p. 1.

5. Jette AM, Becker MC: Nursing, occupational therapy and physical therapy education in rheumatology in the United States and Canada. *Journal of Allied Health* 9(4):268-275, 1980.

6. Katz WA: General approach to the management of rheumatic disease. In WA Katz (ed.), *Rheumatic Disease Diagnosis and Management.* Philadelphia, J. B. Lippincott, 1977, pp. 870-872.

7. White J et al.: Rheumatology nursing. *Nursing 79,* October 1979, pp. 108-112.

8. American Nurses Association: *Standards for Rheumatology Nursing Practice.* Kansas City, Mo., Division of Medical/Surgical Nursing Practice and the Arthritis Health Professionals Association, 1983.

9. Figley BA: The roles of allied health professionals in the management of arthritis. *Clinical Rheumatology in Practice* 1:43-45, 1983.

10. Pigg JS: Nursing care of the hospitalized patient with rheumatic disease. In GE Erlich (ed.), *Rehabilitation Management of Rheumatic Conditions.* Baltimore, Williams and Wilkins, 1980, pp. 76-103.

11. McCaffery M: *Nursing Management of the Patient with Pain,* 2nd Ed. Philadelphia, J. P. Lippincott, 1979.

12. McCaffery M: Understanding your patient's pain. *Nursing* 80:26-31, 1980.

13. Baker GH: Psychological management. *Clinics and Your Rheumatic Diseases* 7(2):455-467, 1981.

14. McCarty DJ: *Arthritis and Allied Conditions,* 9th Ed. Philadelphia, Lea and Febiger, 1979, p. 137.

15. Redmon B: Curriculum and patient education. *American Journal of Nursing* 78:1363-1366, 1978.

16. The Arthritis Foundation: *Arthritis: Diet and Nutrition.* Atlanta, 1982.

17. Fries JF, Lorig K: *The Arthritis Help Book.* Redding, MA, Addison-Wesley, 1980, pp. 125-138.

18. Weiner CL: The burden of rheumatoid arthritis. In AL Stroud and BG Glazer (eds.), *Chronic Illness and the Quality of Life.* St. Louis, C. V. Mosby, 1975, pp. 71-80.

19. Erlich GE: Arthritis and its problems. *Clinics in Rheumatic Diseases* 7(2): 305-320, 1981.

20. Kolodony RC, Masters WH, Johnson VE: *Textbook of Sexual Medicine.* Boston, Little, Brown and Company, 1979, pp. 353-380.

21. Arthritis Foundation: *Living and Loving.* Atlanta, 1982.

22. Pigg JS, Gall EP: Arthritis health professionals family tree. *AHPA Newsletter* 3(1):6-7, 11, 1983.

23. Swezey RL: *Arthritis: Rational Therapy and Rehabilitation.* Philadelphia, W. B. Saunders, 1978.

24. Melvin JL: *Rheumatic Disease: Occupational Therapy and Rehabilitation,* 2nd Ed. Philadelphia, F. A. Davies, 1982.

25. Arthritis Foundation: *Instructional Guide Arthritis Teaching Slide Collection.* Atlanta, 1980, p. 124.

Chapter 6

PSYCHOLOGICAL ASPECTS OF ARTHRITIS

Karen O. Anderson, Ph.D., Laurence A. Bradley, Ph.D.,
Larry D. Young, Ph.D., and Lisa K. McDaniel, M.A.

Treatment of the rheumatic disease patient traditionally has focused upon the medical and physical consequences of the disease process. Until recent years, relatively little attention had been paid to the possibility of altering the psychological and behavioral effects of rheumatic disorders such as rheumatoid arthritis. A sizeable literature had accumulated by 1970, however, indicating that arthritis can have significant adverse effects on a patient's affective, behavioral, and social functioning. Moreover, research and clinical reports developing from the psychosomatic tradition had suggested that psychological factors might play a role in the onset of arthritis.

In the 1970's a renewed interest in the psychological aspects of arthritis and other rheumatic diseases became apparent. This trend was facilitated by the development of the interdisciplinary field of behavioral medicine, which advocates the use of behavioral science knowledge and techniques in the prevention, evaluation, and treatment of physical disease (1). Behavioral scientists began to collaborate with physicians in the assessment and treatment of medical patients, including rheumatic disease patients.

In the case of rheumatology, interdisciplinary collaboration may be especially important. Many rheumatic disorders are chronic conditions that cannot be cured but must be managed over an extended time period. Adjunctive health care professionals (e.g., medical psychologists, occupational therapists) can help patients cope with the psychological and behavioral effects of a chronic disease such as rheumatoid arthritis (2). Behavioral scientists can also use their research and statistical expertise to aid in the continuing assessment of the psychosocial consequences of rheumatic illness and in the critical evaluation of medical and nonmedical treatment efficacy. As rheumatologists have begun to emphasize the importance of addressing psychological and behavioral as well as physiological outcomes of the disease process (3, 4), they have focused attention upon functional outcomes that are amenable to psychological interventions.

The purpose of the present chapter is to review the relevant research reports on the psychological aspects of rheumatoid arthritis (RA), juvenile chronic arthritis, osteoarthritis, and fibrositis. The rationale for limiting the scope to these four rheumatic diseases is the striking lack of research pertaining to the psychological aspects of other rheumatic diseases. In fact, most of the literature to date has focused on psychological factors involved in the onset and course of RA. Relatively little attention has been paid to juvenile arthritis, osteoarthritis, and fibrositis. In the case of fibrositis, only recently has this disorder been recognized as a disease entity with specific symptoms and a proposed etiology (5). As affective disturbance is postulated to play a role in the onset and/or course of primary fibrositis, its inclusion in the chapter seems appropriate.

The chapter will begin with a consideration of possible psychological factors involved in the etiology of RA (adult and juvenile), osteoarthritis, and fibrositis. This section will include an analysis of the literature on the arthritic personality, a concept developed in the psychoanalytic tradition that suggests a specific personality pattern is at least partially responsible for the onset of RA. The possible role of psychological stress in the development of arthritis, including its effects on the immunologic system, also will be considered. The next major section will summarize the relevant research on the various psychological and behavioral effects of RA, osteoarthritis, and fibrositis. Assessment techniques for measuring each effect will be discussed, as well as emerging trends in the measurement of psychosocial and functional consequences of rheumatic disease.

The subsequent section will address psychological treatment strategies designed to supplement traditional medical therapy for rheumatic disease patients. Approaches considered will include traditional psychotherapy, social support interventions, and the more recent cognitive-behavioral treatments. Strategies designed to improve adherence to medical regimens also will be reviewed. In addition, emerging trends in psychologically-oriented interventions will be identified. The chapter will conclude with a summary of the preceding sections and a discussion of future directions in the research on psychological aspects of rheumatic disease.

Etiology

Arthritic Personality

Although RA generally had been considered as one of the major psychosomatic diseases, the early research failed to document consistent personality variables that were antecedent to disease onset and specific to RA (e.g., 6). This search for the "arthritic personality" was plagued by numerous methodological and conceptual problems (7). Many of the earliest studies lacked control groups for comparison (e.g., 8). When control groups have been utilized, investigators often have failed to report patient characteristics (e.g., age, socioeconomic status) and disease parameters (e.g., duration of illness, type of medication) that may have affected their results. Additional methodological problems that may have produced inconsistent results in the research on the arthritic personality have included the retrospective nature of the research and differences in theoretical orientations (e.g., psychoanalytic vs behavioral) and measures employed (e.g., projective tests vs objective measures) across studies.

On the basis of existing research, there is little or no support for the existence of a specific arthritic personality that predates the disease. Several recent studies have suggested that much of the psychological disturbance reported in patients with RA may be the result of living with a chronic disease as opposed to being part of the cause of the disease. For example, Spergel, Ehrlich, and Glass (9) reported highly similar MMPI profiles for patients with RA, multiple sclerosis, gastric ulcers, and low back pain. In sum, the research evidence to date suggests that the "arthritic personality" is an unproven concept.

Role of Psychological Stress in the Development of Arthritis

Much of the older personality research does suggest that many patients experience considerable psychological stress prior to the initial manifestation of the symptoms of RA. Emerging as potentially important are consistent reports of distressed family relationships characterized by parental strife and parental loss, particularly by death or divorce (e.g., 10). Additionally, protracted stressful marital relationships and a high divorce rate in samples of RA patients have been reported by several investigators (e.g., 11). Although the quality of the data is variable, the literature does highlight the recurring theme of disturbed interpersonal relationships, both parental and marital, as major stressors in the lives of RA patients.

An important contribution to our understanding of the possible role of stress in the onset of RA has been the identification of two subgroups of patients that differed with regard to the relationship between psychological factors and the course of the disease (12, 13). The first subgroup presented a clear association of disease onset and psychodynamic conflict. Their disease began suddenly and progressed rapidly; also, their family history of RA was negative. This subgroup contrasts with a second subgroup of patients who had no apparent psychological conflict related to disease onset. They tended to report a slow disease onset, delayed symptom progression, and a much higher incidence of RA in their relatives. These findings are dramatically paralleled by similar findings with juvenile RA patients (12). Future research into the role of psychological stress in the etiology of RA is very promising in light of the evidence regarding individual differences among patients.

Potential Psychophysiological Mechanisms in the Development of Arthritis

Several lines of investigation have examined potential mechanisms whereby psychological stress may be translated into physiological pathogenetic change. Psychophysiological research has consistently demonstrated that patients with RA manifest elevated tonic levels of electromyographic (EMG) activity, an index of the tension level of the muscles at or near affected joints (e.g., 14). Moreover, RA patients have responded to psychological stress with a stereotypic excessive increase in EMG activity which subsides more slowly than normal (15). Each of these factors would function to place patients' joints under increased strain.

In a second arthritis-relevant area of psychophysiological investigation, Horvath and Hollander (16) reported that states of fear and apprehension in RA patients were associated with increases in intra-articular temperature. This interesting observation awaits replication and extension. If such a relationship proves reliable and is specific to RA, then it could prove to be associated with the mechanism involved in inflammatory reactions in the joints.

A third area of psychophysiological investigation which has attempted to examine the precise mechanisms by which psychological stress may contribute to the development of RA is systemic in its orientation and has been labelled psychoneuroimmunology. While recent research has documented widespread immunosuppressive effects of psychological stress, it has simultaneously revealed the intricacies of these relationships (for a review, see 17). These results are likely to be increasingly important in our understanding of the role that psychological stress may play in the development of arthritis. At the present time, however, these findings serve primarily a heuristic function of guiding the development of our hypotheses and research.

Finally, it should be noted that research concerning the role of psychological factors in the etiology of arthritis has focused almost exclusively upon RA to the exclusion of both osteoarthritis and fibrositis. In view of the evidence that psychological factors may contribute to the development of RA, it is important to investigate whether they might play similar roles in the development of either osteoarthritis or fibrositis.

Summary

The existing research provides little or no support for the concept of an arthritic personality that predates the disease and contributes to disease onset. Several lines of investigation do suggest that psychological stress may play a role in the etiology of RA in some patients. Future research should focus on the identification of the patient subgroups for whom psychological stress either does or does not contribute etiologically.

The conclusion that psychological stress may be involved in the onset of RA in some patients raises the question of possible psychophysiological mechanisms involved. Encouraging results have been reported in research using EMG, intra-articular temperature, and immune system responses to stress. It is important that these findings be clarified, refined, and extended in both the psychological and physiological domains.

Psychological and Behavioral Effects

A multitude of clinical and research reports have examined the psychological and behavioral effects of RA. The impact of this chronic disease appears to be multifaceted, with affective, cognitive, behavioral, and social consequences. Unfortunately, most of the research to date has serious methodological problems that complicate interpretation of the results. In the following section the relevant, better-controlled research reports will be examined in an attempt to understand the potentially devastating consequences of this chronic disease. The psychological and behavioral effects of juvenile RA, osteoarthritis, and fibrositis also will be critically evaluated. A lack of research on the psychosocial impact of these disorders limits the conclusions that can be drawn. In addition to examining the psychological and behavioral effects of each disease, assessment techniques for measuring the effects will be addressed. Furthermore, emerging trends in the assessment of psychological and behavioral effects of rheumatic disease will be discussed.

Affective Changes

Rheumatoid Arthritis

Many studies have attempted to measure possible emotional concomitants of rheumatic disease. Although early studies relied on projective tests and semistructured interviews of questionable reliability and validity, more recent investigations have utilized objective standardized tests. When the MMPI has been administered to RA patients, one fairly consistent finding has been an elevation on the Depression scale. In a large sample of hospitalized RA patients, scores on the Depression scale were significantly higher than the scores of control groups of general medical patients and healthy individuals (18). Samples of outpatients with RA have also demonstrated elevated Depression scores that have tended to fall between one and two standard deviations above the mean (e.g., 19). Scores in this range typically indicate mild depression that is reactive in nature. Several authors have suggested that this dysphoria represents one reaction to having a chronic, disabling illness (e.g., 9). Indeed, when the MMPI Depression scale scores of RA patients have been compared to those of patients with other chronic illnesses, similar mild elevations have been noted (9).

Studies using the Beck Depression Inventory (BDI, 20), and Zung Self-Rating Depression Scale (SDS, 21) also have demonstrated significant depression in samples of RA patients (e.g., 22). Clinical reports have suggested that increased anxiety levels may also result from RA, but there is little research to support this claim. In studies using Cattell's 16 PF (23), a factor-analytically constructed personality test, arthritis patients have scored above average on measures of emotionality, apprehension, and tension (e.g., 24). Their overall profiles were similar to those of other chronic disease groups.

Juvenile Rheumatoid Arthritis and Osteoarthritis

There has been an unfortunate paucity of research pertaining to possible affective changes in patients with other types of arthritis. In descriptive studies of hospitalized children with juvenile RA, marked depression and anxiety have been noted in many subjects (e.g., 12). The lack of control groups and reliable assessment measures in such studies prevents conclusions regarding affective changes. Assessment of the parents' affective state also may be an important factor to consider. Psychiatric interviews with mothers of arthritic children have suggested that the mothers may often feel depressed, pessimistic, and/or guilty (25).

Although it has been suggested that patients with osteoarthritis suffer from psychological maladjustment (26), there is a lack of research to document any affective effects of osteoarthritis. A recent paper addressing quality of care in osteoarthritis concluded that assessment of possible anxiety and depression should be included in future outcome measures on these patients (27).

Fibrositis

Although anxiety and depression have been described as important symptoms in the fibrositis syndrome (e.g., 28), the research to date has provided conflicting evidence. In an analysis of 50 fibrositis patients, Yunus and colleagues (29) found that 70% of the patients reported anxiety. Unfortunately, no standardized assessment of anxiety was included. In sleep studies of patients with fibrositis, an observer adjective checklist was used to assess subjects' mood (28). The fibrositic patients were described as anxious, irritable, and sluggish, but no scores or statistics were reported to verify this claim. In a subsequent study, Campbell, Clark,

Tindall, Forehand, and Bennett (30) found that fibrositic subjects did not differ from a matched control group of medical patients on either the BDI or the Spielberger State-Trait Anxiety Inventory (31). Although the authors did not report actual scores or analyses, these preliminary results indicate that fibrositis patients may not differ from other patients on standardized measures of mood.

In one study, however, fibrositis patients did differ from certain patient groups on standardized personality tests (32). As compared to groups of RA and nonrheumatoid arthritis patients, fibrositis subjects had higher mean scores on six of the 10 clinical scales of the MMPI. Clinically significant elevations (two standard deviations above the mean) for the fibrositis patients occurred on the Hypochondriasis and Hysteria scales. Subjects who have high scores on these scales endorse items reflecting physical symptoms and somatic concerns.

Pain

Chronic pain of varying intensity is generally considered to be a major effect of RA, osteoarthritis, and fibrositis. Certainly, it is a symptom of major concern to patients and probably the most likely to precipitate visits to a physician (33). Although the subjective nature of pain makes objective assessment of this symptom difficult, recent advances in pain measurement have led to greater understanding of the role of pain in the rheumatic diseases.

Rheumatoid Arthritis

Patients with RA may experience pain from a variety of sources, including local pain in joints due to inflammation, local pain on movement due to chronic changes in articular tissues, complications of the arthritis, affective changes, medication side effects, and systemic illness (34). Due to increased awareness of the importance of pain in the health status of arthritis patients, health professionals have included pain measures in several recent questionnaires designed to assess patient outcome in the rheumatic diseases (4, 35). The Health Assessment Questionnaire (HAQ) developed by Fries and his colleagues includes a pain scale composed of a rating of pain severity and pain trend (better, same, worse) (35). Similarly, the Arthritis Impact Measurement Scales (AIMS) developed by Meenan and colleagues contains a pain scale composed of four items assessing pain severity, frequency, duration of morning stiffness, and frequency of pain in two or more joints (4). In a small sample of RA patients, scores on the pain scales of the AIMS and HAQ were significantly correlated, suggesting the two instruments are measuring similar concepts of pain (35).

The internal reliability and relevance of the AIMS pain scale has been well documented. In a study of patients with various rheumatic diseases, the total pain scale score correlated significantly with disease-related criteria such as ARA functional class and joint count (36). In a subsequent report of rheumatic disease patients, 60% of whom had RA, the mean pain scale score was reported to be 5.8 on a 10-point scale (33). The authors developed explanatory regression models to explore the contribution of pain in assessments of overall health, medication usage, and changes in health status over time. Pain was more important than physical or psychological disability in explaining medication usage. Pain also made a highly significant contribution to explaining physician and patient assessments of general health, as well as subsequent pain and physical disability. These results confirm the importance of assessing pain as a major factor in the overall health status of rheumatic disease patients.

Indeed, one study of hospitalized RA patients found that pain ratings were significantly related to mood patterns (37). Mood was assessed using an observer adjective checklist, and pain was measured via dolorimeter readings required to produce joint tenderness. Two pain-mood patterns were identified: a synchronous state in which mood changes either preceded or were accompanied by changes in pain readings, and a paradoxical state in which pain readings were inversely related to intensity of mood disturbance. Patients with a paradoxical pattern demonstrated a significantly less favorable outcome following medical treatment.

Thus, the assessment of pain in arthritis patients has important implications for treatment. In patients with RA, pain threshold, as measured by dolorimeter pressure, has been negatively correlated with ratings of pain severity and duration (38). Moreover, patients with a low pain threshold tended to take more analgesic medication. Pain threshold did not correlate with objective measures of disease severity and did not appear to affect the course of the disease in any way. Huskisson and Hart (38) concluded, therefore, that measures to raise pain threshold can safely form part of the treatment of RA.

Juvenile Rheumatoid Arthritis and Osteoarthritis

Several studies have demonstrated that children with juvenile RA report less pain and less pain variability than adults with RA (e.g., 39). Thus, pain is probably not a good indication of disease severity or treatment outcome in young children. An interview study with children of varying ages demonstrated that the younger patients reported less severe pain and less unpleasantness of sensations than older children, as measured by visual analogue scales (40). Interview data suggested that the older children may have attributed a more negative meaning to their sensations because of an unnecessarily pessimistic view of their illness. Correcting such misperceptions may be one way to reduce pain in older children with juvenile RA.

When the AIMS and HAQ were used to assess health status in subjects with osteoarthritis, these patients reported as much pain as RA patients (33, 35). On the HAQ, pain ratings of both RA and osteoarthritis patients tended to average 0.8 on a 0–3.0 scale (3). Pain was the single most important predictor of medication usage in osteoarthritis subjects and also made a significant contribution to physician and patient estimates of overall health (33).

Fibrositis

The presence of prominent localized tenderness in specific anatomic sites is a diagnostic criterion for fibrositis (5). In research trials, these tender points have been assessed using a dolorimeter or palpation (29, 30). Fibrositis patients have demonstrated more areas of localized tenderness than other medical patients but similar pain thresholds and tolerance. Self-report of pain in fibrositis has been assessed using Likert-type rating scales of questionable reliability (28). In order to assess possible overnight changes in pain perception, a visual analogue or verbal descriptor scale might be a more sensitive measure (41). Additional research is needed to assess the severity and nature of pain in fibrositis patients.

Functional Impairment

Functional impairment in activities of daily living is a frequent consequence of arthritis and other rheumatic diseases. The importance of assessing functional disability in arthritis has long been recognized (42). The American Rheumatism Association (ARA) Functional Classification provides a valuable global assessment of functional capacity but is not sensitive enough to detect less than major changes in functional status that may result from therapeutic interventions (43). The need to document such changes has led to the development of measures of functional ability that are specific to arthritis or similar chronic conditions. These measures are usually questionnaires that assess problems with activities of daily living such as dressing, grooming, and ambulation.

Table 6.1 summarizes the functional assessment instruments used in rheumatology for which reliability and validity data have been published (4, 44-51). As can be seen in the table, some of the instruments focus solely on functional assessment (IFI, PDI, Keitel, Index of ADL, Activity diary). Others include scales that measure additional dimensions of health status, such as pain and psychosocial adjustment (AIMS, HAQ, SIP, FSI).

Three of these instruments seem particularly appropriate for use in clinical or research trials. The Sickness Impact Profile (SIP) includes a scale for assessment of physical dysfunction that has correlated significantly with measures of functional ability in RA patients such as grip strength and walking time (50). In a sample of RA outpatients, dysfunction was reported by a majority of subjects in the subcategories of ambulation, body care, and movement (52). One advantage of the SIP is that it provides a patient profile in subcategories of physical function that can provide targets for intervention.

The AIMS and HAQ are easily administered measures of health status that include scales for physical disability. Construct validity of these disability scales has been demonstrated by significant correlations with such external measures as functional class and joint count (35, 36). In a large sample of rheumatic disease patients, the mean disability value on the AIMS was 2.8 on a 10-point scale (33). On the HAQ, patients with RA tended to have an average disability score of 1.1 on a 4-point scale that rose approximately 0.08 per year (3). In samples of patients with osteoarthritis, the disability index has averaged around 0.4, with a significant relationship to age of the patient rather than duration of disease (35).

Most of the functional assessment tools described in Table 6.1 have not as yet been applied to patients with juvenile RA or fibrositis. Modifications in the scales may be necessary to make them relevant to the functional activities of children. Since fibrositis patients do not usually report major functional disability, an activity diary might be an appropriate assessment tool for these patients (51).

Psychosocial Changes

Rheumatoid Arthritis

In addition to affective changes, pain, and physical disability, many arthritis patients have to adjust to psychosocial changes that can result from chronic disease. Impairment has been reported on such factors as self-esteem, life satisfaction, social activities, and family functioning (e.g., 53). Recently, investigators have attempted to document these psychosocial changes using standardized assessment techniques. When psychosocial adjustment was measured using five attitude scales, RA patients expressed lower self-esteem, less work satisfaction, and a greater sense of meaninglessness than healthy controls (54). Similarly, when the Tennessee Self-Concept Scale (TSCS) was used to assess self-esteem in a sample of hospitalized RA patients, low scores on a subscale assessing body image or physical self-esteem were noted (9).

The Sickness Impact Profile (SIP) also has been used to assess psychosocial changes in RA (52). Under the psychosocial dimension, significant percentages of arthritis patients have reported dysfunction in social interaction, communication,

TABLE 6.1 Functional Assessment Scales for Rheumatic Disease Patients

Instrument	Type of Administration	Administration Time	Scales
Arthritis Impact Measurement Scales (AIMS) (4)	Self-report	20 min	Physical disability Psychological disability Pain
Functional Status Index (FSI) (44)	Self-report or interview	20-30 min	Physical mobility Personal care Home chores Transfers Kitchen chores (dependence, pain, and difficulty ratings in each category)
Health Assessment Questionnaire (HAQ) (45)	Self-report	5 min 30 min (cost scales)	Disability Discomfort Side effects Medical costs
Index of ADL (46)	Interview/observation	Not reported	Bathing Dressing Going to toilet Transfer Continence Feeding
Index of Functional Impairment (IFI) (47)	Self-report or interview	10 min	Functional index

Keitel Functional Test (48)	Observer ratings of exercises	15 min	Functional index
Polyarticular Disability Index (PDI) (49)	Interview	15 min	Daily living skills Mobility
Sickness Impact Profile (SIP) (50)	Self-report or interview	20-30 min	Physical dysfunction Psychosocial dysfunction Independent categories
Activity Diary (51)	Self-report	20 min/day	11 types of activities (e.g., sleep, recreation, passive)

and emotional behavior. Moreover, the physical dimension correlated positively with the psychosocial dimension, suggesting that impaired physical function is accompanied by psychosocial disability. The authors recommended using the SIP to identify psychosocial problems and to facilitate referral to appropriate rehabilitative services.

A chronic disease such as RA has an inevitable impact upon the patient's family (2). In a study of patients with advanced RA, approximately 60% reported at least one major psychosocial change related to family functioning (55). In other studies of marital status in RA, conflicting results have been found. Several studies have reported an increased incidence of divorce in RA patients as compared to normal controls (e.g., 11). Other reports found no relationship between RA and divorce (e.g., 56). Using an appropriate control group of patients with chronic rheumatic disease other than RA, Medsger and Robinson (57) found a greater incidence of divorce and a lower rate of remarriage in female RA patients.

Juvenile Rheumatoid Arthritis and Osteoarthritis

Psychosocial problems have frequently been demonstrated in samples of children with juvenile RA. For example, a comprehensive assessment of arthritic children revealed more abnormal behavioral symptoms in the children, as compared to healthy controls (58). An overall school adjustment rating indicated poor adjustment in one-third of the arthritic children, as compared to 9% of the controls. Surprisingly, children with no physical disability (ARA functional class 1) demonstrated the worst school adjustment. The authors speculated that teachers are less likely to make allowances for children without visible stigmata. The children with arthritis also demonstrated lower self-esteem than their healthy peers. In this case, the children with greater physical disability tended to show the poorer self-concept.

Psychosocial problems have not been studied sufficiently in fibrositis or osteoarthritis patients for conclusions to be drawn (27). In a small sample of outpatients with osteoarthritis of the hip, psychosocial events did appear to be related to patients' self-report of physical symptoms (59). Patients who reported a large number of unpleasant events over a 6-month period also tended to report high symptom-disability levels. A time-lag analysis revealed that a decrease in negative events often was followed by a symptom increase, suggesting that for some patients the negative events served as a distraction from focusing on physical symptoms.

Sexual Problems

Possible sexual consequences of the rheumatic disorders have received little attention in clinical or research reports. Yet as Ehrlich (60) has pointed out, a disease that causes pain and interferes with motion must have some effect on sexual functioning. Chronic pain and illness can adversely affect sexual desire and/or ability for arousal and release (61). And physical disability can obviously interfere with attempted motions during sexual activity. In addition, psychological changes such as depression and lowered self-esteem can serve to further reduce libido and energy levels required for optimal sexual performance. Specific sexual problems may also develop following complications of the rheumatic disease (60).

Several recent studies suggest that sexual concerns are common in arthritis patients. In a sample of 79 patients with RA, 36 reported decreased sexual activity since disease onset (52). A questionnaire sent to 121 patients with osteoarthritis of the hip joint revealed that 81 experienced some degree of sexual difficulty due to their arthritis (62). Pain and stiffness were reported more frequently than loss of libido as the cause of sexual difficulty. Among the patients with sexual problems, 64% wanted some form of advice from a health professional.

Patients with juvenile RA also may be at risk for the development of sexual disability. When 58 adults were interviewed approximately 15 years after the onset of juvenile RA, 38% expressed a need for sexual counseling (63). Moreover, nearly all the patients stated that they could have benefited from sexual counseling as adolescents. As a delay in sexual maturation can result from juvenile arthritis, adolescent patients' sexual concerns need to be addressed by health care professionals.

The limited research to date on sexuality in arthritis patients indicates that sexual dysfunction is not uncommon and that many patients have sexual concerns. Assessment of sexuality and possible sexual problems should be included in the patient's medical evaluation. As many patients are reluctant to bring up sexual issues, the health professional can initiate the discussion. Assessment of the patient's premorbid sexual adjustment is needed to determine the sexual preferences of the patient (61). An awareness of the possible role of medical, psychological, mechanical, and pharmacologic factors in sexual dysfunction should facilitate treatment and possible referral to other health care professionals.

Sleep Disturbance

The presence of a significant sleep disturbance has been documented in patients with fibrositis. Sleep studies of patients with fibrositis syndrome have revealed the presence of anomalous alpha-rhythms in the nonrapid-eye-movement (NREM) sleep EEG (28). This NREM sleep disturbance was accompanied by overnight increases in dolorimeter scores used to assess musculoskeletal tenderness at the specified anatomic sites involved in fibrositis. Moldofsky and his colleagues have suggested that fibrositis be considered a "non-restorative sleep syndrome" that can be triggered by either physical trauma or emotional disturbances (28). A deficiency in brain serotonin metabolism has been hypothesized as the physiological factor underlying the sleep disorder. This hypothesis is supported by research indicating that subjective pain ratings in fibrositis patients are inversely related to levels of plasma-free tryptophan, a component necessary for the synthesis of brain serotonin (64).

Some evidence exists that patients with RA are at risk for the development of a sleep disturbance similar to that found in fibrositis patients (65). In a small sample of RA patients experiencing an acute flare, an alpha frequency EEG sleep anomaly during NREM sleep was demonstrated. Overnight increases in dolorimeter-assessed tenderness in joints and at fibrositic points also were found. In addition, patients tended to show overnight decreased energy and increased weakness. Moldofsky and colleagues (65) postulated that arthritic pain can serve as an internal stimulus disrupting NREM sleep.

Sleep problems are typically reported by a majority of patients with fibrositis (29, 30) and a substantial proportion of patients with RA (52). Additional research is needed to confirm the presence of a NREM sleep disturbance in these populations. Larger patient samples and assessment by investigators blind to patient diagnosis would lead to more definitive conclusions. In clinical settings, an awareness of possible sleep problems in arthritis patients should facilitate assessment and appropriate interventions.

Nonadherence

Patients with RA, osteoarthritis, or fibrositis are typically prescribed medications, physical therapy regimens, and/or additional therapeutic interventions. Evaluation of treatment efficacy is frequently made on the assumption that patients have adhered to the prescribed therapies. Unfortunately, the research available indicates that patient cooperation with arthritis treatment recommendations is often lacking. Estimates of nonadherence with medication in arthritis patients have ranged from 22 to 67% (66).

Wide variations in reported nonadherence rates are probably related to numerous methodological problems in the studies to date (66). Estimates of nonadherence often have relied on patient self-report, a measure of questionable reliability (67). Such measures as serum drug levels or percent of intended refills may provide more reliable indications of adherence (e.g., 68). When Deyo, Inui, and Sullivan (68) assessed percent of drug refills within 6 months, they obtained a mean adherence rate of 64%. Adherence varied significantly, however, according to type of medication and type of rheumatic disorder. For instance, RA patients were more compliant than patients with osteoarthritis. Several studies have found low adherence rates for aspirin and indomethacin, whereas adherence rates for prednisone and penicillamine were high (e.g., 68). Thus, in assessing or predicting adherence, it is important to consider the specific medication and diagnosis involved.

Duration and severity of illness are also important factors to consider. Patients with more severe arthritic disease or longer duration of illness may be more likely to be nonadherent (e.g., 69). However, evidence to the contrary also exists (68). Such factors as frequency of physician contact, type of medication, and presence of side effects have not been controlled for in most of the previous research.

Adherence rates for physical therapy have generally been lower than those for medication, with cooperation estimates ranging from 34 to 62% (66). As studies generally have relied on patient self-report and/or health professional estimates, these rates may be overestimates of adherence. Moreover, the research to date has addressed frequency and duration of practice but not quality of exercises performed.

Adherence to medication or physical therapy regimens may be related to patients' beliefs about the efficacy of the treatment. For example, Arluke (70) found that some RA patients believed a drug's efficacy would decline over time and stopped their medication when improvement occurred so as not to "use up a good thing." Thus, when assessing possible adherence problems, it is important to determine patients' beliefs and attitudes regarding both their illness and the treatment prescribed (66).

In summary, monitoring adherence in arthritis patients is obviously essential when evaluating reasons for therapeutic failures or successes. Patient self-report, serum drug levels, pill counts, and number of prescription refills can all be used to assess adherence. As each technique has methodological problems, Deyo (71) suggests using at least two measures as a cross-validation check. This approach is certainly indicated for research trials but may be difficult to implement in clinical practice. One simple, if unvalidated, way to check on patient self-report is to independently ask family members about a patient's adherence (72).

Costs

The direct and indirect costs of a potentially chronic illness are major financial effects of RA, osteoarthritis, and fibrositis. Accurate assessment of the financial impact of chronic illness can facilitate appropriate management of medical costs and referral to social rehabilitative services.

A recent survey of patients with anatomic stage III RA revealed that the direct medical costs for this group were three times the national average (73). Moreover, only 58% of the costs were covered by insurance. The patients with the highest costs due to hospitalization did tend to have the highest percentage of coverage. Physician visits, medications, and laboratory fees were the largest components of outpatient costs. Patients tended to visit physicians about 12 times per year, with eight of those visits to a rheumatologist (55). In contrast, visits to other health care professionals were infrequent, averaging between three and four per year.

In studies assessing medical costs using patient self-report on questionnaires, the cost for medical care has been estimated by applying unit prices for the various services (e.g., 73). When records of medical bills were compared to patient self-report, the actual costs agreed with the reported costs over 80% of the time (45). Thus, patient self-report can be an accurate assessment technique for determining the financial impact of health care services.

In addition to the direct costs of medical care, many arthritis patients have to cope with indirect costs due to vocational disability. A recent survey of RA patients revealed that 59% of the sample who had held jobs when their disease began were no longer working (74). A discriminant analysis of vocational disability indicated that workplace factors (e.g., autonomy, self-employment) and disease factors (e.g., duration, radiographic stage) were both important in predicting disability. Patients who were still working earned on the average only 50% of their expected income, a conservative estimate based on premorbid income. The effects of RA on work status were found in all occupational and sociodemographic classes. The results are particularly striking given that 70% of the sample was classified as functional stage I or II.

Given the pervasive impact of RA on vocational status, the low rate of referral to social-rehabilitative services is surprising (74). An awareness of the direct and indirect costs for individual patients should facilitate appropriate referrals. In addition, documented cost data can be used to evaluate the economic efficacy of treatment interventions. Research on the costs of chronic illness is also important for shaping social policies on services available for disabled patients (75). Although RA appears to cause greater disability than other types of arthritis (3), at least one recent report suggests that osteoarthritis can also have a major financial impact on patients (76). Additional research is needed, however, before conclusions regarding the costs of osteoarthritis or fibrositis can be made.

New Trends in Assessment

A major trend in the assessment of arthritis is the growing awareness of the importance of analysis of multimodal effects: affective, cognitive, and behavioral, as well as the more commonly assessed medical or physiological consequences. When evaluating patient outcome, health care providers are beginning to consider the whole constellation of effects of chronic disease. As Fries (3) has pointed out, outcome criteria such as pain or functional impairment are apt to be more important to patients than more traditional disease criteria (i.e., grip strength, antibody levels). Moreover, outcome measures in each category of change can be assessed using instruments that meet accepted standards of reliability and validity.

A growing trend in the assessment of affective and psychosocial changes is the use of such standardized psychometric instruments. Many of these tests are short self-administered questionnaires that can be used to screen for affective disturbance in clinical and research trials. In the area of functional assessment, psychometric instruments specific for rheumatic disease have recently been developed. The majority of the instruments listed in Table 6.1 are easily administered, reliable questionnaires that are very cost-effective means of assessing functional impact. Future research is expected to further document their validity and sensitivity to changes following therapeutic interventions.

An additional trend in the assessment of arthritis patients is the analysis of possible sexual or sleep-related disorders. Growing interest in the sexual concerns of patients with chronic disease should lead to more comprehensive assessment techniques. Similarly, concern about the role of sleep disturbance in the course of fibrositis and RA should facilitate further assessment in this area.

A realization of the importance of detecting nonadherence to medical regimens has led to critical examination of various assessment techniques for measuring nonadherence. Future work in this area is necessary to develop operational definitions of adherence that allow meaningful comparisons between studies. As Deyo (71) suggests, investigators need to quantify adherence on a continuous scale rather than dichotomize patients as "adherent" or "nonadherent." It is also anticipated that innovative techniques for measuring nonadherence such as medication monitors will be developed to supplement methods already employed (67).

An expected future trend in the area of assessment is an attempt to measure patients' strengths as well as weaknesses. Some of the functional assessment questionnaires allow identification of areas in which patients are coping well. Future work should also assess the patients' cognitive coping strategies, through the use of such instruments as the Health Locus of Control Scale (77) and the Arthritis Helplessness Index (78). These measures of subjects' covert experiences assess the extent to which patients believe that they can control their general health and arthritis symptoms, respectively. A final area of assessment for future investigations is the identification of psychological and behavioral correlates of remissions and flare-ups in arthritis patients. As arthritis is a chronic disease, it is important to follow patients longitudinally in order to determine variations in psychological effects over time that may correlate with disease fluctuations.

Summary

The preceding section indicates that RA often has pervasive psychological and behavioral effects in a patient's life. Reactive depression, chronic pain, psychosocial changes, and major direct and indirect costs are typically reported. Patients with RA may also be at risk for the development of sexual and sleep problems. Given this constellation of effects, as well as the uncertain course of RA, a large number of patients may suffer from a type of learned helplessness which leads to reduced efforts to cope with their uncontrollable illness (79). The limited amount of research on psychological effects of juvenile RA, osteoarthritis, and fibrositis prevents definitive conclusions regarding the impact of these disorders. Children with RA have demonstrated more frequent psychosocial problems, impaired school performance, and family dysfunction than healthy peers. Adults with osteoarthritis tend to report significant functional disability and chronic pain. Although an EEG sleep disturbance has been documented in small samples of fibrositis patients, additional research is needed to assess the effects of the disease. It is expected that future research will more fully explore the psychological and behavioral effects of these other rheumatic diseases, as well as RA.

A general trend in the assessment of rheumatic disease effects is the use of standardized assessment techniques of demonstrated reliability and validity. A number of such instruments specific for arthritis have been developed to measure functional impairment and are currently being used to assess treatment outcome. Nonadherence, sexual dysfunction, and sleep disorders are relatively new targets for assessment in the rheumatic disorders.

The emerging theme in the assessment literature is an awareness of the importance of addressing the multimodal effects of illness. Dealing with traditional medical criteria alone is no longer acceptable and has been supplemented with psychological, behavioral, and social data. Multimodal assessment is needed in order to fully assess treatment outcome. In addition, thorough assessment delineates targets for intervention by physicians and other health care professionals.

Treatment Strategies

In contrast to the large number of investigations that have appeared regarding the psychological and behavioral effects of arthritis, few empirical studies have been published concerning the relative efficacy of psychologically-oriented treatment interventions for rheumatic disease. This dearth of intervention studies may be attributed in large part to two factors. First, it has only been within the past 10-15 years that psychologists interested in health care research have been able to form strong working relationships with physicians involved in the care of the chronically ill (80). Furthermore, as noted in the preceding discussion, it has only been within the past 5 years that a great deal of effort has been directed toward the measurement of functional (i.e., behavioral) disabilities among rheumatic disease patients that might be amenable to psychologically-oriented treatments (cf. 3, 43).

The following discussion will critically examine the empirical literature regarding the efficacy of traditional psychotherapy and social support interventions for patients suffering primarily from RA. The discussion then will present a detailed examination of six recent investigations that have employed "cognitive-behavioral" or "self-control" strategies for enhancing patients' abilities to reduce the pain and suffering associated with RA and hemophilic arthropathy. This will be followed by a brief review of the literature regarding the enhancement of arthritis patient adherence to medical and physical therapy regimens. The discussion will conclude with a summary of emerging trends in research concerning the psychological treatment of patients with rheumatic disease.

Traditional Psychotherapy

The literature concerning the use of traditional, psychodynamically-oriented psychotherapy with arthritis patients consists only of a few descriptive reports. This may seen surprising given that the rheumatology literature emphasizes the difficulties that many patients face in coping with the physical, emotional, social, and economic sequelae of rheumatic disease (e.g., 73, 74). However, the lack of a sophisticated psychotherapy literature may be due in part to patients' reluctance to accept the traditional mental health model as appropriate in the treatment of arthritis (81) and physicians' reluctance to consult with behavioral specialists unless patients display signs of major psychiatric illness (82).

Two of the reports regarding the use of traditional psychotherapy with arthritis patients described group therapy programs for RA patients attending an outpatient rheumatology clinic (83) and inpatients suffering primarily from RA and osteoarthritis (84). Although both reports noted that positive outcomes were found, the reports suffered from the lack of control groups and the use of any standard outcome measures.

Rimón (85), however, used the Beck Depression Inventory (BDI, 20) to assess pre- to posttreatment changes in depression among 40 female RA patients who were treated with brief (3-8 sessions), supportive psychotherapy and one of two antidepressant medications (chlorimipramine or sulpiride). A significant association was reported between reductions in BDI scores and the author's judgment of decreases in disease activity (based upon measures such as the joint exam, erythrocyte sedimentation rate, etc.). Nevertheless, the absence of appropriate controls for the attention provided to patients, the confounding of pharmacotherapy with psychotherapy, and the subjective rating of improvements in disease activity levels preclude any valid conclusions regarding the outcome of the investigation.

In summary, only three studies have been reported concerning the use of traditional, psychodynamically-oriented psychotherapy with arthritis patients. These investigations primarily have been descriptive in nature. No valid statements may be made, then, regarding the efficacy of traditional psychotherapy for patients with rheumatic disease.

Social Support Interventions

The results of several correlational investigations have suggested that there may be complex interactions among rheumatic disease activity, social support, and patients' coping abilities. For example, Meenan and his colleagues (73, 74) found that the majority of patients in two independent samples suffered at least one negative psychosocial consequence of RA. It also was reported that income loss due to RA was significantly associated with psychosocial change. These psychosocial changes are quite important given that two independent investigations have provided evidence that social adjustment (86) and degree of social support (87) are significantly and positively associated with patients' functional status. Indeed, it has been suggested (87) that a stable, positive, marital relationship may serve as a "marker" of social support given that marital strain was a significant predictor of disabilities in self-care, mobility, and work after the effects of age, sex, and health status were statistically controlled.

Two empirical investigations regarding the efficacy of education and support programs for arthritis patients have appeared in the past 5 years. Kaye and Hammond (88) assessed changes in 48 RA patients' knowledge of the disease and self-reports of behavioral changes following participation in a brief education and social support program. The patients showed a significant pre- to posttreatment increase in scores on an arthritis knowledge questionnaire. The great majority of patients (80-85%) indicated that the program a) aided in family communication; b) helped them communicate better with their physicians; c) increased their understanding of the importance of adhering to their medication regimens; and d) led them to make one or more behavioral changes following participation in the program (e.g., resting more frequently). However, the lack of a control group and reliance solely upon self-report of patient change make it impossible to draw firm conclusions regarding the value of the program.

Potts and Brandt (89) recently reported negative evidence regarding the efficacy of an education and support program for RA patients. Nineteen patients who lived within a 1-hour drive from a university-based arthritis center participated in four weekly, 1½-hour meetings. The control group consisted of 19 patients who could not easily drive to the arthritis center on a weekly basis. The patients completed questionnaires concerning their knowledge of RA and attempts to cope with the disease at pretreatment, posttreatment, and a 6-month follow-up. Neither of the two patient groups reported any changes across assessment periods with regard to their attempts to cope with RA. Only the patients who received education and social support showed a significant increase in RA knowledge from pre- to posttreatment; however, this increase was not maintained at follow-up. It was reported, nevertheless, that at each assessment patients' self-reports of coping were positively and significantly related to their perceptions of their families' attitudes and behavior. Thus, although the brief education and social support intervention failed to affect patients' knowledge and self-reports of coping efforts, it did suggest that the positive support communicated by family members (i.e., their attitudes and behavior) was related to patients' reports of relatively effective coping. As with the other reports examined thus far, however, this positive finding must be regarded with caution due to the potential biases associated with self-report data.

In summary, the correlational literature regarding the value of social support for RA patients suggests that patients' reports of relatively effective coping and low levels of psychological distress are associated with perceived social (e.g., marital) support. There are no data, however, concerning the value of social support to patients with osteoarthritis, fibrositis, or other rheumatic conditions. The education and social support intervention studies have produced conflicting results that may be attributed in part to methodological deficiencies associated with the investigations. There remains a great need for well-controlled research concerning the efficacy of education and social support interventions for patients with various forms of arthritis. If these interventions do show positive effects, it will be necessary for future investigators to attempt to determine the relative contributions of education and social support to the outcomes that are achieved.

Cognitive-Behavioral Interventions

Several investigators recently have attempted to use "cognitive-behavioral" or "self-control" interventions to alleviate pain and disability among patients with RA and hemophilic arthropathy. The assumption underlying cognitive-behavioral therapy is that persons' expectations and other appraisals of life events influence their emotional and behavioral reactions to those events (90). Thus, in order to help patients make the behavioral changes necessary to better cope with arthritis, it is necessary to increase patients' perceptions of self-efficacy or their beliefs in their ability to control pain and other displays of disability (cf. 91). Cognitive-behavioral intervention strategies, therefore, include techniques designed to promote adaptive cognitions concerning life events (e.g., information provision, promotion of the belief that one has potentially successful coping strategies within one's repertoire of skills) as well as behavioral interventions to facilitate improved coping skills such as relaxation training, biofeedback, modeling of appropriate coping behavior, and provision of rewards (e.g., verbal praise, social attention) for appropriate coping behavior (90).

Bradley (92) recently provided a detailed review of the literature regarding the use of cognitive-behavioral interventions with arthritis patients. Consistent with this review, the following discussion first will examine several programmatic studies concerning the efficacy of a cognitive-behavioral treatment package for persons suffering from hemophilic arthropathy. This will be followed by a summary of several independent investigations that have used a variety of cognitive-behavioral interventions and other self-control techniques with RA patients.

Hemophilic Arthropathy

Varni (93) has noted that "chronic, severe degenerative arthritis represents the most frequent problem confronting the physician who manages the care of adult hemophiliacs, with an estimated 75% of adult hemophiliacs demonstrating one or more affected joints" (p. 183). On the basis of a survey of hemophiliacs with severe arthritis pain and a review of the medical literature regarding arthritis pain management, Varni developed a three-part treatment protocol consisting of progressive muscle relaxation, meditative breathing exercises, and imagery training (i.e., vivid imagination of scenes that patients previously experienced as warm and pain-free). The protocol also involved home practice of warming imagery at least twice each day for 15 minutes and verbal feedback regarding patients' abilities to increase peripheral skin temperature at the sites of their most severe pain (as measured by a thermal biofeedback unit).

Table 6.2 shows that Varni's treatment protocol produced substantial decreases in the pain ratings and analgesic medication intake of six adults and one pediatric patient (93-96). It also should be noted that the Varni (94) study demonstrated that patients' control of their chronic pain was not merely an artifact of decreased acute bleeding episodes or altered perceptions of the intensity of acute bleeding pain. Thus, it appears warranted to empirically assess the efficacy of the protocol (or a similar protocol) with persons suffering from other forms of arthritis that are not secondary to hemophilia. This conclusion, however, is made with the caution that the patients who volunteered for the studies may have been unusually motivated to use the cognitive-behavioral procedures and thus may not have been representative of the population of hemophiliacs with arthritic pain.

Rheumatoid Arthritis

Three investigations have been performed concerning the use of cognitive-behavioral therapy interventions with RA patients. Table 6.3 shows that the results of all three studies indicated that providing RA patients with training in deep muscle relaxation and other adjunct procedures may allow them to increase their physical activity levels. However, only two of the investigations (97, 98) showed that relaxation training produced significant reductions in patients' self-reports of pain intensity. It also should be noted that all of the studies suffered from various methodological flaws such as a) failure to demonstrate that instructions to increase or decrease peripheral skin temperatures using thermal biofeedback produced reliable changes in peripheral skin temperature levels (97, 98); b) reliance upon self-report of outcome (99); and c) inadequate follow-up assessment procedures (97-99).

Nevertheless, the results have been sufficiently positive to warrant the development of well-controlled investigations of the long-term effects of cognitive-behavioral interventions with RA patients. All future investigations should include follow-up periods of at least 6 months; a 12-month follow-up, however, would be more desirable as it would allow the assessment of fluctuations in perceived pain, physical activity, and peripheral skin temperature due to seasonal changes. Finally, since it is posited that cognitive-behavioral interventions positively alter patients' perceptions of their self-efficacy in coping with pain and other disabilities, it is important to attempt to monitor patients' perceptions of self-efficacy prior to and during treatment as well as at follow-up (cf. 92).

In summary, the literature described above strongly indicates that cognitive-behavioral intervention strategies appear to offer greater promise for pain reduction and functional status improvements among patients with hemophilic

TABLE 6.2 **Capsule Summary of Outcome Studies Using Varni's Treatment Protocol for Hemophilic Arthropathy**

Authors	Patients	Skin Temperature Changes	Pain Rating Changes	Other Functional Changes
Varni (93)	2 males (ages 19 and 27)	One patient increased temperature at most affected site from 84.8°F at baseline to 90.1°F at 8-month follow-up (other patient did not undergo biofeedback assessment)	Average number of days with pain at most affected site during 1-wk baseline were 6 and 4, respectively; at follow-up the means were 0.5 and 0.2, respectively	Review of pharmacy records during treatment and follow-up showed both patients reduced use of analgesic medications; one patient reported cessation of morning stiffness
Varni (94)	3 adults (ages 19, 26, and 28; gender not provided)	Increased average temperature at most affected site from 84.4°F at baseline to 88.5°F at 7-14 month follow-up	Average pain rating at most affected site decreased from 5.1 at baseline to 2.2 at follow-up (on 10-point scale)	Review of pharmacy records showed average decrease in number of analgesic tablets from 7.6 at baseline to 2.6 at follow-up; plasma protein factor replacement requirements and patients' reports of bleeding frequency and acute bleeding pain intensity did not change following treatment; the finding above indicated that increased control of chronic pain was not an artifact of decreased acute bleeding or altered perceptions of acute bleeding pain intensity.

TABLE 6.2 (Cont'd)

Authors	Patients	Skin Temperature Changes	Pain Rating Changes	Other Functional Changes
Varni and Gilbert (95)	1 male (age 31)	Increased temperature at most affected site from 85°F at baseline to 88.2°F at 5-month follow-up	Average pain rating at most affected site decreased from 5.4 at baseline to 2.2 at follow-up (on 10-point scale)	Review of pharmacy records showed reduction in monthly propoxyphene usage from 17,550 mg at baseline to 7670 mg at follow-up
Varni, Gilbert, and Dietrich (96)	1 male (age 9)	Not reported	Average pain rating at most affected site decreased from 7.0 at baseline to 2.0 at 1-yr. follow-up (on 10-point scale)	Reduced meperidine (50 mg) intake from 74 tablets for baseline year to 0 tablets for follow-up yr.; reduced acetaminophin/codeine elixir (24 mg) intake from 438 doses for baseline yr. to 78 doses for follow-up yr.; reduced hospitalizations and school absences from 11 and 33 days, respectively, for baseline yr. to 0 and 6 days, respectively, for follow-up yr.

TABLE 6.3 Capsule Summary of Outcome Studies Using Cognitive-Behavioral Intervention for Rheumatoid Arthritis

Authors	No.	Interventions	Results	Methodological Weaknesses
Achterberg, McGraw, and Lawlis (97)	23	Relaxation training, finger temperature biofeedback, home exercise program, and education regarding proper body mechanics and posture; physiotherapy, home exercise program, and education regarding proper body mechanics and posture	Both treatments produced significant and positive changes in 50-ft walking time, self-reports of performance of activities of daily living and erythrocyte sedimentation rate; only the patients who received relaxation training and biofeedback showed significant and positive changes in number of nighttime awakenings due to pain, disability-related work changes, number of involved joints, and self-reports of physical activity and pain severity	Some patients were instructed to use biofeedback to increase skin temperature and others were instructed to attempt to decrease skin temperature; the skin temperature increases that were recorded were due to relaxation training rather than biofeedback instructions; no follow-up assessment of maintenance of treatment gains
Denver, Laveault, Girard, Lacourciere, Latulippe, Grove, Preve, and Doiron (98)	12	Hand-temperature biofeedback and relaxation training; relaxation training only; no-treatment control	Patients who received biofeedback and relaxation training a) significantly reduced variability of peripheral skin temperature and electromyographic (EMG) levels; b) significantly increased pain tolerance; and c) showed reduction in 50-ft walking time	Since patients who received biofeedback and relaxation training did not produce reliable skin temperature increases, the results may have been due to nonspecific factors; no follow-up assessment of maintenance of treatment gains

TABLE 6.3 (Cont'd)

Authors	No.	Interventions	Results	Methodological Weaknesses
Randich (99)	44	Stress inoculation training (deep-muscle relaxation training, imagery training and cognitive strategy training); social support; no-treatment control	Stress-inoculation training produced significant and positive changes from pretreatment to 8-wk follow-up assessment in self-reports of daily work, leisure, social and functional activities	All outcome data were based upon patient self-reports and thus could not be verified; follow-up assessment was not sufficiently long to assure stability of treatment gains

arthropathy and RA than do traditional psychotherapy and social support interventions (cf. 81). It is likely, then, that additional controlled outcome studies will be produced in the future involving patients with RA and other forms of arthritis. In addition to heeding the present authors' suggestions for methodological improvements, future investigators should focus greater attention upon the amelioration of pain and disability displayed by arthritic children. It also might be useful to attempt to develop and evaluate a cognitive-behavioral treatment protocol that would be appropriate for patients with fibrositis. Smythe (5) has suggested that treatment of fibrositis should include components such as education, minimal administration of salicylates, changes in lifestyle (e.g., gradual increase in exercise), support for the cervical spine during sleep, and alteration in patients' attitudes (e.g., reduce patients' needs to assume undue responsibilities). These factors clearly could be incorporated into a cognitive-behavioral intervention package similar to those used by Achterberg et al. (97) and Randich (99). Indeed, a description of the use of EMG biofeedback with fibrositis patients already has been presented at a meeting of the Biofeedback Society of America (100).

Improving Adherence to Medical Regimens

Jette (66) recently has suggested that nonadherence to or noncooperation with medical regimens may be classified as either voluntary or nonvoluntary. Voluntary nonadherence is defined as the patient's deliberate failure to undertake the recommendations of health care providers. Jette (66) has attributed this phenomenon in large part to patient motivation and perceptions of the relevance of the providers' recommendations. Nonvoluntary nonadherence, however, is defined as failure to undertake therapeutic recommendations due to "incongruity between what the patient thinks he or she is supposed to do and what the provider thinks the patient is doing" (p. 452).

In order to reduce nonadherence that is nonvoluntary, Jette has offered the following guidelines:

1. All regimen instructions to patients should be provided in legible written form.
2. Medical jargon should be avoided in both verbal and written instructions.
3. Nonmedical professionals (e.g., psychologists, pharmacists, social workers) may be used to help patients learn the skills necessary to perform some regimens.
4. Patients should be given the opportunity to provide feedback to medical personnel regarding prescribed regimens to ensure the instructions are fully understood.
5. Family members and other persons in patients' support networks may be used to help patients maintain high levels of adherence.

With respect to reducing voluntary nonadherence, Jette (66) has provided these suggestions:

1. Physicians should be trained to assess patients' attitudes regarding disease severity, treatment efficacy, personal susceptibility to complications secondary to treatment, and barriers to adherence.
2. Physicians should attempt to gear their educational interventions to patients' attitudes.
3. Treatment regimens should be simplified as much as possible.

4. Attention should be given to the unique psychological needs of patients in order to maximally enhance the patient-physician interaction (e.g., gauge the extent to which patients wish to be "directed" by an authoritative physician versus desire a "relaxed" relationship with the physician).

Jette's (66) suggestions are consistent with those provided by compliance investigators in medical areas other than arthritis (cf. 67). However, the arthritis literature contains no well-controlled intervention studies regarding the long-term efficacy of implementing the suggestions described above.

Automated monitors and self-monitoring techniques have been shown to hold a great deal of promise for enhancing patient adherence to medication regimens (see 67 for a complete review). This technology has not received a great deal of attention from rheumatologists. Nevertheless, Waggoner and LeLieuvre (101) recently demonstrated that adding an automated electronic counter with a visual display to a hand exercise device substantially enhanced the adherence of 12 RA patients with their exercise regimens. Prior to giving patients access to the visual display, the electronic counter recordings showed a mean percentage of nonadherence across three baseline periods of 17%. Allowing patients access to the visual display reduced mean nonadherence to 2.85%. It should be noted, however, that the investigation failed to adequately control for the effects of increased attention and other nonspecific factors on the patients' adherence levels. The study also did not include a long-term follow-up assessment of patient adherence with their exercise regimens.

In summary, only one study regarding the efficacy of an intervention for enhancing arthritis patient adherence has been performed. Based upon reviews of the adherence literature in areas other than rheumatology, it appears that Jette's (66) suggestions for reducing both nonvoluntary and voluntary nonadherence should be of value to physicians. However, Jette's suggestions have not been empirically demonstrated to be of value with arthritis patients and, in some cases, may be difficult for many current physicians to operationalize (e.g., assessing patients' attitudes regarding barriers to adherence).

Emerging Trends

The present review has examined the empirical literature regarding interventions designed to help patients better cope with the pain and functional disabilities associated with arthritis and to increase patients' adherence to their medical regimens. These areas of the literature have been of interest for many years to rheumatologists and other professionals who deal with arthritis patients. There also are several new areas of interest in the arthritis literature that are beginning to attract the attention of rheumatologists and psychologists alike. These emerging areas of interest will be reviewed briefly below.

Multidisciplinary Approaches to Treatment

The past 10 years have been characterized by an increased level of collaboration among physicians and nonmedical health professionals (e.g., psychologists, epidemiologists, biomedical engineers) in the prevention, assessment, and treatment of disease as well as the rehabilitation of persons afflicted with chronic disorders (1, 2). This general trend also has been reflected in the arthritis literature. For example, Vignos et al. (86) used a clinical psychologist in their comprehensive treatment program only for the purpose of assessing patients' intelligence, motivation for treatment, and personal as well as social adjustment. The current review, however, has shown that a growing number of psychologists are developing and empirically evaluating interventions for arthritis patients that may be provided as adjunct treatments in addition to their medical therapies. Indeed, two rheumatologists have called for increased collaboration with psychologists and other behavioral scientists in order to promote the development of reliable and valid outcome measures (3) and to reduce nonadherence to medical regimens (66). It is quite likely that collaborative efforts between rheumatologists and behavioral scientists will increase in the next 5 years given that a) a high level of expertise in behavioral measurement and psychometrics may be found among behavioral scientists (cf. 102); and b) there currently exists a great deal of interest among behavioral scientists in improving the quality of care provided to the growing number of Americans who suffer from chronic diseases such as arthritis (cf. 2).

Treatment of Sexual Dysfunction

Similar to the growing emphasis on multidisciplinary approaches to the care of arthritis patients described above, there has been increased interest within the past 10–15 years on the sexual dysfunction often experienced by persons with chronic disease (e.g., 61). Until recently, however, little attention was directed toward the alleviation of sexual dysfunction among arthritis patients.

Ehrlich (60) and other authors (e.g., 103) have offered helpful suggestions that may be communicated to arthritis patients concerning appropriate planning for sexual activity, use of medication to reduce pain during and after intercourse, positioning, surgery for improved joint mobility, and the benefits of psychological counseling regarding sexual difficulties. Unfortunately, no empirical investigations have been published regarding the efficacy of behavioral or psychological interventions for sexual dysfunction experienced by arthritis patients.

It should be noted that empirical investigations of the efficacy of behavioral and psychological interventions for sexual dysfunction among persons with chronic diseases other than arthritis recently have begun to appear. The spinal cord injury literature (see 104 for a complete review) is particularly worthy of examination given that many of the sexual difficulties associated with spinal cord injury are also associated with the rheumatic diseases. These difficulties include "emotional responses to physical losses, negative attitudes, and lack of information concerning sexual functioning as well as specific adaptive devices and techniques" (104, p. 299). It is anticipated that as behavioral scientists increase their collaborative efforts with rheumatologists, there will appear within the next 5 years controlled evaluations of behavioral and psychological treatments for sexual dysfunction among arthritis patients.

Use of Cognitive-Behavioral Interventions and the Involvement of the Family in Treatment

F.D. Hart (34) anticipated the use of cognitive-behavioral interventions with arthritis patients in 1974: "It would seem legitimate to attempt to raise pain threshold as part of the therapeutic programme when and if this is possible. This would presumably include encouragement of the patient to lead a life of maximum fulfillment within a certain therapeutic framework, a positive rather than a negative programme of controlled activities" (p. 65). The cognitive-behavioral interventions described in this chapter were designed to increase patients' beliefs in their abilities to control their pain and reduce their functional disabilities as well as to provide them with the requisite behavioral skills to do so. The cognitive-behavioral intervention studies have shown very promising results. Thus, it is anticipated that cognitive-behavioral interventions will be used and empirically evaluated with greater frequency during the next 5 years.

The use of cognitive-behavioral interventions with arthritis patients developed as a natural extension of the literature concerning the application of such interventions to patients suffering from chronic benign pain with no demonstrable organic pathology (cf. 92). There appears to be a consensus that it is necessary to include the family members of chronic benign pain patients in treatment and in posttreatment planning in order for cognitive-behavioral therapy to be maximally effective (92). Family members are used to encourage patients to practice the self-control skills learned during treatment, maintain the use of these skills, and to develop other healthy behaviors following treatment. However, the cognitive-behavioral intervention studies currently available in the arthritis literature have not included descriptions of families' involvement in treatment.

There is disagreement within the arthritis literature concerning the degree to which family members may positively influence patients' compliance with medical regimens (e.g., 72, 105). Nonetheless, the present authors' experience in the use of cognitive-behavioral interventions with RA patients suggests that family members may be used effectively to reinforce patients' home practice of self-control skills and to help patients set attainable behavioral goals with respect to increasing functional abilities (105). It is anticipated that future investigators will begin to empirically evaluate the benefits of including family members in cognitive-behavioral treatment programs during the next 5 years.

Long-Term Evaluation of Treatment Efficacy

There currently exists a great deal of interest in developing the most appropriate methods for measuring the outcomes produced by arthritis intervention packages (e.g., 3, 4, 35, 43, 45). Although the measurement techniques used in the arthritis literature have become increasingly sophisticated during the past several years, the outcome studies reviewed in the present chapter generally have used very short follow-up periods or have failed entirely to assess the maintenance of treatment gains. Future investigators will have to include follow-up assessments of at least 6 months in their investigations of treatment outcome.

Summary

The preceding discussion has shown that psychologists have become increasingly involved in the treatment of arthritis patients during the past 10 years. The most promising treatments for RA patients appear to be the cognitive-behavioral treatment interventions that have included various combinations of biofeedback training, deep muscle relaxation, and techniques for increasing patients' perceptions of self-efficacy as well as their functional abilities. Although these interventions currently appear to be superior to traditional psychotherapy and to educational and social support interventions, it is necessary to empirically determine the extent to which large numbers of arthritis patients may maintain their positive outcomes over extended periods of time.

The literature regarding the enhancement of arthritis patients' adherence to their medical regimens is less sophisticated than that concerning arthritis treatment interventions. There are few controlled studies on adherence enhancement, although there is some evidence (101) that the development of automated monitoring systems may increase adherence with physical therapy regimens. Psychologists may prove to be of value in helping rheumatologists to better evaluate the levels of adherence exhibited by arthritis patients and to more precisely assess patients' attitudes that might be related to adherence.

With respect to emerging trends in the arthritis literature, it is expected that the next 5 years will be characterized by a) increased collaboration between rheumatologists, psychologists, and other behavioral scientists; b) greater emphasis upon treating sexual dysfunction associated with arthritis; c) increased use of cognitive-behavioral treatment interventions with arthritis patients; and d) greater involvement of family members in the treatment of arthritis patients. It is essential, however, for psychologists to consistently and carefully assess the long-term benefits of their treatment interventions.

Summary

The authors have attempted to provide an overview of what is currently known about the psychological aspects of arthritis. Due to a lack of research on many rheumatic diseases, the discussion has been restricted to RA, juvenile arthritis, osteoarthritis, and fibrositis. Although the psychological research to date is characterized by many methodological problems, psychological factors do appear to play an important role in the course of these disorders.

The proposed role of psychological variables in the etiology of arthritis remains controversial. The literature on the arthritic personality provides little support for this concept and suggests instead that psychopathology may result from a chronic disease such as RA. The research on the role of psychological stress in the onset of RA is plagued by serious methodological problems, including determination of when the disease process actually begins. The research does suggest, however, that psychological stress may play a role in the onset of adult and juvenile RA in some patients.

Several psychophysiological processes have been postulated as the mechanism that mediates the role of stress in the etiology of RA. Elevated EMG levels at rest and in response to psychological stress have been found in RA patients. Thus, one possible mechanism is an elevated level of muscle tension producing chronic joint strain. Other proposed mechanisms are changes in intra-articular temperature and alteration of the immunological system in response to stress. More rigorous clinical and laboratory research in psychophysiology and psychoneuroimmunology is needed to further analyze these possible mechanisms. The role of psychological factors in the onset of osteoarthritis and fibrositis also requires additional research efforts. Although anxiety and depression have been discussed as etiological factors in fibrositis (5), no research to date has supported this claim.

Multimodal psychological and behavioral effects of RA have been repeatedly documented. The potentially devastating consequences of this chronic disease can include affective disturbances, chronic pain, psychosocial changes, functional impairment, sexual problems, noncompliance with medical regimens, and direct as well as indirect financial costs. The effects of juvenile RA, osteoarthritis, and fibrositis appear substantial but are not well researched. Perhaps the most important trend in the assessment of psychological and behavioral effects is the use of standardized objective measurement techniques that provide meaningful data and allow comparisons between studies. Promising instruments specific for arthritis have been developed to assess functional impairment.

More thorough assessment of arthritis patients has facilitated the development of psychological treatment strategies designed to alleviate the negative effects of rheumatic disease. The most promising treatments for RA patients appear to be cognitive-behavioral interventions designed to reduce pain, improve functional ability, and enhance perceived coping ability. Psychological treatments for patients with juvenile RA and fibrositis have not, as yet, been evaluated empirically. The psychosocial problems of juvenile RA patients and the symptom complex of fibrositis patients suggest that cognitive-behavioral interventions may be beneficial to these patient populations.

The increasing use of adjunct psychological treatment for rheumatic disease reflects the growing collaboration among rheumatologists and nonmedical health professionals. As sexual, family, and compliance issues in rheumatic disease are beginning to receive attention, this multidisciplinary collaboration will become increasingly important. Such collaboration should also facilitate comprehensive evaluation of medical and nonmedical treatment efficacy. Longitudinal studies that assess long-term benefits of treatment interventions are particularly needed.

In conclusion, the comprehensive care of rheumatic disease patients necessitates thorough analysis of psychological factors involved in the onset, course, and outcome of the disease process. It is anticipated that future research will further delineate the role of psychological variables in arthritis and other rheumatic conditions. Collaboration with nonmedical health professionals is expected to increase as further validation is provided for the measurement and intervention techniques being developed by psychologists and other behavioral scientists.

Acknowledgements

Preparation of this chapter was supported by Robert Wood Johnson Foundation Grant No. 8236 to Laurence A. Bradley.

We gratefully acknowledge the assistance of Nan Hartman, Beverly McClellan, and Vicky Raulerson in the preparation of this chapter.

References

1. Bradley LA, Prokop CK: The relationship between medical psychology and behavioral medicine. In CK Prokop, LA Bradley (eds.), *Medical Psychology: Contributions to Behavioral Medicine.* New York, Academic Press, 1981, pp. 1-4.

2. Burish TG, Bradley LA: Coping with chronic disease: Definitions and issues. In TG Burish, LA Bradley (eds.), *Coping with Chronic Disease: Research and Applications.* New York, Academic Press, 1983, pp. 3-12.

3. Fries JF: Toward an understanding of patient outcome measurement. *Arthritis Rheum* 26:697-704, 1983.

4. Meenan RF, Gertman PM, Mason JH: Measuring health status in arthritis: The Arthritis Impact Measurement Scales. *Arthritis Rheum* 23:146-152, 1980.

5. Smythe HA: "Fibrositis" as a disorder of pain modulation. *Clin Rheum Dis* 5:823-832, 1979.

6. Booth GC: Organ function and form perception: Use of the Rorschach method with cases of chronic arthritis, Parkinsonism, and arterial hypertension. *Psychosom Med* 8:367-385, 1946.

7. Moos RH: Personality factors associated with rheumatoid arthritis: A review. *J Chronic Dis* 17:41-55, 1964.

8. Thomas GW: Psychic factors in rheumatoid arthritis. *Am J Psychiatry* 93: 693-710, 1936.

9. Spergel P, Ehrlich GE, Glass D: The rheumatoid arthritic personalilty: A psychodiagnostic myth. *Psychosomatics* 19:79-86, 1978.

10. Baker GHB: Life events before the onset of rheumatoid arthritis. *Psychother Psychosom* 38:173-177, 1982.

11. Cobb S, Miller M, Wieland M: On the relationship between divorce and rheumatoid arthritis. *Arthritis Rheum* 2:414-418, 1959.

12. Rimón R, Belmaker RH, Ebstein R: Psychosomatic aspects of juvenile rheumatoid arthritis. *Scand J Rheumatol* 6:1-10, 1977.

13. Rimón R: A psychosomatic approach to rheumatoid arthritis: A clinical study of 100 patients. *Acta Rheum Scand Suppl* 13, 1969.

14. Moos RH, Engel BT: Psychophysiological reactions in hypertensive and arthritic patients. *J Psychosom Res* 6:227-241, 1962.

15. Anderson CD, Stoyva JM, Vaughn LJ: A test of delayed recovery following stressful stimulation in four psychosomatic disorders. *J Psychosom Res* 26: 571-580, 1982.

16. Horvath SM, Hollander JL: Intraarticular temperature as a measure of joint reaction. *J Clin Invest* 28:469-473, 1949.

17. Ader R (ed.): *Psychoneuroimmunology.* New York, Academic Press, 1981.

18. Polley HF, Swenson WM, Steinhilber RM: Personality characteristics of patients with rheumatoid arthritis. *Psychosomatics* 11:45-49, 1970.

19. Nalven F, O'Brien J: On the use of the MMPI with rheumatoid arthritis patients. *Arthritis Rheum* 7:18-29, 1964.

20. Beck AT: Depression inventory. Philadelphia, Center for Cognitive Therapy, 1978.

21. Zung W: A self-rating depression scale. *Arch Gen Psychiatry* 12:63-70, 1965.

22. Zaphiroporelos G, Burry HC: Depression in rheumatoid disease. *Ann Rheum Dis* 33:132-135, 1974.

23. Cattell RB: *The Scientific Analysis of Personality.* Chicago, Aldine, 1965.

24. Robinson H, Kirk RF, Frye RL: A psychological study of rheumatoid arthritis and selected controls. *J Chronic Dis* 23:791-801, 1971.

25. Cleveland SE, Reitman EE, Brewer EJ Jr: Psychological factors in juvenile rheumatoid arthritis. *Arthritis Rheum* 8:1152-1157, 1965.

26. Lihn H, Menninger K, Mayman M: Personality factors in osteoarthritis. *Assoc Res Nervous Men Dis* 29:744-749, 1949.

27. Greenfield S, Solomon NE, Brook RH, Davies-Avery A: Development of outcome criteria and standards to assess the quality of care for patients with osteoarthrosis. *J Chronic Dis* 31:375-388, 1978.

28. Moldofsky H, Scarisbrick P, England R, Smythe H: Musculoskeletal symptoms and non-REM sleep disturbance in patients with "fibrositis syndrome" and healthy subjects. *Psychosom Med* 37:341-351, 1975.

29. Yunus M, Masi A, Calabro J, Miller K, Feigenbaum S: Primary fibromyalgia (fibrositis): Clinical study of 50 patients with matched normal controls. *Seminars in Arthritis Rheum* 11:151-171, 1981.

30. Campbell S, Clark S, Tindall E, Forehand M, Bennett R: Clinical characteristics of fibrositis. *Arthritis Rheum* 26:817-824, 1983.

31. Spielberger CD, Gorsuch RL, Lushene RE: *Manual for the State-Trait Anxiety Inventory.* Palo Alto, Consulting Psychologist Press, 1970.

32. Payne TC, Leavitt F, Garron DC, Katz RS, Golden HE, Glickman PB, Vanderplate C: Fibrositis and psychologic disturbance. *Arthritis Rheum* 25: 213-217, 1982.

33. Kazis LE, Meenan RF, Anderson JJ: Pain in the rheumatic diseases. *Arthritis Rheum* 26:1017-1022, 1983.

34. Hart FD: The control of pain in the rheumatic disorders. In FD Hart (ed.), *The Treatment of Chronic Pain.* Philadelphia, F. A. Davis, 1974, pp. 63-96.

35. Fries JF, Spitz PW, Young DY: The dimensions of health outcomes: The Health Assessment Questionnaire, disability and pain scales. *J Rheumatol* 9:789-793, 1982.

36. Meenan RF, Gertman PM, Mason JH, Dunaif R: The Arthritis Impact Measurement Scales: Further investigations of a health status measure. *Arthritis Rheum* 25:1048-1053, 1982.

37. Moldofsky H, Chester WJ: Pain and mood patterns in patients with rheumatoid arthritis: A prospective study. *Psychosom Med* 32:309-318, 1970.

38. Huskisson EC, Hart FD: Pain threshold and arthritis. *Br Med J* 4:193-195, 1972.

39. Scott PJ, Ansell BM, Huskisson EC: Measurement of pain in juvenile chronic polyarthritis. *Ann Rheum Dis* 36:186-187, 1977.

40. Beales JG, Keen JH, Holt PJ: The child's perception of the disease and the experience of pain in juvenile chronic arthritis. *J Rheumatol* 10:61-65, 1983.

41. Bradley LA, Prokop CK, Gentry WD, Van der Heide LH, Preito EJ: Assessment of chronic pain. In CK Prokop, LA Bradley (eds.), *Medical Psychology: Contributions to Behavioral Medicine.* New York, Academic Press, 1981, pp. 91-117.

42. Steinbrocker O, Traeger CH, Battman RC: Therapeutic criteria in rheumatoid arthritis. *JAMA* 140:659-662, 1949.

43. Liang MH, Jette AM: Measuring functional ability in chronic arthritis: A critical review. *Arthritis Rheum* 24:80-86, 1981.

44. Jette AM: Functional status index: Reliability of a chronic disease evaluation instrument. *Arch Phys Med Rehab* 61:395-401, 1980.

45. Fries JF, Spitz P, Kraines RG, Holman HR: Measurement of patient outcome in arthritis. *Arthritis Rheum* 23:137-145, 1980.

46. Katz S, Downs TD, Cash HR, Grotz RC: Progress in development of the Index of ADL. *Gerontologist* 10:20-30, 1970.

47. Lee P, Jasani MK, Dick WC, Buchanan WW: Evaluation of a functional index in rheumatoid arthritis. *Scand J Rheumatol* 2:71-77, 1973.

48. Ebert DR, Fasching V, Rahlfs V, Schleyer I, Wolf R: Repeatability and objectivity of various measurements in rheumatoid arthritis: A comparative study. *Arthritis Rheum* 19:1278-1286, 1976.

49. Convery FR, Minteer MA, Amiel D, Connett KL: Polyarticular disability: A functional assessment. *Arch Phys Med Rehabil* 58:494-499, 1977.

50. Bergner M, Bobbitt RA, Carter WB, Gilson BS: The Sickness Impact Profile: Development and final revision of a health status measure. *Med Care* 19: 787-805, 1981.

51. Skevington SM: Activities as indices of illness behavior in chronic pain. *Pain* 15:295-307, 1983.

52. Deyo RA, Inui TS, Leininger J, Overman S: Physical and psychosocial function in rheumatoid arthritis: Clinical use of a self-administered health status instrument. *Arch Intern Med* 142:879-882, 1982.

53. Cobb S, Kasl SV, Chen E, Christenfeld R: Some psychological and social characteristics of patients hospitalized for rheumatoid arthritis, hypertension, and duodenal ulcer. *J Chronic Dis* 18:1259-1278, 1965.

54. Earle JR, Perricone PJ, Maultsby DM, Perricone N, Turner RA, Davis J: Psychosocial adjustment of rheumatoid arthritis patients from two alternative treatment settings. *J Rheumatol* 6:80-87, 1979.

55. Yelin E, Feshbach DM, Meenan RF, Epstein WV: Social problems, services and policy for persons with chronic disease: The case of rheumatoid arthritis. *Soc Sci Med* 13:13-20, 1979.

56. Hellgren L: Marital status in rheumatoid arthritis. *Acta Rheum Scand* 15:271-276, 1969.

57. Medsger AR, Robinson H: A comparative study of divorce in rheumatoid arthritis and other rheumatic diseases. *J Chronic Dis* 25:269-275, 1972.

58. McAnarney ER, Pless B, Satterwhite B, Friedman SB: Psychological problems of children with chronic juvenile arthritis. *Pediatrics* 53:523-528, 1974.

59. Lunghi ME, Miller PM, McQuillan WM: Psychosocial factors in osteoarthritis of the hip. *J Psychosom Res* 22:57-63, 1978.

60. Ehrlich GE: Sexual problems of the arthritic patient. In GE Ehrlich (ed.), *Total Management of the Arthritic Patient.* Philadelphia, J. B. Lippincott, 1973, pp. 193-208.

61. Wise TN: Sexual dysfunction in the medically ill. *Psychosomatics* 24:787-805, 1983.

62. Currey HL: Osteoarthrosis of the hip joint and sexual activity. *Ann Rheum Dis* 29:488-493, 1970.

63. Herstein A, Hill RH, Walters K: Adult sexuality and juvenile rheumatoid arthritis. *J Rheumatol* 4:35-39, 1977.

64. Moldofsky H, Warsh JJ: Plasma tryptophan and musculoskeletal pain in non-articular rheumatism ("fibrositis syndrome"). *Pain* 5:65-71, 1978.

65. Moldofsky H, Lue FA, Smythe HA: Alpha EEG sleep and morning symptoms in rheumatoid arthritis. *J Rheumatol* 10:373-379, 1983.

66. Jette AM: Improving patient cooperation with arthritis treatment regimens. *Arthritis Rheum* 25:447-453, 1982.

67. Masur FT: Adherence to health care regimens. In CK Prokop, LA Bradley (eds.), *Medical Psychology: Contributions to Behavioral Medicine.* New York, Academic Press, 1981, pp. 441-470.

68. Deyo RA, Inui TS, Sullivan B: Compliance with arthritis drugs: Magnitude, correlates, and clinical implications. *J Rheumatol* 8:931-936, 1981.

69. Litt IF, Cuskey WR: Compliance with salicyclate therapy in adolescents with juvenile rheumatoid arthritis. *Am J Dis Child* 135:434-436, 1981.

70. Arluke A: Judging drugs: Patients' conceptions of therapeutic efficacy in the treatment of arthritis. *Hum Org* 39:84-87, 1980.

71. Deyo RA: Compliance with therapeutic regimens in arthritis: Issues, current status, and a future agenda. *Sem in Arthritis Rheum* 12:233-244, 1982.

72. Oakes TW, Ward JR, Gray RM, Klauber MR, Moody PM: Family expectations and arthritis patient compliance to a hand resting splint regimen. *J Chronic Dis* 22:757-764, 1970.

73. Meenan RF, Yelin EH, Henke CJ, Curtis DL, Epstein WV: The costs of rheumatoid arthritis: A patient-oriented study of chronic disease costs. *Arthritis Rheum* 21:827-833, 1978.

74. Meenan RF, Yelin EH, Nevitt M, Epstein WV: The impact of chronic disease: A sociomedical profile of rheumatoid arthritis. *Arthritis Rheum* 24: 544-549, 1981.

75. Yelin E, Meenan R, Nevitt M, Epstein W: Work disability in rheumatoid arthritis: Effects of disease, social, and work factors. *Ann Intern Med* 93: 551-556, 1980.

76. Muller CF, Kayaalp O, Kaplan D, Forman M: Costs and impact of arthritis in a low income population. *Arthritis Rheum* 25:S149, 1982. (Abstract)

77. Wallston BS, Wallston KA, Kaplan GD, Maides SA: Of the Health Locus of Control (MHLC) Scale. *J Consult Clin Psychol* 44:580-585, 1976.

78. Wallston KA, Pincus TP, Nicassio P, Woodward N, Dodd MA: Correlates of functional capacity in patients with rheumatoid arthritis. Paper presented at the meeting of the Society of Behavioral Medicine, Baltimore, March 1983.

79. Garber J, Seligman MEP (eds.): *Human Helplessness: Theory and Applications.* New York, Academic Press, 1980.

80. Gentry WD, Matarazzo JD: Medical psychology: Three decades of growth and development. In CK Prokop, LA Bradley (eds.), *Medical Psychology: Contributions to Behavioral Medicine.* New York, Academic Press, 1981, pp. 5-15.

81. Achterberg-Lawlis J: The psychological dimensions of arthritis. *J Consult Clin Psychol* 50:984-992, 1982.

82. Rogers MP, Liang MH, Partridge AJ: Psychological care of adults with rheumatoid arthritis. *Ann Intern Med* 96:344-348, 1982.

83. Schwartz LH, Marcus R, Condon R: Multidisciplinary group therapy for rheumatoid arthritis. *Psychosomatics* 19:289-293, 1978.

84. Udelman HD, Udelman DL: Team therapy in a rheumatology unit. *Psychosomatics* 18:42-46, 1977.

85. Rimón R: Depression in rheumatoid arthritis. *Ann Clin Res* 6:171-175, 1974.

86. Vignos PJ, Thompson HM, Katz S, Moskowitz RW, Frick S, Svec KH: Comprehensive care and psychosocial factors in rehabilitation in chronic rheumatoid arthritis: A controlled study. *J Chronic Dis* 24:457-467, 1972.

87. Kaplan GA, DeLongis A: Psychosocial factors influencing the course of arthritis: A prospective study. Paper presented at the meeting of the American Psychological Association, Anaheim, California, August 1983.

88. Kaye RL, Hammond AH: Understanding rheumatoid arthritis: Evaluation of a patient education program. *JAMA* 239:2466–2467, 1978.

89. Potts M, Brandt KD: Analysis of education–support groups for patients with rheumatoid arthritis. *Patient Counsel Health Educ* 4:161–166, 1983.

90. Tan S-Y: Cognitive and cognitive-behavioral methods for pain control: A selective review. *Pain* 12:201–228, 1982.

91. Grzesiak RC: Cognitive and behavioral approaches to management of chronic pain. *NY State J Med* 82:30–38, 1982.

92. Bradley LA: Coping with chronic pain. In TG Burish, LA Bradlet (eds.), *Coping With Chronic Disease: Research and Applications.* New York, Academic Press, 1983, pp. 339–379.

93. Varni JW: Behavioral medicine in hemophilia arthritis pain management: Two case studies. *Arch Phys Med Rehabil* 62:183–187, 1981.

94. Varni JW: Self-regulation techniques in the management of chronic arthritic pain in hemophilia. *Behav Ther* 12:185–194, 1981.

95. Varni JW, Gilbert A: Self-regulation of chronic arthritic pain and long-term analgesic dependence in a haemophiliac. *Rheumatol Rehabil* 21:171–174, 1982.

96. Varni JW, Gilbert A, Dietrich SL: Behavioral medicine in pain and analgesia management for the hemophilic child with Factor VIII inhibition. *Pain* 11:121–126, 1981.

97. Achterberg J, McGraw P, Lawlis GF: Rheumatoid arthritis: A study of relaxation and temperature biofeedback training as an adjunctive therapy. *Biofeedback Self Regul* 6:207–223, 1981.

98. Denver DR, Laveault D, Girard F, Lacourciere Y, Latulippe L, Grove RN, Preve M, Doiron N: Behavioral medicine: Biobehavioral effects of short-term thermal biofeedback and relaxation in rheumatoid arthritis patients. *Biofeedback Self Regul* 4:245–246, 1979. (Abstract)

99. Randich SR: Evaluation of pain management program for rheumatoid arthritis patients. *Arthritis Rheum* 25:511, 1982. (Abstract)

100. Fritz G, Fehmi L: Primary fibrositis: A skeletal muscle disorder treated with biofeedback-assisted attention training. *Biofeedback Self Regul* 8: 332–333, 1983. (Abstract)

101. Waggoner CD, LeLieuvre RB: A method to increase compliance to exercise regimens in rheumatoid arthritis patients. *J Behav Med* 4:191–201, 1981.

102. Prokop CK, Bradley LA: Methodological issues in medical psychology and behavioral medicine research. In CK Prokop, LA Bradley (eds.), *Medical Psychology: Contributions to Behavioral Medicine.* New York, Academic Press, 1981, pp. 485–496.

103. Richards JS: Sex and arthritis. *Sex Disab* 3:96-104, 1980.

104. Brucker BS: Spinal cord injuries. In TG Burish, LA Bradley (eds.), *Coping With Chronic Disease: Research and Applications.* New York, Academic Press, 1983, pp. 285-311.

105. Carpenter JO, Davis LJ: Medical recommendations — Followed or ignored? Factors influencing compliance in arthritis. *Arch Phys Med Rehabil* 57:241-246, 1976.

Chapter 7

THE SURGICAL MANAGEMENT OF ARTHRITIS

Anthony G. Gristina, M.D. and
Lawrence X. Webb, M.D.

The preeminent goal of surgical procedures for the treatment of arthritis is the alleviation of pain. The arthritic joint is a biological linkage in functional deficit because the naturally smooth, lubricated surfaces have been destroyed by inflammation. The surgical remedies attempt to 1) inhibit or forestall the process by removing the synovium, loose bodies, or frayed cartilage; 2) smooth the bearing surfaces of the joint; 3) redistribute the intrinsic load-bearing characteristics of the joint; or 4) remove completely or replace the joint surfaces. The specific operative procedures, therefore, are synovectomy, joint debridement, osteotomy, joint arthroplasty, joint replacement, and arthrodesis.

Historically, osteotomy and joint arthroplasty were pioneered more than a century ago by J. Rhea Barton (1). The first report of a synovectomy is credited to Volkmann(2), and the earliest report of an implanted artificial joint is that of Péan (a shoulder, in 1893) (3).

The modern era of total joint replacement (1950 to date) was exponentially expanded by the innovations of Sir John Charnley (4), although his contributions were based on and preceded by the work of Austin Moore (5) and of Smith-Petersen (6) in the earlier decades of this century.

These advances were made possible by the development of new biomaterials such as advanced stainless steel and cobalt-chrome alloys, high-density polyethylene, and acrylic cements. It was only a matter of time before well-understood engineering principles could be applied to joint surgery. A key factor in total joint replacement was the discovery that a form of acrylic cement (methylmethacrylate) enhanced the binding of the prosthetic device to the adjacent osseous matrix (4). Once the total hip replacement was successful, the principles used were applied to other joints, the result being today's bewildering array of interpositional joint replacement devices. A recent development is coating the stem of the prosthesis with a porous material that allows ingrowth of new bone; by this means the loosening that often occurs with methylmethacrylate may be avoided.

Surgical Methods and Procedures

Arthroscopy

Arthroscopy is a technique with low morbidity and minimal time in the hospital. Early reports of its use (7-10) show that it was successful in the debridement of joints involved in early inflammatory and degenerative disease. Subjectively, at least, the patients so treated have improved, with diminution of pain and enhanced motion over 1-2 years of follow-up. Whether the disease itself has been significantly arrested, as is the case with an open surgical synovectomy, remains debatable.

Arthroscopy has also been used for abrasion chondroplasty, a technique that debrides the residual traumatized cartilaginous surfaces and is believed to encourage replacement by smooth fibrocartilage. The results of this technique are early and are not yet proven. For anatomical and practical reasons, arthroscopy is currently best suited for large joints with adequate capsule-to-articular contact surface ratios, such as the knee and the shoulder.

Synovectomy

Synovectomy, or the removal of the inflamed joint lining, whether performed arthroscopically or through a surgical incision, may be indicated in the early stages of rheumatoid arthritis before erosion of the cartilage has taken place (11). In actual clinical practice, arthroscopic debridement appears to achieve temporary symptomatic relief even in the more advanced stages of disease.

Osteotomy

Osteotomy is a surgical technique used to redistribute the basic stresses upon damaged joint surfaces by cutting and realigning the bones on one or both sides of the involved joint. Most frequently, proximal tibial osteotomy is used as a relatively early operative procedure for knee deformities, when the arthritic process is localized to one anatomic compartment of the joint. Its use in the management of hip joint degeneration, although still advocated by some (12), has diminished markedly since the advent of total hip arthroplasty.

Joint Arthroplasty

Joint arthroplasty generally refers to resection of the damaged surfaces with the interposition of biological tissues. This type of procedure is generally reserved for joints that are not suitable for prosthetic devices for one reason or another.

Total Joint Arthroplasty

Total joint replacement is by far the single most important and successful new surgical method for treating arthritic and traumatized joints. Its success rate is relatively high, and, based on the last 15 years' experience, it is appropriately indicated for progressive painful arthritis that cannot be resolved by medical methods. Total joint replacement is most common in the hip, knee, and hand, but is increasingly being used in the shoulder.

Arthrodesis

Arthrodesis involves the removal of residual joint surfaces and the bridging of the joint interval with solid bone. Arthrodesis is usually accomplished by a simple resection of residual joints and the attachment of a compression device for a period of time. It represents a very reliable, long-term surgical procedure that offers complete relief of pain, but, by its very nature, no further movement of the joint. Most patients, when given a choice between total joint replacement and arthrodesis, will choose total joint replacement. Arthrodesis, however, has very definite indications in significant arthritis of the ankle, subtalar joints, and certain small joints of the hand. It is also the procedure of choice, especially at the knee, whenever total joint replacement fails and cannot be revised.

Perioperative Considerations

Preoperative

Patients with severe long-term rheumatoid arthritis are less medically robust than the group of patients requiring elective orthopedic surgery on the whole (13-16). This group of patients either has been unresponsive to medical management of their arthritis or has been affected by their disease for a number of years with resultant architectural alterations in the joints despite the medical management. When these architectural aberrations infringe on the patient's ability to care for himself or herself—whether due to pain, restricted motion, or a combination of the two—surgical correction may be considered. In addition, there are some surgical procedures that may be indicated to forestall the development of the painful end-stage joint with its attendant, coincident restriction of patient mobility and comfort. A careful weighing of benefits and risks must be undertaken by the surgeon in consultation with the patient. The likelihood of success or failure of the proposed procedure as well as an alternative plan in the event of failure should be discussed, understood, and agreed upon by both the surgeon and the patient. An enhanced susceptibility to infection exists in patients with severe rheumatoid disease, and it is thought that many of these patients may have an altered immune mechanism (17), or diminished host defense mechanisms secondary to steroid usage (15, 18). Prophylactic perioperative antibiotics and avoidance of unnecessary soft tissue dissection and devitalization of tissue are of paramount importance in these patients. These measures are especially applicable to the skin, which is often paper-thin and of marginal vascularity in rheumatoid patients who have been taking steroids (15, 18). In the patient with psoriatic arthritis with skin lesions in the vicinity of a proposed surgical procedure, it may be important to treat and minimize the skin lesions preoperatively (19).

Anesthetic considerations include micrognathia in those with severe juvenile rheumatoid arthritis, which often makes an intubation difficult (20). A rigid or subluxing cervical spine may also make intubation difficult and potentially dangerous (21). Because of the high incidence (30-40%) of cervical spine involvement in patients with rheumatoid arthritis (21-23), current preoperative roentgenograms of the cervical spine are indicated in the patient with severe rheumatoid arthritis. Patients with ankylosing spondylitis have diminished chest expansion and are more prone to postoperative atelectasis. Preoperative studies in these patients should include pulmonary function tests, including an arterial blood gas measurement and incentive spirometry.

Patients with ankylosing spondylitis, calcified spinal ligaments, and fixed deformities of the spine may be particularly difficult to anesthetize by spinal anesthesia. One should suspect an increased incidence of heterotopic ossification in these patients, especially subsequent to total hip replacement (24). Methods for minimizing heterotopic ossification in these patients should be considered: for example, the preoperative and intraoperative administration of prostaglandin inhibitors, irradiation, or the administration of etidronate disodium (25-27).

In general, patients with systemic involvement of rheumatoid disease have osteoporotic bone, which provides a relatively weak anchorage for the prosthesis or for the methylmethacrylate bonding the bone to the prosthesis. This fact leads to long-term failure due to periprosthetic fracture and loosening, and it is of particular concern when the arthritis involves major weight-bearing joints in the lower extremities of the young patient with monoarticular disease, as well as the young patient with polyarthritic juvenile rheumatoid arthritis. The replaced joint in such patients may be protected from increased wear because the pain in neighboring joints restricts the patients' activities (28).

Postoperative

Postoperative considerations include minimized immobilization of adjacent joints and early involvement of a physical therapist to supervise active range of motion exercises, gait training, and, if needed, training in the use of aids for activities of daily living (29).

There is evidence that all patients with artificial joints continue to be at some risk of hematogenous infection (30, 31), and that patients with rheumatoid arthritis and artificial joints are particularly prone to develop septic arthritis (13). With these considerations in mind and being aware of the long-term hazard of prosthetic loosening in these patients with osteoporotic bone, the rheumatoid patient who complains of pain or discomfort in the area of an orthopedic prosthesis warrants careful monitoring and appropriate investigations to exclude infection or loosening. Also, these patients should be advised to take prophylactic antibiotics before, during, and for several days after other bacteriogenic procedures, however minor. These procedures include dental extractions and urological, dermatological, and gynecological procedures.

Anatomic Categories

Shoulder

The shoulder is unusual when compared to other joints, in that it places a high demand on its soft tissue restraints for stability. Many of the muscle tendon units that bring about shoulder movement are in close anatomical proximity to the affected glenohumeral joint capsule and bone. Specifically, in the early stages of inflammatory arthritis, the rotator cuff complex is subject to painful inflammatory processes that ultimately lead to a nonfunctional cuff and perhaps even to partial or complete rupture of the cuff mechanism.

The cuff mechanism may be best understood as the muscular complex consisting of the supraspinatous, infraspinatous, teres minor, and subscapularis, which in addition to other roles, functions to position the humeral head dynamically on the glenoid during shoulder movement. Without the precise functioning of this complex and the major assistance from the deltoid muscle, all shoulder motion becomes painful; the rotator cuff itself is subject to inflammation, and its insertion into the greater tuberosity may become entrapped beneath the acromion and the coracoacromial ligament. These mechanical and inflammatory processes may lead to both anatomical and physiological disruption of the cuff mechanism. Early extraarticular surgical treatment may include debridement with release of the impinging coracoacromial ligament and removal of a small portion of the anterior acromion (32). Quite often such procedures are effective in diminishing the rate of wear of the cuff and in relieving pain. Additional soft tissue debridement may be carried out on the acromioclavicular joint. The biceps tendon is also commonly involved in the inflammatory process and may be treated by tenodesis (33). Arthroscopy shows significant promise (34, 35) when used to provide early debridement and synovectomy for inflammatory processes or avascular necrosis of the shoulder. Arthrotomy of the shoulder may be used for a more thorough synovectomy and for debridement of osteophytes, with good results in those cases that do not have degeneration severe enough to warrant more radical procedures. New developments in total joint replacement have now made available several prosthetic replacements for the humeral head and glenoid (36-39) (Figure 7.1).

The most widely used current total shoulder prosthetic designs consist of 1) a humeral head replacement that is fixed to the humerus by means of an intramedullary stem and methylmethacrylate, and 2) a glenoid component that consists of a

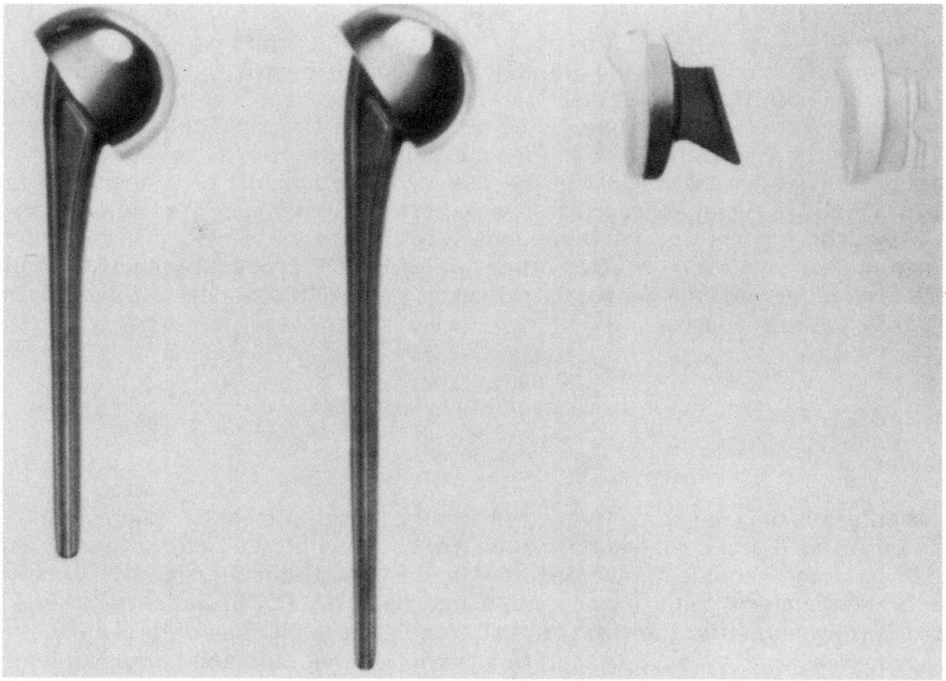

FIGURE 7.1 A total shoulder replacement of current design (monospherical). The humeral components (left) are variably sized and composed of cobalt-chrome alloy. The glenoid components (right) are composed of high-molecular-weight polyethylene and are backed with metal.

low-friction, high density polyethylene socket with or without a metal back and a central fin to enhance its fixation with methylmethacrylate to the glenoid portion of the scapula (40) (Figure 7.1). Results over the past 6 years suggest a reasonable degree of success with these devices and a high degree of patient satisfaction (39).

Arthrodesis of the shoulder may be considered as an alternative for end-stage arthritis of the shoulder. A study by Rybka et al. (41) of 41 patients with severe rheumatoid arthritis who underwent arthrodesis showed 68% with good to excellent results. In certain occupational groups such as laborers, shoulder arthrodesis remains a procedure worth considering. It is usually accomplished by resection of the cartilaginous surfaces and compression of the shoulder by means of external or internal fixation until fusion is achieved (42). Most reported rates of fusion are relatively high.

Elbow

A functioning elbow joint is essential for positioning the hand in space. It permits the movements of flexion and extension through an arc of 160°, as well as supination and pronation of the forearm through an arc of 180°. Arthritic restriction of elbow function can be compensated for, to some extent, by normal neighboring joints, which are usually present if the elbow arthritis was caused by trauma. When, however, there is also some restriction of the shoulder and wrist, the ability to position the hand in space is severely compromised. Synovectomy with or without radial head resection has had mixed results (43–45). Arthroscopic surgery and osteotomy are seldom used in the arthritic elbow. Resectional arthroplasty with or without interposition can give good relief of pain but stability and range of motion are compromised. Total joint replacement for the elbow is still very much in an early phase of development and there are multiple prosthetic designs currently under study (46–52); to date, most early reports show good relief of pain and a greater degree of stability and range of motion than that following resection-arthroplasty, but deep wound sepsis, dislocation, and ulnar nerve palsies have been frequent enough to be discouraging (46–52).

Elbow arthrodesis, if successful, provides stability and complete relief of pain. It is not advisable in the patient whose neighboring joints are also restricted, for example, in the rheumatoid arthritic patient; it is best suited for the younger patient with monoarticular disease who wishes to place normal power demands on the arm. Arthrodesis in 90° flexion is probably the most functional position and can be accomplished by any of several techniques (53–55).

Wrist

For severe arthritic involvement of the radiocarpal joint, either an arthrodesis or total wrist replacement may be indicated. An arthrodesis is the more time-proven of the two. When successful, it reliably relieves pain and provides a stable base for hand and finger movement. The operative techniques of Millender and Nalebuff (56) or of the AO-Group (55) are commonly used.

The selection of an arthrodesis versus a joint replacement at the wrist is influenced by the following factors:

1. Poor bone stock.
2. History of infection in or about the wrist.
3. Rupture or impending rupture of surrounding wrist flexors or extensors.
4. A mobile opposite wrist.

5. A young patient.
6. Involvement of lower extremity joints requiring or projected to require the use of a cane or crutch.

The disadvantage of an arthrodesis is loss of wrist motion and, in suitable candidates, the silicone arthroplasty of Swanson's design (57), as well as Volz's metallo-polyethylene type (58), has performed adequately.

Hand and Wrist

Partial synovectomy in the wrist for patients with symptoms consistent with early rheumatoid arthritis may, in addition to relieving symptoms, prevent rupture of the involved flexor tendons (59). This synovectomy can be done in combination with carpal tunnel release where needed. When a rheumatoid synovitis has resulted in rupture of an extensor tendon, tenosynovectomy is a therapeutic measure that should be undertaken relatively early (60, 61). Patients with dorsal prominence of the distal ulna are thought to be particularly prone to extensor tendon rupture, because the rupture is the result of combined attrition and synovitis. In this situation the procedure should include an excision of the distal ulna; replacement with a silastic prosthesis is advocated by some (62, 63) (Figure 7.2). Ideally, a dorsal synovectomy should be carried out in patients with synovitis of the extensor compartment before rupture of the tendon occurs (64). The principles of early synovectomy also apply on the volar aspect of the wrist: minimizing or eliminating the compression on the median nerve and of joint contractures, and avoidance of flexor tendon rupture (65). If the synovitis involves the hand, there may be palpable crepitus in the palm with active finger flexion (63). Flexor tenosynovectomy at the fingers with an aim toward avoidance of joint contractures is

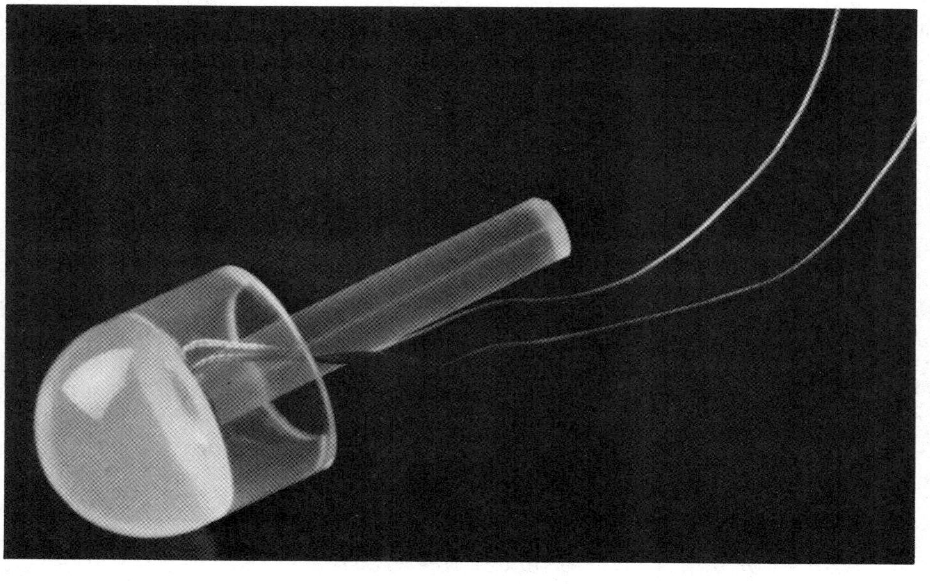

FIGURE 7.2 Silastic replacement for the distal ulna (courtesy Dow Corning Company).

indicated when there is a discrepancy between the active and passive range of motion (65). Flexor tenosynovectomy should be carried out in patients who present with flexor tendon rupture, and if the cause is thought to be partly attritional with changes secondary to an osteophyte, that osteophyte should be removed, the tendon should be repaired or grafted, and a synovectomy should be carried out (65). If the flexor tendon is ruptured in the wrist, a tendon graft can be used for the flexor pollicis longus and side-to-side suture of the flexor digitorum profundis can be used. If a single tendon rupture is diagnosed within the digit or palm, tenodesis or arthrodesis of the distal interphalangeal joint in addition to the flexor tenosynovectomy can be performed if the profundis is involved, or one may excise the tendon if the sublimis is involved (66).

The results of synovectomy of the joints of the fingers, carpus, and wrist are difficult to evaluate, but synovectomy seems to alleviate pain, slow the erosive process and hence the progress of deformity, and lessen the likelihood that the neighboring tendons will rupture. When medical management is unsuccessful, synovectomy is carried out either alone or in combination with other procedures such as release of the carpal tunnel.

Hand and Fingers

Although resection arthroplasty (64) is an option, replacement of the severely diseased metacarpophalangeal joint with a flexible silastic prosthesis has enjoyed great success in recent years (67) (Figure 7.3). Candidates are patients with severe arthritic involvement of fixed or stiff metacarpophalangeal joints with architectural deformities (e.g., ulnar drift) unresponsive to splinting (65). When metacarpophalangeal joint replacement is executed properly, one can expect excellent

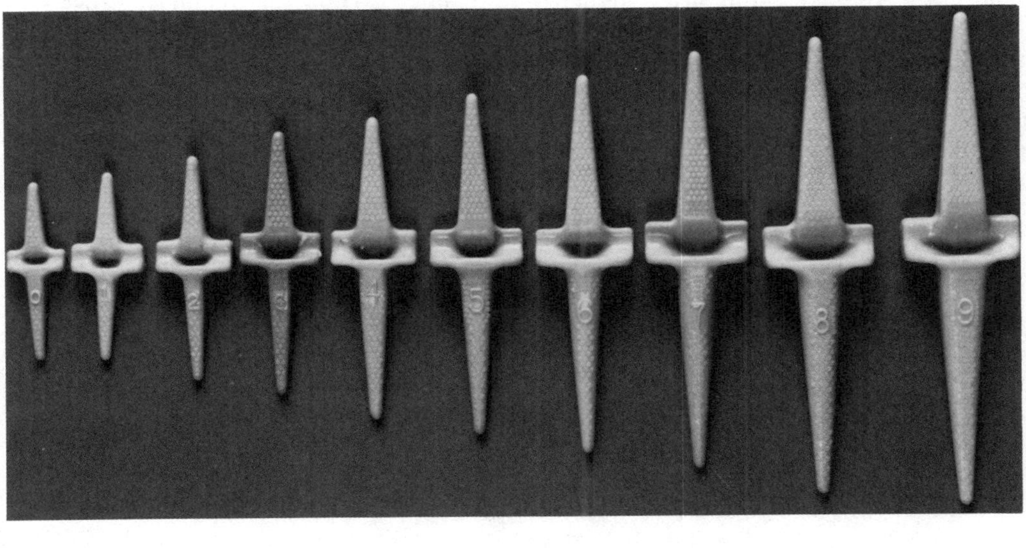

FIGURE 7.3 Flexible silastic implants used to replace the metacarpophalangeal joints and occasionally the proximal interphalangeal joints.

relief of pain, a reasonable restoration of alignment, and a functional range of motion. Correction of soft tissue laxity and tightness is important. Splinting to neutralize the tendency toward recurrence of malalignment and assurance of early active joint motion are essential postoperatively for a good result (68). The incidence of infection is low (69), and long-term functional results are encouraging (67).

Arthrodesis is usually indicated for severely affected proximal interphalangeal joints, especially the joint of the index finger of a manual laborer (67, 70). Silastic implants are occasionally indicated for arthritis involving the proximal interphalangeal joints. They do fairly well in the ulnar three digits of patients with osteoarthritis (71) or posttraumatic arthritis (72); they are less successful in patients with rheumatoid arthritis for several reasons: stretching of the central slip with flexion deformity of the joint can be secondary to synovitis of the proximal interphalangeal joint; hyperextension deformity can be secondary to synovitic involvement of the volar plate with secondary stretching aggravated by rupture of the flexor sublimis tendon; and integrity of the proximal interphalangeal collateral ligament is necessary for a satisfactory silastic arthroplasty, and often this is not the case in rheumatoid arthritis.

The distal interphalangeal joint, when the arthritic process causes pain, deformity, or rupture of the flexor profundis tendon, is best managed by arthrodesis. The ideal position for arthrodesis of the distal interphalangeal joint is either in full extension or in slight flexion. A careful evaluation of the proximal interphalangeal joint and correction of any pathological condition (for example, boutonnière deformity or swan neck deformity) at that level is advisable before any formal procedure on the distal interphalangeal joint is done.

Thumb

The most common rheumatoid arthritic deformity of the thumb consists of hyperflexion deformity at the metacarpophalangeal joint level and secondary hyperextension deformity at the interphalangeal joint level (73). This latter deformity is corrected by fusion of the interphalangeal joint, and a motion-preserving joint arthroplasty of the resectional or implant type can be utilized at the metacarpophalangeal joint (74). If the secondary deformities at the interphalangeal joint are not severe, an arthrodesis of the metacarpophalangeal joint can be used.

Hip

The hip is a major weight-bearing joint with large muscle forces acting across it. Arthritic changes, once underway, are alleviated to a certain extent by efforts to diminish these forces (for example, by limping or by using a cane or crutch) or by medical measures, but, in time, the changes usually progress despite those efforts.

Synovectomy of the hip, although reported to be efficacious by some (75), is seldom used, and arthroscopy is not well suited to the hip joint for anatomical reasons: the small, narrow joint space and the large amounts of soft tissue between the skin and the capsule.

Osteotomy is still used by some surgeons in the management of localized coxarthrosis, usually that due to traumatic or early osteoarthritis (12, 75-77). The procedure may be a reasonable alternative to total joint replacement in the young patient with localized monoarticular disease and, if it is done for femoral head containment or coverage, it may make a future total hip replacement more likely to succeed by providing a more correctly oriented bony anchor for seating of the acetabular component (78, 79).

Total joint replacement of the hip is the operation that has introduced a new surgical era. It has gained well-deserved public and professional approval and is indicated for most patients with severe coxarthrosis. The results provide good motion with almost complete pain relief in most patients. Surgeons wary of the development of late loosening prefer to offer this procedure only to patients over 60 years of age. The exception is the patient with polyarthritis, whose restricted neighboring joints leave few viable therapeutic alternatives (and will restrict the patient's activities overall); thus the patient with severe juvenile rheumatoid arthritis may also be a candidate for a total hip replacement as early as his second or third decade of life.

Hip arthrodesis is well suited for the young male patient with quiescent monoarticular infectious arthritis. The hip is usually positioned in slight (10°) adduction, neutral rotation, and slight (15-20°) flexion, and most techniques employ internal fixation (80, 81).

Resectional arthroplasty, popularized in 1923 by Girdlestone (82), is currently used as a salvage procedure for patients with failed hip replacements or infections. In the wheelchair-bound patient with a painful arthritic hip, or the nonambulatory patient who has sustained severe trauma to the hip area with fracture, a resectional arthroplasty is a reasonable option.

Knee

The goals of surgical therapy of the arthritic knee are first to relieve pain and second to preserve function as a major weight-bearing joint. Rheumatoid arthritis or its variants most commonly involve all three knee compartments (patellofemoral, lateral, and medial) and, in long-standing rheumatoid arthritis, there is characteristically a valgus angulation with some external rotation and lateral subluxation of the tibia on the femur. In osteoarthritis, on the other hand, a varus angulation is more common because the arthritis is most commonly initially confined to the medial compartment. Flexion contractures are also quite common in joints affected by rheumatoid arthritis; they are not commonly associated with osteoarthritis.

Synovectomy of an arthritic knee may afford the patient some relief of pain, alleviation of swelling, and some restoration of joint motion/function (83, 84).

Arthrodesis is a suitable procedure for young men affected by a severe monoarticular arthrosis. Arthroscopy and joint debridement with arthroscopic synovectomy and chrondroplastic shaving are being used more frequently now. This technique has the advantage of minimizing the surgical wound; it may afford temporary pain relief and an attendant increase in knee function, and it may forestall the need for a more extensive reconstruction of the knee.

Osteotomy of the proximal tibia for isolated medial compartment arthritis has been shown to unweight the medial compartment effectively. It can provide excellent pain relief and restoration of knee function provided that, preoperatively, the knee is stable, there is less than 15° varus, and the lateral compartment is free of arthritis, and provided that, postoperatively, correct alignment in slight valgus (10°) is obtained (85, 86). For several reasons, this procedure is less satisfactory when isolated lateral compartment arthritis is present, perhaps the most important reason being the resultant obliquity of the knee joint, which causes medial subluxation of the femur and varus deformity. Also, the higher incidence of peroneal nerve complications following high tibial varus osteotomy makes this procedure less than desirable. For these reasons, an osteotomy for lateral compartment arthritis should be done on the femoral side, but here again there are potential complications with higher morbidity, more frequent nonunion, and occasional knee stiffness due to postoperative tethering of the quadriceps mechanism.

Total knee replacement is indicated in patients with severe arthritis of the knee whose symptoms of pain and limitation of motion justify the risks of the operation. Correction of soft tissue contractures by appropriately designed releases is necessary in the more severely deformed knees. Knees with flexion contractures may require manipulation of the contractures under anesthesia combined with a posterior capsulotomy. Subperiosteal release of the pes anserinus, periosteum, and deep medial collateral ligament at the level of the proximal tibia may be necessary for knees with severe varus deformity. Release of the fascia about the peroneal nerve combined with subperiosteal release of the iliotibial band and lateral intermuscular septum at the level of the distal femur and longitudinal release of the patella retinaculum may be necessary for knees with severe valgus deformity. Most currently used total knee prostheses are metal on high-molecular-weight polyethylene surface replacements. Most current designs have a central fixation peg for the metal (usually cobalt-chrome alloy) portion of the tibial component; a high-molecular-weight polyethylene tibial component rests on the metal tray anchored in the tibia. The femoral component is made of cobalt-chrome alloy. Most current designs also have a high-molecular-weight polyethylene button that replaces the articular surface of the patella (Figure 7.4). Fully constrained, hinged prostheses of the Walldius, Shiers, and Guepar designs suffer for biomechanical reasons (rotatory stresses generated at the bone cement interface with flexion and extension of the knee) and their use has been followed by high rates of loosening, breakage, and infection (87). In addition, because of the considerable magnitude of bone resected during insertion, future revision—either replacement with a second prosthesis or an attempt at arthrodesis—is a formidable undertaking.

Current prosthetic designs that can bypass the need for methylmethacrylate anchorage in the bone by the use of a porous coating along portions of the metallic implant exposed to the surface of the bone may help alleviate the long-term problem of component loosening. But long-term results of clinical trials with this type of prosthesis in the knee are not yet available.

Ankle

The ankle is a major weight-bearing joint with a low capsule-to-articular cartilage contact surface ratio; it is not well suited to arthroscopic debridement and synovectomy. Open surgical debridement is also seldom effective, and there is little to be gained from soft tissue reconstruction or osteotomy once the arthritic process is underway. The use of a patella-tendon-bearing brace may help alleviate pain while relieving the ankle of the brunt of its weight-bearing role. Enthusiasm for total ankle replacement in rheumatoid patients has been mixed (88-91). The progression of radiolucent lines and clinical loosening has been a problem, and the procedure is reserved, therefore, for selected cases.

An effective surgical procedure for significant arthritis of the ankle is arthrodesis of the ankle joint. This procedure offers a high degree of reliability and relative freedom from complications such as infection and loosening. There are many reported techniques of ankle arthrodesis. The ideal position for arthrodesis is neutral and 0° or slight valgus alignment after the joint surfaces are resected (92). Immobilization is required for 6-12 weeks. Nonunion may occur in 10-20% of cases, but, in our experience, even in such cases good relief of pain is accomplished. Ankle joint arthrodesis can be successfully combined with total knee and total hip replacement in the panarthritic patient.

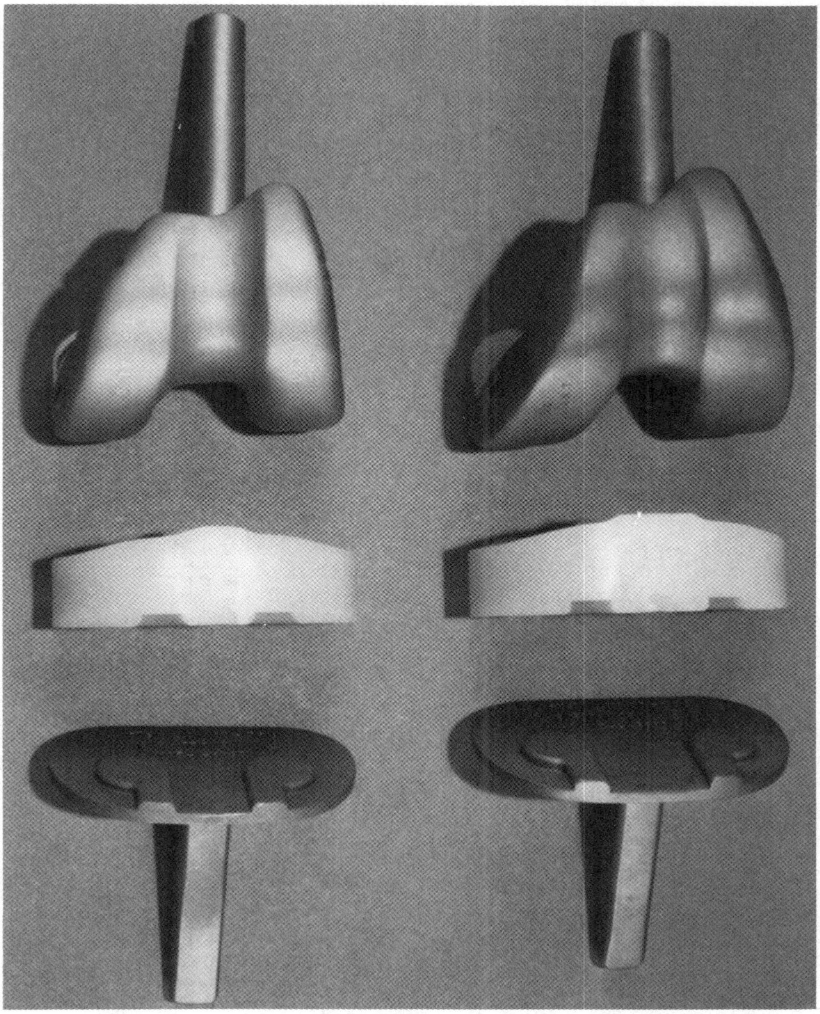

FIGURE 7.4 Trial total knee replacement components of a current design. The femoral component (above) and the tibial component (below) are made of implantable metal (usually cobalt-chrome alloy). The tibial surface component is made of high-molecular-weight polyethylene. Most manufacturers produce a range of component sizes. The button of high-molecular-weight polyethylene that replaces the articular surface of the patella is not shown.

Foot

The majority of the 5 million patients who suffer from rheumatoid arthritis in this country have some involvement of the joints of their feet (93, 94), most commonly, the forefoot joints (95). Initially, this arthritis manifests itself as synovitis with swelling, tenderness, and some erythema. Movement of the joints as well as lateral compression of the distal metatarsals elicits tenderness. As the condition progresses, the intermetatarsal ligaments become lax and the forefoot splays. In these early stages, as the disease characteristically progresses, there is a valgus deformity of the first toe at the metatarsophalangeal joint, the lateral four toes progressively sublux dorsally at the metatarsophalangeal joint level, and the interphalangeal joints develop a flexion deformity, which leads to either a claw toe or a hammer toe deformity. The forefoot's plantar fat pad gradually shifts distally (96). This shift, in combination with compromised biomechanics resulting in increased load transmission through the metatarsal heads when the deformed toes are unable to participate in the toe-off phase of gait, results in painful secondary callosities typically over the heads of the second and third metatarsals.

Surgical management of these deformities is indicated when nonoperative methods, including modification of shoe wear, fail to afford relief of symptoms. In these early stages, as forefoot deformity progresses, the Hoffman procedure (97) can be employed. When the first metatarsal is short (that is, no longer than the metatarsal neck of the second ray), a Keller procedure (98) can be used for the first ray instead of resection of the metatarsal head.

When the joints of the midfoot are involved, a limited arthrodesis is often satisfactory, for example, talonavicular fusion for localized talonavicular joint involvement or local arthrodesis for metatarsal cuneiform arthritis (99, 100). When the hindfoot is affected by rheumatoid arthritis, the most common secondary deformity is a valgus deformity. If the deformity is mild, it can be managed with shoes modified with a one-eighth of an inch inner heel wedge or sometimes a Thomas heel. If there is greater valgus deformity of the hindfoot, which can still be corrected passively, a short-leg orthosis with an outer upright bar and an inner T-strap will be enough to control the deformity. If the ankle is also involved, a double upright bar, ankle foot orthosis (AFO) may be required. If the deformity cannot be corrected passively and there is multiple joint involvement, or if orthotic management is unacceptable, the problem is best solved by an arthrodesis. A triple arthrodesis usually suffices (101, 102), but if the ankle is also involved with arthritis and participates in the valgus deformity of the hindfoot, a pantalar arthrodesis may be considered (93). Other options include a talectomy (103) or a triple arthrodesis combined with a joint arthroplasty for the ankle.

The role of surgical treatment of the arthritic foot is not to restore the foot to normal function but to achieve pain relief and restoration of foot architecture compatible with wearing shoes and providing support for ambulation.

Other surgical procedures that are occasionally required in the arthritic foot are resection of rheumatoid nodules, shaving of painful callosities, repair of ruptured tendons secondary to chronic tenosynovitis, resection of painful bursae, and release of the tarsal tunnel when symptoms of tarsal tunnel syndrome are the result of the arthritic process, for example, the result of hypertrophic synovitis.

Spine

The role of surgery in the management of spinal arthritis is largely confined to the cervical spine. Synovitis can weaken structures of the cervical spine so that secondary subluxation can and often does result. As Winfield et al. (104) have pointed out, cervical instability may manifest itself rather early in the course of the disease (greater than 80% of cases within 2 years). It resulted in atlantoaxial subluxation in 12%, atlantoaxial impaction in 3%, and subaxial subluxation in 20% of 100 patients studied prospectively with annual cervical roentgenograms from the onset of their disease.

Atlantoaxial subluxation is most common anteriorly, although posterior and lateral subluxations are also possible. Anterior subluxation greater than 3.5 mm in an adult is regarded as abnormal (105). Subaxial subluxations can be found at multiple levels in patients with rheumatoid arthritis. Although these subluxations alone do not constitute an indication for surgical intervention, as they progress they may jeopardize the anatomical and physiological integrity of the spinal cord as well as the vertebral artery.

Neurological involvement is the major indication for surgical treatment. A period of skull traction is advisable preoperatively to reduce the cervical spine and alleviate the impingement.

Computed tomography and plain tomography are useful studies that clearly delineate these architectural aberrations as well as their relation to vital structures. Clinically, neurological changes can be vague and may include occipital neuralgia, upper motor neuron signs, abnormal reflexes, vertebrobasilary insufficiency, bulbar disturbances, and severe pain in a radicular distribution.

Posterior spinal fusion of the involved levels, supplemented by internal fixation to allow early mobilization is the procedure most commonly used for stabilizing the involved cervical spine. The role of anterior fusion as well as laminectomy for the arthritic cervical spine has not yet been delineated clearly (106).

Trends

The indications are that total joint replacement will continue to be the mainstay of definitive treatment for significantly involved arthritic joints. There continues to be some expanding promise that early arthroscopic synovectomy may result in several years of symptomatic relief but not necessarily in long-term suppression of the disease. There will be expansion of early interventional soft-tissue operations about the shoulder for relief of soft tissue, rotator cuff, and biceps tendon disease, as these interventions become more and more familiar to practicing surgeons.

A significant body of study has been devoted to the use of allografts, and while they show some promise in the reconstruction of joints following removal of tumors, there is as yet little indication for their use in the management of arthritis.

Various arthroscopic techniques are being investigated for replacement of surface cartilage. Those techniques involving abrasion chondroplasty seem to yield only transient relief of pain and secondary replacement by fibrocartilage without significantly intervening in the course of the disease. Some experimental work is being performed in the transfer of cellular surface cartilaginous elements, but no definitive information is available on the results at this time. Surface allograft transplants remain in an experimental stage of investigation.

In summary, despite the exciting experimental work mentioned above, a look at the history of the surgical management of arthritis shows that many of the surgical procedures performed on arthritic joints years ago are still being used today. One would surmise that tomorrow's surgical options for the patient with severe arthritis will not be all that different from today's, although our ability to predict and thereby forestall the advance of arthritis in a predisposed patient may reach new levels of sophistication.

References

1. Barton JR: On the treatment of anchylosis, by the formation of artificial joints. Reproduced in *Clin Orthop* 182:4-13, 1984.

2. Volkmann R von: Die Synovektomie unter besonderer Berucksichtigung der an der Erlanger Chirurgischen Universitatsklinik erzielten Erfolge. Dissertation, Erlangen, 1952 [cited by Gschwend R (55)].

3. Lugli T: Artificial shoulder joint by Péan (1893): The facts of an exceptional intervention and the prosthetic method. *Clin Orthop* 133:215-218, 1978.

4. Charnley J: Anchorage of the femoral head prosthesis to the shaft of the femur. *J Bone Joint Surg* 42B:28-30, 1960.

5. Moore AT: Metal hip joint: A new self-locking vitallium prosthesis. *South Med J* 45:1015-1019, 1952.

6. Smith-Petersen MN: Treatment of fractures of the neck of the femur by internal fixation. *Surg Gynecol Obstet* 64:287-295, 1937.

7. Keller CS, Stulberg SD: The principles and results of arthroscopic surgical treatment of rheumatoid arthritis of the knee (abstract). *Orthop Trans* 6: 425, 1982.

8. Bray T, Glick J, Gordon R: Arthroscopic management of the osteoarthritic knee (abstract). *Orthop Trans* 6:98, 1982.

9. Zarins B: Arthroscopic resection of osteophytes of the knee (abstract). *Orthop Trans* 6:108, 1982.

10. Del Pizzo W, Quante W, Fox J, Friedman M, Snyder S, Seagraves R: Operative arthroscopy for treatment of fibroarthrosis of the knee (abstract). *Orthop Trans* 8:67-68, 1984.

11. Jakubowski S, Pongowska J: Indikationen zur synovektomie bei pcP. *Orthopade* 2:6, 1973.

12. Bombelli R, Santore RF, Poss R: Mechanics of the normal and osteoarthritic hip: A new perspective. *Clin Orthop* 182:69-78, 1984.

13. Gristina AG, Rovere GD, Shoji H: Spontaneous septic arthritis complicating rheumatoid arthritis. *J Bone Joint Surg* 56A:1180-1184, 1974.

14. Kellgren JH, Ball J, Fairbrother RW, Barnes KL: Suppurative arthritis complicating rheumatoid arthritis. *Br Med J* 1:1193-1200, 1958.

15. Garner RW, Mowat AG, Hazleman BL: Wound healing after operations on patients with rheumatoid arthritis. *J Bone Joint Surg* 55B:134-144, 1973.

16. Schorn D, Mowat AG: Penicillamine in rheumatoid arthritis: Wound healing, skin thickness and osteoporosis. *Rheumatol Rehabil* 16:223-230, 1977.

17. Harris ED Jr: Pathogenesis of rheumatoid arthritis. *Clin Orthop* 182:14–23, 1984.

18. Antisecretory/Antiulcer Agents/Antispasmodics/Urinary Agents. In ES Greffner (ed.), *Compendium of Drug Therapy.* New York, Biomedical Information Corporation, 17, 1–31, 1982.

19. Lambert JR, Wright V: Surgery in patients with psoriasis and arthritis. *Rheumatol Rehabil* 18:35–37, 1979.

20. Conway WA, Bower GC, Barnes ME: Hypersomnolence and intermittent upper airway obstruction. Occurrence caused by micrognathia. *JAMA* 237: 2740–2742, 1977.

21. Crellin RQ, Maccabe JJ, Hamilton EBD: Severe subluxation of the cervical spine in rheumatoid arthritis. *J Bone Joint Surg* 52B:244–251, 1970.

22. Rana NA, Hancock DO, Taylor AR, Hill AGS: Upward translocation of the dens in rheumatoid arthritis. *J Bone Joint Surg* 55B:471–477, 1973.

23. Nakano, KK: Neurologic complications of rheumatoid arthritis. *Orthop Clin North Am* 6:861–880, 1975.

24. Taylor AR, Kamdar BA, Arden GP: Ectopic ossification following total hip replacement (abstract). *J Bone Joint Surg* 58B:134, 1976.

25. Finerman GAM, Brooker AF Jr, Coventry MB, Krengel WF Jr, McRoberts RL, Salvati EA, Volz RG: The Carmel Symposium on Heterotopic Ossification Following Total Hip Replacement (Monograph). Distributor: Procter and Gamble, 1981, pp. 1–28.

26. Ritter MA, Gioe TJ: The effect of indomethacin on paraarticular ectopic ossification following total hip arthroplasty. *Clin Orthop* 167:113–117, 1982.

27. Coventry MB, Scanlon PW: The use of radiation to discourage ectopic bone. A 9-year-study in surgery about the hip. *J Bone Joint Surg* 63A:201–208, 1981.

28. Scott RD, Sledge CB: The surgery of juvenile rheumatoid arthritis. In WN Kelley, ED Harris, S Ruddy, CB Sledge (eds.), *Textbook of Rheumatology.* Philadelphia, W. B. Saunders, 1981, pp. 2014–2019.

29. Melvin JL: *Rheumatic Disease: Occupational Therapy and Rehabilitation,* 2nd Ed. Philadelphia, F. A. Davis, 1982, pp. 109–111.

30. D'Ambrosia RD, Shoji H, Heater R: Secondarily infected total joint replacements by hematogenous spread. *J Bone Joint Surg* 58A:450–453, 1976.

31. Gristina AG, Kolkin J: Total joint replacement and sepsis. *J Bone Joint Surg* 65A:123–134, 1983.

32. Neviaser TJ, Neviaser RJ, Neviaser JS, Neviaser JS: The four-in-one arthroplasty for the painful arc syndrome. *Clin Orthop* 163:107-112, 1982.

33. Dines D, Warren RF, Inglis AE: Surgical treatment of lesions of the long head of the biceps. *Clin Orthop* 164:165-171, 1982.

34. Caspari RB: Shoulder arthroscopy: A review of the present state of the art. *Contemp Orthop* 4:523-531, 1982.

35. Johnson LL: Arthroscopy of the shoulder. *Orthop Clin North Am* 11:197-204, 1980.

36. Post M, Jablon M: Constrained total shoulder arthroplasty. Long-term follow-up observations. *Clin Orthop* 173:109-116, 1983.

37. Gristina AG, Webb LX: The trispherical total shoulder replacement. In I Bayley, L Kessel (eds.), *Shoulder Surgery,* New York, Springer-Verlag, 1980, pp. 153-156.

38. Ranawat CS, Warren R, Inglis AE: Total shoulder replacement arthroplasty. *Orthop Clin North Am* 11:367-373, 1980.

39. Cofield RH; Unconstrained total shoulder prostheses. *Clin Orthop* 173:97-108, 1983.

40. Gristina AG, Webb LX: Shoulder and humerus: Reconstruction. In *Orthopaedic Knowledge Update-I, Home Study Syllabus,* Chicago, American Academy of Orthopedic Surgeons, 1984, pp. 125-132.

41. Rybka V, Raunio P, Vainio K: Arthrodesis of the shoulder in rheumatoid arthritis: A review of 41 cases. *J Bone Joint Surg* 61B:155-158, 1979.

42. Cofield RH: Arthrodesis and resectional arthroplasty of the shoulder. In C McC Evarts (ed.), *Surgery of the Musculoskeletal System.* New York, Churchill Livingstone, 1983, pp. 109-124.

43. Inglis AE, Ranawat CS, Straub LR: Synovectomy and debridement of the elbow in rheumatoid arthritis. *J Bone Joint Surg* 53A:652-662, 1971.

44. Taylor AR, Mukerjea SK, Rana NA: Excision of the head of the radius in rheumatoid arthritis. *J Bone Joint Surg* 58B:485-487, 1976.

45. Ferlic DC, Clayton ML, Parr PL: Surgery of the elbow in rheumatoid arthritis (abstract). *J Bone Joint Surg* 58A:726, 1976.

46. Hass J: Functional arthroplasty. *J Bone Joint Surg* 26:297-306, 1944.

47. Dickson RA, Stein H, Bentley G: Excision arthroplasty of the elbow in rheumatoid disease. *J Bone Joint Surg* 58B:227-229, 1976.

48. Dee R: Total replacement of the elbow joint. *Orthop Clin North Am* 4:415-433, 1973.

49. Dunn HK, Carson RW: Total replacement of the elbow (abstract). *J Bone Joint Surg* 56A:196, 1974.

50. Ewald FC: Nonconstrained metal to plastic total elbow arthroplasty in rheumatoid arthritis (abstract). *Orthop Trans* 1:110, 1977.

51. London JT: Resurfacing total elbow arthroplasty (abstract). *Orthop Trans* 2:217, 1978.

52. Rosenberg GM, Turner RH: Nonconstrained total elbow arthroplasty. *Clin Orthop* 187:154-162, 1984.

53. Steindler A: *Reconstructive Surgery of the Upper Extremity.* New York, D. Appleton and Company, 1923.

54. Brittain HA: *Architectural Principles in Arthrodesis.* Edinburgh, Livingston, 1952, pp. 161-167.

55. Muller ME, Allgower M, Schneider R, Willenegger H: Arthrodesis of the elbow and of the wrist. In J Shatzker (translator), *Manual of Internal Fixation: Technique Recommendations by the AO-Group,* 2nd Ed. New York, Springer-Verlag, 1979, pp. 386-387.

56. Millender LH, Nalebuff EA: Arthrodesis of the rheumatoid wrist. An evaluation of 60 patients and a description of a different surgical technique. *J Bone Joint Surg* 55A:1026-1034, 1973.

57. Swanson AB: Flexible implant arthroplasty for arthritic disabilities of the radiocarpal joint. A silicone rubber intramedullary stemmed flexible hinge implant for the wrist joint. *Orthop Clin North Am* 4:383-394, 1973.

58. Volz RG: Total wrist arthroplasty. *Clin Orthop* 189:112-120, 1984.

59. Gschwend N: Synovectomy. In WN Kelley, ED Harris, S Ruddy, CB Sledge (eds.), *Textbook of Rheumatology,* Vol. II. Philadelphia, W. B. Saunders, 1981, pp. 1874-1899.

60. Linscheid RL: Surgery for rheumatoid arthritis—timing and techniques: The upper extremity. *J Bone Joint Surg* 50A:605-613, 1968.

61. Nalebuff EA, Potter TA: Rheumatoid involvement of tendon and tendon sheaths in the hand. *Clin Orthop* 59:147-159, 1968.

62. Cracchiolo A III, Marmor L: Resection of the distal ulna in rheumatoid arthritis. *Arthritis Rheum* 12:415-422, 1969.

63. Swanson AB: The ulnar head syndrome and its treatment by implant resection arthroplasty (abstract). *J Bone Joint Surg* 54A:906, 1972.

64. Nalebuff EA: Surgical treatment of tendon rupture in the rheumatoid hand. *Surg Clin North Am* 49:811-822, 1969.

65. Millender LH, Nalebuff EA: Preventive surgery—Tenosynovectomy and synovectomy. *Orthop Clin North Am* 6:765-792, 1975.

66. Nalebuff EA, Millender LH: Reconstructive surgery and rehabilitation of the hand. In WN Kelley, ED Harris, S Ruddy, CB Sledge (eds.), *Textbook of Rheumatology,* Vol. II. Philadelphia, W. B. Saunders, 1981, pp. 1900-1920.

67. Swanson AB: Flexible implant arthroplasty for arthritic finger joints. Rationale, technique, and results of treatment. *J Bone Joint Surg* 54A:435-455, 1972.

68. Swanson AB: Flexible implant resection arthroplasty. *Hand* 4:119-134, 1972.

69. Millender LH, Nalebuff EA, Hawkins RB, Ennis R: Infection after silicone prosthetic arthroplasty in the hand. *J Bone Joint Surg* 57A:825-829, 1975.

70. Granowitz S, Vainio K: Proximal interphalangeal joint arthrodesis in rheumatoid arthritis. A follow-up study of 122 operations. *Acta Orthop Scand* 37:301-310, 1966.

71. Burton RI: The arthritic hand. In C McC Evarts (ed.), *Surgery of the Musculoskeletal System.* New York, Churchill Livingstone, 1983, pp. 621-692.

72. Strickland JW, Dustman JA, Stelzer L, Stromberg WB, Steichen JB, Bell JL: Posttraumatic arthritis of the proximal interphalangeal joint. *Orthop Rev* 11:75-83, 1982.

73. Nalebuff EA: Diagnosis, classification and management of rheumatoid thumb deformities. *Bull Hosp Joint Dis* 29:119-137, 1968.

74. Swanson AB, Herndon JH: flexible (silicone) implant arthroplasty of the metacarpophalangeal joint of the thumb. *J Bone Joint Surg* 59A:362-368, 1977.

75. Lipscomb PR: Surgery for rheumatoid arthritis—timing and techniques: Summary. *J Bone Joint Surg* 50A:614-617, 1968.

76. Chiari K: Medial displacement osteotomy of the pelvis. *Clin Orthop* 98:55-71, 1974.

77. Mueller KH: Resection of the femoral head and neck and resection-angulation osteotomy. In RG Tronzo (ed.), *Surgery of the Hip Joint.* Philadelphia, Lea and Febiger, 1973, pp. 644-656.

78. Coleman SS: *Congenital Dysplasia and Dislocation of the Hip.* St. Louis, C. V. Mosby Company, 1978, pp. 209-248.

79. Hoffman DV, Simmons EH, Barrington TW: The results of Chiari osteotomy. *Clin Orthop* 98:162-170, 1974.

80. Muller ME, Allgower M, Schneider R, Willenegger H: Arthrodesis of the hip with the cobra plate. Technique of R. Schneider. In J Shatzker (translator), *Manual of Internal Fixation. Technique Recommendations by the AO-Group,* 2nd Ed. New York, Springer-Verlag, 1979, pp. 386-389.

81. Liechti R: *Hip Arthrodesis and Associated Problems,* PA Casey (translator), Berlin, Springer, 1978, p. 269.

82. Girdlestone GR, et al.: In Discussion on treatment of unilateral osteoarthritis of the hip-joint, section of Orthopedics. *Proc R Soc Med* 38:363-368, 1945.

83. Mori M, Ogawa R: Anterior capsulectomy in the treatment of rheumatoid arthritis of the knee joint. *Arthritis Rheum* 6:130-137, 1963.

84. Gschwend N, Winer J, Boni A: *Clinical Results of Synovectomy in Rheumatoid Arthritis.* Darmstadt, D. Steinkopff-Verlag, 1977, pp. 1-45.

85. Coventry MB: Upper tibial osteotomy. *Clin Orthop* 182:46-52, 1984.

86. Insall J, Shoji H, Mayer V: High tibial osteotomy. A 5-year-evaluation. *J Bone Joint Surg* 56A:1397-1405, 1974.

87. Deburge A: Guepar hinge prosthesis. Complications and results with 2 years' follow-up. *Clin Orthop* 120:47-53, 1976.

88. Lachiewicz PF, Inglis AE, Ranawat CS: Total ankle replacement in rheumatoid arthritis. *J Bone Joint Surg* 66A:340-343, 1984.

89. Stauffer RN: Total joint arthroplasty. The ankle. *Mayo Clin Proc* 54:570-575, 1979.

90. Demottaz JD, Mazur JM, Thomas WH, Sledge CB, Simon SR: Clinical study of total ankle replacement with gait analysis. A preliminary report. *J Bone Joint Surg* 61A:976-988, 1979.

91. Newton St E III: Total ankle arthroplasty. Clinical study of 50 cases. *J Bone Joint Surg* 64A:104-111, 1982.

92. Stauffer RN: Intraarticular ankle problems. In C. McC Evarts (ed.), *Surgery of the Musculoskeletal System.* New York, Churchill Livingstone, 1983, pp. 115-142.

93. Rana NA: Rheumatoid arthritis, other collagen diseases, and psoriasis of the foot. In MH Jahss (ed.), *Disorders of the Foot,* Vol. II, Philadelphia, W. B. Saunders, 1982, pp. 1024-1063.

94. Vainio K: The rheumatoid foot. A clinical study with pathological and roentgenological comments. *Ann Chir Gynaecol* (Suppl. 1)1:1-107, 1956.

95. Thomas WH: Reconstructive surgery and rehabilitation of the ankle and foot. In WN Kelley, ED Harris, S Ruddy, CB Sledge (eds.), *Textbook of Rheumatology.* Philadelphia, W. B. Saunders, 1981, pp. 1999-2013.

96. Kates A, Kessel L, Kay A: Arthroplasty of the forefoot. *J Bone Joint Surg* 49B:552-557, 1967.

97. Hoffman P: An operation for severe grades of contracted or clawed toes. *Am J Orthop Surg* 9:441-449, 1912.

98. Keller WL: The surgical treatment of bunions and hallux valgus. *NY Med J* 80:741, 1904.

99. Jones WN: Treatment of rheumatoid arthritis of the foot and ankle. In RL Druess, NS Mitchell (eds.), *Surgery of Rheumatoid Arthritis.* Philadelphia, J.B. Lippincott, 1971, pp. 87-92.

100. Clayton ML: Surgical treatment of the rheumatoid foot. In NJ Giannestras (ed.), *Foot Disorders: Medical and Surgical Management,* 2nd Ed. Philadelphia, Lea and Febiger, 1973, pp. 444-466.

101. Benson GM, Johnson EW Jr: Management of the foot in rheumatoid arthritis. *Orthop Clin North Am* 2:733-744, 1971.

102. Clayton ML: Surgery of the lower extremity in rheumatoid arthritis. *J Bone Joint Surg* 45A:1517-1536, 1963.

103. Murray WR, Inman VT: Vascular and metabolic disorders affecting the foot. In VT Inman (ed.), *DuVries' Surgery of the Foot.* St. Louis, C. V. Mosby Company, 1973, pp. 282-288.

104. Winfield J, Cooke D, Brook AS, Corbett M: A prospective study of the radiological changes in the cervical spine in early rheumatoid disease. *Ann Rheum Dis* 40:109-114, 1981.

105. Lipson SJ: Rheumatoid arthritis of the cervical spine. *Clin Orthop* 182: 143-149, 1984.

106. Conaty JP, Mongan ES: Cervical fusion in rheumatoid arthritis. *J Bone Joint Surg* 63A:1218-1227, 1981.

Part II

RHEUMATOLOGIC DISEASES

Chapter 8

RHEUMATOID ARTHRITIS

Robert A. Turner, M.D.

The first descriptions of polyarticular synovitis leading to deformities and disability are in an ancient Indian text with source material dated from the sixth century B.C. and revisions dated from the first century A.D. (1). There has been much controversy as to whether rheumatoid arthritis is the disease described by many subsequent observers (2). Sydenham (1624-1689) probably described some of the main features of rheumatoid arthritis under the heading Rheumatismus (2). Recent articles have suggested that several of the Flemish painters (1400-1700), Botticelli (1445-1510) and Rubens (1577-1640), have depicted the features of this disease in their paintings (3-5). Over the years it has been difficult but necessary to separate patients with this symmetrical, chronic, inflammatory, polyarticular, and extraarticular disease from patients with other types of arthritis. In 1859 Garrod proposed the name rheumatoid arthritis with subsequent eminent clinicians such as Still in 1896 and Felty in 1924 expanding our concepts of the clinical manifestations of this important disease in children and in patients with associated hematologic and infectious problems.

Epidemiology

The prevalence of rheumatoid arthritis appears to be between 0.1 and 7% depending on the stringency of the criteria utilized and the population studied (6). In general the disease appears to have peaks at middle age and again in the elderly and is more common in women than in men (7). Prevalence figures necessarily depend on the criteria utilized in making the diagnosis and these will be discussed more fully in later portions of this text. Diagnostic criteria can range from those labelling any chronic polyarthritis rheumatoid arthritis to more stringent criteria requiring characteristic clinical and laboratory as well as, in some cases, x-ray findings. As the joints are involved with the chronic inflammatory process characteristic erosions appear which can be helpful in making the diagnosis. The mortality from this disease seems to be similar in Western Europe and the United States amounting to about 5/1,000,000/annum in white males and 9/1,000,000/annum in females (7). In the aging population, for example, those over 74 years of age, the mortality reaches 33 in males and 81/1,000,000/annum in females (7). Mortality after adjustment for age is less in nonwhites but varies in different parts of the United States. Geographic as well as racial variations may occur and surveys using tests for rheumatoid factor have found this test to be positive 5-10 times as often in Central African as in European populations (7). Racial factors may also be important in that certain populations such as the Pima Indians in Arizona seem to have a high prevalence of this disease. Although hard data are lacking it has been suggested that the peak of the epidemiologic curve for rheumatoid arthritis may have been seen in the 1960's and the disease might be expected to decrease in future generations (8).

Etiopathogenesis

Etiology

Since rheumatoid arthritis is a chronic polyarthritis involving primarily the joints but also extraarticular tissues with lymphoid infiltration and the production of several autoantibodies, an autoimmune etiology of this disease has been sought by numerous investigators. Genetic factors have also been sought to attempt to explain the development of this disease in individual patients and families.

The reporting in 1976 by Stastny utilizing mixed lymphocyte cultures of an increased prevalence of an HLA D locus determinant in patients with rheumatoid arthritis has stimulated interest in the possibility that rheumatoid arthritis occurs through the interaction of several etiologic factors in a genetically predisposed host (9). Subsequent work has utilized microlymphocytotoxicity testing with well-defined antigens and confirmed the association between rheumatoid arthritis and an HLA antigen termed DR4 (10). While this antigenic marker occurs in varying numbers within different populations the association always seems higher in patients with rheumatoid arthritis than in those without (11). There is controversy regarding whether this marker is also associated with seropositive disease. One study found 65% of seropositive rheumatoid arthritis patients to be DR4 positive in comparison to 27% of normal controls (10). This association has been confirmed in testing of several ethnic groups and an increased prevalence of this marker has been found in Chippewa Indians who have an increased prevalence of clinically manifested rheumatoid disease (12). There has been recent interest in leukocyte stimulation to produce anticollagen antibodies and a recent study has shown that HLA DRW_4 positive individuals tend to be collagen responders and non-DRW_4 individuals tend to be nonresponders (13). Figure 8.1 represents a highly simplified scheme for the development of rheumatoid arthritis in which a patient who may be genetically predetermined to the development of this disease may come in contact with an etiologic agent in the environment which initiates the immunopathologic response leading eventually to the clinical expression of rheumatoid disease. One candidate for an initiating agent is the Epstein-Barr virus (14). Antibodies to cell lines produced through infection with this virus (termed rheumatoid arthritis precipitan or antirheumatoid arthritis nuclear antigen) have been found in a high percentage of patients with rheumatoid arthritis but also in a high percentage of patients without this disease (14). Because of the latter and because rheumatoid

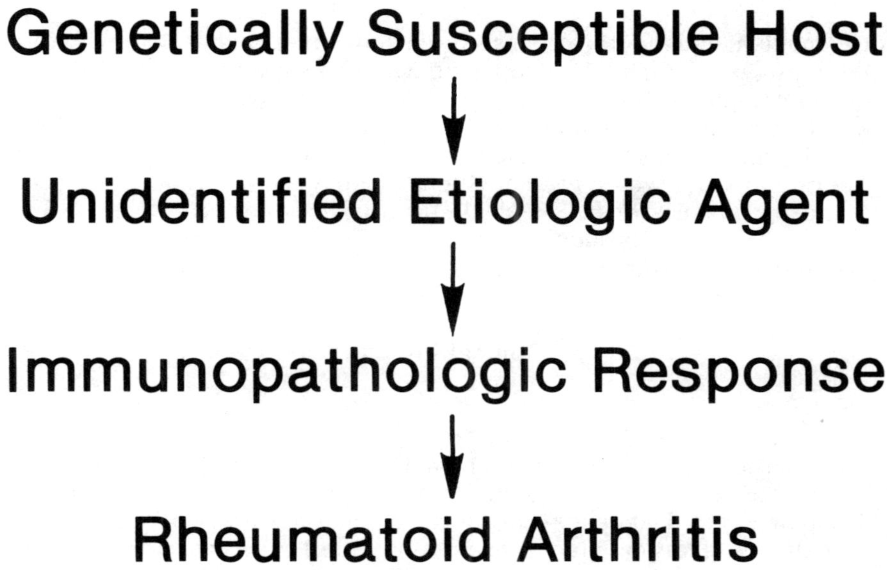

FIGURE 8.1 Scheme for the etiopathogenesis of rheumatoid disease.

arthritis nuclear antigen and Epstein-Barr virus specific antigens have not been identified with any regularity in tissues and/or cells from patients with rheumatoid arthritis, it appears likely that other etiologic agents may be more important in initiating the polyclonal immunopathologic response occurring in patients with rheumatoid arthritis (15).

Pathogenesis

Stimulation of the immune system results in the production of numerous autoantibodies, the classic one being rheumatoid factor which has been discussed in a previous chapter. Rheumatoid factor combines with immunoglobulin G and produces complexes which may further stimulate effector cells to cause lymphoproliferation, synovial proliferation, and/or proliferation of endothelial cells with formation of a tumor-like pannus capable of invading bone or cartilaginous tissue leading to the erosions and tissue destruction seen in rheumatoid arthritis. While these events are occurring in the synovial tissue larger complexes are formed in the synovial fluid and the interaction of these complexes with neutrophils and macrophages may lead to the release of mediators capable of furthering the inflammatory process occurring within the synovial cavities of these patients (16). Such mediators include complement- and noncomplement-derived chemotactic factors capable of calling in additional cellular inflammatory elements, prostaglandins capable of furthering the inflammatory process, and enzymes capable of destroying cartilage.

Large numbers of polymorphonuclear leukocytes accumulate in the synovial fluids of patients with rheumatoid disease. These cells may be attracted by the chemotactic factors released after antigen antibody complex interactinons trigger the complement cascade. Both C5A and cell-derived chemotactic factors have been described in these patients' synovial fluids. These chemotactic factors are capable of activating arachidonic acid metabolic pathways. Products of these pathways may in themselves be chemotactic as well as acting as mediators of polymorphonuclear leukocyte response to various immunopathologic factors existing in the joint fluid milieu. Neutrophils have been shown to respond to contact with immune complexes by release of several types of granular enzymes (17). Enzymes which may be released include the neutral proteases: elastase, collagenease, and cathepsis G, all of which are present in synovial fluid neutrophils and macrophages and all of which are capable of destroying articular tissues such as collagen and ground substances. Multiple interactions between cellular and humeral agents combine to produce the proliferative synovial and exudative phases of the rheumatoid inflammatory process.

Clinical Features

Articular

Rheumatoid arthritis is characterized by articular involvement which may be transient or which may persist with the gradual development of deformities and physical impairment. The hands and wrists are characteristically involved with swelling at the metacarpophalangeal joints especially the second and third, being the earliest sign of involvement in many patients. The proximal interphalangeal joints are also commonly involved but not the distal interphalangeal joints. With continued involvement, marked deformities of the hands and wrists can develop (Figure 8.2) making it difficult to perform many of the integral hand functions necessary for the proper performance of the patient's occupation or at times even the usual activities of daily living. Wrist disease may progress to subluxation of

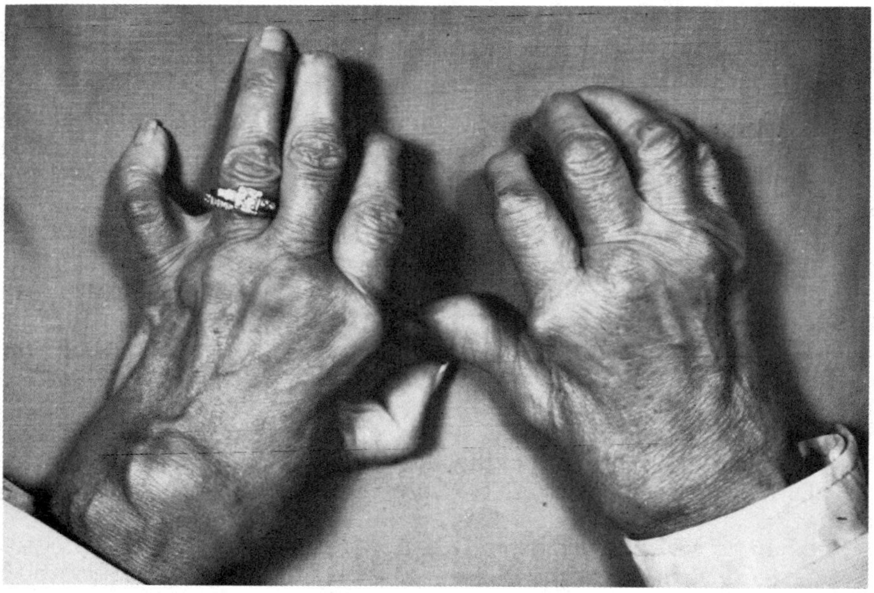

FIGURE 8.2 Deformities of the hands with sustained progression of rheumatoid arthritis. Note synovial protrusion at the dorsum of the left wrist, synovial thickening at metacarpophalangeal joints, and chronic deformities of the thumbs and fingers of both hands.

the carpal bones and the proliferative synovium may involve the median nerve at the carpal tunnel leading to the classic carpal tunnel syndrome with numbness over the thumb, index, and middle fingers of the hands. These patients may have wasting at the thenar eminance and may also have difficulty with abduction and opposition of the thumb. Ulnar nerve entrapment may occur at the wrist producing wasting of the interossei and muscles of the hypothenar eminance and numbness over the ring and fifth fingers. Synovial swelling may occur along the extensor tendons on the dorsum of the wrist and involvement of these tendons may produce rupture with an inability to extend the fourth and fifth fingers. Prolonged involvement at the metacarpophalangeal joints with synovitis, stretching of the tendons and ligaments, and weakening of the interosseous muscles may produce the classic symmetrical ulnar deviation of the digits which has long been one of the hallmarks of rheumatoid joint deformity. With advanced disease a swan neck deformity may develop with hyperextension of the proximal interphalangeal joint and flexion of the terminal interphalangeal joint. The proximal interphalangeal joint may protrude upward through the lateral extensions of the extensor tendon giving rise to the boutonnière deformity in some patients. Volar displacement of the thumb with metacarpophalangeal joint flexion and hyperextension of the distal phalanx may produce the so-called Z-shaped deformity of the thumb. With unrelenting chronic inflammation severe deformities may occur with the so-called opera glass hand resulting from severe destruction of the bones and cartilage.

The elbows are also frequently involved in rheumatoid arthritis with flexion contractures occurring early in the course of this disease. The area just distal to the elbows is a common site for the finding of subcutaneous rheumatoid nodules. These nodules are firm, rounded, and are loosely bound to the subcutaneous tissue. They are usually associated with the presence of rheumatoid factor in the serum and may occur over the extensor surfaces of other joints or tendons and in extraarticular deep structures. The periolecranon grooves may be obliterated by hypertrophied synovial tissue or by the occurrence of a synovial effusion at the elbow.

The shoulder may also be involved with pain or limitation of motion occurring in this important joint. Swelling is usually not appreciated on physical examination but an associated bursitis may be found to be a contributing factor to the patient's overall shoulder problems.

Involvement of the spine is rare in rheumatoid arthritis except in the cervical area (18). Cervical spine involvement is a frequent cause of pain and disability with the most common symptom being occipital or temporal headaches. Atlantoaxial subluxation may occur with or without weakness of the arms and legs. Paresthesia or quadraplegia may develop in severely affected patients. Patients may also have a sense of weakness in the neck and a clicking sensation on movement of the head. In addition to atlantoaxial subluxation, subluxation of C2-3, C3-4, C4-5, and/or C5-6 may also occur in patients with severe, long-standing disease. Platybasia may also occur with basalar invagination at the foramen magnum. The odontoid itself may show loss of cortex, erosions, pointing, sclerosis, or diminution in size. Narrowing of the disc spaces, erosion of the vertebrae, or osteoporosis of the cervical spine may also occur. These abnormalities and apophyseal joint erosion are usually diagnosed during x-ray studies and may or may not be clinically significant in a given patient. It is probably wise to obtain flexion-extension views of the cervical spine in all of these patients in whom surgery is contemplated since induction of general anesthesia with manipulation of the cervical spine is an especially hazardous undertaking in patients with atlantoaxial problems.

Hip involvement in rheumatoid arthritis seems less common than involvement of the more peripheral joints. As is usually the case with the shoulder joint, detection of swelling at the hip joint is not clinically possible on physical examination. Late in the course of the disease pain and limitation of motion may occur and in some patients destruction of the acetabulum may lead to protrusio acetabuli with severe pain and limitation of function. Avascular necrosis of the femoral head may occur in rheumatoid arthritis especially in patients being treated with corticosteroids and this may lead to accelerated destruction and increased disability. Trochanteric bursitis may lead to tenderness over the greater trochanter in the presence or absence of intrinsic hip disease. Asymptomatic radiologic changes, usually best detected by tomography, may occur in the sacroiliac joints or at the symphysis pubis (19).

Knee involvement is common in rheumatoid arthritis and synovial effusions or hypertrophy are usually relatively easily detected on physical examination. Joint effusions may be detected by balotting the patella or by the observance of a bulging posterior to the patella. A bulging may also occur in the popliteal space from a Baker's cyst and extension of synovial inflammation may occur into the gastrocnemius with the patient presenting acutely with symptoms and signs mimicking thrombophlebitis. Flexion contractures, valgus or varus deformities, and ligamentous instability may also occur.

Because the ankle joint has relatively little synovial tissue rheumatoid involvement of this joint is uncommon. Pain about the ankle joint, however, is common in rheumatoid arthritis since tenosynovitis of the tendons about the ankle is common during acute phases of the disease. Inflammation at the insertion of the Achilles tendon into the calcaneus may cause pain on walking. Subtalar or talocalcaneal joints may frequently be involved in rheumatoid arthritis as may the talonavicular joints leading to painful valgus deformities of the feet. Involvement of the metatarsophalangeal joints may occur with the first and more lateral joints undergoing a progressive valgus deformity as shown in Figure 8.3. Cocking up of the toes may occur as may protrusion of the metatarsal heads producing pain at the plantar surface over the forefoot.

Although we have discussed the major joint involvement with rheumatoid arthritis, this disease can affect any of the diarthrodial joints including the acromioclavicular, coracoclavicular, sternoclavicular, manubriosternal, costovertebral and costatransverse, and (perhaps more commonly and more characteristically) the temporomandibular joints (20). Involvement of these joints may lead to limitation in opening the mouth, stiffness, referred pain, crepitus, and tenderness on palpation of the joints.

Extraarticular Clinical Features

Although rheumatoid arthritis is characteristically an articular disease, it may have widespread systemic manifestations thought to be at least in part related to the autoimmune nature of this disease. Individual variations in the production, transport, and deposition of autoantibodies and complexes have been thought to be important in helping to determine the clinical pattern of the extraarticular involvement which can occur in individual patients with rheumatoid arthritis (21). The major extraarticular organ system involvement in rheumatoid arthritis is summarized in Table 8.1.

A cutaneous vasculitis may occur in many patients and may take the form of nail fold or digital pulp lesions, purpuric lesions over the extremities, livedo reticularis, or in some patients progression to large ischemic ulcerations or areas of frank gangrene. Vasculitis type lesions may appear in many tissues in rheumatoid arthritis with no characteristically specific clinical picture. The pathogenesis of these vasculitic lesions is probably multifactoral but much evidence points to

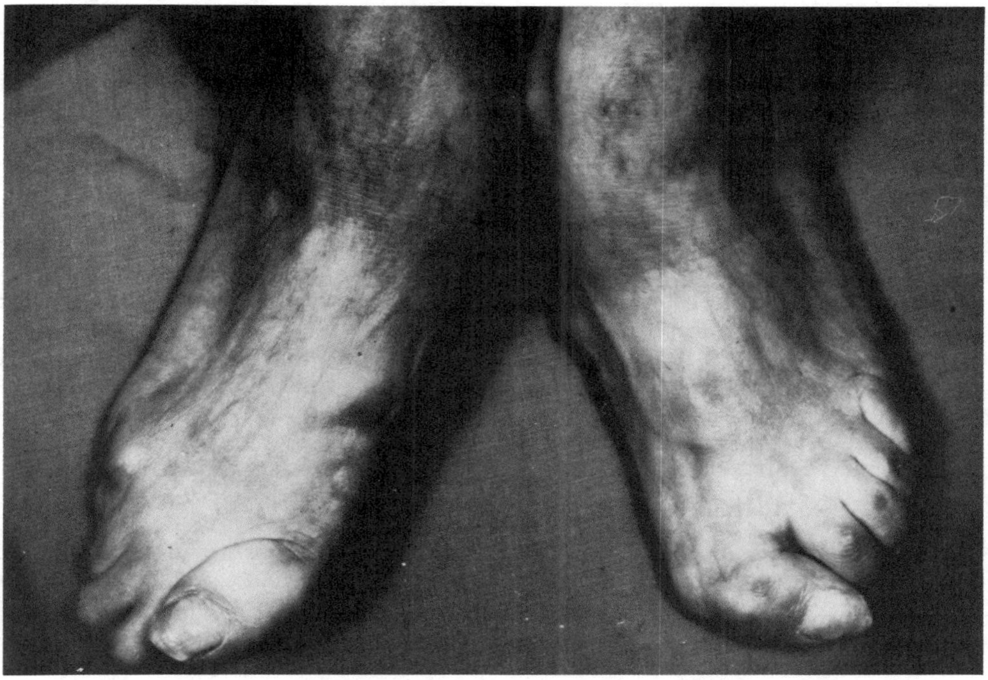

FIGURE 8.3 Deformities of the feet in the same patient shown in Figure 8.2. Note hallux valgus deformities bilaterally and evidence of cocking up of the toes on the left.

TABLE 8.1 Major Extraarticular Organ System Involvement in Rheumatoid Arthritis

NEUROVASCULAR	PULMONARY
Cutaneous	Nodular
Subcutaneous	Pleural
Neuropathic	Interstitial
Synovialpathic	Vascular
CARDIAC	HEMATOLOGIC
Pericardial	Iron deficiency anemia
Myocardial	Anemia of chronic disease
Vascular	Megaloblastic anemia
Nodular	Felty's syndrome
	Lymphoid hyperplasia

immune complex mediated mechanisms as important elements in their development. Patients with vasculitis generally have high titers of rheumatoid factor, decreased complement, and deposition of IgG, IgM and complement in their vascular lesions. A fulminating systemic vasculitis may occur in some rheumatoid arthritis patients and is associated with a high mortality. An interesting characteristic of this vasculitic syndrome is the relative lack of renal involvement as opposed to the occurrence of vasculitis in other collagen diseases such as systemic lupus erythematosus and polyarteritis nodosa. Patients without other skin manifestations may, as illustrated in Figure 8.4, develop large ulcerative lesions over the malleoli which seem rather uniquely likely to occur in rheumatoid arthritis.

Patients who develop frank vasculitis with cutaneous manifestations may also develop a peripheral neuropathy. The most common peripheral neuropathy in rheumatoid arthritis is a digital neuropathy which may be minimally symptomatic. Some patients, however, may develop a sensory-motor neuropathy with marked neurologic changes. In others, hypertrophic synovium at the wrist may involve the median nerve producing a classic carpal tunnel syndrome or, as previously discussed, hypertrophic synovium at the cervical spine may involve the ligaments maintaining the position of the atlantoaxial joint allowing ligamentous laxity and/or odontoid erosion with atlantoaxial subluxation.

Since the pericardium is a serosal tissue similar to the synovium it is not surprising that pericarditis occurs commonly in this disease (22). This manifestation was first detected in autopsy studies being present in 40% of rheumatoid arthritis patients undergoing this procedure. A similar prevalence has now been detected in asymptomatic ambulatory rheumatoid arthritis patients using sensitive echocardiographic methods (22). An interesting additional finding has been that whereas pericardial effusions tend to be evanescent, pericardial thickening tends to

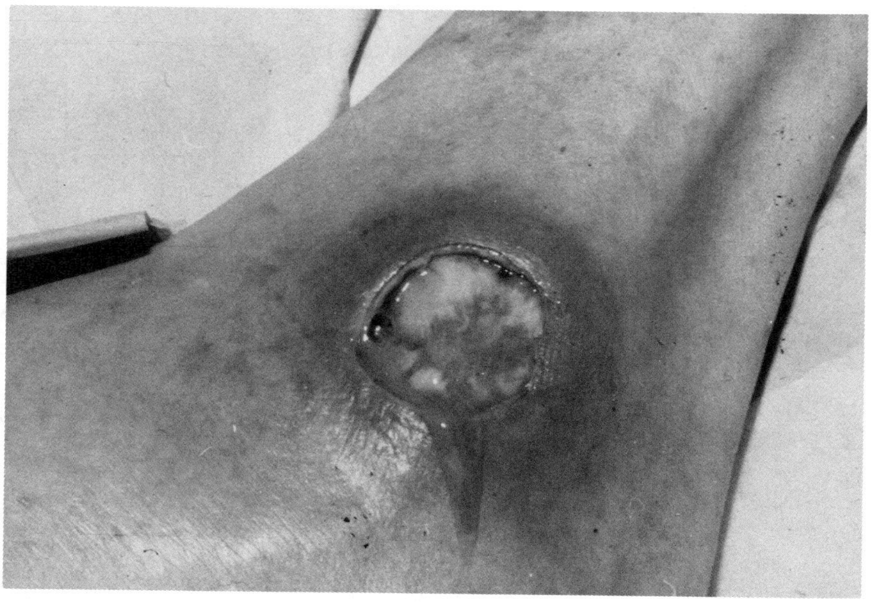

FIGURE 8.4 Left lateral malleolar ulcer in rheumatoid arthritis patient without other cutaneous manifestations of this disease.

persist in some patients (23). Although pericardial lesions are usually asymptomatic, marked inflammation and/or fibrosis can lead to cardiac decompensation in 1% or less of patients. When hemodynamic compromise occurs, pericardidectomy is the treatment of choice. Although dysfunction of the mitral valve has been reported in echocardiographic studies, the hemodynamic and clinical significance of this remains uncertain (22). Of greater significance is the occurrence of a myopathic process resembling viral myocarditis leading to arrhythmias in patients so affected. Another uncommon rheumatoid cardiac lesion is coronary artery vasculitis which may lead to myocardial infarction. Rheumatoid nodules in the myocardium may also occur and may lead to conduction abnormalities.

Nodular lesions in the pulmonary parenchyma may also be present in some patients. These may be seen in two settings: 1) in the absence of any occupational exposure to silica or other noxious agents, or 2) in association with a pneumoconiosis (Caplan's syndrome). In either case, these nodules closely resemble the subcutaneous nodules of rheumatoid arthritis in their histologic appearance. The nodules occurring alone usually have a discrete radiographic appearance and those occurring with Caplan's syndrome usually have a shaggy border. Solitary nodules may cavitate suggesting neoplasia or tuberculosis. Biopsy may be required to make the differential diagnosis. Pleuritis and pleural effusions are probably the most prevalent clinically significant pleuropulmonary manifestations directly related to rheumatoid arthritis (21). Evidence of these manifestations has been found in autopsy studies in the majority of patients with rheumatoid arthritis; however, few patients (approximately 5%) develop clinically detectable effusions. These effusions are usually relatively noninflammatory and share biochemical and laboratory characteristics with synovial and pericardial effusions as will be discussed later in this chapter. Less frequent manifestations include interstitial fibrosis, which is more common with scleroderma, and a reticulonodular pattern on x-ray, which may correlate with the presence of significant rheumatoid factor titers in some patients (24). Widespread pulmonary vasculitis is uncommon although pulmonary arterial lesions may occur and may be an important contributing factor to the pathologic picture noted above. Obstructive lung disease is a common finding with or without rheumatoid arthritis and many rheumatoid arthritis patients may exhibit evidence on pulmonary function testing of small airways obstruction (24).

Hematologic manifestations of rheumatoid arthritis may occur with iron deficiency anemia developing secondary to gastrointestinal blood loss induced by many of the medications utilized. Rheumatoid arthritis patients may also exhibit the anemia of chronic disease with a low serum iron and a high iron binding capacity thought to be secondary to increased uptake of iron by and deposition in the reticuloendothelial system. Macrocytic anemia may occur usually secondary to folate deficiency. Splenomegaly and leukopenia may develop and this combination of problems has been called Felty's syndrome. These patients usually have deforming arthritis and high titers of rheumatoid factor. The white blood counts may range from 4500 cells/mm^3 down to as low as 500 cells/mm^3 in some patients. The greatest part of the reduction is in the neutrophilic series. There may be an associated reduction in lymphocytes and an associated anemia which is usually hypochronic. There also may be accelerated red cell destruction in some patients. The etiology of these abnormalities remains uncertain although there clearly is accelerated neutrophil destruction in the spleen and reticuloendothelial systems. Patients with Felty's syndrome may develop chronic leg ulcers and recurrent infections. Immunomodulating agent therapy has been shown to reverse the hematologic abnormalities in conjunction with ameliorating the clinical and laboratory signs of inflammation in some patients. The results of splenectomy are difficult to assess and this form of therapy cannot be recommended except in extreme circumstances. Lymphadenopathy may occur in up to 10% of patients with rheumatoid arthritis with or without Felty's syndrome. Biopsy of the involved lymph nodes may suggest malignancy, and careful pathologic differentiation between the hyperplasia associated with rheumatoid arthritis and the lymphoid proliferation associated with a lymphatic malignancy is necessary.

Other organ systems also may be involved in the rheumatoid process. Rheumatoid nodules may involve the ocular tissue with progressive scleritis occurring and in some patients leading to a thinning of the sclera or to scleromalacia perforans. Ulceration of the cornea may occur and may lead to perforation. A tenovaginitis has been described leading to lateral gaze palsy. Sjögren's syndrome may occur in some patients with rheumatoid arthritis as described in Chapter 15. Although decreased tear production has been reported in a high percentage of asymptomatic rheumatoid arthritis patients (25), most of these patients do not develop the same degree of lacrimal gland involvement as that classically described for Sjögren's syndrome.

The middle ear may be involved in rheumatoid arthritis since the incudomalleal and incudostadedial articulations are synovial joints with cartilaginous articular discs. Such involvement may lead to conductive or sensorineural hearing loss. Dentition may be poor perhaps because of inflammation of the supporting tissues. Cricoarytenoid joint involvement may lead to inspiratory strider and respiratory decompensation. Rheumatoid nodules may also occur in the vocal cords leading to hoarseness or respiratory problems.

Gastrointestinal involvement is more likely to be due to drugs than to the disease itself, although rheumatoid patients are thought to be unusually susceptible to the development of gastric ulcers. Various liver function abnormalities have been reported but these also may be related more to drugs than to the disease. Esophageal involvement appears to occur more commonly in other collagen diseases than in rheumatoid arthritis (26). Renal involvement also is more likely to be related to drugs than to the rheumatoid disease process, although periodically, glomerular hyperplasia is reported in renal biopsy studies. No regularly recognized endocrine abnormalities are reported although juxtaarticular osteoporosis certainly occurs and is probably related to local factors or to corticosteroid therapy. Muscular weakness may occur with a frank polymyositis picture occurring in some patients. Corticosteroid therapy may also lead to a noninflammatory myopathic process. Because of the multisystem nature of this disease, numerous case reports will continue to document new systemic findings in rheumatoid arthritis patients.

Differential Diagnosis

The classic criteria for rheumatoid arthritis are summarized in Table 8.2 from the criteria delineated by the American Rheumatism Association Criteria Committee (27).

These criteria make use of some of the systemic and articular manifestations of the disease described in previous sections along with laboratory, pathologic, and radiographic findings. The American Rheumatism Association criteria also exclude patients with the diagnoses of other collagen diseases likely to mimic rheumatoid arthritis. Morning stiffness may occur in this and other rheumatic diseases but in rheumatoid arthritis it should last more than 30 minutes. Tenderness or pain on motion should be observed by a physician and should have a history of recurrence or of persistence for at least 3 weeks. Swelling should consist of soft tissue thickening or fluid accumulation and not bony overgrowth alone. This finding also should be observed by a physician. To satisfy the fourth criterion

TABLE 8.2 **Summary of ARA Criteria for Rheumatoid Arthritis**

Morning stiffness	Roentgenographic changes
Pain or tenderness	Rheumatoid factor
Swelling and/or fluid	Inflammatory synovial fluid
Polyarticularity	Hypertrophic and inflammatory synovial histopathology
Symmetry	Characteristic nodule histology
Clinical nodularity	

of polyarticularity, swelling should be observed in one additional joint and the interval between joint symptoms in the two joints should not be more than 3 months. Simultaneous involvement of the same joint on both sides of the body constitutes symmetry. Terminal phalangeal joint involvement will not satisfy this criterion. Subcutaneous nodules must be observed by a physician over bony prominences on extensor surfaces or in juxtaarticular regions. X-ray changes typical of rheumatoid arthritis must include at least bony decalcification localized to or greatest around the involved joints. Any positive test for rheumatoid factor is acceptable if accomplished by a method which in two laboratories has been positive in not more than 5% of normal controls. In the original criteria, an inflammatory synovial fluid was believed to be demonstrated by a poor mucin precipitate from the synovial fluid. Decreased viscosity and/or a polymorphonuclear leukocytosis has now been substituted for this criterion in some clinical settings. Characteristic synovial histopathology must consist of at least three or more of the following: marked villus hypertrophy; proliferation of superficial synovial cells often with palisating, marked infiltration with chronic inflammatory cells; and deposition of compacted fibrin either on the surface or interstitially and/or foci of cell necrosis. Characteristic nodule histology is represented by granulomatis foci with central zones of cell necrosis surrounded by proliferated fixed cells and proliferative fibrosis with chronic inflammatory cell infiltration predominantly perivascular.

Categories of diagnosis under these criteria have been delineated. The diagnosis of classic rheumatoid arthritis requires seven, definite five, and probable three of these criteria. Exclusions have been incorporated into the criteria for disorders such as other collagen diseases, crystal deposition diseases, rheumatic fever, infectious arthritis, Reiter's syndrome, neuropathic arthropathies, hypertrophic pulmonary osteoarthropathy, metabolic arthropathies, neurogenic arthopathy, hematologic abnormalities, and erythema nodosum. A more strenuous set of criteria termed the New York criteria have been reported (28) and compared to the American Rheumatism Association criteria (29). These criteria, which emphasize the joint manifestations of rheumatoid arthritis, are summarized in Table 8.3.

The New York criteria do not include guidelines for summation of individual items although some studies have required the presence of the second item for making the initial diagnosis of rheumatoid arthritis in study patients (29). With the first of these criteria, there must be a history, past or present, of an episode of joint pain involving three or more limb joints without stipulations as to duration. The joints on either side shall count separately but joints that occur in

TABLE 8.3 New York Criteria for Rheumatoid Arthritis

Three painful limb joints
Three swollen or deformed characteristic joints
Erosive x-ray changes
Rheumatoid factor

groups such as the proximal interphalangeal joints or the metacarpal-phalangeal joints on one side shall count only as a single joint. Swelling, limitation, subluxation, or ankylosis of at least three limb joints including one hand, wrist, or foot with symmetry of at least one joint pair are required for meeting the second criterion. Excluded from consideration for this criterion are: distal interphalangeal joints, fifth proximal interphalangeal joints, first carpometacarpal joints, hips and the first metatarsalphalangeal joints. X-rays of the joints must show erosions as discussed later in this chapter and in Chapter 3. Rheumatoid factor must be present as in the American Rheumatism Association criteria. The use of the New York criteria seems to lend more specificity for the diagnosis of rheumatoid arthritis in population studies (29). Both sets of criteria, however, should serve only as a guide to the clinical manifestations and laboratory parameters which can help the clinician in making the diagnosis in an individual patient.

It is important to differentiate rheumatoid arthritis from other autoimmune or collagen diseases which share similar spectrums of involvement in many instances. Many of the collagen diseases described in other sections of this text can mimic rheumatoid arthritis through either articular or extraarticular manifestations so that a familiarity with these diseases and their clinical diagnostic criteria remains the best route toward reaching the correct diagnosis. Particularly bothersome diagnostic problems are diseases such as mixed connective tissue disease which produce joint deformities overlapping with those of rheumatoid arthritis. Also difficult to diagnose is early rheumatoid arthritis which may present with transient joint involvement which mimics and blends into a syndrome termed palindromic rheumatism. The systemic form of juvenile rheumatoid arthritis (Still's disease described in Chapter 19) may occur in adults producing a febrile illness with at times difficult and confusing diagnostic signals for the clinician.

Laboratory Features

Laboratory Findings

Many of the general and more specific laboratory abnormalities occurring in rheumatoid arthritis have been discussed earlier in this chapter and in Chapter 2 on laboratory abnormalities in the rheumatic diseases. The anemia of chronic disease may be present in rheumatoid arthritis as may an iron deficiency anemia or a megaloblastic anemia as previously discussed. White blood counts may be normal, elevated, or depressed depending on the stage of the disease. Thrombocytosis has been reported and the extent of this may vary with the activity of the disease. In patients with ongoing active disease, the acute phase reactants such as the sedimentation rate or C reactive protein may be moderately elevated.

Automated chemistry panels may show elevated gammaglobulin with decreased albumin. Liver function studies and tests for renal function such as creatinine and BUN usually are normal. Immunologic studies may demonstrate rheumatoid factor with varying specificity and sensitivity depending on the methods used. Antinuclear antibodies may be present as may circulating immune complexes. Elevated levels of these immune factors may suggest that the patient has more highly expressed disease with more severe articular and extraarticular manifestations (21). Analysis of effusions from the joints, pericardium, and pleura share interesting characteristics. The synovial fluid leukocyte count may vary from 5 to 20,000 or higher with a predominance of polymorphonuclear leukocytes in most cases. The cell counts in the pleural or pericardial fluids are usually somewhat lower. All of these serosal fluids share a low glucose concentration in rheumatoid arthritis even in the absence of a striking leukocytosis. Rheumatoid factor and immune complexes may be detected in a large percentage of these fluids. A high protein concentration often exceeding 3 g% may occur with a decreased total hemolytic complement activity.

Pathological Findings

As discussed in previous sections, the synovium proliferates from a single cell layer to a mass of granulation tissue containing blood vessels and synovial fibroblast and mononuclear cell infiltrates. This mass of tissue invades centrally articular cartilage and subchondral bone leading to the erosions seen on x-ray. Late in the disease the granulation tissue may form adhesions leading to ankylosis. Deformities may occur due to destruction of bones and remodeling of articular surfaces. Tendon lysis and contractures also contribute to the chronic deformities occurring in some patients.

The hallmark of articular rheumatoid pathology is the inflammation involving the synovium. Early in rheumatoid inflammation, exudation of fluid from the small blood vessels occurs along with the migration of polymorphonuclear leukocytes into the synovial cavity. Mononuclear cells follow and invade the synovial membrane. Within the extravascular spaces there is congestion, edema, and extravasation of large molecular components of the blood plasma. There also appears to be an increased lymphatic drainage and an increase in regional blood flow. Fibrin is laid down over the synovial membrane and may contribute to the synovitis there (30).

With persistence of the synovitis, damage to the avascular hyaline articular cartilage may occur. This damage usually begins at the cartilage synovial junction. There is degeneration within the marginal articular cartilage with disorganization and loss of intracellular matrix. There is also an early ingrowth of buds of young capillaries and attenuated fibroblasts from the synovial border into the cartilaginous tissue. A mass of granulation tissue forms a pannus which can invade both the cartilage and the subchondral bone. Periarticular tissues such as bursae and tendons may also be sites for rheumatoid synovitis. Infiltration with neutrophils, fibroblasts, and lymphocytes may occur and healthy structures may be replaced with granulation tissue. Focal tendinitis and necrosis may result in spontaneous tendon rupture in severe long-standing cases. Gross changes may evolve in the joints with exuberant pannus and fibrous tissue covering the articular surfaces. As the disease progresses, striking deformities may develop with narrowing of the joint space progressing to frank ankylosis in some patients. Cartilaginous tissue may undergo hyalinization and be detached as rice bodies. The appendages may become shortened if marked erosions develop and loss of bone occurs.

Pathological differentiation of rheumatoid synovitis from that associated with other articular diseases may be difficult. In general, diseases such as systemic lupus erythematosus cause less synovial destruction while the more exuberant synovial disease, pigmented villonodular synovitis, may produce more aggressive lesions with more staining with hemosiderin. Other systemic and articular diseases such as early psoriasis and the spondyloarthropathies may present even more challenging pathologic diagnostic problems making reliance on the accompanying clinical and laboratory findings essential for determining the correct final diagnosis in a given patient.

The extraarticular lesion most frequently examined pathologically in patients with rheumatoid arthritis is the subcutaneous nodule. These nodules may occur in various locations in up to 20% of patients with this disease. Wherever their location, be it synovial membrane, sclera, dura mater, lung, or heart, the histologic picture is remarkably similar. The nodules range in size from a few millimeters to 2-3 cm in diameter and they usually have a firm binding through fibrous tissues to nearby structures. On microscopic examination there is pallisading of histiocytes radiating from a necrotic center containing a mesh-work of fibrin, fragments of cells and partially degraded collagen fibrils.

Vascular derangement has been postulated as of basic importance in the pathogenesis of rheumatoid arthritis (32). While the significance of this pathogenic theory remains unproven, it is clear that widespread blood vessel involvement may occur and may be severe in many patients with this disease. A necrotizing arteritis may be present which may be indistinguishable from polyarteritis nodosa (Chapter 18). Renal, cerebral, and mesenteric arteries may be involved with perivascular lymphocytic infiltration and medial necrosis. A subacute arteritis may also occur especially in skeletal muscles (33). Blood flow is usually not impaired and there is usually no consequent ischemia or infarction. Fibromuscular hyperplasia may also occur in long-standing disease with obstruction of the digital arteries. These vessels may show a bland thrombosis leading to ischemia or recanilization. Common vascular diseases such as venous thrombosis and atherosclerosis may occur in patients with rheumatoid arthritis just as they do in patients without this disease.

Lymphoreticular tissue may be involved perhaps due to the autoimmune nature of the disease. Clinical lymphadenopathy occurs in many patients. Histologically there is cortical follicular hyperplasia with fibroblastic infiltration of the capsule of the lymph node. There also may be edema and neutrophilic infiltration into the lymph nodes. The spleen may be enlarged and the histologic changes there may closely mirror those of the regional lymph nodes. There may be accumulation of amyloid tissue in the spleen and other organs. An enlarged spleen may occur in the absence of amyloidosis in Felty's syndrome. The serosal tissue of the heart may be inflamed leading to pericarditis with mononuclear cell infiltration and fibrosis. A similar picture may be seen in the lungs with pleuritis and a subsequent fibrosis or with pleural effusions. Other organ system involvement may occur with myositis mimicking that seen in polymyositis, pulmonary interstitial fibrosis being indistinguishable from that seen with scleroderma or Hammand Rich syndrome, and epithelial cell proliferation in the salivary glands in the presence or absence of Sjögren's syndrome.

Radiographic Findings

The roentgenographic features of rheumatoid arthritis have been detailed in Chapter 3. Roentgenographic criteria have been used as a guide for the anatomical staging of rheumatoid arthritis (34). As seen in Table 8.4 stages range from juxtaarticular osteoporosis through characteristic erosion of cartilage and bone to frank deformity and ankylosis. Soft tissue swelling although not listed in the staging process is one of the hallmarks of the roentgenographic findings in rheumatoid arthritis. It develops early in the disease and precedes other x-ray changes. The soft tissue swelling follows the symmetrical and clinical distributive patterns described in previous sections on the clinical manifestations of this disease. Osteopenia may accompany the soft tissue swelling around the joints. The periarticular regions contain predominantly trabecular bone which seems to respond rapidly to the increased blood flow or other aspects of the inflammatory process causing the development of this roentgenographic manifestation of rheumatoid arthritis. These x-rays show increased radiolucency and may show relative accentuation of the primary trabeculae. Later in the disease, narrowing of the interosseous spaces may occur reflecting cartilage loss. Weight-bearing views of the larger joints of the lower extremities may be helpful in demonstrating these findings. As more distinctive evidence of cartilage and bone destruction appears articular erosions develop because of bone resorption along the surface of the subchondral compact bone. These erosions generally begin at the joint margins in the region of the synovial reflection and progress as the pannus proliferates. In late disease large erosions may develop and bizarre deformities may be seen. Problems in alignment may occur which alter joint mechanics along with flexion deformities which result from chronic inflammation and secondary fibrosis. Bony ankylosis also may occur in approximately 10% of the cases involving especially the small peripheral joints.

Roentgenographic findings of extraarticular disease may range from relatively specific such as the discrete rheumatoid nodule occurring in the lung to relatively nonspecific such as the shaggy Caplan's syndrome nodule seen with pneumoconiosis with rheumatoid arthritis. Even less specific are lesions such as pleural opacities or enlarged pericardial silhouettes seen with pleural or pericardial effusions in some patients. Specialized radiologic studies such as arthrography to identify dissecting Baker's cysts, or computed tomography to identify sacroililac or pubic abnormalities have been discussed previously. Experience with the use of routine and specialized roentgenologic testing is necessary for full utilization of these potentially worthwhile procedures.

TABLE 8.4 Summary of Anatomical Stages of Rheumatoid Arthritis

No radiologic changes other than juxtaarticular osteoporosis
No more than slight bone destruction without deformities
Radiographic evidence of cartilage and bone destruction with deformities
Fibrosis or bony ankylosis

Outcome

General Management

The overall prognosis in rheumatoid arthritis is quite good for most patients (35). General management utilizing physical therapy, occupational therapy, psychosocial counseling, and the team approach to general management can be quite helpful. Use of surgical procedures has been discussed (Chapter 7) and specific indications such as synovectomy at the wrist in the presence of carpal tunnel compression or incipient lysis of extensor tendons have obvious advantages. In general, pain relief, correction of deformities, and restoration of movement and stability seem to be the major clinical indications for surgical procedures. Synovectomy, arthroplasty, and arthrodesis are the major types of procedures. Local factors along with risk/benefit considerations for individual patients must be carefully weighed to determine the procedure to be utilized for a given patient. It is important, for example, to combine synovectomy of the dorsum of the wrist with synovectomy of the related extensor tendon sheaths to prevent incipient extensor tendon rupture in some patients. Total joint replacements such as those at the fingers and hips have shown remarkably improved results in recent years. As shown in Figure 8.5, the optimal overall management of rheumatoid arthritis involves a combination of physical, psychosocial, surgical, and medical techniques. The team approach to arthritis and the importance of psychological support for these patients have been discussed in Chapters 5 and 6. Rest has long been recognized as important both in general terms and for specific joints. Hospitalization

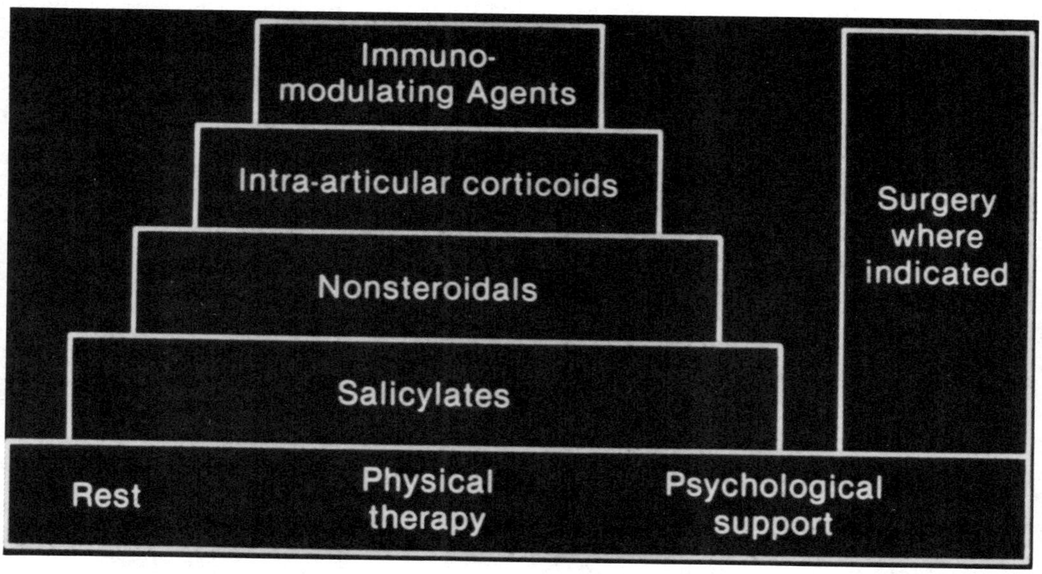

FIGURE 8.5 Scheme for the overall management of rheumatoid arthritis.

for rest alone has been thought to play an important part in leading to a good overall prognosis (35). An initial hospitalization for the patient with rheumatoid arthritis may be a good maneuver in order to bring the full medical and surgical team together to focus on the patient's problems. Hospitalization also provides the opportunity for beginning to teach joint protection, modified rest, and other techniques which can be helpful in allowing the patient to manage his disease. Graded exercise may be helpful in some patients as may physical modalities of therapy such as moist heat or in some cases immersion of the extremities in the whirlpool or of the entire patient in devices such as the Hubbard tank. The patient must work closely with the physical therapist to develop the best balance between rest and exercise along with applying the physical modalities available in the best possible manner. The occupational therapist can provide training for managing daily living activities and for prevocational assessment to help the patient function better at home and on the job. As the pain of the acute inflammatory process is brought under control and the patient learns more about his disease, psychological counseling can be utilized as discussed in Chapter 6 to help the patient to adjust to his chronic problems. Functional assessment can be accomplished in the patient's home and working conditions assessed. Various assistive devices may be prescribed to help the patient with his tasks of daily living.

Medical Management

The medical management of rheumatoid arthritis has been reviewed in several recent publications (36, 37) and is outlined elsewhere in this text. The pharmacology of aspirin is discussed in detail in Chapter 4. This drug remains the cornerstone of many practitioners' therapeutic programs. It is the cheapest of the nonsteroidal antiinflammatory agents available and remains efficacious in many patients with rheumatoid arthritis. Because of its ulcerogenic properties which can be related in part to a surface erosive effect, the drug is probably best given with meals and at bedtime with a snack. Newer formulations of aspirin such as the zero order release preparation (Zorprin) may be given at less frequent intervals but it remains to be seen whether they offer any advantage in efficacy or side effects to offset their increased cost over standard aspirin preparations. Enteric coated preparations have a slower onset of action and longer half-life than regular aspirin and although they alleviate surface erosive problems in the stomach, they may cause problems through their prostaglandin E_2 inhibition and subsequent loss of the mucosal barrier cytoprotective effect in the stomach.

Nonacetylated salicylates are available which show little if any prostaglandin inhibition. These preparations may be used in patients with aspirin allergies and do seem to be less ulcerogenic than aspirin. The newest of these agents is calcium magnesium trisalicylate (Trilisate) which may be given in the dose of 1000 mg with each meal. Other preparations such as magnesium salicylate (Magan) and choline salicylate (Arthropan) may also be efficacious. Salsalicylate (Disalsid) may also be effective in a dose of 3.5 g/day. Additional careful studies of both efficacy and side effects will be necessary to determine the value of the many available nonacetylated nonprostaglandin-inhibiting salicylate compounds. A newer salicylate compound diflunisal (Dolobid) adds a difluorophenyl group to the basic salicylate molecule. This compound seems to be a somewhat selective prostaglandin inhibitor with some competitive inhibition of platelet cycloxygenase but with a sparing effect on PGE_2 production by the gastric mucosa. It has been shown to be efficacious in the therapy of rheumatoid arthritis (38) and is more closely aligned to the newer nonsteroidal antiinflammatory agents than to the other nonacetylated salicylates. Salicylates remain the preferred initial antiinflammatory agent of many practitioners although newer nonsteroidal antiinflammatory agents show increasing promise when compared with aspirin (39) and with each other (40).

Propionic acid derivatives constitute one of the major classes of nonsteroidal antiinflammatory agents. In this group, ibuprofen (Motrin) and fenoprofen (Nalfon) have relatively short half-lives and therefore probably are best used in a dosage regimen similar to that for aspirin giving the medication with meals and at bedtime with a snack. Utilization of this type of regimen for all of these shorter acting nonsteroidal antiinflammatory agents may be useful in decreasing gastrointestinal irritation and also in teaching the patient a uniform dosing schedule which can be used with many of these agents. The maximum dose for ibuprofen is 2400 mg/day and for fenoprofen is 3000 mg/day. Naproxen (Naprosyn) has a longer half-life and may therefore be given twice a day. As with the other agents in this class, the maximum dose has been extended beginning at 750 mg and now being 1000 mg/day. There is some evidence that higher doses may produce increased efficacy with no increase in side effects (41).

Indole derivatives constitute another large class of nonsteroidal antiinflammatory agents. Indomethacin (Indocin) has been a useful agent over the years for treating rheumatoid arthritis and, perhaps to an even greater extent, the spondyloarthropathies and crystal deposition diseases (Chapters 10, 11). Although this preparation may be given in bid dosages the existence of 50 mg tablets and a maximum dose of 200 mg again suggest that a dosage regimen with meals and at bedtime may be the most conveniently learned by the patient. A sustained release preparation (Indocin-SR) is available which may be given on a bid dosage schedule. Tolmetin (Tolectin) may also be given in a qid schedule with a maximum dose of 2000 mg/day. Although some evidence exists that a combination of this drug with aspirin may be more efficacious than aspirin alone (42), combination therapy involving several nonsteroidal antiinflammatory agents (as discussed in Chapter 4) cannot be recommended at this time since the increased propensity for side effects has not clearly been shown to be outweighed by an increased efficacy in treating rheumatoid arthritis. Sulindac (Clinoril) is a relatively long-acting agent which may be used in a twice a day dosage. This agent is reduced from the inactive sulfoxide to the active sulfide which has a longer half-life allowing the drug to be given in the dosage of 200 mg bid. Recent studies have suggested a sparing of renal prostaglandin inhibition since the kidney is rich in oxidizing agents and thus converts the drug back to its inactive form (43). Much work remains to confirm these findings in multiple laboratories and to determine their clinical relevance in the appropriate studies.

The pyrazolone, phenylbutazone (Butazolidin), may be efficacious for short-term therapy in rheumatoid arthritis. The use of phenylbutazone for up to 3 months in this disease has been suggested (36), but with the advent of many newer agents and the known propensity for hematologic problems with this agent other medications are usually prescribed by most practitioners. Meclofenamic acid (Meclomen) is an anthrinilic acid derivative which has been used in treating rheumatoid arthritis. This drug in the maximum dose of 100 mg 4/day may be equal in efficacy to aspirin but has a disquieting propensity for causing diarrhea in some patients. The oxicam derivative, piroxicam (Feldene), is another newer agent which has proven itself useful in the treatment of rheumatoid arthritis (44). This drug's 40-hour half-life allows it to be given in the dose of 20 mg once per day. Combination with aspirin and higher dosage of this agent are not to be recommended, especially with patients who are prone to develop duodenal ulcers (45).

Systemic corticosteroids have been advocated for the treatment of refractory rheumatoid arthritis but cannot be recommended at this time for articular manifestations alone since the propensity for side effects may outweigh the efficacy in most patients (36). Intraarticular steroids may be efficacious although much controversy surrounds their use also. Hollander has outlined (46) his indications and contraindications for the use of these agents. Injection may be indicated when one or only a few peripheral joints are inflamed, as adjacent to systemic therapy for control of resistant joints, and to assist rehabilitation and attempt to mobilize and reassure the patient regarding the possibility of efficacious therapeutic intervention in this chronic disease. Contraindications for intraarticular corticosteroid injection include the presence of infection either systemically or near the joint, active disease in multiple joints, severe destruction with uncorrected deformities and previous injection with little or no benefit. Controversy also exists as to the number of times a single joint should be injected and one reasonable program would advocate injecting no more than 3-4 times in a single joint at no greater than yearly intervals. Hollander has suggested the use of a long-acting agent such as triamcinolone acetonide t-butyl acetate (Aristospan) in the dose of 20 mg for the knee or hip and in relatively scaled down dosages for smaller joints to provide a long local antiinflammatory effect in patients with rheumatoid arthritis (47).

Gold remains the standard immunomodulating agent for the treatment of rheumatoid arthritis (48) although penicillamine (49) and the cytotoxic agents are also being used (50). Careful monitoring of patients on these agents is important and the risk to benefit ratio remains to be determined especially in view of a recent report (51) suggesting that only the gold compounds have been shown in a convincing way to decrease the x-ray progression of rheumatoid arthritis. One useful regimen for giving the injectable gold compounds, gold sodium thiomalate (Myocrysine) or gold thioglucose (Salganol), would include a stepwise graduated dose over 3-4 weeks to reach a 50 mg/week dose and then continuation of this dose for 6 months until 1 g of the medication has been given. At that time the injections can be given less frequently perhaps in a monthly schedule. Careful monitoring of either the most sensitive indicator which is the platelet count or the next most sensitive which is the white blood cell count or the obtaining of a complete blood count at each injection should minimize the possibility of not detecting a severe hematologic problem. The urine should be checked for protein at each administration of the medication since development of the nephrotic syndrome is another possible complicating problem. Since cutaneous problems may occur, careful inspection for a rash is necessary at each therapeutic visit. The practitioner should be aware that 3-6 months may be required before efficacy may be demonstrated with this potentially useful but also potentially toxic form of therapy.

Penicillamine (Depen, Cuprimine) shares with the gold compounds the propensity for cutaneous, renal, and hematologic side effects. Many different regimens have been proposed but one reasonable approach is to give 250 mg/day for 3 months, increase this to 500 mg/day for 3 months and continue increasing up to 1 g/day at the same slow rate for up to 1 year. Since this agent shares the propensity for cutaneous, renal, and hematologic side effects with gold a similar monitoring schedule should be set up to that described for gold-treated patients. Important differences may exist in that the onset of a late rash may herald the development of pemphigus so the development of bullus eruptions and fever associated with the rash after several months of therapy should result in discontinuation of the drug with no rechallenge. Proteinuria of less than 2 g/day may be well tolerated by the patient and continued therapy may be attempted as opposed to patients on gold who should be stopped when significant proteinuria develops. As with gold, significant thrombocytopenia or leukopenia should result in discontinuation of the drug. Patients may respond to this agent later than with gold even up to 1 year of initiating the drug on the slow increase regimen previously described.

Azathioprine (Imuran) may be one of the easiest of the immunomodulating agents to use (50). A dose-related leukopenia is the major common side effect so careful monitoring of complete blood counts on a schedule similar to that used for gold is appropriate in patients treated with this agent. Since disease-modifying efficacy has not been unequivocally proven (51) and since the potential for onchogenesis has not been disproved (50) gold or penicillamine should probably be utilized prior to initiating therapy with this agent.

The antimalarial agent hydroxycholoquine (Plaquenil) has been advocated in the dose of up to 200 mg twice a day for the long-term treatment of rheumatoid arthritis (36). Since an unequivocal disease-modifying effect of this agent is even more difficult to prove than with the other long-acting compounds (51) and since the potential for rash, retinal toxicity, and neuromuscular problems remains a threat, many practitioners have moved away from the utilization of this agent in the therapy of rheumatoid arthritis. It does remain, however, an agent which may be useful in some patients and probably has an overall side-effect incidence which is less than that of the other more commonly used agents (36).

It is expected that there will be a continued proliferation of newly developed drugs along with continued development of experimental agents and procedures such as lymphoplasmaphoresis (52) and total lymphoid irradiation (53, 54) for the management of the occasional patient whose disease progresses despite exposure to optimal regimens with existing antirheumatic agents. Numerous new nonsteroidal antiinflammatory agents are awaiting approval by the FDA. Many of these drugs are similar to the major classes now being utilized. Some may offer advantages in dosing, lower side-effect potential, and perhaps in the future greater efficacy in suppressing both the inflammatory components and the long-term tissue destructive elements of rheumatoid disease. The oral gold compound auranofen (Ridura) has recently been approved by the FDA for use in rheumatoid arthritis. Continuing research should produce interesting new immunomodulating agents which may strikingly modify the underlying disease process in rheumatoid arthritis. The next decade should be an exciting period in the history of rheumatoid arthritis with the discovery of new insights into its pathogenesis and the development of new specific and effective agents for its treatment.

References

1. Sturrock RD, Sharma JN, Buchanan WW: Evidence of rheumatoid arthritis in ancient India. *Arthritis Rheum* 20:42-44, 1977.

2. Short CL: The antiquity of rheumatoid arthritis. *Arthritis Rheum* 17:193-205, 1974.

3. Dequeker J: Arthritis in Flemish paintings (1400-1700). *Br Med J* 1:1203-1205, 1977.

4. Alarcon-Segovia D, Laffon A, Alcocer-Varela J: Probable depiction of juvenile arthritis by Sandro Botticelli. *Arthritis Rheum* 26:1266-1268, 1983.

5. Appelboom T, DeBoelpaepe C, Ehrlich GE, Famaey JP: Rubens and the question of antiquity of rheumatoid arthritis. *JAMA* 245:483-486, 1981.

6. Allander E, Bjelle A: Developments in epidemiologic studies on rheumatoid arthritis. *Scand J Rheumatol* 10:257-261, 1981.

7. Lawrence JS: Rheumatoid arthritis. In JS Lawrence (ed.), *Rheumatism in Populations.* London, William Heinemann Medical Books Limited, 1977, pp. 156-271.

8. Buchanan WW, Murdoch RM: Hypothesis: That rheumatoid arthritis will disappear. *J Rheumatol* 6:324-329, 1979.

9. Stastny P: Mixed lymphocyte cultures in rheumatoid arthritis. *J Clin Invest* 57:1148-1157, 1976.

10. Gran JT, Husby G, Thorsby E: The association between rheumatoid arthritis and the HLA antigen DR4. *Ann Rheum Dis* 42:292-296, 1983.

11. Ueno Y, Iwaki Y, Terasaki PI, Park MS, Barnett EV, Chia D, Nakata S: HLA-DR4 Negro and Mexican rheumatoid arthritis patients. *J Rheumatol* 8:804-807, 1981.

12. Harvey J, Lotze M, Arnett FC, Bias WB, Billingsley ML, Harvey E, Hsu SH, Sutton JD, Zizic TM, Stevens MB: Rheumatoid arthritis in a Chippewa band. II. Field study with clinical serologic and HLA-D correlations. *J Rheumatol* 10:28-32, 1983.

13. Solinger AM, Bhatnagar R, Stobo JD: Cellular, molecular, and genetic characteristics of T cell reactivity to collagen in man. *Proc Nat Acad SC USA* 78:3877-3881, 1981.

14. Depper JM, Zvaifler NJ: Epstein-Barr virus - Its relationship to the pathogenesis of rheumatoid arthritis. *Arthritis Rheum* 24:755-761, 1981.

15. Alspaugh MA, Shoji H, Nonoyama M: A search for rheumatoid arthritis - Associated nuclear antigen and Epstein-Barr virus specific antigens or genomes in tissues and cells from patients with rheumatoid arthritis. *Arthritis Rheum* 26:712-720, 1983.

16. Hollander JL, McCarty DJ Jr, Astorga G, Castro-Murillo E: Studies on the pathogenesis of rheumatoid joint inflammation. I. The "RA cell" and a working hypothesis. *Ann Intern Med* 62:271-280, 1965.

17. Treadway W, Colins RL, Turner RA, DeChatelet L: Polymorphonuclear leukocyte secretory and metabolic responses in immunoglobulin aggregates. *J Rheumatol* 6:636-644, 1979.

18. Bland JH: Rheumatoid arthritis of the cervical spine. *J Rheumatol* 1:319-342, 1974.

19. Wilkinson M, Meikle JAK: Tomography of the sacroiliac joints. *Ann Rheum Dis* 25:433-440, 1966.

20. Chalmers IM, Blair GS: Rheumatoid arthritis of the temporomandibular joint. *Q J Med* (XLII):369-386, 1973.

21. Turner R, Collins R, Nomeir AM: Extraarticular manifestations of rheumatoid arthritis. *Bull Rheum Dis* 29:986-991, 1978-79.

22. Nomeir AM, Turner R, Watts E, Smith D, West C, Edmonds J: Cardiac involvement in rheumatoid arthritis. *Ann Intern Med* 79:800-806, 1973.

23. Nomeir AM, Turner RA, Watts LE: Cardiac involvement in rheumatoid arthritis. Follow-up study. *Arthritis Rheum* 22:561-564, 1979.

24. Collins RL, Turner RA, Johnson AM, Whitley NO, McLean RL: Obstructive pulmonary disease in rheumatoid arthritis. *Arthritis Rheum* 19:623-628, 1976.

25. Pisko EJ, Turner RA, Yeatts RP, Burch PG, McKinley PH, Collins RL: Ocular pathology, tear production, and tear lysozyme in rheumatoid arthritis. *J Rheumatol* 9:708-711, 1982.

26. Turner R, Lipshutz W, Miller W, Rittenberg G, Schumacher HR, Cohen S: Esophageal dysfunction in collagen disease. *Am J Med Sci* 265:191-199, 1973.

27. Ropes MW, Bennett GA, Cobb S, Jacox R, Jessar RA: 1958 revision of diagnostic criteria for rheumatoid arthritis. *Bull Rheum Dis* 9:175-176, 1958.

28. Bennett PH, Burch TA: New York Symposium on Population Studies in the Rheumatic Diseases: New diagnostic criteria. *Bull Rheum Dis* 17:453-458, 1967.

29. O'Sullivan JB, Cathcart ES: The prevalence of rheumatoid—Follow-up evaluation of the effect of criteria on rates in Sudbury, Massachusetts. *Ann Intern Med* 76:573-577, 1972.

30. Glyn LE: The chronicity of inflammation and its significance in rheumatoid arthritis. *Ann Rheum Dis* 27:105-121, 1968.

31. Schumacher HR, Kitridou RC: Synovitis of recent onset. A clinicopathologic study during the first month of disease. *Arthritis Rheum* 15:465-485, 1972.

32. Kulka JP: Vascular derangement in rheumatoid arthritis. In AGS Hill (ed.), *Modern Trends in Rheumatology,* 1st Ed. London, 1966, pp. 49-69.

33. Cruickshank B: The arteritis of rheumatoid arthritis. *Ann Rheum Dis* 13: 136-146, 1954.

34. Steinbrocker O, Traeger CH, Batterman RC: Therapeutic criteria in rheumatoid arthritis. *J Am Med Assoc* 140:659-662, 1949.

35. Duthie JJR, Brown PE, Truelove LH, Baragar FD, Lawrie AJ: Course and prognosis in rheumatoid arthritis—A further report. *Ann Rheum Dis* 23:193-204, 1964.

36. Turner R: Medical management of rheumatoid arthritis. Rec Adv Clin Ther Vol III: In JZ Yetiv, JR Bianchine (eds.), *Antivirals and Antimicrobials Anticancer Agents Cardiovascular Therapy.* New York, Grune and Stratton, 1983, pp. 279-294.

37. Turner R: Aspirin and newer antiinflammatory agents in rheumatoid arthritis. *Fam Physician* 16:110-115, 1977.

38. Turner RA, Whipple JB, Shackleford RW: Diflunisal (500-750 mg) versus aspirin (2600-3900 mg) in the treatment of rheumatoid arthritis. *Pharmacotherapy* 4:151-157, 1984.

39. Davis JD, Turner RA, Collins RL, Ruchte IR, Kaufman JS: Fenoprofen, aspirin, and gold induction in rheumatoid arthritis. *Clin Pharmacol Ther* 21:52-61, 1977.

40. Turner R, April PA, Robbins DL: Double-blind multicenter study comparing piroxicam and ibuprofen in the treatment of rheumatoid arthritis. *Am J Med* S34-S538, 1982.

41. Day RO, Furst DE, Dromgoole SH, Kamm B, Roe R, Paulus HE: Relationship of serum naproxen concentrate to efficacy in rheumatoid arthritis. *Clin Pharm Ther* 31:733-740, 1982.

42. Chalmers A, Offer R, Robinson HS: A double-blind controlled study comparing the use of ASA and tolmetin with ASA and placebo in the treatment of rheumatoid arthritis. *Curr Ther Res* 24:517-523, 1978.

43. Ciabattoni G, Cinotti GA, Pierucci A, Simonetti BM, Manzi M, Pugliese F, Barsotti P, Pecci G, Taggi F, Patrong C: Effects of sulindac and ibuprofen in patients with chronic glomerular disease. *NEJM* 310:279-283, 1984.

44. Turner R: Review of the management of rheumatoid arthritis with piroxicam. *Postgrad Med Special Report,* April, 1982, pp. 42-49.

45. Semble E, Metcalf D, Turner R, Agudelo C, Pisko E, Johnson AM, Heise E: Genetic predictors of patient response and side effects in the treatment of rheumatoid arthritis with a high dose nonsteroidal antiinflammatory drug regimen. *Arthritis Rheum* 25:370-374, 1982.

46. Hollander JL: Intrasynovial corticosteroid therapy in arthritis. *MD State Med J* 19:62-66, 1970.

47. Hollander JL, Jessar RA, Restifo RA, Fort HJ: A new intraarticular steroid ester with longer effectiveness. *Arthritis Rheum* 4:422, 1961.

48. Sharp JT, Lidsky MD, Duffy J: Clinical responses during gold therapy for rheumatoid arthritis. *Arthritis Rheum* 25:540-549, 1982.

49. Metcalf DL, Turner RA, Agudelo CA: Penicillamine in rheumatoid arthritis: A clinical guide. *South Med J* 73:1053-1057, 1980.

50. Davis JD, Muss HB, Turner RA: Cytotoxic agents in the treatment of rheumatoid arthritis. *South Med J* 71:57-64, 1978.

51. Iannuzzi L, Dawson N, Zein N, Kushner I: Does drug therapy slow radiographic deterioration in rheumatoid arthritis? *NEJM* 309:1023-1028, 1983.

52. Wallace D, Goldfinger D, Lowe C, Nichols S, Wiener J, Brachman M, Klinenbert JR: A double-blind, controlled study of lymphoplasmapheresis versus sham apheresis in rheumatoid arthritis. *N Engl J Med* 306:1406-1410, 1982.

53. Kotzin BL, Strober S, Engleman EG, Calin A, Hoppe RT, Kansas GS, Terrell CP, Kaplan HS: Treatment of intractable rheumatoid arthritis with total lymphoid irradiation. *N Engl J Med* 305:969-976, 1981.

54. Trentham DE, Belli JA, Anderson RJ, Buckley JA, Goetzl EJ, David JR, Austen KF: Clinical and immunological effects of fractionated total lymphoid irradiation in refractory rheumatoid arthritis. *N Engl J Med* 305:976-982, 1981.

Chapter 9

OSTEOARTHRITIS

John F. Benson, M.D., Edward J. Pisko, M.D.,
and Christopher M. Wise, M.D.

General

Introduction

Osteoarthritis is an illness characterized by cartilage degeneration and new bone (osteophyte) formation. In addition, there is sclerosis and cyst formation in subchondral bone and variable synovial changes consisting primarily of fibrosis. Symptomatically, patients develop pain, swelling, and stiffness in their joints which can be followed by joint laxity, decreased joint motion, and deformity. A large variety of pathologic and pathogenetic processes can lead to osteoarthritis of a joint and conceptually osteoarthritis should be thought of as a final common pathway for which multiple causes are responsible for the late findings. Osteoarthritis can be divided into primary and secondary forms in which the etiology of the disease is either unknown or secondary to known inflammatory, biochemical, or mechanical factors. The prevalence of osteoarthritic joint changes at autopsy can approach 100% by age 80. Thus it has been postulated that osteoarthritis is merely a part of the aging process in which there is selective senescence manifested in the joints. The stereotype of osteoarthritis as an unfortunate and relatively benign concomitant of aging belies the complex events which underly its pathogenesis. Recent work has shown that excessive enzyme activity, synovitis, crystal deposition, and/or immunoglobulin deposition may be important in the pathogenesis of this disease. Osteoarthritis is responsible for considerable morbidity throughout the world. There are profound economic effects from this illness in terms of decreased productivity secondary to work absences and early retirement because of disability.

Historical Aspects

Osteoarthritis is a widespread disease of man and other vertebrates. There is evidence that suggests that early man and dinosaurs suffered from this condition. The development of this illness in seagoing mammals emphasizes the importance of factors other than weight-bearing in the pathogenesis of this disease. Despite its long history (1), osteoarthritis is a relatively newly described (twentieth century) clinical entity. Throughout the nineteenth century and even much of the twentieth century, osteoarthritis was lumped with other forms of arthritis, particularly rheumatoid arthritis, in papers describing chronic deforming arthritis. The process of splitting off osteoarthritis from rheumatoid arthritis was greatly aided by Goldthwait's 1904 classification of osteoarthritis as atrophic and rheumatoid as hypertrophic arthritis. In 1802, Heberden described the characteristic firm nodular swelling of the distal interphalangeal joints that bear his name and osteoarthritic changes of the proximal interphalangeal joints were described by Bouchard in 1884. However, it was not until 1907 that Garrod related these nodes to osteoarthritic involvement of the distal interphalangeal and proximal interphalangeal joints. In recent decades, attempts have been made to subdivide osteoarthritis into more specific categories enabling clinicians and researchers to better define these entities. Kellgren's description of generalized osteoarthritis is such an attempt. However, further work will be necessary before the usefulness of splitting up patients with osteoarthritis into specific subsets can be demonstrated to clinicians and researchers.

Definitions

Osteoarthritis, osteoarthrosis, and degenerative joint disease are all names for the same disease entity. Osteoarthritis is a term popular in the United States. This term has been criticized because it suggests that this disease is a primary inflammatory disorder. While inflammatory arthritis can predispose to osteoarthritis and inflammation is a common secondary event in osteoarthritis, the British may be correct in suggesting that osteoarthrosis is a better term. This term refers to the overproduction of new bone which is quite characteristic of this disease. The term degenerative joint disease is unacceptable because it suggests that this illness is merely part of the overall aging process.

Clinical criteria for osteoarthritis have not been formulated by the American Rheumatism Association as they have for many other rheumatic diseases. For the purposes of clinical trials, three major criteria are needed to diagnose this illness. These include roentgenographic changes and clinical symptoms suggestive of this illness in a setting where other joint diseases have been excluded. The roentgenographic features include cartilage loss, osteophyte formation, bony sclerosis, and/or cyst formation. Characteristic symptoms include resting pain, night pain, and pain on motion. Joint pain occurring in a patient with roentgenographic features of the disease is a good working definition of this illness. It is important to note that patients may have roentgenograms consistent with osteoarthritis, but joint pain attributable to other causes such as trauma, tendonitis, infection, and crystal-induced disease. In addition, patients may have no symptoms and typical, sometimes advanced, changes of osteoarthritis on roentgenogram.

As summarized in Table 9.1, osteoarthritis may be classified as either primary or secondary. The terms primary and secondary osteoarthritis refer to osteoarthritis of idiopathic etiology or secondary to a known inflammatory, biomechanical, or biochemical insult to the joint. The terms are artificial because etiologic

TABLE 9.1 Classification of Osteoarthritis (OA)

Primary

- Primary generalized OA
- Erosive OA

Secondary

- Congenital and developmental abnormalities (especially in hips)
- Posttraumatic [including neuropathic (Charcot's) arthropathy]
- Postinflammatory (RA, infectious arthritis, gout, pseudogout, psoriatic arthritis)
- Other localized bone and joint disorders (Paget's disease, avascular necrosis)
- Endocrine/metabolic disorders (acromegaly, diabetes, hypothyroidism, hemochromatosis, recurrent hemarthrosis (hemophilia), ochronosis, Wilson's disease)

factors can be found in most cases of osteoarthritis. Osteoarthritis with Heberden's nodes, which most likely is under hereditary and sex-linked influence because of its frequent occurrence in women with a positive family history, is considered part of primary osteoarthritis.

Various subsets of osteoarthritis have been described, although these do lead to similar pathological changes. The term primary generalized osteoarthritis has been used to describe a group of patients with widespread disease who have involvement of the usual sites such as the distal interphalangeal, proximal interphalangeal, and first carpal-metacarpal joints of the hand as well as the hip, knees, and first metatarsal-phalangeal joints. These patients can occasionally have mild systemic involvement with their disease and a slight elevation of the sedimentation rate is occasionally found. Erosive osteoarthritis is another subset of osteoarthritis that is occasionally difficult to differentiate from rheumatoid arthritis. The sedimendation rate may also be slightly elevated and the synovium may be more inflamed than is usually seen in osteoarthritis. A cardinal feature of erosive osteoarthritis is marked joint destruction with extensive cystic change and erosions that are found on roentgenogram. This disease is less likely to be generalized and the proximal and distal interphalangeal joints are characteristically involved. The metacarpophalangeal joints and/or the carpal joints are occasionally also involved. When this occurs, there can be more confusion as to whether or not the patient has rheumatoid arthritis. However, erosive osteoarthritis does not usually involve the shoulders, elbows, or ankles. In general, joint involvement in joints other than the distal and proximal interphalangeal joints tends to be relatively minor.

Diffuse idiopathic skeletal hyperostosis, or DISH syndrome, is considered a form of spinal osteoarthritis and is discussed later in the chapter. Osteophytes formed in this disease tend to flow from one vertebral body to the next. Studies suggesting that these patients may have hyperinsulinemia point to a possible metabolic defect leading to marked periosteal change. Chondromalacia patellae, a specialized cartilage degeneration problem of the knee, often occurs in younger individuals in the absence of other evidence of osteoarthritis.

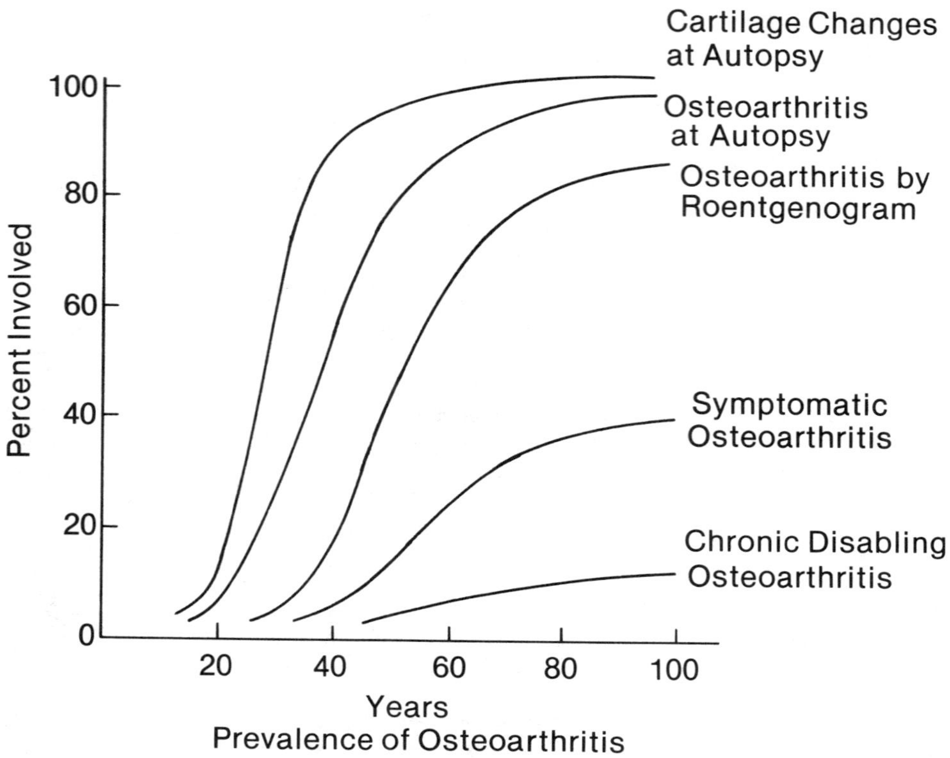

FIGURE 9.1 Prevalence of osteoarthritis. Osteoarthritis can be defined by cartilage change at autopsies suggestive of osteoarthritis, definite osteoarthritis at autopsy, roentgenogram, or by symptomatic disease in individuals with roentgenographic findings. The prevalence of disease at autopsy rises rapidly during the third decade. The prevalence of disease on roentgenograms and symptomatic disease rises rapidly between ages 40 and 60. Chronic disabling osteoarthritis may affect 10% of older individuals.

Epidemiology

As noted in the previous section, osteoarthritis can be difficult to define and statements about the prevalence of this disease are therefore also difficult. Figure 9.1 pictorially shows the prevalence of osteoarthritis using various criteria. Cartilage changes consistent with early osteoarthritis can be found in autopsy by the early 20's and osteoarthritis at autopsy is not uncommon by the end of the second decade. Autopsy studies suggest that osteoarthritis is almost universal by age 80. By age 60, about half of all individuals will have roentgenographic evidence of osteoarthritis. However, symptomatic osteoarthritis is much less common and chronic osteoarthritis leading to permanent disability is relatively rare.

The high frequency of osteoarthritis on autopsy and roentgenograms in the elderly is responsible for the widespread belief that osteoarthritis is an unavoidable effect of aging. These data are more accurately interpreted in terms of accumulated episodes of osteoarthritis over time. Since complete healing is rare in this disease, there will be cumulative disease by roentgenogram or histologic examination. By using roentgenographic and histological criteria, the high prevalence of osteoarthritis in the elderly is therefore a reflection of the relatively high incidence of this disease during middle age. Symptomatic osteoarthritis begins in the late 30's and the incidence rises rapidly to age 60 before the incidence rate may even fall after age 60. The likelihood of developing osteoarthritis in the aged may be less than in middle age. Osteoarthritis of the large joints affects men more commonly by age 50 and osteoarthritis with Heberden's and Bouchard's nodes tends to be more of an illness of women over age 50. Both of these forms of osteoarthritis tend to be well established by retirement.

Etiopathogenesis

Normal Cartilage

Osteoarthritis is primarily a disease of cartilage disintegration (2-5). The balance between cartilage synthesis and degradation is shifted towards cartilage destruction. Changes in the synovium, joint capsule, and underlying bone are secondary to the cartilage changes. Normal cartilage as well as subchondral bone and accessory structures such as muscle and the joint capsule are responsible for absorbing impact loads. When cartilage is altered or lost, increased force is transmitted to bone and the accessory structures. Since these areas are innervated by pain fibers, pain may result. Cartilage is a body structure that is ideally suited to its function. When intact, it performs superbly, but when altered, it can lead to decreased function and pain. In a normal joint, the articular cartilage is smooth and glistening. There is an extremely low coefficient of friction (one/fifth of ice on ice). Joint lubrication depends in part on the synovial fluid and to some extent on the rapid transfer of water in and out of the cartilage to form a boundary lubrication system. These "beads of water" are compressed out of the gel-like cartilage, and we "walk on water." The cartilage matrix is hyperhydrated (70-80% water) with a pressure of over 1000 mmHg.

Articular cartilage appears to be ideally adapted for friction-free movement of the synovial joints and at the same time it transmits impact load energy to the underlying cancellous bone which is well adapted to absorb it. The structure of cartilage is responsible for its unique properties. Cartilage consists of an intertwined mesh of type II collagen and proteoglycan. Proteoglycans have a complex structure in which a protein core is surrounded by bottlebrush-like negatively charged glycose-aminoglycan side chains. These consist of chondroitin and keratan sulfate. The proteoglycans form aggregates in cartilage and are attached by a link protein to a hyaluronic acid core.

Cartilage Changes

The earliest changes in osteoarthritis can be osberved in cartilage, where there is an increase in water content and an alteration in the structure of the proteoglycan molecules. Histological changes of osteoarthritis are shown in Table 9.2.

With the onset of degenerative changes, the proteoglycan content decreases overall despite increased synthesis by the chondrocytes. In addition, there is a shift in the ratio of chondroitin-4 to chondroitin-6 sulfate accompanied by a decrease in the keratan sulfate. It is important to note that these changes in matrix composition are the reverse of those seen in aging. The collagen content of osteoarthritic cartilage is basically unchanged, but there is a shift in its com-

TABLE 9.2 Histological Changes in Osteoarthritis

Loss of proteoglycan in the superficial layers
Irregularity of the surface layer produced by tangential fissures
Replication of chondrocytes
Vertical-oriented clefts in cartilage
Replication of the "tide-mark" or boundary area between calcified and noncalcified cartilage with vascular invasion
Subchondral bone sclerosis with microfractures of trabecular bone and cyst formation
Formation of marginal osteophytes
Synovial changes consistent with low-grade inflammatory changes

position to include type I collagen (bone and tendon type collagen). This change in collagen content may represent fibrocartilaginous repair, although its exact significance remains to be demonstrated. As previously noted, the process whereby osteoarthritic cartilage is destroyed is a very dynamic process in which senescence plays little or no role. The metabolic and chemical changes that occur during the pathogenesis of osteoarthritis are seen in Table 9.3.

It is not surprising that the changes in cartilage reflected by the histological changes and metabolic and chemical changes lead to a marked alteration in the mechanical properties of cartilage. The altered biochemical changes of cartilage are seen in Table 9.4.

General Pathogenetic Factors

Aging

As previously mentioned, the aging process has been believed to be important in the pathogenesis of osteoarthritis. However, the prevailing evidence suggests that aging factors may be of little or no importance in the pathogenesis of this illness. Perhaps the most important evidence suggesting that aging is of little importance in this illness is that aging leads to an increase in the ratio of keratan to chondroitin sulfate in cartilage and this is opposite to the changes that occur in osteoarthritis.

Mechanical Factors

Mechanical factors are believed by some authors to be the major pathogenetic factor in the development of osteoarthritis (3,6). Mechanical factors primarily affect subchondral bone and cartilage is affected only indirectly. Repetitive impulse loading causes tensile fatigue and microfractures within the subchondral bone. As a result of this, callus and vascularization develop. As the physical

TABLE 9.3 Metabolic and Chemical Changes in Osteoarthritis

Increased thymidine uptake indicative of DNA synthesis and cell replication
Increased water content of cartilage
Increased radiolabelled sulfate uptake indicative of increased proteoglycan synthesis
Decreased aggregation of proteoglycans
Slight increase in collagen synthesis
Abnormalities in link protein
Increased amount of degradative enzymes found in synovial fluid and cartilage including proteases such as the cathepsins
Increased hyaluronidase and collagenase are found in the synovial fluid
Increased amounts of prostaglandin are found in synovial fluid
Immunoglobulins are found in cartilage bound to antigenic products of matrix injury

TABLE 9.4 Biomechanical Changes in Osteoarthritis

Diminished compliance of cartilage related to loss of proteoglycan
Increased stiffness of subchondral bone transferring more load impact stress to articular cartilage
Increased friction secondary to surface irregularity
Synovitis occasionally associated with calcium hydroxyapatite and/or pyrophosphate crystals

characteristics of subchondral bone change, there is more impulse load absorbed by the cartilage. Cartilage is better equipped to transmit energy than to absorb it and the changes in the subchondral bone therefore lead to cartilage damage as the cartilage can no longer withstand the normal impulse loading of everyday life.

It is thought by some authors that the early changes in subchondral bone consist of interruption of the microvascular supply to subchondral bone. When the microvascular supply to the subchondral bone is compromised, a resultant microosteonecrosis may be followed by the typical microfractures that can occur in this illness. These mechanical factors may lead to the release of proteoglycan into synovial fluid and increased water content of the cartilage which in turn alters the properties of the cartilage and makes it much less efficient.

Chondrocyte Changes

Increases in the numbers of chondrocytes and increases in chondrycyte metabolic activity may be of prime importance in the pathogenesis of osteoarthritis. As previously noted, a large variety of factors may lead to the osteoarthritic process, and it has been proposed that the factors primarily operate by activating chondrocytes. This process is summarized pictorially in Figure 9.2. Complex changes in the microenvironment of the chondrocyte may be responsible for chondrocyte activation and these activated chondrocytes may begin to mitose, increase in number, and synthesize cartilage as well as degradative enzymes (7). The insulted chondrocyte becomes a powerhouse, increasing in numbers and showing a sixfold increase in synthetic activity (6). This remodeling process can lead to overproduction of collagen and proteoglycans, as well as new bone (osteophytes). In general, the chondrocyte is unable to compensate for cartilage destruction by making sufficient new cartilage. The mechanical properties of the new cartilage that is formed are not as adequate as the previously normal cartilage. Fibrocartilage formed after cartilage damage may be of some benefit in terms of maintaining joint function. However, the altered biochemical properties of this cartilage may help to perpetuate the osteoarthritis disease process.

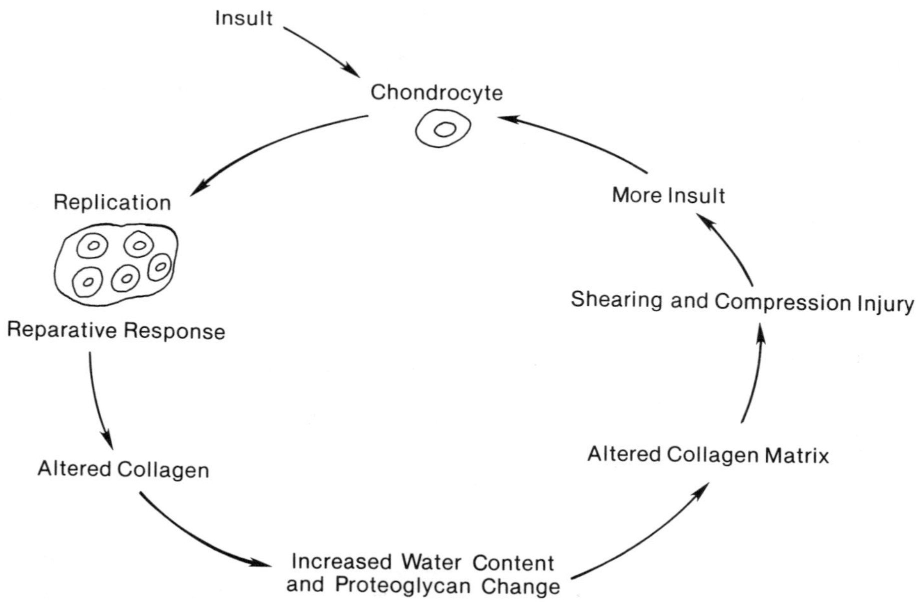

FIGURE 9.2 The pathogenesis of osteoarthritis. The chondrocyte may play an essential role in the pathogenesis of osteoarthritis. Insults such as trauma, infections, inflammatory conditions, or biochemical changes may lead to chondrocyte proliferation with ineffective cartilage remodeling that predisposes to further chondrocyte injury. This process perpetuates the cycle and leads to further osteoarthritis.

Synovial Changes

It is possible that proteolytic enzymes contained within the macrophage-like or type A synovial lining cells are capable of digesting the core protein of chondroitin sulfate. These type A lining cells can be activated by a large variety of processes. Inhibitory factors produced by the type B or fibroblast-like cells in the joint may inhibit proteolytic enzymes, and insults occurring during the osteoarthritic disease process may operate by blocking the release of such inhibitory factors. Alterations in the proteoglycan molecule caused by proteolytic enzymes may lead to adverse mechanical factors which in turn may either activate chrondrocytes or lead to increased stress on the subchondral bone.

Specific Pathogenetic Factors

Acute Trauma

Acute trauma is generally not considered to be associated with inflammation, but acute trauma is followed by an inflammatory reaction which in turn can lead to bony proliferation about the damaged joint.

Chronic Trauma

Minor occupational trauma of a chronic nature can lead to osteoarthritic changes of the spine and knees such as those found in coal miners. The toes of dancers, the shoulders of bus drivers, and the hands of jack hammer operators may also be affected. More severe repeated injuries such as those in the knees of football players and the spine of ice hockey players can also lead to osteoarthritic changes.

Neuropathic Joint Disease

Neuropathic joint disease is an extreme example of traumatic arthritis in which loss of sensation and proprioception leads to loss of joint protection and secondary osteoarthritis. Syphilis is the classic cause of neuropathic joint disease (the Charcot joint). However, diabetes is more likely to cause neuropathic joint disease and syringomyelia is also frequently implicated. Trauma to the spinal cord or peripheral nerves may also lead to neuropathic joint disease and a variety of inflammatory and metabolic conditions causing peripheral damage may lead to a neuropathic joint. Changes seen on roentgenogram often enable one to distinguish the neuropathic joint from other joints involved with osteoarthritis. There is marked cartilage loss and quite dramatic new bone formation. The neuropathic process leads to a severe derangement of the joint with marked deformities on roentgenogram.

Congenital Defects

Congenital defects, particularly in the hip, have frequently been implicated in the pathogenesis of osteoarthritis. Acetabular abnormalities ranging from idiopathic protrusion acetabuli to shallow acetabulus have been implicated. Epiphyseal dysplasias such as those of the hip and knee may also be implicated in the pathogenesis of this disease.

Osteonecrosis

Conditions such as aseptic necrosis of the hip, which in turn may be secondary to a variety of factors, will often lead to secondary osteoarthritis. The osteochondritides such as that of the knee may also lead to secondary osteoarthritis.

Inflammatory Arthritides

Infectious and idiopathic inflammatory forms of arthritis such as rheumatoid arthritis, septic arthritis, and psoriatic arthritis may lead to a secondary osteoarthritis, particularly when there is relative inactivity of the inflammatory joint disease process. Joint injury caused by crystals such as those seen in gout, pseudogout, or apatite disease may also lead to osteoarthritis (8).

Chondrocalcinosis

Chondrocalcinosis, pseudogout, and osteoarthritis are all related to each other, but the exact nature of this relationship remains unknown (8).

Endocrine Diseases

Acromegaly is frequently associated with osteoarthritis. Osteoarthritic changes are felt secondary to increases in the number of chondrocytes as well as thickening of articular cartilage. These changes in turn are secondary to increases in growth hormone and somatomedin. Patients with diabetes mellitus are at increased risk for developing osteoarthritis. It is possible that the relative unavailability of insulin may block the cartilage repair process. Conversely, in the DISH syndrome, hyperinsulinemia may lead to increased metabolic activity and bony proliferation.

Wilson's Disease

Wilson's disease may be associated with premature osteoarthritis. The occurrence of the joint findings is apparently unrelated to the other manifestations of this disease. Pseudogout and chondromalacia patellae are also associated with Wilson's disease.

Hemochromatosis

The articular manifestations of hemochromatosis resemble those of osteoarthritis, although the pattern of joint involvement differs (as discussed in Chapter 23). Hemochromatosis is also associated with chondrocalcinosis and pseudogout. The relationship between these entities and associated osteoarthritic-like changes have not been totally clarified.

Ochronosis (Alkaptonuria)

Patients with ochronosis have increased urinary excretion of homogentisic acid and this pigment is responsible for darkening of cartilage and vertebral calcification. The binding of homogentisic acid to connective tissue is responsible for the secondary osteoarthritis that is seen in this condition. Osteoarthritis of the spine and pseudogout are characteristic findings in this illness.

Clinical Features

Symptoms and Signs

Because osteoarthritis is such a common condition, it is not surprising that the clinical presentation may be very different from one patient to another, depending on the pattern of joint involvement, duration, and severity of the process. Pain is usually localized to a particular joint or to a general area of the body near the joint. In osteoarthritis, there may often be a discrepancy between pathologic and radiographic findings and the intensity of the pain. Although the mechanisms for this inconsistency are not entirely clear, it is probable that most of the pain results from irritation of pain receptors in areas around the affected joint (such as fibrous capsule, ligaments and periosteum), rather than from the diseased cartilage itself (9). Pain in osteoarthritis is usually of a deep, aching quality. Although it is usually localized to the joint, pain may be referred to a nearby area, such as pain in the knee resulting from OA of the hip.

Morning stiffness and "gel phenomenon" during the day frequently occur in osteoarthritis, but are seldom generalized, and usually only last 15-30 minutes. Prolonged or generalized stiffness, constitutional symptoms such as weight loss, fever, and fatigue should not be present in osteoarthritis and, if present, should suggest another disease process (such as rheumatoid arthritis or polymyalgia rheumatica) to the clinician.

Typical physical findings in osteoarthritis include localized tenderness, joint enlargement (either soft tissue or bony), and crepitus (grating and crackling sensation within the joint felt on passive movement). Synovial effusions may be detected but tend to be smaller than those seen in inflammatory disorders, and mild warmth may be present. As the disease becomes more progressive, loss of movement and deformity may be seen.

The joints most commonly affected by osteoarthritis are the distal and proximal interphalangeal (DIP and PIP) joints of the hands, the first carpal-metacarpal (CMC) joints, the knees and hips, cervical and lumbar spine, and the first metatarsal phalangeal joint (MTP) in the foot (10). Involvement of other joints by osteoarthritis is relatively unusual, and should suggest a secondary cause (see discussion below), such as in the case of metacarpal-phalangeal (MCP) joints in the hands (seen in hemochromatosis), or when the shoulders, elbows, wrists, or ankles are involved (usually resulting from trauma).

Clinical Patterns of Osteoarthritis

Primary Osteoarthritis

Primary generalized osteoarthritis, first described by Kellgren and Moore (11), is considered to be a heritable form of osteoarthritis which occurs most frequently in middle-aged and elderly females. There is usually a family history of the condition in one or both parents, and it appears to be inherited in a dominant form in women, and recessively in men. As shown in Figure 9.3 the small joints of the hands are most typically involved as bony enlargement of the DIP joints (Heberden's nodes) and PIP joints (Bouchard's nodes). The other joints typically involved are noted above. This condition is generally slowly progressive, but may have an episodic course with inflammatory exacerbations associated with mild elevations of sedimentation rates (10).

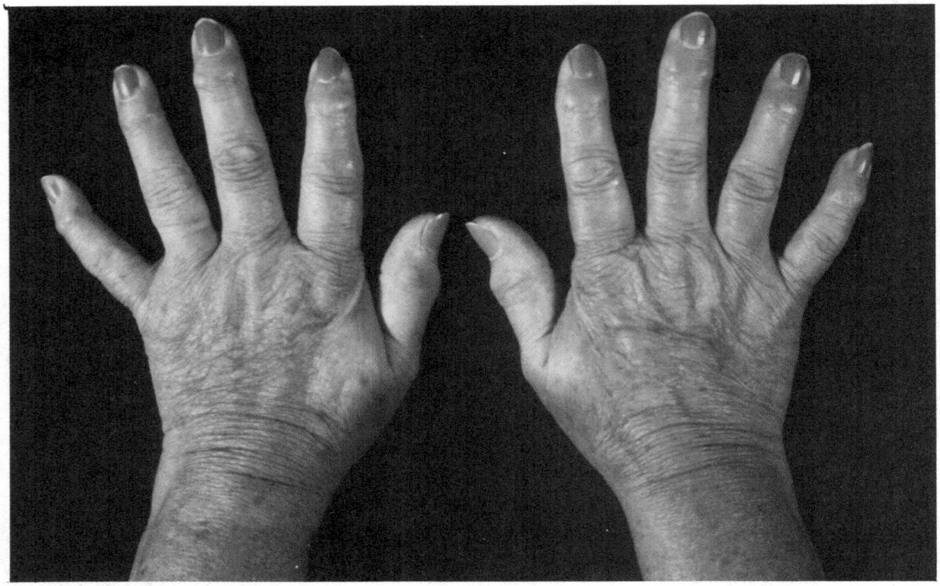

FIGURE 9.3 The hands of a patient with primary osteoarthritis, demonstrating bony enlargement of most of the distal interphalangeal joints (Herberden's nodes). There is also enlargement of the proximal interphalangeal joints of both index fingers (Bouchard's nodes).

Erosive osteoarthritis is a variant of the above, with disease confined to the DIP and PIP joints. It is characterized by acute episodes of inflammation followed by severe destructive changes, bony erosions, and osteophytes. In general, this syndrome tends to involve the small joints of the hands intermittently in sequence and leads eventually to deformity and ankylosis of these joints (12).

Secondary Forms of Osteoarthritis

As listed in Table 9.1, osteoarthritis may occur in secondary forms. Although the distinctions between primary and secondary forms of osteoarthritis may sometimes be difficult, there are several situations in which the clinical and pathologic changes of osteoarthritis can be attributed to an underlying process.

Congenital and developmental abnormalities that result in alteration of alignment and mechanical forces that act across the joints are frequent causes of secondary osteoarthritis. This is particularly true in the hip, where a long list of abnormalities is associated with the later development of osteoarthritis (10). Congenital hip dysplasia, slipped capital femoral epiphysis, and Legg-Calve-Perthes disease are conditions seen in the pediatric age group which are associated with osteoarthritis of the hip in adults. Joint hypermobility, as seen in Ehler's-Danlos syndrome and related conditions, may also predispose to osteoarthritis because of loss of ligamentous support. Valgus and varus deformities of the knees and unequal leg lengths, as well as subtle abnormalities in angulation of the femoral neck are also thought to predispose to osteoarthritis.

Posttraumatic osteoarthritis can occur after any injury in which the articular surfaces of the bone are injured and do not heal properly (13). This sometimes is related to occupational overuse, such as osteoarthritis in the elbows and shoulders seen in pneumatic drill workers, or ankle disease in ballet dancers and soccer players. Sports participation in general, though, does not necessarily predispose to the development of osteoarthritis unless there has been a specific injury (14). Neuropathic arthropathy (Charcot joint) may occur in a wide variety of conditions in which there are abnormalities of proprioception and other sensory mechanisms. This entity is distinct from other forms of osteoarthritis in the severity of the destructive and hypertrophic bone changes, as well as the relative paucity of associated pain. Neuropathic arthropathy may involve the shoulders, elbows, knees, ankles, and small joints of the feet. In the past, syphilitic tabes dorsalis was the most common cause of this, but in recent years, chronic diabetic neuropathy and syringomyelia have been more frequently associated with this syndrome.

The end-stage of almost any inflammatory arthritis will have most of the clinical, radiographic, and pathologic features of osteoarthritis. Rheumatoid arthritis, in particular, is a very common cause of postinflammatory osteoarthritis. Infectious arthritis, when inadequately treated, may result in loss of joint space, cartilage degeneration, osteophyte formation, and ankylosis. Gout, pseudogout, and psoriatic arthritis may also result in secondary osteoarthritis, but there are usually features of these conditions that allow easy distinction from primary osteoarthritis. In some cases, distinguishing between primary osteoarthritis and postinflammatory osteoarthritis may be difficult, as in the case of "burned out" rheumatoid arthritis when it affects the knees and hips. Careful review of the clinical history, pattern of other joint involvement, and radiographic features usually make the separation of these entities possible.

Almost any other localized disorder of bone or joint space that results in altered joint space mechanics can lead to a secondary osteoarthritis. Paget's disease, which results in remodeling of bone, may result in reshaping of the joint space with subsequent altered mechanics and degenerative changes, particularly in the hip. Avascular necrosis of bone (ischemic necrosis, osteonecrosis, aseptic necrosis) may occur anywhere, particularly in the femoral head or in the bones about the knee and may be associated with trauma or multiple systemic diseases, including hemoglobinopathies, caisson worker's disease, alcoholism, chronic pancreatitis, liver disease, rheumatoid arthritis, SLE, or chronic corticosteroid therapy. This localized area of ischemic bone will often result in remodeling of the articular surface of the affected joint and result in osteoarthritis.

A large number of endocrine and metabolic disorders are associated with secondary osteoarthritis. The clinical features of these are discussed earlier in this chapter and in Chapter 23 in more detail. In some situations, as in the case of diabetes, there is an increased association with typical osteoarthritis, while in others, such as acromegaly, hypothyroidism, or hemochromatosis, the pattern of joint involvement and certain radiographic features distinguish these forms from typical primary osteoarthritis.

Regional Involvement in Osteoarthritis

Hand

Hand involvement in primary osteoarthritis is relatively predictable. The distal interphalangeal (DIP) joints are the most commonly involved in the hands with proximal interphalangeal (PIP) being the next most common, occurring in about 40% of those with DIP involvement. Typically, patients will experience pain and stiffness in these joints with gradual bony enlargement over many years, and moderate loss of function. These enlargements, termed Heberden's nodes (DIP) and Bouchard's nodes (PIP), are very characteristic and radiographically show loss of cartilage with lateral bony overgrowth. As noted previously, there is a strong hereditary component to the development of these nodes, particularly in women. The other joint frequently involved in the hand is the carpal-metacarpal (CMC) joint at the base of the thumb, which is thought to be subjected to excessive stress in many hand functions. Involvement of this joint is manifest by pain, loss of grip strength, and local tenderness, with occasional swelling. Later destruction and subluxation will lead to the "square thumb" that is typical of the osteoarthritic hand.

The major differential diagnostic problem in the hand is distinguishing between rheumatoid arthritis and osteoarthritis. In general, rheumatoid arthritis tends to involve the wrist and metacarpal-phalangeal (MCP) joints along with the PIP's. Osteoarthritis, on the other hand, may involve the PIP's, but rarely involves the MCP's. Radiographic evidence of osteoarthritis at the MCP joints, particularly the second and third, should suggest an alternative diagnosis such as hemochromatosis or pseudogout. The hand changes of psoriatic arthritis may be quite similar to that of osteoarthritis, involving the PIP and DIP joints, but asymmetric involvement and skin and nail changes should allow the clinician to make this distinction. DeQuervain's tenosynovitis of the thumb, discussed in Chapter 12, may cause pain in the area of CMC joint and should be considered when physical findings and radiographs are not compatible with a diagnosis of osteoarthritis.

Knee

Osteoarthritis of the knee is a common problem, particularly in patients over the age of 50. The typical patient complains of a gradually increasing pain that is worse with weight-bearing and associated with limping, difficulty climbing stairs, or getting out of low chairs. Pain at rest occurs rarely. Physical examination may reveal a very small or moderate effusion. Crepitus can usually be detected, and symptoms may be reproduced by passively moving the knee. Genu varum (bow-leg) or genu valgum (knock-knee) can be detected clinically and may reflect the compartment (medial or lateral) most affected by joint space narrowing. In general, the medial compartment is more commonly involved and genu varum is a more likely physical finding. The diagnosis of osteoarthritis of the knee should be confirmed radiographically, with typical findings as noted below. The differential diagnosis should include a meniscal tear or internal derangement, particularly when symptoms of locking or instability are prominent. The various forms of inflammatory arthritis should always be considered, and synovial fluid examination is usually indicated to rule out inflammation, infection, or crystal-induced arthritis. Spontaneous osteonecrosis of the knee (SONK) must also be considered in the differential diagnosis of the painful knee in elderly individuals. In this condition, routine radiographs are usually unremarkable and a radionuclide scan is often required to confirm the diagnosis (15).

Hip

Osteoarthritis of the hip (coxarthrosis) is a frequent cause of pain and disability. It occurs more often unilaterally than bilaterally and is considered by many to be the result of subtle developmental defects in the majority of cases (10). Hip pain in OA may be localized to the groin, anterior thigh or knee, or may be felt in the lateral buttocks or in the area of the greater trochanter. Pain is seldom referred to the medial or posterior buttocks or down the back of the leg, or to any point below the knee. Thus, pain in these areas should suggest pain referred from the lumbar spine. Symptoms often begin spontaneously and are followed by a gradually progressive increase in discomfort. Pain is usually made worse with activity and is relieved by rest. Physical examination will reveal loss of range of motion, with the earliest findings being loss of internal and external rotation. Comparison with the unaffected side is often helpful in distinguishing subtle abnormalities, and pain will usually be reproduced at the extremes of motion. Abnormalities in gait, particularly antalgic gait, where weight-bearing is avoided on the affected hip, may be seen if the patient is carefully observed while walking. The diagnosis of osteoarthritis should be confirmed by radiographs, and comparison with the opposite side is often helpful. The typical radiographic findings of osteoarthritis are also seen in the hip, with joint space narrowing being present more superiorly rather than medially. Since some patients with radiographic evidence of osteoarthritis in the hip do not have symptoms or limitation of activity, correlation of physical findings with radiographs is important, since referred pain or pathology in nonarticular structures about the hip may also cause hip pain.

Cervical Spine

The cervical spine is a frequent site of radiographic and clinical osteoarthritis. The term spondylosis is a nonspecific term denoting a disease process affecting the spine. This term has been commonly used to imply hypertrophic and degenerative changes along the vertebral column, particularly when osteophytes are present.

Cervical spondylosis (OA of the cervical spine) is not an acute process, but is a gradual degenerative change in one or more intervertebral discs. The process is thought to begin with loss of tissue turgor and resilience, with subsequent shrinkage and narrowing of the disc space. Normal cervical curvature is altered, followed by minimal degrees of vertebral subluxation. The stress of these changes and daily activity promotes the formation of osteophytes in the articular facets (zygoapophyseal joints) which form the posterior wall of the intervertebral foramen. The annulus fibrosus will protrude and this protrusion in combination with spur formation and disc narrowing results in a transverse bony ridge across the posterior aspect of this space, which may encroach on the intervertebral foramina and spinal canal (16).

The clinical presentation of cervical spondylosis is highly variable. Many patients will have radiographic changes, sometimes quite severe, and be totally asymptomatic. Early symptoms include stiffness, restriction of movement, and pain with movement. Some patients may have an acute onset of symptoms, while some may have gradual worsening of symptoms over many years. Symptoms of radiculopathy occur when nerve roots are entrapped or irritated as they pass through narrowed foramina. Myelopathy may occur rarely when there is sufficient narrowing of the spinal canal to produce spinal cord compression.

The typical radiographic changes of cervical spondylosis are shown in Figure 9.4, and include narrowing of intervertebral disc spaces, alteration of the normal lordotic curve of the cervical spinal, facet joint subluxation, marginal osteophytes and, occasionally, narrowing of the vertebral canal. Oblique views of the cervical spine are usually necessary to see narrowing of the intervertebral foramina. Since radiographic changes are seen in increasing numbers with age, and in virtually all patients by the age of 70, it is important that the clinician correlate radiographic findings to the clinical syndrome, and investigate symptoms further when they do not fit the typical clinical picture.

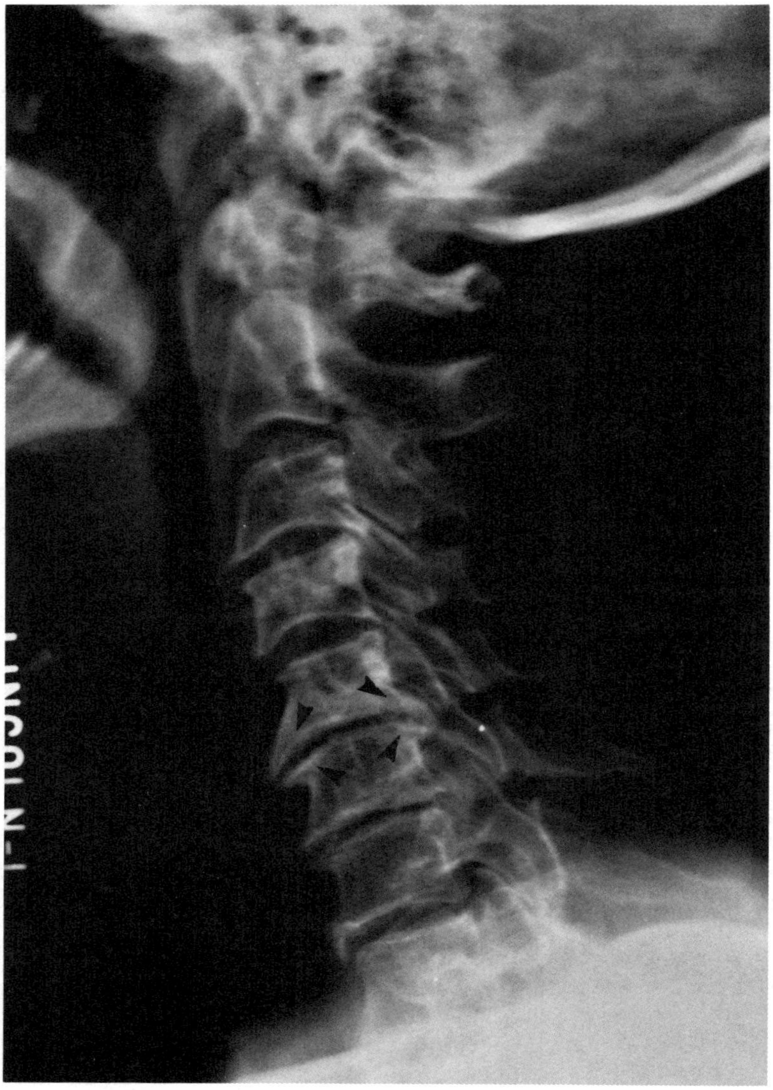

FIGURE 9.4 A lateral radiograph of the cervical spine in osteoarthritis (cervical spondylosis). Disc space narrowing and osteophytes are present at several levels, particularly at the level of C_5-C_6, where large osteophytes are present anteriorly and posteriorly.

Lumbosacral Spine

Osteoarthritis affects the lumbar spine in two basic areas, the posterior "facet" joints or the intervertebral discs. As in the cervical spine, the frequency of radiographic changes increases with age, and a majority of persons over the age of 40 will have abnormalities either in the intervertebral discs or posterior elements. Since acute back pain affects such a large proportion of the population at some time and usually occurs in an intermittent self-limited pattern, it seems that these superimposed episodes probably represent irritation of other pain-sensitive areas within the vertebral unit, and do not always correspond to radiographic changes (17). Back pain may also be associated with peripheral nerve root irritation and results from acute or chronic intervertebral disc herniation, or osteophytes. In examining patients with low back pain, a careful evaluation of range of motion and attempts to detect evidence of nerve root involvement are essential, as outlined in Chapter 1. X-rays will confirm the presence of changes either in the disc space or posterior elements. Typical findings, shown in Figures 9.5 and 9.6, include narrowing of the disc space with marginal osteophyte formation. Posteriorly, narrowing, sclerosis, and osteophytes may be seen. In general, symptoms of chronic osteoarthritis of the lumbar spine are chronic pain associated with moderate stiffness and loss of movement. Symptoms tend to be worse with movement and get better with rest.

Lumbar Spinal Stenosis

This disorder has been recognized increasingly as a cause of chronic back pain associated with radiculopathy. The typical history is of mild to moderate backache that gradually worsens and is associated with numbness and weakness of the lower extremities. Typically, the pain will get worse with walking, particularly when the patient is walking down inclines, and tends to get better with sitting or bedrest.

Because of the relationship to activity, the symptoms will often suggest vascular insufficiency, and are referred to as neurogenic claudication or pseudoclaudication. Physical examination of the back may be relatively normal, with only minor limitations of movement or straight-leg raising, and inconsistent abnormalities in sensation, strength, and reflexes may be seen in the lower extremities. Lumbar spinal stenosis may occur in young people, in whom the spinal canal is congenitally narrowed. In older individuals, particularly over the age of 50, lumbar spinal stenosis typically results from osteoarthritic spurs from chronic disc degeneration and facet joint arthritis. Although changes may be seen on routine x-rays, definitive diagnosis may require CT scanning or myelography (as seen in Figure 9.5) to confirm the extent and location of lumbar canal narrowing (18,19).

Diffuse Idiopathic Skeletal Hyperostosis (DISH)

This entity, characterized by radiographic evidence of hypertrophic ossification along the anterolateral aspect of the vertebral column, was first described by Forestier and Rotes-Querol in 1950 (20). This condition is actually relatively common and probably occurs in 5-10% of the general population. It is much more frequently seen in males, particularly over the age of 50, and there is an association with obesity and diabetes. Clinically, patients may be entirely asymptomatic or experience varying degrees of aching and stiffness in the area affected. There is also a tendency for formation of new bone around certain joints and in the areas of ligamentous attachment, leading to painful peripheral joints. Radiographically, there is a characteristic "flowing" osteophyte formation, usually anteriorly and laterally on the right side of the spinal column, as shown in Figure 9.7. The thoracic and lumbar spine are most often involved, with the cervical spine being affected slightly less commonly. This syndrome may be distinguished from typical osteoarthritis of the spine by the absence of degenerative disc changes and preservation of disc height. The large hypertrophic syndesmophytes may suggest anky-

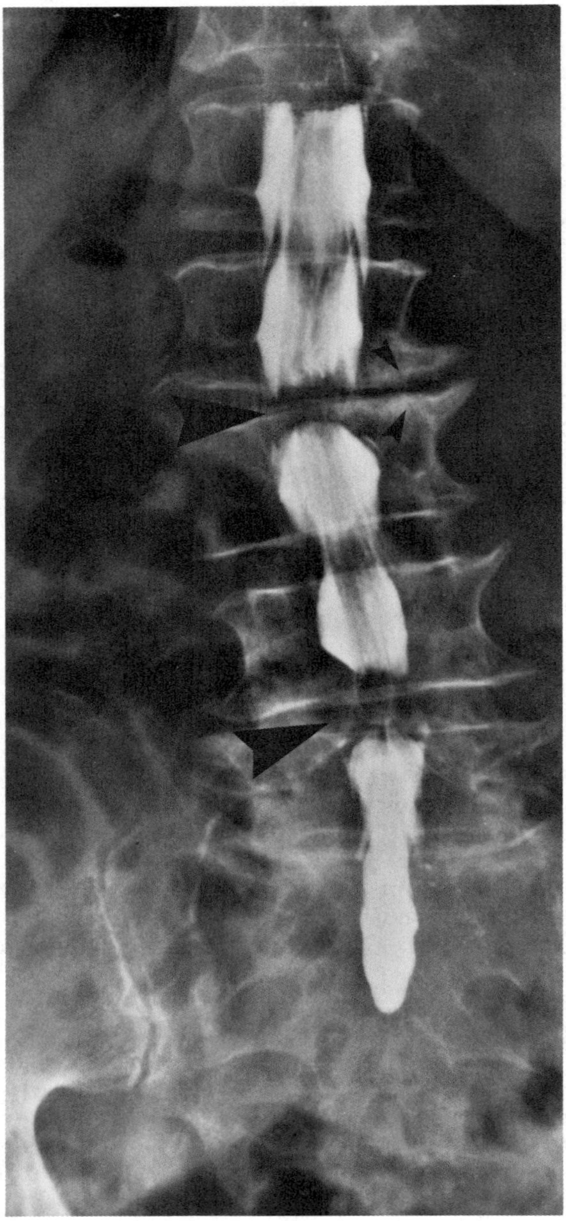

FIGURE 9.5 An anteroposterior (AP) radiograph after myelography of the lumbar spine in a patient with osteoarthritis and lumbar spinal stenosis. Disc space narrowing and lateral osteophytes are present at several levels, particularly at L_2-L_3 (small arrows). Large "bar" defects are demonstrated in the myelographic contrast at L_2-L_3 and L_4-L_5 (large arrows), diagnostic of spinal stenosis.

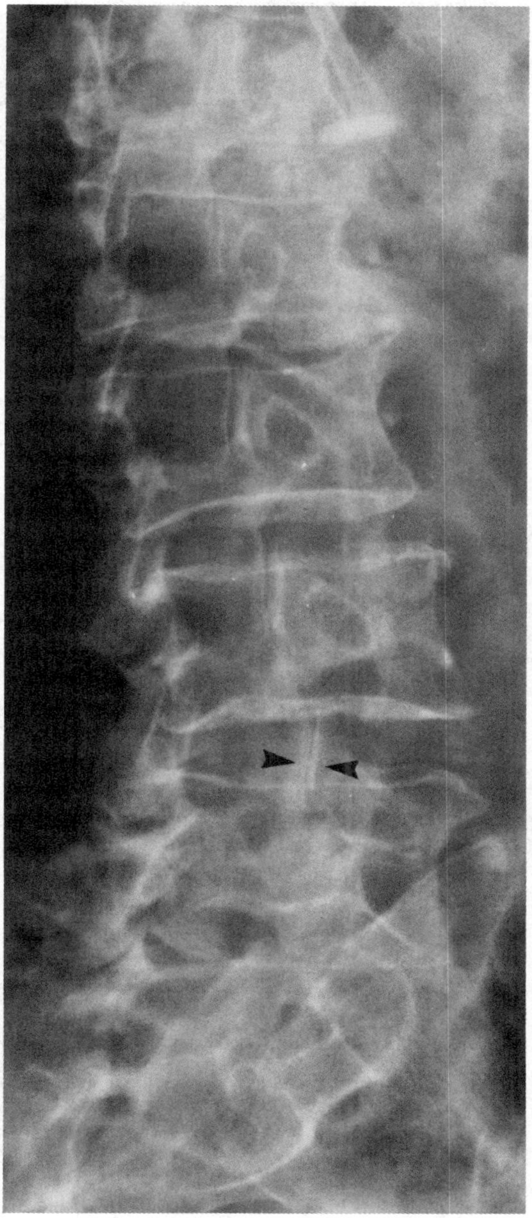

FIGURE 9.6 An oblique view of the lumbar spine in osteoarthritis, demonstrating joint space narrowing and mild bony sclerosis in a posterior "facet" joint at the level of L_4–L_5 (arrows).

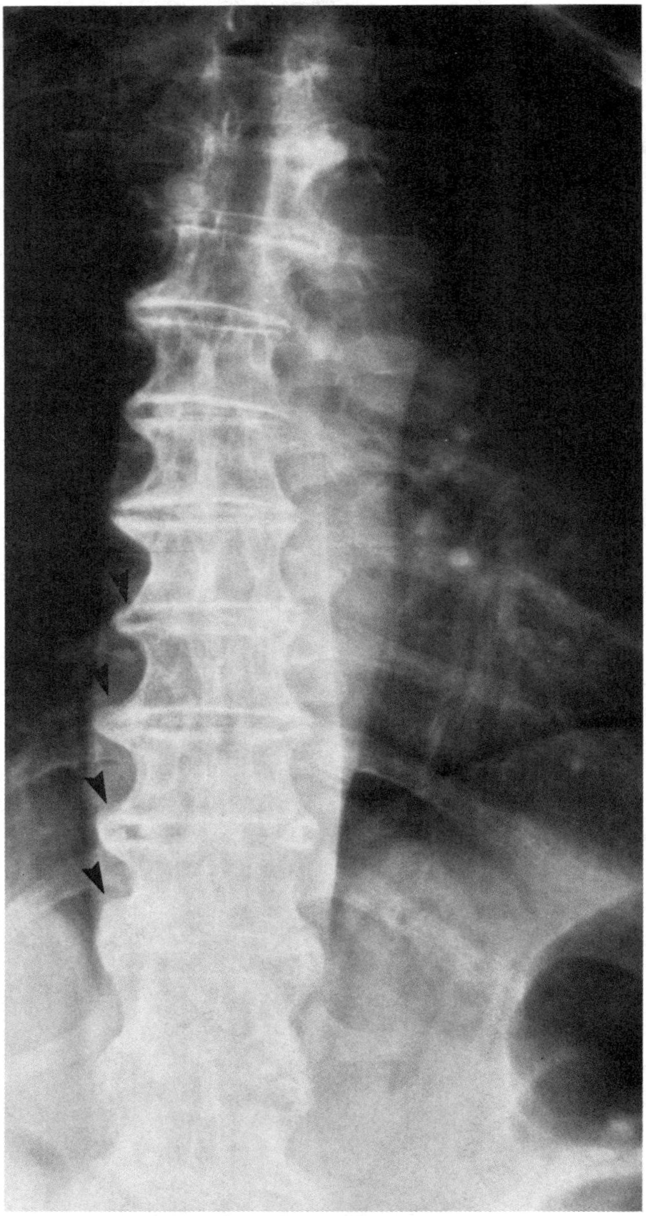

FIGURE 9.7 An AP radiograph of the lower thoracic and upper lumbar spine in a patient with diffuse idiopathic skeletal hyperostosis (DISH). "Flowing" lateral osteophytes (arrows) are demonstrated predominantly on the right side. The intervertebral disc spaces are preserved, differentiating this syndrome from typical osteoarthritis of the spine.

losing spondylosis, but there is usually some separation of these calcifications from the vertebral elements, and sacroiliac changes are absent in this condition. Although it is usually classified among forms of degenerative arthritis, there is little pathologic evidence of cartilage degeneration, and there are no inflammatory changes seen. Thus, the etiology of DISH remains an enigma (21).

Osteoarthritis of the Sacroiliac Joint

Although this joint can be affected by typical changes of osteoarthritis, the exact incidence of this is unknown (10). OA in this location may be confused with the sacroilitis of ankylosing spondylosis or other related conditions. OA generally occurs in an older age group and the pain and limitation of movement are usually less severe. Radiographic changes should include increased subchondral bone, sharp defined joint margins, and osteophyte formation.

Diagnosis of Osteoarthritis

Establishing a diagnosis of osteoarthritis requires careful review of the patient's history, physical findings, and radiographic findings. As noted below, the initial radiographic criteria which are still in use today were set forth by Kellgren and Lawrence in 1957 (22). Although these are useful, the poor correlation of the clinical syndrome with radiographic findings has prompted formation of a committee by the American Rheumatism Association to set forth clinical criteria for diagnosis of osteoarthritis (23). In general, the diagnosis of osteoarthritis requires a history of pain in a given joint, with stiffness that does not last more than 30 minutes on arising in the morning. Physical findings of crepitus, bony enlargement, and limitation of motion should usually be present, and as noted below, most routine laboratory studies, including sedimentation rate, should be normal. Synovial fluid should be of a noninflammatory nature (see Chapter 2) and show no evidence of crystals by polarized microscopy. Radiographic changes should be present to confirm the diagnosis (see below).

Laboratory Features

There are no laboratory features that are typical for osteoarthritis. Routine hematologic and blood chemistry studies should be normal. The sedimentation rate is usually normal, although mild elevations may occur, probably reflecting the elderly population in which this condition is seen. Specific tests for associated conditions such as hypothyroidism, hemochromatosis, or diabetes should be performed when other clinical features suggest these conditions. Rheumatoid factors should be negative in the majority of patients with osteoarthritis, but again, because of the elderly age group in which this is seen, a low-titer positive rheumatoid factor may be detected in a minority of patients. Blood studies are usually done in osteoarthritis to exclude other forms of muscoloskeletal disease, and significant abnormalities such as anemia or marked elevation of sedimentation rates should alert the physician to an alternative diagnosis. Synovial fluid in osteoarthritis should be noninflammatory. Effusions are usually small, although very large effusions are occasionally seen in certain joints, such as the knees. Synovial fluid usually has less than 300 white cells/mm^3, although mild elevations to 1000-2000 may be seen on occasion. Synovial fluid glucose is slightly below that of serum, as in other noninflammatory effusions. The fluid should be examined for the presence of crystals by polarized microscopy to exclude the possibility of gout or pseudogout. Electron microscopic study of synovial fluid has demonstrated calcium hydroxyapatite crystals in some synovial fluids from patients with osteoarthritis, but the significance of this finding in relationship to pathogenesis has yet to be resolved (8) (see Chapter 11).

Radiographic findings of osteoarthritis are often diagnostic. Radiographs may appear normal early in the course of osteoarthritis, but the diagnosis is extremely difficult to make without at least some abnormalities. The typical radiographic findings of osteoarthritis are seen in Chapter 3 and include the following: 1) joint space narrowing, usually asymetric and irregular, 2) subchondral bony sclerosis, 3) subchondral cysts, and 4) osteophytes or extra bone formation around the margins of the joint. Erosions and ankylosis of the joints are uncommon in osteoarthritis and osteoporosis should not be a typical radiographic feature of the disease. In the end stage, distortion or angulation of the joint may be seen. Joint space narrowing occurs as the result of a loss of hyaline cartilage, and subchondral bony sclerosis (eburnation) usually represents new bone deposition in this region, which is probably a reparative process. The general characteristics of radiographic changes in osteoarthritis tend to be the same regardless of the region or joint involved except in the spine, where the changes are also seen involving the disc space (not a true synovial joint). As discussed in the section on etiopathogenesis, the pathologic changes of osteoarthritis are seen primarily in the articular cartilage, where focal softening of the surface, fibrillation, chondrocyte proliferation, and finally fissuring and loss of cartilage are seen. The changes in the synovium may include inflammation and hypertrophy, but are not present to the extent seen in rheumatoid arthritis.

Prognosis and Management

Natural History of Osteoarthritis

Osteoarthritis is generally considered to be a progressive process in which symptoms and radiographic changes evolve over a period of several months to years. It is not uncommon, however, for symptoms to improve after an initial period of pain, although radiographic changes seldom revert to normal. There have been isolated case reports and animal models in which spontaneous reversal of the degenerative process in the cartilage has been demonstrated, but the clinical applicability of these observations is unclear (5). A recent study of osteoarthritis of the knee in a large number of elderly patients demonstrated that the frequency and severity of disease does not increase between the ages of 60 and 90, again suggesting that osteoarthritis is not inevitably progressive (24). In general, though, accurate epidemiologic information on the natural history of osteoarthritis is lacking, and would require very long and costly studies to determine, because of the slowly progressive nature of the condition.

Therapeutic Modalities

General Considerations

Current management of osteoarthritis is symptomatic, directed primarily toward the relief of pain and secondary inflammation (25). The treatment of osteoarthritis is briefly discussed and outlined in Chapter 4, and involves a combination of rest, physical and occupational therapy, and psychological support, as well as medical and surgical intervention. Therapy should be tailored to the complaints and needs of the individual patient; thus, aggressive therapy is not warranted where symptoms are minimal or the affected joint is very rarely used. The patient should be educated about the natural history of the disease and the goals of therapy, which should be to relieve pain and preserve function.

Physical and Occupational Therapy

Since biomechanical abnormalities play an important role in the development of osteoarthritis and because symptoms are usually made worse with certain activities, adequate rest should be encouraged, not only to improve symptoms but possibly to slow the degenerative articular process. The use of supportive braces, canes, or crutches, as discussed in Chapter 5, can be particularly helpful in relieving stresses on weight-bearing joints. Obese patients should be encouraged to lose weight, since this will also help to reduce stress on weight-bearing joints. Exercise should be encouraged, both to maintain range of motion and strengthen muscles. Passive range of motion exercises are particularly helpful in the hand, and are often facilitated by the prior use of local heat. For strengthening, isometric exercises are generally preferred, since these do not put the joint through a painful range of motion. Swimming is also considered a good exercise for those patients who are able, since very little weight-bearing is involved. Any exercise program should begin gradually, and increase over a period of several weeks, and patients should be advised to take a common sense approach to exercise by avoiding or decreasing the amount of an activity that worsens pain for more than a few minutes after stopping.

Specific measures may be helpful in certain joints to lessen pain and to improve function. In the hand, such measures as trying to use the other hand, the use of heavy gloves at work, alteration of tools, and the use of self-help devices may allow reduction of stress on tendons and joints. Some patients report the improvement of symptoms by the use of nighttime stretch gloves. Local heat application and passive range of motion are also helpful in improving symptoms in the hand. Splinting may be very effective for an intermittently symptomatic area, particularly when the PIP or CMC joint at the base of the thumb is involved. In the cervical spine, the use of a soft or hard plastic cervical collar may provide temporary stabilization of areas of nerve root irritation. In the symptomatic low back, education to avoid aggravating stresses and therapeutic exercises are often helpful, as discussed in Chapter 12.

Drug Therapy

When a basic program of rest, avoidance of stress, and physical therapy do not provide the relief desired by the patient, analgesics and antiinflammatory agents are indicated (25). The primary goal of drug therapy in osteoarthritis is to provide analgesia. Since there is some evidence that inflammation plays a role in both pathogenesis and clinical symptomatology of the condition, however, the antiinflammatory effects of these drugs may be important as well. Acetaminophen and aspirin should be tried initially in moderate doses. Other nonsteroidal antiinflammatory agents (NSAID's) may be used when one of these agents is not helpful. Almost any of the currently available NSAID's may be utilized in the management of osteoarthritis, much as they are used for the relief of pain and inflammation in rheumatoid arthritis. In general, lower doses of these agents should be tried first, and then gradually increased. A more extensive review of the NSAID's may be found in Chapter 4.

In certain situations, such as acute cervical or lumbosacral strain superimposed on osteoarthritis, muscle relaxants help relieve pain and spasm. Although systemic corticosteroid therapy is never indicated in the management of osteoarthritis, locally injected corticosteroids are often very useful in relieving pain and inflammation. Intraarticular steroid injections may be utilized in the management of pain in an individual joint, but should not be used repeatedly, particularly in weight-bearing joints, since there is some evidence that frequently injected steroids may accelerate the degenerative process (26). In addition, local injection of periarticular tendons and ligamentous structures may provide great relief when these areas cause an exacerbation of pain around the joint, as in anserine bursitis at the knee.

Research into other drugs for the relief of pain and inflammation in osteoarthritis is continuing, and further understanding of the etiology and pathogenesis of this disorder may be helpful in uncovering other effective therapies, particularly those that might promote the healing of cartilage. Among the many agents being investigated are Orgotein (a superoxide dismutase inhibitor), growth hormone, new intra-articular corticosteroids, or other new nonsteroidal antiinflammatory agents (25).

Surgical Intervention

Surgery in osteoarthritis is usually reserved for patients severely afflicted in whom there is loss of function and inadequate response to drug therapy and other conservative measures. This is reviewed more extensively in Chapter 7. Arthroscopic debridement of cartilage or bone may be very helpful in providing pain relief and improving movement, particularly in the knee. Osteotomy (removing a wedge of bone) can be helpful in correcting the forces of weight-bearing in the hip and knee. Joint fusion (arthrodesis), previously the only modality available for surgical management of damaged joints, is still used on occasion, and although the relief of pain is good, joint motion is always sacrificed. Recently, improvements in technology have made total joint replacement a very effective means of managing refractory osteoarthritis in specific joints. This is particularly true in the hip, but great advances have also been made in total knee replacement.

Decisions regarding surgical intervention in cervical spondylosis should be individualized, but in general, indications for surgery include painful radiculopathies that result in neurologic impairment or are unresponsive to conservative measures. In the lumbar spine, surgery (usually laminectomy) is usually indicated for obvious herniated nucleus pulposus with nerve root impingement, or when there is no response to nonsurgical measures. In lumbar spinal stenosis, wide debridement of osteophytes is usually required, and results are not uniformly positive. However, surgery should be considered in this condition, particularly in younger patients, or in older patients with refractory pain unresponsive to rest, physical therapy, and medical management.

References

1. Benedek TG, Rodnan GP: A brief history of the rheumatic diseases. *Bull Rheum Dis* 32:59-68, 1982.

2. Brandt KD: Pathogenesis of osteoarthritis (OA). In WN Kelley, ED Harris Jr, S Ruddy, CB Sledge (eds.), *Textbook of Rheumatology*. Philadelphia, W.B. Saunders, 1981, pp. 1457-1470.

3. Radin EL: Aetiology of osteoarthritis. *Clin Rheum Dis* 2:509-522, 1976.

4. Altman RD: Osteoarthritis: Pathogenesis, differential diagnosis, treatment. *Orthop Rev* 13:256-266, 1984.

5. Bland JH: The reversibility of osteoarthritis: A review. *Am J Med* (Symposium, June 14):16-26, 1983.

6. Mankin HJ: The response of articular cartilage to mechanical injury. *J Bone Joint Surg* 64A:460-466, 1982.

7. Pelletier J-P, Martel-Pelletier J, Altman RD, Ghandur-Mnaymneh L, Howell DS, Woessner FJ Jr: Collagenolytic activity and collagen matrix breakdown of the articular-cartilage in the Pond-Nuki dog model of osteoarthritis. *Arthritis Rheum* 26:866-874, 1983.

8. Schumacher HR, Gibilisco P, Reginato A, Cherian V, Gordon G: Implications of crystal deposition in osteoarthritis. *J Rheumatol* (suppl. 9) 10:40-41, 1983.

9. Kellgren JH: Pain in osteoarthritis. *J Rheumatol* (suppl. 9) 10:108-109, 1983.

10. Bland J, Stulberg SD: Osteoarthritis: Pathology and clinical patterns. In WN Kelly, ED Harris, S Ruddy, CB Sledge (eds.), *Textbook of Rheumatology.* Philadelphia, W.B. Saunders, 1981, pp. 1471-1490.

11. Kellgren JH, Moore R: Generalized osteoarthritis and Heberden's nodes. *Br Med J* 1:181-187, 1952.

12. Crain DC: Interphalangeal osteoarthritis characterized by painful inflammatory episodes resulting in deformity of the proximal and distal articulations. *JAMA* 175:1049-1053, 1961.

13. Radin EL: Mechanical aspects of osteoarthritis. *Bull Rheum Dis* 26:862-865, 1975.

14. Adams ID: Osteoarthrosis and sport. *Clin Rheum Dis* 2:523-541, 1976.

15. Houpt JB, Pritzker KPH, Alpert B et al.: Natural history of spontaneous osteonecrosis of the knee (SONK): A review. *Semin Arth Rheum* 13:212-227, 1983.

16. Long EF: Cervical spondylosis. Postgrad Medicine 33:58-64, 1963.

17. Cailliet R: *Low Back Pain Syndrome,* 3rd Ed. Philadelphia, F.A. Davis, 1981.

18. Kirkaldy-Willis WH, Paine KW, Couchoix J, McIvor G: Lumbar spinal stenosis. *Clin Orthop* 99:30-50, 1974.

19. Rosenthal DI, Manken HJ, Bauman RA: Musculoskeletal applications for computed tomography. *Bull Rheum Dis* 33:3, 1983.

20. Forestier J, Rotes-Querol J: Senile ankylosing hyperostosis of the spine. *Ann Rheum Dis* 9:321-330, 1950.

21. Dwosh IL: Diffuse idiopathic skeletal hyperostosis: Degenerative disease or metabolic disturbance. *J Rheumatol* (suppl. 9) 10:101-102, 1983.

22. Kellgren JH, Lawrence JS: Radiological assessment of osteoarthritis. *Ann Rheum Dis* 16:494-501, 1957.

23. Altman RD, Meenan RF, Hochberg MC et al.: An approach to developing criteria for the clinical diagnosis and classification of osteoarthritis. *J Rheumatol* 10:180-183, 1983.

24. Forman MD, Malamet R, Kaplan D: A survey of osteoarthritis of the knee in the elderly. *J Rheumatol* 10:282-287, 1983.

25. Moskowitz RN: Management of osteoarthritis. *Bull Rheum Dis* 31:31-35, 1981.

26. Moskowitz RW, Goldberg VM, Schwab W et al.: Effects of intraarticular corticosteroids and exercise in experimental models of inflammatory and degenerative arthritis. *Arthritis Rheum* 18:417, 1975.

Chapter 10

Seronegative Spondyloarthropathies

Christopher M. Wise, M.D.

Ankylosing Spondylitis

General

Historical Aspects

Ankylosing spondylitis is a chronic inflammatory arthropathy primarily involving the axial skeleton, particularly the spine. Its name derives from the Greek term "ankylos" (meaning bent or crooked) and "spondylos" (meaning vertebrae). The condition has been recognized in pathologic specimens dating back as far as 3000 years, while clinical descriptions of the disease and our understanding of it as a separate disease entity have evolved over the last four centuries (1). The first definite description of ankylosing spondylitis probably came from Bernard Conner in 1695, who described the typical bony findings in a skeleton from a cemetery. During the nineteenth century, more detailed descriptions of the disorder became available. The separate clinical descriptions by von Bechterew, Marie, and Strumpell generally promoted the clinical recognition of the disease. Over the years, this condition has been known under a variety of names, including spondylitis deformans, atrophic spondylitis, von Bechterew's disease, Marie-Strumpell disease, and eventually rheumatoid spondylitis. As more has been learned about the pathologic, clinical, laboratory, and genetic features of this condition, it has become apparent that ankylosing spondylitis is not a variant of rheumatoid arthritis, but is an entirely separate disease. Ankylosing spondylitis is now considered the prototype of a family of diseases, known as the seronegative spondyloarthropathies. Other closely related syndromes within this category include Reiter's syndrome, psoriatic arthritis and spondylitis, and enteropathic arthritis.

Epidemiology and Genetic Aspects

Ankylosing spondylitis has traditionally been considered a disease of young white males. Early studies suggested that the disease occurred in about 1 in 2000 members of the general population with a male to female ratio of 10 to 1. More recent studies have suggested that the condition is somewhat more common than this, with a prevalence in the general population of 0.1%-1% (2,3). Underrecognition of the condition in less symptomatic patients, and differences in study design probably account for most of the discrepancies between studies.

The prevalence of ankylosing spondylitis varies widely between racial groups, being far more common in Caucasian populations, exceedingly rare in the Japanese, and almost unheard of in black Africans. Certain American Indian groups, on the other hand, seem to have an even higher prevalence than whites (4).

With increasing recognition of ankylosing spondylitis as a specific disease entity in the 1950's, several observations and genetic studies noted an increased incidence of the condition in first-degree relatives of those known to have spondylitis. In 1973, two separate investigators reported a high incidence of the genetic marker, HLA-B27, in patients with ankylosing spondylitis (5,6). This white cell surface antigen, coded for by a gene at the B locus of the major histocompatibility complex on the sixth human chromosome, occurs in approximately 8% of Caucasians. Several studies in the last 10 years have confirmed the high degree of association of this marker with ankylosing spondylitis and have also indicated a higher than expected incidence in many of the other seronegative spondyloarthropathies. In addition, it has been shown that this antigen is not nearly as prevalent in black and Japanese populations, and that the association with ankylosing spondylitis in these populations is not nearly as strong (see Table 10.1). It appears that the genetic marker HLA-B27 is found more frequently in white patients with this group of diseases, particularly when accompanied by sacroiliitis. Nevertheless, HLA-B27 is not always a marker for sacroiliac disease, since many patients with Reiter's syndrome carry the gene but do not have sacroiliitis.

Etiopathogenesis

Ever since the discovery of the association of HLA-B27 with ankylosing spondylitis, there has been speculation that this disease might be caused by an hereditary immunogenetic mechanism. Because of clinical similarities to Reiter's syndrome and the arthritis following enteric infection, a great deal of attention has been focused on trying to find an infective agent that might trigger an immunologic response. It has been thought that such an infectious agent might have determinants which cross-react with those of the B27 antigen, resulting in an immune response which causes damage to host tissue.

Along these lines some studies have shown increased serum IgA levels (7), increased incidence of fecal colonization with certain Klebsiella species (8), and altered immunity to Klebsiella in groups of patients with ankylosing spondylitis. Subsequently, however, there has been conflicting data in regard to all of these associations. Thus, although the hypothesis is attractive, there is still no convincing evidence that a specific microbe plays a role in triggering the disease in a genetically susceptible host (9).

TABLE 10.1 HLA-B27 Prevalence and Disease Association in Different Ethnic Groups

		Prevalence %
Healthy Populations		
	Caucasians (U.S.)	8
	Blacks (U.S.)	3-4
	Blacks (Africa)	<1
	Japanese	<1
Disease Associations		
Whites:	Ankylosing Spondylitis	90-100
	Reiter's Syndrome	80
	Psoriasis (all patients)	8
	Psoriatic Arthritis (without sacroiliitis)	20
	Psoriatic Arthritis (with sacroiliitis)	50-60
	Inflammatory Bowel Disease (IBD)	8
	IBD with peripheral arthritis	8
	IBD with spondylitis	60
	Reactive Arthropathy (post Shigella, Salmonella, Yersinia)	80
Nonwhites:	Ankylosing Spondylitis (black)	60
	Reiter's Syndrome (black)	50
	Ankylosing Spondylitis (Japanese)	60

Clinical Features

Clinical Presentation

Ankylosing spondylitis is a chronic disease with symptoms beginning typically in late adolescence or early adulthood (10). The earliest symptom is usually low back pain which is usually diffuse with an insidious onset. Pain is sometimes localized to the buttocks or may radiate into the legs. In the rare patient with acute pain, there can be confusion with mechanical injury or a herniated disc. The back pain of ankylosing spondylitis is usually of an inflammatory nature, and thus associated with morning stiffness (often lasting several hours) and improved with exercise. Pain in the upper thorax may also be present, and occasionally patients will complain of pleuritic chest pain.

The principal findings on physical examination early in the disease consist of tenderness in the sacroiliac joints and limitation of movement in the lumbar and thoracic spine. Sacroiliac tenderness may be elicited either by direct percussion over the joint, or by maneuvers such as iliac crest compression, to elicit pain in this area. Loss of motion in the lumbar spine is usually evident when the patient attempts to bend forward and touch the floor (forward flexion deficit), and also may be measured by estimation of the separation of the bony prominences of the lumbar spine (Schober test, see Chapter 1). Loss of movement in the thoracic spine may be evident on rotation, lateral flexion, or may be measured as a decrease in chest expansion resulting from involvement of the costovertebral joints.

As the disease progresses over many years, spinal involvement may progress from the lumbar to the thoracic and cervical spines. Over this period of time, the pain itself may become less severe while permanent stiffness and deformity become more obvious. The end-stage spondylitic will show classic signs of a "bamboo spine." Complete loss of lumbar lordosis, accentuation of thoracic kyphosis, and a fixed straight cervical spine results in a patient with a classic stooped forward posture and upward gazing eyes requiring rotation of the entire body to look from side to side (see Figure 10.1). Such patients usually have almost no chest expansion and will be obvious abdominal breathers. A high frequency of hip and knee disease may result in other characteristic postural changes.

Diagnostic Criteria

The diagnosis of ankylosing spondylitis may be made utilizing elements of a careful history and physical examination, along with radiographic views of the sacroiliac joints. Diagnostic criteria were first established at a symposium held in Rome in 1961 and were subsequently revised in New York in 1966 (11) (see Table 10.2). The radiographic demonstration of sacroiliitis is an absolute necessity when using these criteria. It may be very difficult to make a diagnosis early in the disease without definite radiographic changes, while the diagnosis of ankylosing spondylitis may be made with minimal symptomatology if radiographic changes are obvious.

The diagnostic value of HLA-B27 testing in ankylosing spondylitis has been a matter for much recent debate in the medical literature. Since the vast majority of patients are positive for this genetic marker, it would appear on the surface that this test could be very useful in establishing a diagnosis of ankylosing spondylitis. On the other hand, the high prevalence of this marker in the general population would result in a large number of false-positive tests, if the test were used indiscriminantly. Histocompatibility testing is probably of clinical use in certain specific situations, such as young Caucasian men with atypical findings, females with undiagnosed peripheral joint disease, atypical seronegative rheumatoid arthritis, or pediatric patients with late-onset seronegative pauciarticular joint disease.

Differential Diagnosis

Ankylosing spondylitis must be differentiated from other syndromes which cause back pain and radiographic changes that mimic those of ankylosing spondylitis (Table 10.3). Mechanical causes of low back pain usually have a more acute onset, usually after some sort of activity. Pain in these situations is usually made worse with activity and gets better with rest, in marked contrast to the pain of inflammatory spondylitis. Although limitation of motion may be present in lumbar disc disorders, lateral spinal flexion is usually preserved, while this is invariably abnormal in patients with spondylitis. Referred pain should be suspected when examination of the back shows full range of motion and no specific tenderness. Osteoarthritis of the apophyseal and intervertebral joints in the lumbar spine is common. This should be suspected when the onset of pain is at an older age. The sacroiliac joints may show changes of osteoarthritis as well, but these are usually limited to a lower part of the joint. Ankylosing hyperostosis (Forestier's disease, DISH) may cause large flowing syndesmophytes across several vertebral bodies,

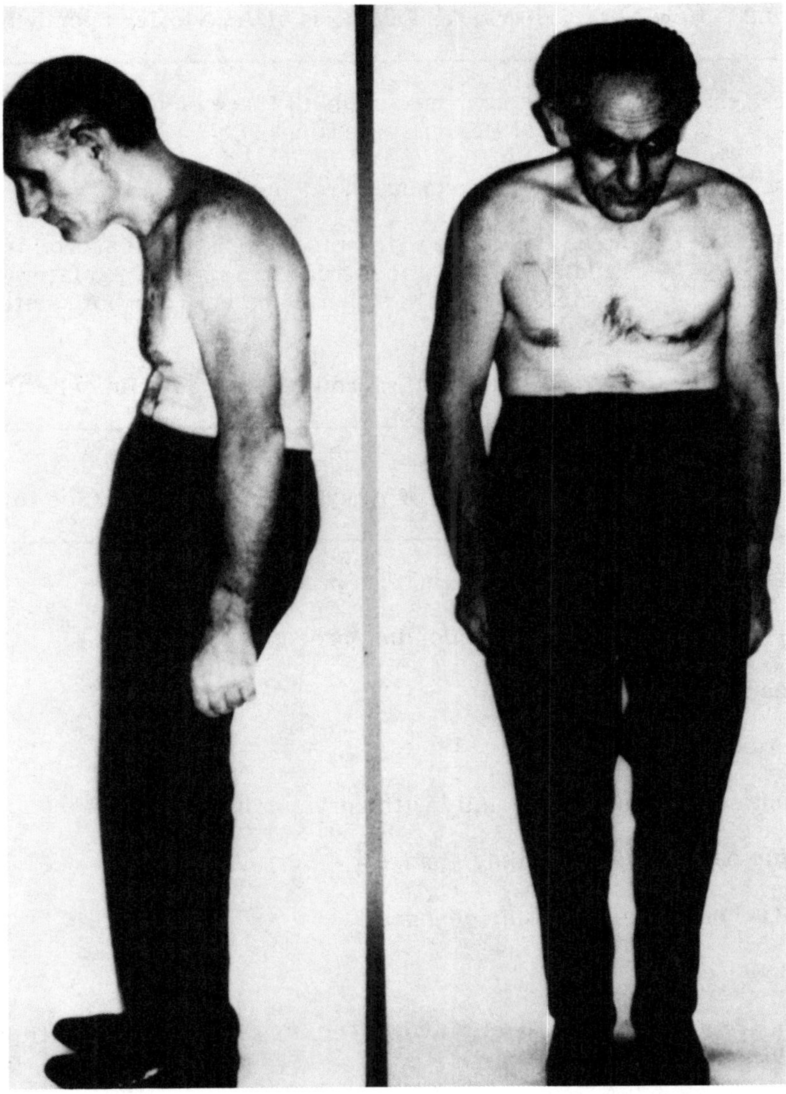

FIGURE 10.1 The classic postural changes of chronic ankylosing spondylitis (reprinted from the *Revised Slide Collection on the Rheumatic Diseases,* Copyright 1981, used by permission of the Arthritis Foundation).

but this disease usually occurs in older individuals and seldom involves the sacroiliac joints radiographically.

Involvement of the cervical spine in rheumatoid arthritis may mimic that of ankylosing spondylitis radiographically. The presence of peripheral joint disease and rheumatoid factor should make this distinction easier, but the two diseases may coexist. The presence of paravertebral ossification and sacroiliac fusion has been described in several patients chronically immobilized due to paraplegia and should not be confused with ankylosing spondylitis. Osteitis condensans ilii is

TABLE 10.2 New York Criteria for Diagnosis of Ankylosing Spondylitis (11)

Clinical criteria:	Limited lumbar motion in all three planes: anterior flexion, lateral flexion, extension Lumbar pain Limited chest expansion (<1 inch)
Definite AS:	One of the above with grade 3–4 bilateral sacroiliitis Grade 3–4 unilateral sacroiliitis or grade 2 bilateral sacroiliitis with either criterion 1, or both criteria 2 and 3
Probable AS:	Grade 3–4 bilateral sacroiliitis without clinical criteria

TABLE 10.3 Differential Diagnosis of Ankylosing Spondylitis (See text)

Mechanical low back pain - strain, disc prolapse

Referred pain - pelvic, intraabdominal process

Osteoarthritis

Forestier's disease (DISH)

Rheumatoid arthritis (especially with cervical disease)

Chronic paraplegia (sacroiliac changes)

Osteitis condensans ilii (iliac changes)

Paget's disease

Secondary ankylosing spondylitis with Reiter's syndrome, psoriatic arthritis, enteropathic arthritis

Infectious sacroiliitis (bacterial, tuberculous)

manifest by sclerosis of iliac subchondral bone and is seen primarily in women of child-bearing age or men who have experienced trauma. This condition is more often unilateral, and careful examination of x-rays will show that the sacroiliac joints themselves as well as the sacrum are normal. Pelvic involvement in Paget's disease can cause radiographic confusion with ankylosing spondylitis, but seldom occurs in younger individuals and is usually associated with an elevation in alkaline phosphatase.

Ankylosing spondylitis may occur in its primary form without any associated disease, but may also occur in association with the other seronegative spondyloarthropathies. In Reiter's disease and psoriasis, sacroiliitis is more characteristically asymmetric and spinal involvement may often be discontinuous. The spondylitis associated with inflammatory bowel disease is virtually indistinguishable radiographically from that of primary ankylosing spondylitis. The arthropathy of Behcet's disease may cause erosions of the sacroiliac joints, but other clinical features should suggest this diagnosis. Finally, infectious involvement of the spine should be suspected when there is associated fever or other systemic signs. Intravenous drug abusers seem particularly prone to hematogenous seeding of the sacroiliac joints with bacteria, and needle aspiration of the joint should be carried out if this is suspected.

Late Spinal Complications

Erosive and destructive lesions of the vertebral body and disc spaces may be found in some patients with ankylosing spondylitis (12,13). These lesions, termed spondylodiscitis, may occur in up to 25% of patients, and are usually limited to patients with long-standing disease. These may cause localized pain or may be asymptomatic, and must be distinguished from localized disc space infection. Some controversy exists over whether these are caused by microfractures through osteoporotic bone or whether they represent an extension of the primary inflammatory process, but most authors agree that conservative management usually results in spontaneous healing and that neurologic complications are uncommon.

Spinal fractures are an uncommon but serious and potentially fatal complication of long-standing ankylosing spondylitis (14,15). These occur most frequently in the lower cervical region, usually after minor trauma or an automobile accident. Often the patient will not remember the specific trauma but will present with localized increased pain. Increased movement (pseudoarthrosis) may be noted in an area of the spine that was previously immobile. Radiographic visualization of fractures is sometimes difficult, with tomography or bone scans sometimes necessary to define specific lesions. Management of spinal fractures in ankylosing spondylitis requires careful immobilization and observation for neurologic deterioration. Cervical traction will usually result in healing of the fracture, but neurologic deterioration often requires surgical stabilization.

Extraspinal Articular Manifestations

Extraspinal joint disease probably occurs at some point during the course of the disease in 50-60% of patients. The frequency with which this occurs in specific joints is summarized in Table 10.4. The axial joints (hips, shoulders, and temporomandibular joints) tend to be the most frequently involved (16). Disease in the hips can become particularly severe and lead to significant morbidity (17). In general, peripheral arthritis tends to be asymmetric and to involve the lower extremities. Erosive changes are usually much less severe than those in rheumatoid arthritis, and bony ankylosis is much more common. A small number of patients may develop peripheral joint disease after the spondylitis has become inactive. In these cases, the peripheral arthritis tends to be a little more severe and results in more disability (18).

TABLE 10.4 Extraspinal Joint Involvement in Ankylosing Spondylitis

	Percent Frequency
Hips	35-40
Shoulders	32
Knees	25-30
Hands/wrists	25-30
Feet	15
Elbows	12
TMJ	12
Ankles	8

Enthesopathic lesions (inflammation at tendon insertions) occur in ankylosing spondylitis as in the other seronegative spondyloarthropathies. Many patients develop achilles tendonitis, intercostal muscle insertion tenderness, and plantar fasciitis. These lesions may be recurrent but cause little bone or joint destruction, and are usually self-limited.

Extraarticular Complications

Although ankylosing spondylitis has been traditionally viewed as a disease confined to the back with little or no systemic involvement, there has been increasing recognition in the past several years that this is a systemic disease. Extraarticular manifestations do not usually become as prominent or occur as frequently as in rheumatoid arthritis, but there are several well-described complications associated with this disease that often pose diagnostic and therapeutic problems.

Pleuropulmonary involvement may take several forms. Ankylosis of the costovertebral junctions may cause marked limitation of chest expansion. Although this results in restricted ventilation, there is rarely any impairment of gas exchange. The best known pulmonary complication is a characteristic upper lobe fibrosis which may mimic tuberculosis, and occurs in about 1% of patients (19). On occasion, superinfection with fungi or atypical mycobacteria may occur. Rarely, patients will develop pleuritis or pleural effusions.

Cardiovascular disease is now well recognized, and occurs in up to 20% of patients, especially those with long-standing disease. Aortic insufficiency, cardiomegaly, and conduction defects are the usual clinical manifestations of cardiac involvement, although up to half of patients may have no abnormalities detected before death. The characteristic pathologic lesion is an adventitial scarring and intimal proliferation affecting the aortic wall, aortic valve cusps, and extending below the valve into the ventricular septum and conducting system (20). In addition, ankylosing spondylitis, often undiagnosed or asymptomatic, has been recognized with increased frequency in studies of large numbers of patients requiring permanent pacemakers for complete heart block (21).

Neurologic complications of ankylosing spondylitis include spinal cord compression, resulting from spinal fractures or atlantoaxial subluxation and cauda equina syndrome (resulting from diverticuli in the lumbar arachnoid) (22).

In the genitourinary tract, chronic prostatitis has been reported in up to 80% of patients at some time during their course (23). Although renal disease has been considered exceedingly rare in ankylosing spondylitis, an increased mortality from nephritis has been noted in large series of patients (24). Recent reports of an association with IgA nephropathy provide a possible explanation for this (25). Conjunctivitis and anterior uveitis occur in about 25% of patients (10). Although this can be severe and cause loss of vision, the eye lesions in ankylosing spondylitis usually are self-limited and much less severe than those seen in Reiter's syndrome.

As with many chronic inflammatory diseases, secondary amyloidosis may occur as a complication of ankylosing spondylitis. This is usually an autopsy finding and rarely of clinical significance, although some cases with progressive renal failure have been reported.

Clinical Variants

Ankylosing Spondylitis in Women

Comparisons of female to male patients have shown several differences in disease expression (26,27). Women with ankylosing spondylitis often go much longer (average of 10 years) before diagnosis than men. Women will more often have peripheral joint disease initially and on subsequent follow-up. In the spine and axial skeleton, back pain is often milder and spinal involvement is usually less severe and progressive. In addition, women are more likely to have cervical spine symptoms and inflammatory lesions of the pubic symphysis (osteitis pubis). Because of these differences, many women with ankylosing spondylitis probably are diagnosed as having seronegative rheumatoid arthritis and are followed with this diagnosis for many years. Pregnancy is well tolerated in women with ankylosing spondylitis, although a minority will experience a postpartum flare of joint disease and/or anterior eye disease (28).

Juvenile-Onset Ankylosing Spondyitis

Among the many subsets of juvenile rheumatoid arthritis is a group that is considered to have juvenile-onset ankylosing spondylitis. This is a group of older children, predominantly male, with a pauciarticular peripheral arthritis. Spinal complaints and radiographic sacroiliitis may take several years to develop. Compared to adults, this group has a higher incidence of peripheral arthritis and, in particular, hip disease (29,30). Closely related is the newly described seronegative enthesopathy and arthropathy of childhood, characterized by oligoarthritis, low back symptoms and limitation of motion, enthesopathic lesions, and a high incidence of HLA-B27. Many of these patients can be diagnosed as having ankylosing spondylitis or another seronegative spondyloarthropathy, but many can be given no specific diagnosis and may eventually develop more definable disease (31). Further discussion of juvenile-onset spondylitis can be found in Chapter 20.

Relationship to the Other Spondyloarthropathies

The striking clinical, radiographic, and genetic similarities between ankylosing spondylitis and other diseases in this group may often lead to some diagnostic confusion. A high incidence of anterior eye disease, enthesopathy, and urogenital disease may make the differentiation between ankylosing spondylitis and Reiter's syndrome particularly difficult, depending upon when the manifestations become evident. Studies showing examples of two or more different diseases within the same pedigree lend further evidence that the distinction between these conditions may sometimes be artificial (4). Because of this, it is often useful to view this group of diseases as a spectrum and allow sufficient time for disease patterns to evolve before making more specific diagnoses in confusing cases.

Laboratory Features

Clinical Laboratory

Routine laboratory abnormalities are infrequent and generally nonspecific. Anemia occurs in only a small number of patients (15–20%) and is usually mild, normocytic, and normochromic. The erythrocyte sedimentation rate is probably elevated at some time during the course of disease in most patients, but there is no general agreement as to whether the sedimentation rate correlates with disease activity. Mild elevation in serum globulin may be seen, but rheumatoid factors and antinuclear antibodies should be absent. Mild elevations in serum creatinine phosphokinase and alkaline phosphatase of bone origin have been reported in a few patients.

Pathologic Features

In contrast to rheumatoid arthritis, which is primarily a disease of synovium, ankylosing spondylitis is manifest initially by pathologic changes at the sites of insertion of ligaments and capsules into bone (the entheses) (32). Biopsies of these areas will show nonspecific inflammation which results in destruction of the calcified part of the ligament and replacement by granulation tissue with infiltration by lymphocytes and plasma cells (Figure 10.2). A localized osteitis may be seen in bone near the entheses. These erosive and early healing phases have been observed at the attachment of the outer fibers of the annulus fibrosus along the anterior and lateral aspects of the vertebral bodies. These eventually lead to small erosive lesions around the circumference of the vertebral bodies. The repair process results in calcification of the annulus fibrosus and formation of a syndesmophyte, or bony bridge between vertebral bodies. Similar lesions may be seen at other attachments of ligament and joint capsule to bone throughout the body.

A synovitis of diarthrodial joints also occurs in ankylosing spondylitis. Pathologically, this is similar to that seen in rheumatoid arthritis, although the density of inflammatory cells and extent of necrosis are generally much less. The end result is usually fibrosis and ossification rather than joint destruction and instability.

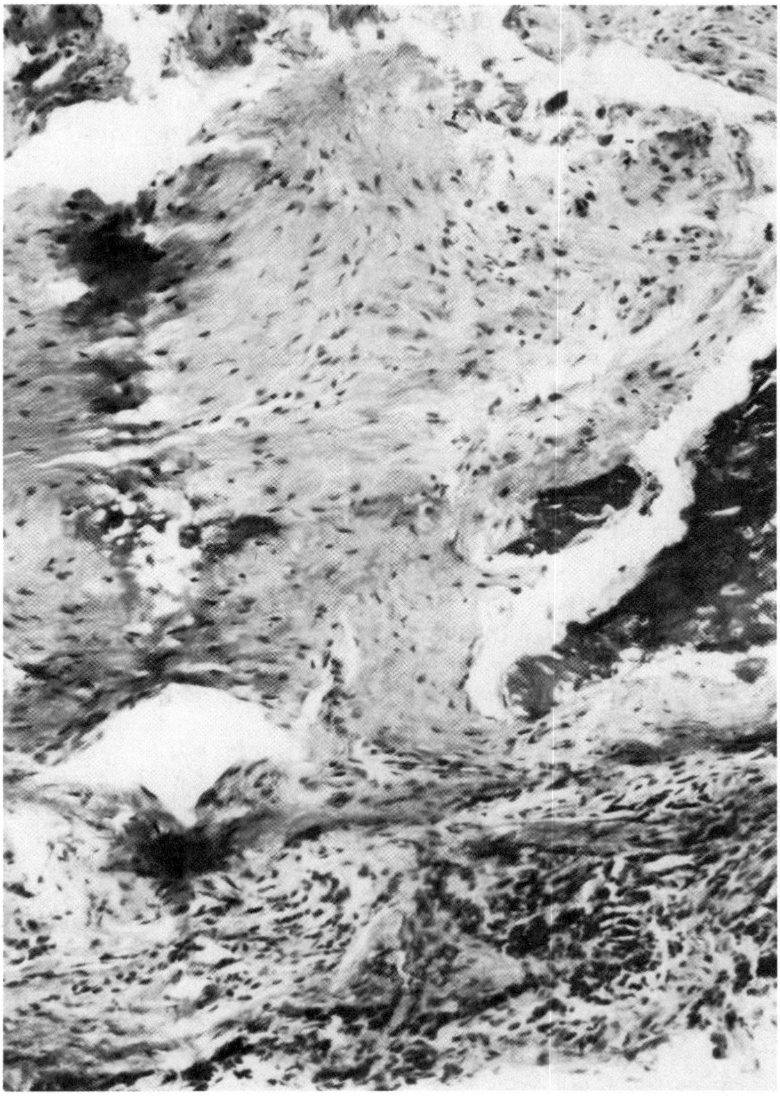

FIGURE 10.2 A focus of lymphocytic infiltration near a ligamentous insertion on bone. This specimen was obtained from an inflammatory disc space lesion. Similar pathology is seen at other sites of tendon and ligament insertion.

Radiologic Features

Although ankylosing spondylitis may have radiographic changes in virtually any joint, initial changes are invariably seen in the axial skeleton, particularly the sacroiliac joints. Evaluation of the sacroiliac joints may be difficult because of the undulating nature of their surfaces. A single anterior-posterior radiograph of the pelvis usually is sufficient to recognize sacroiliac disease (9), although special views with cephalad angulation of the beam or oblique views may be necessary. Recently, computed tomography has been shown to be helpful in equivocal cases (33). Sacroiliac involvement is usually bilateral and symmetric. Initial changes include erosion and sclerosis of bone with widening of the joint space followed by joint space narrowing and bony ankylosing of the joint. As the disease progresses, margins of the bones become less distinct.

Involvement of the spine usually is first seen in the lumbar region. Early, the vertebral bodies will lose their concave anterior configuration. This is followed by calcification of the spinal ligaments, syndesmophyte formation, and finally the classical "bamboo spine" appearance. Similar changes may be seen in the thoracic and cervical spines, and occasionally atlantoaxial subluxation is seen in patients with long-standing disease. Typical radiographs of sacroiliac and spinal involvement are shown in Chapter 3.

In the peripheral joints, bony erosions or spurs may be seen at the attachment of ligaments to bone. This is particularly common in the Achilles tendon. Soft tissue swelling, demineralization, joint space narrowing, and erosions may be seen in peripheral joints, but eventual bony ankylosis occurs which is more characteristic.

Prognosis and Management

Natural History

Ankylosing spondylitis, although sometimes a devastating disease, is rarely life-threatening. In spite of this, one large study has shown a higher mortality when compared to the general population due to gastrointestinal disease, accidents, suicide, vascular disease, nephritis, and respiratory disease (24). Nevertheless, long-term follow-up suggests that 80-92% of patients will be able to function normally throughout their life and maintain employment (34). Approximately two-thirds of patients will continue to have symptoms into late adulthood, but only about 40% will develop severe spinal restriction. Complications that cause the most disability seem to be iritis and peripheral joint involvement, particularly in the hips. Most of these complications tend to occur within the first 10 years of disease if at all. In general, a predictable pattern of disease severity will develop within the first 10 years while a minority of patients will develop worse spinal and peripheral joint disease after that time.

Management

General Considerations

Careful evaluation, early diagnosis, counseling, patient education, and participation of the patient in the management of his own disease are all essential components of the comprehensive management of patients with ankylosing spondylitis (35). Education of the patient and family about the chronic nature of the disease and generally good prognosis is important. The systemic nature of the disease should be emphasized. Common sense advice about maintenance of normal weight, discontinuation of smoking, and good posture should be given.

An active exercise program and avoidance of prolonged immobility should be encouraged. Patients should use a hard mattress and no more than one pillow if possible. An exercise program should be initiated early, since many authors feel that this may be as important as anything in preventing spinal deformities. Exercises should be designed to promote thoracic spine extension, active range of motion of the shoulders and hips, and lumbar flexion and mobility. Good posture should be encouraged throughout the day, and occupational adjustments should be considered to avoid prolonged immobilization in cramped positions. General conditioning exercises should be encouraged, particularly swimming, which enhances muscle tone and avoids unnecessary trauma. In regard to genetic counseling, patients should be told that their offspring have a 50% chance of being B27-positive, but that since there is only a 1 in 5 chance of developing disease, only about 10% of children will develop ankylosing spondylitis.

Drug therapy for ankylosing spondylitis is generally empiric, and the nonsteroidal antiinflammatory drugs are the mainstay. Phenylbutazone was long considered the drug of choice, but because of potential bone marrow toxicity, its prolonged use is probably best avoided except in those patients with severe disease unresponsive to other drugs. Indomethacin is now favored by most authors (10,35) and should be given in regular doses of 25-50 mg 3 times daily. Several other nonsteroidal antiinflammatory medications are now available, and many of these have been proven to be of some efficacy in treating this condition. Ibuprofen, tolmetin, fenoprofen, meclofenamate, sulindac, naproxen, or piroxicam all may be of benefit in individual patients and each of these medicines should be considered in those patients not responding to indomethacin. The use of aspirin is somewhat controversial, but most authors believe that it is much less effective than indomethacin or phenylbutazone. Gold, penicillamine, antimalarial, or immunosuppressive drugs have little use in ankylosing spondylitis. Systemic corticosteroids have no demonstrated role in the management of ankylosing spondylitis although these may be useful for local intraarticular or tendon insertion injection and may be required locally for treatment of inflammatory eye disease. In addition, intravenous methylprednisolone "pulse" therapy has been shown to give several months of remission in a few patients with severe relentless disease unresponsive to other agents (36). Radiation therapy was popular during the 1950's and 1960's, but this fell into disrepute when a high incidence of leukemia and other malignancy was reported in patients receiving this form of therapy.

Surgical Management

Total hip and knee arthroplasty as well as spinal surgery may be required in selected patients. This is especially true of pediatric patients who have a higher incidence of hip and peripheral joint disease. An increased incidence of new bone formation and ankylosis has been reported after hip arthroplasty, but this is rarely a significant functional problem (37). Spinal osteotomy may sometimes be useful in patients with severe kyphosis.

Management of Complications

Most of the long-term spinal and extraarticular complications require specific individualized management. Destructive lesions of spondylodiscitis or spinal fractures usually respond to bed rest, but occasionally require surgery for neurologic sequelae. Anterior uveitis may require topical mydriatics and corticosteroids. Cardiac complications may require pacemaker or prosthetic valve insertion. The pulmonary fibrosis rarely causes clinical problems but superinfection requires specific management.

Reiter's Syndrome

General

Historical Aspects

Although the association of arthritis following recently acquired urethritis in males was described as early as the sixteenth century, probably the best known description of this syndrome of urethritis, conjunctivitis, and arthritis following an episode of diarrhea occurred in a Prussian army officer described by Hans Reiter in 1916 (38). Since then, the literature on this syndrome has grown, and large numbers of cases have been reported in isolated forms or as part of large epidemics of infectious diarrhea (39,40). In the last several years, the relationship between Reiter's syndrome, other seronegative spondyloarhtropathies, and a high incidence of the histocompatibility antigen HLA-B27 have stimulated more interest in what was previously thought to be a relatively obscure condition.

Epidemiology and Genetics

The incidence and prevalence of Reiter's syndrome are very difficult to assess (41). The condition is often hard to diagnose because of difficulty in obtaining a history of some of the more mild mucocutaneous symptoms and overlooking nonspecific features. In females in particular, it is extremely difficult to recognize urethritis and cervitis. In spite of this, it is estimated that 1-3% of subjects with nonspecific urethritis or Shigella gastroenteritis will develop Reiter's syndrome (39).

As in ankylosing spondylitis, there is a strong association between the histocompatibility gene HLA-B27 and Reiter's syndrome. In Caucasians, about 80% of patients carry this antigen (42), while in blacks, only 50-60% are positive (43). Overall, approximately 20-25% of HLA-B27-positive individuals will develop Reiter's syndrome after an episode of urethritis or certain enteric infections (41).

Etiopathogenesis

Although no specific disease mechanism is known, it appears that the development of Reiter's syndrome depends on an interrelationship between environmental and genetic factors (44). The role of urethral infection has been investigated as a possible infective event that triggers an immunologic response as in other forms of reactive arthritis. The distinction between urethritis as a precipitating factor and urethritis as a manifestation of the disease remains unclear. Some cases of postvenereal Reiter's syndrome appear to be associated with chlamydia or mycoplasma infection. However, doubt has been cast on the specificity of these findings, since a large number of men with nonspecific urethritis have similar microbiologic findings. Infective agents have been isolated in many cases of epidemic Reiter's syndrome associated with diarrhea, including shigella, salmonella, and yersinia.

The relationship between these infective agents and HLA-B27 is unclear, but it has been speculated that the B-27 antigen has some cross-reactivity with bacterial antigens, or may be involved in the immune response to a specific infective agent (39).

Clinical Features

Clinical Presentation (See Table 10.5)

Arthropathy

Articular involvement usually occurs after an initial episode of urethritis, diarrhea, or conjunctivitis. The arthritis is typically an asymmetric arthritis of large weight-bearing joints. Occasionally, the toes, fingers, and joints of the upper extremity may be involved. There is usually a polyarticular arthritis, but a small minority of patients present with one or a few involved joints. The findings on physical exam are variable, ranging from a mild swelling with minimal objective signs to a tense joint with marked swelling, redness, heat, and severe pain. The arthritis is often progressive, with new joints becoming involved over the course of several days.

Periarticular Disease

Enthesopathic lesions are a hallmark of the disease and much more commonly seen with this disease than ankylosing spondylitis. Back pain, plantar fasciitis, chest wall pain, and Achilles tendonitis ("lover's heels") are frequently seen in Reiter's syndrome. These are often manifest by local tenderness, warmth, redness, and swelling.

Urogenital disease

Urethritis occurs in 80-90% of patients and may be either an initial (precipitating) event or an occurrence after the onset of diarrhea. Urethritis may be mild with minimal symptoms, or may be associated with a mucoid or a mucopurulent discharge. Prostatitis, hemorrhagic cystitis, bladder contraction, and hydronephrosis have been reported as well.

TABLE 10.5 Reiter's Syndrome: Percent Frequency of Initial Manifestations

Arthritis	100
Tendinitis	20-50
Urethritis	85
Conjunctivitis	55
Stomatitis	25
Balanitis	40-45
Keratodermia	20
Diarrhea	15

Ocular Disease

Conjunctivitis is a classic initial manifestation of eye involvement and is often difficult to differentiate from anterior uveitis or iritis, which may coexist. Symptoms are often mild and eye disease may go unnoticed, but chronic eye involvement can become a serious problem.

Mucocutaneous Disease

Typical mucocutaneous lesions include keratodermia blenorrhagica, circinate balanitis, oral ulcerations, destructive nail lesions, and dactylitis. Keratodermia blenorrhagica may begin several weeks after the onset of other manifestations as papular lesions which evolve into pustules and become larger and coalesce (as shown in Figure 10.3). Eventually they may form a thick keratotic crust that is difficult to distinguish from psoriasis both clinically and microscopically. These are most typically found on the soles of the feet, (as shown in Figure 10.4), but have been known to involve all part of the body and become quite severe and generalized. Circinate balanitis begins as painless and superficial erosions around the urethral meatus. These lesions enlarge and coalesce, forming an irregular erythematous lesion around the glans (see Figure 10.5). Mucous membrane lesions are often minimally symptomatic and may go unnoticed. These are usually shallow ulcers on the palate, tongue, buccal mucosa, or lips. Nail changes consist of keratosis under the nails, nail thickening, and onycholysis. Dactylitis (sausage toe) results from inflammation of the skin and enthesopathic lesions in the toe.

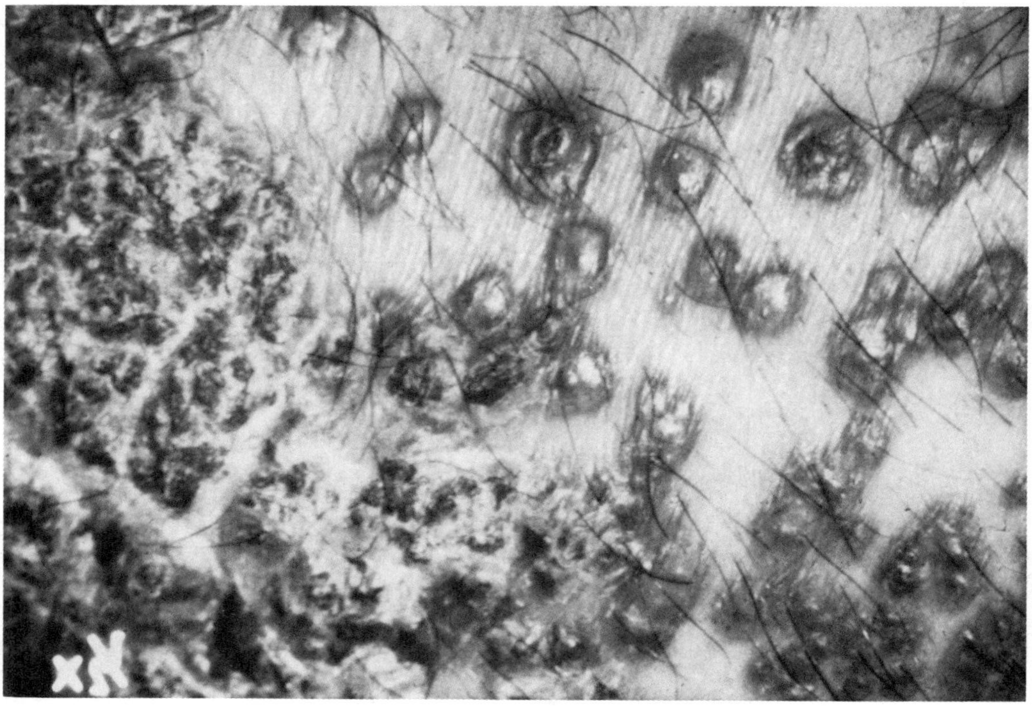

FIGURE 10.3 Early localized lesions of keratodermia blenorrhagica.

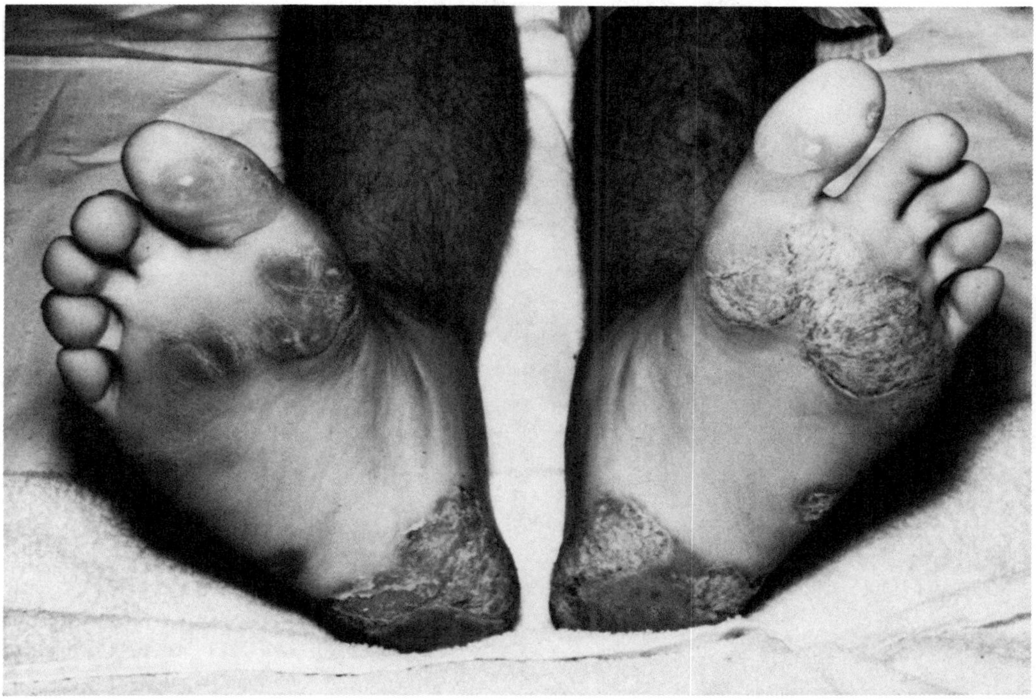

FIGURE 10.4 Extensive keratodermia blenorrhagica involving the soles of the feet.

Systemic Features

Because Reiter's syndrome is a disease involving multiple organ systems, many patients will have signs of systemic illness. Weight loss, fever, and anorexia are common during periods of active disease, but these tend to resolve when other features improve.

Diagnostic Criteria

Reiter's syndrome should be suspected in any young person who presents with an acute or chronic asymmetric arthritis, especially when large weight-bearing joints are involved. Because of a great deal of overlap among the seronegative spondyloarthropathies, recent attempts have been made to set forth criteria for definitive diagnosis of this condition (45). A diagnosis of Reiter's syndrome can be made when there is peripheral arthritis of more than 1 month's duration occurring in association with urethritis and/or cervitis. These criteria were found to be 84% sensitive and 98% specific in differentiating Reiter's syndrome from various other closely related syndromes.

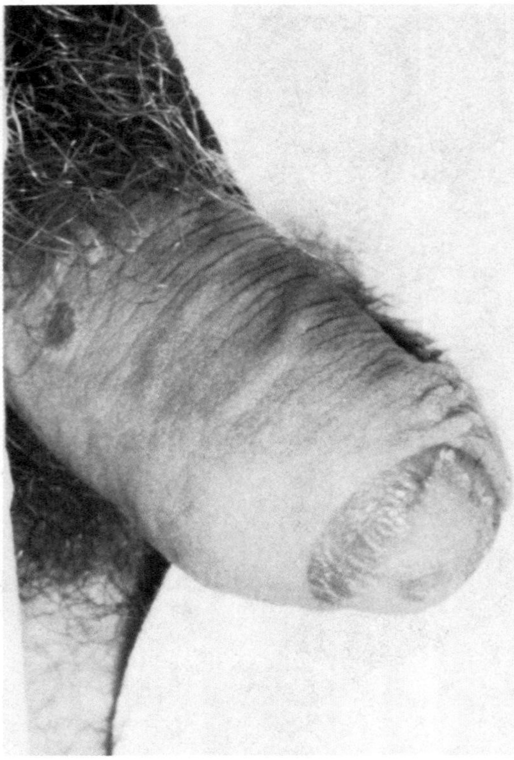

FIGURE 10.5 Circinate balanitis in Reiter's syndrome.

Differential Diagnosis

An acute arthritis in a young male associated with urethritis should always suggest the possibility of gonococcal arthritis. On occasion, urethral cultures will be positive for gonococcus, but the arthritis will not improve with treatment of the urethritis, lending support to a diagnosis of Reiter's syndrome. Reiter's syndrome is much more likely to be associated with skin lesions, stomatitis, or balanitis and enthesopathic lesions, such as achilles tendonitis. Psoriatic arthritis and Reiter's syndrome may be confused, especially since the skin lesions and nail changes may be nearly identical. Eye disease and mucous membrane lesions are less likely to occur in psoriasis. Distinguishing between Reiter's syndrome and ankylosing spondylitis can sometimes be difficult. Although the extraarticular features of these diseases are similar, they tend to be a major part of the presenting illness in Reiter's syndrome, while they are more often late sequelae in ankylosing spondylitis. Sacroiliitis is seen in both conditions, but is more often asymmetric in Reiter's syndrome. Spinal syndesmophytes occur in both, but tend to be large and asymmetric in Reiter's syndrome.

Late Features

Spinal Disease

Roughly 20-30% of patients with Reiter's syndrome develop sacroiliitis and spinal disease similar to ankylosing spondylitis (41). As noted previously, there is a tendency for this to occur more often in patients with severe disease and it tends to be asymmetric (46).

Late Ocular Disease

Progressive iridocyclitis, intraocular hemorrhage, and optic neuritis may occur during the course of the disease and lead to blindness.

Cardiovascular Disease

Cardiovascular complications of Reiter's syndrome are unusual but well recognized. Aortic insufficiency, pericarditis, and various conduction disturbances and arrhythmias have all been described in large series of patients with an overall incidence of about 10% (40,47). Aortic valvular lesions have been described which are identical to those seen in ankylosing spondylitis. Pericarditis tends to occur early in disease. Cardiac conduction abnormalities were recently described in 5 of 19 patients followed for several years. Correlation between these abnormalities and other manifestations of Reiter's syndrome was not noted (48).

Neurologic Disease

A wide range of neurologic manifestations have been attributed to Reiter's syndrome, and probably occur in about 1% of patients. Peripheral neuropathy, transient hemiplegia, and cranial nerve findings are the most frequently described complications.

Pulmonary Disease

Pleurisy, pulmonary infiltrates, and pleuritic chest pain thought to be due to tendonitis of the intercostal muscles have all been described as long-term extra-articular complications of Reiter's syndrome, but are exceedingly rare, and not often associated with significant morbidity.

Laboratory Features

Clinical Laboratory Evaluation

There are few specific laboratory abnormalities in Reiter's syndrome. The sedimentation rate may range from normal to extremely high with little correlation with disease severity or prognosis. Mild anemia and elevated acute phase proteins may be seen. Synovial fluid is typically inflammatory, often with cell counts ranging as high as 50,000. Glucose in synovial fluid is usually normal.

Pathologic Features

Pathologic studies of synovium are nonspecific and show inflammatory changes with edema, vascular congestion, and infiltration with acute and chronic inflammatory cells. During chronic stages, some synovial proliferation may occur and this may be indistinguishable from changes seen in rheumatoid arthritis. Inflammatory lesions at the sites of ligament insertions into bone (enthesopathy) are seen in Reiter's syndrome and are similar to those seen in ankylosing spondylitis.

Radiologic Features

Radiographs are usually normal early in disease. In those patients that do develop progressive disease, juxtaarticular osteoporosis, joint space narrowing, and erosive changes may be seen. Periostitis and ligamentous calcification occur as in the other seronegative spondyloarthropathies. Sacroiliitis may be indistinguishable from that seen in ankylosing spondylitis, but may also be asymmetric. Large discontinuous syndesmophytes and lateral bony bridging between vertebral bodies have also been described (40).

Prognosis and Management

Natural History

The long-term prognosis of Reiter's syndrome has been very difficult to assess for many reasons. Because of the young population group and intermittent and often unpredictable course, long-term follow-up studies have been difficult to perform and have usually been done in academic centers where patients with more aggressive disease are seen. The traditional view that the arthritis of Reiter's syndrome is short-lived and transient has been challenged by a number of long-term follow-up studies over the years. Most recent studies agree that a majority of patients will have persistent and recurrent symptoms, but not all studies indicate significant disability from these. Two recent studies, in which patients were followed for roughly 5-6 years, showed that 17-22% of patients were entirely asymptomatic, while 34-54% of patients had evidence of sustained, more than annoying, symptomatology (42,49). The degree of disability varied between these two studies, however; one study found that 27% of patients were either unemployable or had to change jobs, while in the other study, almost all patients were able to function normally between flares of disease. At present, no consistent patterns have emerged for determining prognostic indicators in this condition. Although there has been some indication that patients positive for HLA-B27 carry a worse prognosis, other data have shown that this has no real prognostic value (42).

Management

There is no curative treatment for Reiter's syndrome, and management of this recurrent, unpredictable, and sometimes severe disease often proves frustrating to both patient and physician (41). General education, as always, is important. Although some authors suggest avoidance of sexual indiscretion or use of condoms, many patients will have recurrences of symptoms without any specific sexual exposure.

Acute episodes are best managed by a combination of analgesics, antiinflammatory agents, and physical therapy. Although antibiotics have been suggested to treat associated nongonococcal urethritis, there is no evidence that this ameliorates the articular manifestations.

Indomethacin and phenlybutazone have been the most frequently used nonsteroidal antiinflammatory agents, although there are no controlled studies to demonstrate their superiority over aspirin or other agents. In general, indomethacin is preferable for long-term use, but phenylbutazone may be extremely useful for acute episodes.

Corticosteroids are often useful locally for ocular inflammation or may be injected for specific joint or tendon problems, but systemic steroids are of little benefit in this disorder. The use of cytotoxic drugs has been advocated for the rare patient with relentless progressive disease. Methotrexate and azathioprine have been among those most frequently used, but well-controlled data regarding their efficacy and safety are lacking.

Psoriatic Arthritis

General

Historical Aspects and Definitions

Although there were several descriptions of arthritis associated with psoriasis during the nineteenth century, the idea of psoriatic arthritis being a separate disease entity was not generally accepted. Recognition of rheumatoid factors and the introduction of criteria for the diagnosis of rheumatoid arthritis have made psoriatic arthritis more easy to recognize and differentiate. Several forms of psoriatic arthritis are now recognized, and this variety of presentation caused a great deal of confusion in the early literature. Currently, psoriatic arthritis is defined as any inflammatory arthritis occurring in association with psoriasis in a patient with a negative rheumatoid factor (50).

Epidemiology and Genetics

It has been difficult to determine a true figure for the frequency of psoriasis and psoriatic arthritis. Much of this may be due to the underrecognition of mild psoriasis. The frequency of arthritis among patients with psoriasis has varied widely from study to study, but is probably in the range of 6-7% (51). The disease tends to occur with almost equal frequency in men and women, with a very slight increased frequency in females.

The tendency for psoriatic arthritis to occur in several members of the same family has been noted for many years, although an exact mode of inheritance has yet to be determined. There is an increased incidence of the histocompatibility antigen HLA-B27 in patients with psoriatic arthritis. While the gene is no more frequent than in the general population in those with skin disease alone, it occurs in approximately 20% of patients with peripheral arthritis and 50-60% of those with psoriatic arthritis associated with sacroiliitis (see Table 10.1) (52). Studies have also shown an increased incidence of HLA-B13 and B17 in psoriasis patients with skin disease alone, and an increase in DR4, DR7, and B38 in those patients with peripheral arthritis (53).

Etiopathagenesis

It is clear from family surveys, individual pedigrees, and histocompatibility typing that heredity plays an important role in the development of psoriasis as well as the arthritis associated with it. Several morphologic, biochemical, and immunologic changes are seen in psoriasis which may have some bearing on the pathogenesis of the arthritis. A generalized capillary abnormality has been considered a possible common mechanism for both skin and articular disease. A relationship to streptococcal or staphylococcal infections has also been noted. Several immunologic abnormalities have been noted in serum and in blood lymphocytes, but intraarticular immune complex formation does not appear to play a major role in the pathogenesis of the arthritis, as it does in rheumatoid arthritis (54).

Clinical Features

Skin Disease

The skin disease in psoriasis has a bimodal peak of onset, with an initial peak in the 16-20 year age group, and a secondary peak in the 45-55 year age group (51). Typical lesions appear on the elbow initially, with subsequent involvement of the legs, scalp, and back. Skin disease precedes the onset of arthritis in the majority of patients, but about 16% of patients will have arthritis before skin lesions. There is no particular pattern of skin involvement that is associated with peripheral or spinal arthritis. The skin disease in psoriatic arthritis may be quite mild and may go unnoticed without a careful history and physical examination. Hidden areas of the scalp or perineum should be carefully examined in all patients presenting with undiagnosed seronegative arthritis, particularly when the pattern of involvement suggests psoriatic arthritis. Pustular psoriasis, with lesions on the palms and soles, may also be associated with psoriatic arthritis. Patients with this form of psoriasis appear to make up a disproportionally large number of the patients with severe arthritis. Although flares in skin and joint disease are usually not closely related, those patients with more extensive psoriasis are more likely to have arthritis than those with less extensive skin disease (55).

Nail Changes

Arthritis is more closely related to nail changes than to skin changes. Although nail changes may be seen in about 30% of all patients with psoriasis, they occur in about 85% of those with arthritis (51). There also appears to be a tendency for arthritis to occur in the same fingers where there are nail changes, although this is not a uniform association. Pitting of the nails, as seen in Figure 10.6, is the most characteristic finding. Transverse ridges, onycholysis, splinter hemorrhages, nail bed erythema, and subungual keratosis may also be seen.

Articular Disease

It is now apparent that psoriatic arthritis is not manifest in any single typical clinical pattern, but rather represents a wide spectrum of presentations which may range from a mild monoarticular process to a rapidly destructive arthritis mutilans. Five broad patterns of clinical joint involvement are generally recognized today (see Table 10.6) (50).

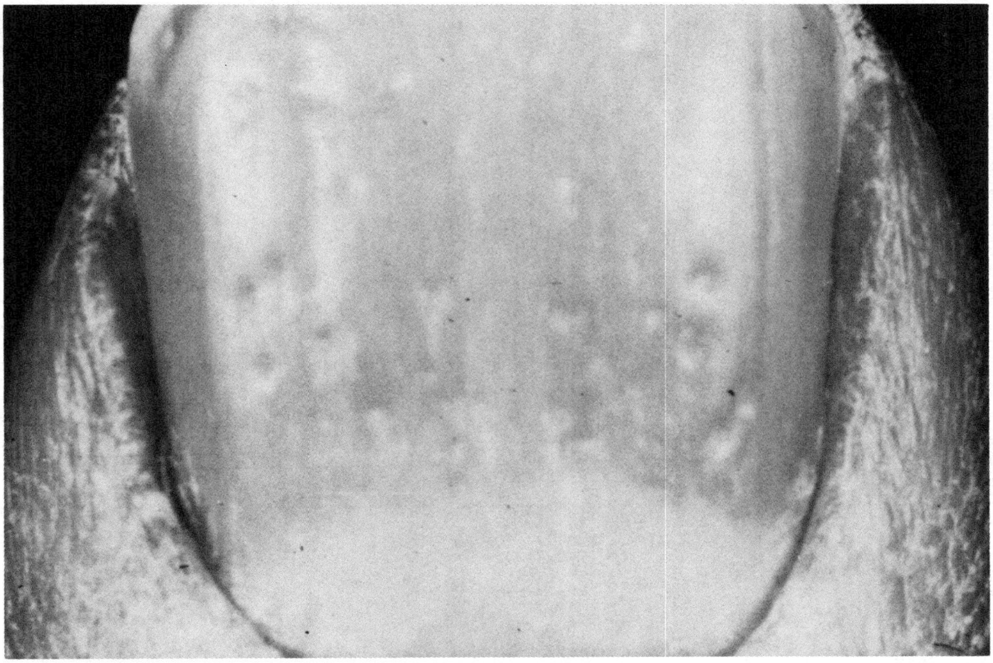

FIGURE 10.6 Typical nail pitting seen in psoriasis. There is a high correlation of this finding with peripheral arthropathy (reprinted from the *Revised Clinical Slide Collection on the Rheumatic Diseases,* copyright 1981, used by permission of the Arthritis Foundation).

TABLE 10.6 Clinical Patterns of Psoriatic Arthritis

	Percentage of Total Group*
Classic distal IP disease	17
Arthritis mutilans	5
Symmetric rheumatoid-like	15
Asymmetric oligoarthritis	70
Ankylosing spondylitis	5

*Totals over 100% because some patients have a combination of forms.

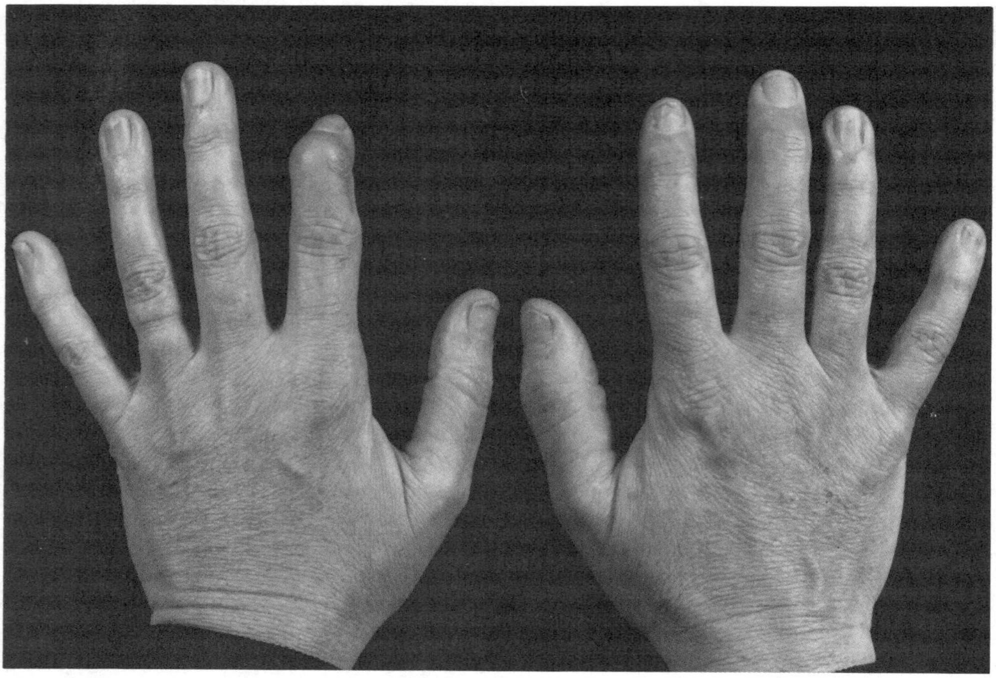

FIGURE 10.7 Classic psoriatic arthritis involving the distal IP joints, most evident in the left second and third DIP's. Several nails demonstrate mild onycholysis (separation from the nail bed).

1. Classic psoriatic arthritis is a disease predominantly of the distal interphalangeal joints, as seen in Figure 10.7. This pattern is most typically associated with nail lesions, often involving the same finger. Although considered the most typical form, large studies have shown that this pattern probably represents only about 17% of all patients (56).
2. Arthritis mutilans is a severely deforming type of arthritis which results from widespread joint space destruction, osteolysis of phalanges and metacarpals, and ankylosis. Deformity may be so striking as to give an "opera glass" appearance to the hand. Fortunately, this condition is relatively uncommon, occurring in about 5% of patients.
3. A symmetrical rheumatoid-like arthritis has been described in about 15% of patients with psoriatic arthritis. The patients in this group have symmetric polyarticular arthritis which is clinically indistinguishable from rheumatoid arthritis. A small percentage of these patients may develop positive rheumatoid factors at some time, and these probably have coexistent rheumatoid arthritis and psoriasis. The majority, however, are seronegative, and tend to have less extensive joint destruction and a more benign course than rheumatoid arthritis.
4. An asymmetric mono- or oligoarthritis is probably the most common form of psoriatic arthritis, accounting for about 70% of all cases. In this form, one or a few joints in the hands and feet may be involved in a scattered, patchy distribution. The joints most commonly affected are the distal interphalangeal, proximal interphalangeal, and metatarsal-phalangeal joints.

5. Ankylosing spondylitis accounts for about 5% of all cases of psoriatic arthritis. There is a tendency for this to occur more often in men who develop psoriasis later in life. Otherwise, however, the spondylitis associated with psoriasis is quite similar clinically to idiopathic ankylosing spondylitis, except for several subtle clinical and radiographic differences. Many patients with psoriatic spondylitis may have a relative lack of back pain and stiffness. Radiographic sacroiliitis is more often asymmetric and thus similar to that seen in Reiter's syndrome. In addition, striking paravertebral ossification, disc calcification, and nonmarginal syndesmophytes are more common than in ankylosing spondylitis (46,57).

The onset of psoriatic arthritis may be gradual or abrupt, and occasionally acute onset in the toes may suggest gout. When compared to rheumatoid arthritis, the disease tends to be much less severe and progressive and tends to remain asymmetric.

Extraarticular Manifestations

Extraarticular involvement is much less commonly seen in psoriatic arthritis than in rheumatoid arthritis. Subcutaneous nodules are almost never seen. Ocular lesions, including conjunctivitis, uveitis, and scleritis, have been described in a minority of patients, with conjunctivitis being the most common, occurring in about 20% of patients (58). Eye involvement appears to be associated with the occurrence of sacroiliitis and a positive test for HLA-B27. Other extraarticular features described in isolated cases of psoriatic arthritis include myopathy, fibrosing alveolitis, aortic insufficiency, and amyloidosis (51,54).

Arthritis Associated with Other Skin Diseases

In recent years, other syndromes have been described which may be related to psoriatic arthritis in that they all appear to be related to idiopathic cutaneous lesions and have clinical features of seronegative spondyloarthropathies.

Sternocostoclavicular hyperostosis (also referred to as pustulotic arthro-osteitis) is a rare syndrome in western countries, but seems to be relatively frequent in Japan. This syndrome is characterized by low grade inflammation and eventual fibrosis and ankylosis of sternoclavicular joints, and is associated with skin lesions known as palmoplantar pustulosis (59).

Spondyloarthropathy associated with hidradenitis suppurativa and acne conglobata has been described in 10 patients, although no association with HLA-B27 was found (60).

Laboratory Features

Clinical Laboratory Evaluation

Laboratory findings in psoriatic arthritis are typically nonspecific and seldom helpful in diagnostic evaluation. Rheumatoid factors have been found in small numbers of patients, and this usually reflects concurrent association of psoriasis with true rheumatoid arthritis. Antinuclear antibodies are typically negative. Mild anemia, elevation of sedimentation rate, and leukocytosis may occur in small numbers of patients. Hyperuricemia has been reported in about 10-20% of patients, and has been attributed to increased epidermal cell turnover (54), but this has been disputed and the elevation attributed to concomitant drug therapy (51).

Pathologic Features

Histologic studies of synovium in psoriatic arthritis show nonspecific changes of chronic synovitis including synovial cell proliferation and mononuclear cell infiltration. Although rheumatoid granulomas are not found, the other inflammatory findings may make the synovial histology indistinguishable from that seen in rheumatoid arthritis. An increase in periarticular fibrosis may be more characteristic of psoriatic than rheumatoid arthritis (61).

Radiographic Features

The radiographic features of psoriatic arthritis are also often indistinguishable from those of rheumatoid arthritis. In general, however, fewer joints tend to be involved, and the distribution is more patchy and asymmetric. Involvement of the distal interphalangeal joints is much more typical of psoriatic arthritis. In some cases, erosion of the terminal phalangeal tufts (acroosteolysis) occurs. Erosive changes in the small joints of the hands and feet may take on a characteristic pencil-in-cup appearance. This results from marginal erosions which progress and may produce apparent widening of the joint space, expansion of the base of the distal phalanx, and whittling of the proximal portion of the joint. This characteristic picture is relatively uncommon, occurring mostly in the arthritis mutilans subgroup.

Although ankylosing spondylitis is clinically apparent in only about 5% of patients, sacroiliac changes may be seen in about 20% of patients (57). As mentioned above, findings may be similar to that of idiopathic ankylosing spondylitis, but asymmetric sacroiliitis, paravertebral ossification, and atypical syndesmophytes are more likely to occur.

Prognosis and Management

Natural History

In spite of severe deforming arthritis that occurs in a small number of patients, the general outlook in psoriatic arthritis is good. The disease is usually mild and tends to have an intermittent course affecting only a few joints. Several long-term studies have confirmed the relatively good overall prognosis, including a recent study which showed that 97% of patients had lost less than 1 year of work over a 10-year period (56).

Management

Since the disease is usually mild, patients should be made aware of this early to allay anxiety. Treatment of the usual patient with mild disease should begin with general principles of rest, splinting, joint protection, and use of adaptive devices as in rheumatoid arthritis. Satisfactory symptomatic relief can usually be obtained with antiinflammatory doses of aspirin or one of the other nonsteroidal antiinflammatory agents. Local corticosteroid injection is often very useful, since a relatively few joints are often involved. Special care should be taken to avoid intraarticular injections in the area of active psoriatic skin lesions, since the potential for contamination with skin bacteria is probably increased in this situation.

In those few patients with progressive and potentially deforming arthritis, more potent and toxic agents may be required. Methotrexate has been one of the most widely used cytotoxic drugs in the treatment of skin disease in psoriasis and has been effective in suppressing the articular manifestations as well, but with a high frequency of side effects (62). Hepatic toxicity appears to be the most frequent side effect in the doses used for psoriasis and hepatic fibrosis may result. Several reports suggest that intermittent high doses are safer, but some authors still recommend annual liver biopsies to monitor for potential toxicity. Azathioprine and other cytotoxic agents have also been used with varying success.

Gold is apparently safe and effective for treatment of severe psoriatic arthritis (63,64). When compared to patients with rheumatoid arthritis receiving gold, psoriasis patients have no increase in adverse reactions and the drug appears to be at least as effective in this condition. Of the other long-acting agents used in rheumatoid arthritis, there is almost no data on D-penicillamine for use in psoriatic arthritis, and antimalarial drugs are discouraged because of the potential for provoking an exfoliative reaction (65).

It is unclear whether successful treatment of the skin disease invariably results in improvement in arthritis. One recent study suggested that patients treated with a PUVA regimen for their skin disease showed improvement in peripheral joint disease, although those with spondylitis were generally unimproved (66).

Enteropathic Arthritis

General

Since the original recognition of arthritis as one of the major extracolonic complications of ulcerative colitis in 1929, a number of studies have described both a peripheral and axial arthropathy associated with this condition, as well as with Crohn's disease (67-69). Arthritis has also been associated with various other inflammatory bowel conditions, including Whipple's disease, after intestinal bypass surgery, and various enteric infections (including salmonella, shigella, yersinia, and campylobacter). Together this group of conditions is best regarded as a family of diseases, known as enteropathic arthropathies. In many ways, the clinical manifestations of these syndromes are quite similar to Reiter's syndrome and many might be considered forms of reactive arthritis.

Although strict definitions for the arthritis associated with these conditions do not exist, the arthritis of ulcerative colitis and Crohn's disease has been previously defined as having four essential characteristics: 1) articular manifestations begin after the onset of intestinal disease; 2) attacks of arthritis are related to flares of bowel disease; 3) attacks of arthritis are followed by complete remission; 4) rheumatoid factor is absent (66). Various genetic associations have been described with this family of diseases, particularly with the HLA-B27 antigen, and these were summarized previously in Table 10.1.

Etiopathogenesis

Genetic factors appear to play a role in the development of various forms of enteropathic arthritis. The high prevalence of the HLA-B27 antigen in those that develop arthritis after enteric infection suggests several possible pathogenetic mechanisms, including cross-reactivity of this antigen with bacterial products, or alterations in immunologic self-recognition. In ulcerative colitis and Crohn's disease, there is an increased incidence of HLA-B27 in those developing spondylitis but not with peripheral arthritis.

Circulating immune complexes, with bacterial antigens playing a role, may well be important in the pathogenesis of the peripheral arthritis associated with these conditions, since immune complexes have been demonstrated in sera and skin lesions of patients with arthritis following intestinal bypass as well as in those with ulcerative colitis and Crohn's disease (70,71).

Clinical Features

Patterns of Articular Involvement

Peripheral Arthritis

The peripheral arthritis associated with inflammatory bowel disease is characteristically an acute, intermittent, self-limited condition involving relatively few joints. In a majority of cases (85%), fewer than four joints are involved, but occasionally more joints may be involved in a migratory pattern. The knees, ankles, and elbows are the most frequent joints involved, with fingers, wrists, and shoulders affected less often. Flares of peripheral arthritis usually last less than a month, but sometimes last up to 2 months. Approximately 20% of patients will have attacks lasting 2-12 months, and a few have chronic problems lasting several years. In most cases, permanent joint damage is not seen. Peripheral arthritis may be seen with any of the types of enteropathic arthritis and, in general, the characteristics are similar among the different conditions. In Whipple's disease joint disease does not tend to correlate with gastrointestinal disease.

Spondylitis

Ankylosing spondylitis occurs in about 4% of patients with ulcerative colitis and Crohn's disease (68, 72). Women are about half as frequently affected as men in ulcerative colitis and about equally affected in Crohn's disease. HLA-B27 is increased in frequency, being positive in 50-60% of those associated with Crohn's disease, and 60-70% of those with ulcerative colitis. Ankylosing spondylitis may precede the symptoms of inflammatory bowel disease in many cases. There is no good correlation of the activity of the spondylitis with that of the inflammatory bowel disease. There are also a group of patients with asymptomatic radiographic sacroiliitis who may never become symptomatic or develop full-blown ankylosing spondylitis (72). Radiographically, the features of spondylitis associated with inflammatory bowel disease are quite similar to those seen in idiopathic ankylosing spondylitis (46).

Specific Disease Associations

Ulcerative Colitis

Arthritis is more frequently seen in patients with more extensive disease and complications of bowel disease. Overall, about 10% of patients develop peripheral arthritis, and about 4% develop spondylitis. Arthritis is more common in patients with other systemic manifestations such as pyoderma gangrenosum and uveitis.

Crohn's Disease

Peripheral arthritis occurs in about 20% and ankylosing spondylitis in 4% of patients with Crohn's disease. Peripheral arthritis is much more frequent in patients with disease of the colon, and less common in those with disease limited to the small bowel. There is no good correlation of the arthritis of Crohn's disease with the complications of bowel disease, such as fistula formation or malabsorption, and the concurrence of arthritis with flares of bowel disease is less predictable than in ulcerative colitis. Arthritis is more common in patients with extraintestinal manifestations such as erythema nodosum and stomatitis.

Intestinal Bypass Arthritis

Since the advent of intestinal bypass surgery for morbid obesity, a high percentage of patients have been found to develop arthritis and other long-term immunologic complications. After the original jejunocolostomies, about one-third of patients subsequently developed arthritis, and with the more recent jejunoileostomy, about 40% of patients have developed articular symptoms (74). The arthritis may occur from a few weeks to several years after surgery and may have a gradual or sudden onset. There is a tendency to be intermittent and migratory, with the knees, shoulders, hips, hands, wrist, and feet most often affected. Other associated features occurring relatively frequently include cutaneous vasculitis, Raynaud's phenomenon, and occasionally erythema nodosum (70).

Arthritis Following Salmonella Infection

Aseptic arthritis, usually occurring 1-2 weeks after enteric symptoms, occurs in approximately 2-4% of patients infected with salmonella (39). Joint involvement may be monoarticular, polyarticular, or migratory and may last from a few days to several months. Fever is usually present early in disease, and other features seen in Reiter's syndrome may be seen. About two-thirds of patients developing arthritis after salmonella infection will be positive for HLA-B27. Salmonella may also cause direct hematogenous seeding of a joint, and this should always be considered in the differential diagnosis.

Arthritis Following Shigella Infection

Approximately 2% of patients with *Shigella flexneri* dysentery develop arthritis, and a large percentage of these develop other features of Reiter's syndrome as well (40). Most patients develop arthritis within 4 weeks of the onset of diarrhea, with the knees and ankles being the most frequently involved joints. Oligoarthritis is most common, with a few patients developing symmetric polyarthritis resembling rheumatoid disease. Most attacks clear within 3 months without residual symptoms.

Arthritis Following Yersinia Infection

This type of arthritis has been reported almost exclusively in Finland and other Scandinavian countries, although a few North American cases probably exist (73). This arthritis usually involves two to four large or small joints and clears completely within 1-3 months, although a few patients with prolonged arthritis have been reported. Back pain and sacroiliitis have been noted during the acute phase and in long-term follow-up, and several cases of full Reiter's syndrome have been observed (73,75). The HLA-B27 antigen is found in 60-90% of patients developing arthritis, and those that carry this antigen tend to have more severe acute disease, and may be more likely to develop chronic sacroiliitis. Yersinia may also cause bacteremia and septic arthritis.

Arthritis Following Campylobacter Infection

Since the recognition of *Campylobacter jejuni* as an infective agent responsible for a diarrheal illness, there have been several case reports of arthritis following this infection. Most of these are acute, and are either monoarticular or polyarticular, and most patients to date have been positive for HLA-B27 (76).

Whipple's Disease

This is a rare multisystem disease of unknown etiology associated with bacteria-like structures seen in small bowel biopsy specimens. Diarrhea and malabsorption are always present at some time during the disease, but arthralgias or arthritis occur in most patients as well. A small percentage of patients will have articular manifestations long before bowel disease becomes apparent. The arthritis is characterized by intermittent acute attacks in a migratory poly- or oligoarticular pattern. There is little correlation with the activity of the diarrhea. Several other systemic features have been reported, including pleuritis, pericarditis, thyroiditis, and central nervous system involvement (73). Peripheral joint disease usually leaves little deformity. Several cases of ankylosing spondylitis have been reported in association with Whipple's disease.

Laboratory Features

The laboratory features of the enteropathic arthropathies are nonspecific. Mild elevations in sedimentation rate are frequently seen, but do not correlate well with disease activity. Synovial fluid analysis usually shows inflammatory fluid, and synovial biopsies show chronic inflammatory changes. There are no specific diagnostic tests for the arthritis of ulcerative colitis, Crohn's disease, or intestinal bypass. Diagnosis requires exclusion of infectious causes of arthritis in the proper clinical setting. A positive stool culture for the suspected infective agent is usually required for the diagnosis of arthritis following enteric infection, although serologic confirmation of recent infection is possible following salmonella, yersinia, or campylobacter infection. Special stool cultures may be necessary to diagnose yersinia or campylobacter infection. In Whipple's disease, a jejunal biopsy, with the demonstration of PAS-positive inclusion bodies in macrophages, is usually the best means of diagnosis. These bodies have also been identified in several other sites, including synovium.

Radiographic changes in most forms of enteropathic arthritis are minimal or nonspecific. Joint destruction is rare in most forms of peripheral arthritis, and spondylitis, when it occurs, is similar to that seen in idiopathic ankylosing spondylitis.

Prognosis and Management

In almost all forms of enteropathic arthritis, chronic disability, joint destruction, and deformity are rare. Most peripheral arthritis tends to follow an acute self-limited course, although chronic peripheral arthropathy may be seen in Whipple's disease and following yersinia infection. Ankylosing spondylitis tends to progress much like idiopathic spondylitis with little relationship to the underlying bowel disease.

Therapy for most forms of enteropathic arthritis is nonspecific. In ulcerative colitis and Crohn's disease, peripheral arthritis seldom requires therapy, but usually responds to aspirin or other nonsteroidal antiinflammatory medications. Spondylitis responds similarly, and chronic therapy with nonsteroidal antiinflammatory agents is usually well tolerated in the absence of peptic ulcer disease. Corticosteroids are often used for the underlying bowel disease, and usually control articular symptoms as well. Arthritis following intestinal bypass has been reported to respond occasionally to tetracycline or other antibiotics, but has required steroids in some patients. Reconstruction of the blind loop of bowel usually results in remission of the arthritis. Arthritis following salmonella infection usually responds to salicylates or other antiinflammatory drugs. Antibiotics, usually ampicillin or chloramphenicol, are used only in cases of bacteremia. In shigella infections, antibiotic therapy is controversial, and is usually reserved for patients who are systemically ill. In addition to antiinflammatory drugs for the arthritis, tetracycline is usually effective for yersinia infections, although septicemia may require other antibiotic therapy determined by susceptibility studies. Arthritis after campylobacter infection usually requires no antibiotics. In Whipple's disease, tetracycline is the mainstay of antibiotic therapy, although combinations of penicillin, streptomycin, and erythromycin have also been used (73).

References

1. Bywaters EGL: Historical introduction. In JMH Moll (ed.), *Ankylosing Spondylitis,* 1st Ed. London, Churchill Livingston, 1980, pp. 1-15.

2. Van der Linden SM, Valkenburg, HA, de Jongh BM, Cats A: The risk of developing ankylosing spondylitis in HLA-B27-positive individuals. A comparison of relatives of spondylitis patients with the general population. *Arthritis Rheum* 27:241-249, 1984.

3. Calin A, Fries JF: The striking prevalence of ankylosing spondylitis in "healthy" W27-positive males and females. *N Engl J Med* 293:835-839, 1975.

4. Calin A: Spondyloarthropathy in Caucasians and non-Caucasians. *J Rheumatol Suppl* 10:16-19, 1983.

5. Brewerton DA, Caffrey M, Hart FD et al.: Ankylosing spondylitis and HL-A27. *Lancet* 1:904-907, 1973.

6. Schlosstein L, Terasaki PI, Bluestone R et al.: High association of an HL-A antigen, W-27, with ankylosing spondylitis. *N Engl J Med* 288:704-706, 1973.

7. Veys EM, Van Laere M: Serum IgG, IgM, and IgA levels in ankylosing spondylitis. *Ann Rheum Dis* 32:493-496, 1973.

8. Ebringer R, Cooke D, Cawdell DR et al.: Ankylosing spondylitis, klebsiella, and HLA-B27. *Rheumatol Rehabil* 16:190-196, 1977.

9. Kinsella TD, Fritzler MJ, McNeil DJ: Ankylosing spondylitis: A disease in search of microbes. *J Rheumatol* 10:2-4, 1983.

10. Calin A: Ankylosing spondylitis. In WN Kelley, ED Harris, S Ruddy, CB Sledge (eds.), *Textbook of Rheumatology,* 1st Ed. Philadelphia, W.B. Saunders, 1981, pp. 1017-1032.

11. Bennett PH, Burch TA: Population studies of the rheumatic diseases. Amsterdam, Excerpta Medica Foundation, 1968, p. 305.

12. Cawley MID, Chalmers TM, Kellgren JH, Ball J: Destructive lesions of the vertebral bodies in ankylosing spondylitis. *Ann Rheum Dis* 31:345-358, 1972.

13. Wise CM, Irby WR: Spondylodiscitis in ankylosing spondylitis - Variable presentations. *J Rheumatol* 10:1004-1006, 1983.

14. Murray GL, Persellin RH: Cervical fracture complicating ankylosing spondylitis. *Am Jour Med* 70:1033-1041, 1981.

15. Hunter T, Dubo JC: Spinal fractures complicating ankylosing spondylitis. A long-term follow-up study. *Arthritis Rheum* 26:751-759, 1983.

16. Resnick D: Patterns of peripheral joint disease in ankylosing spondylitis. *Radiology* 110:523-532, 1974.

17. Dwosh IL, Resnick D, Baker MA: Hip involvement in ankylosing spondylitis. *Arthritis Rheum* 19:683-692, 1976.

18. Cohen MD, Ginsburg WM: Late onset peripheral joint disease in ankylosing spondylitis. *Ann Rheum Dis* 41:574-578, 1982.

19. Rosenow EL, Strimlan CV, Muhm JR, Fergusen RH: Pleuropulmonary manifestations of ankylosing spondylitis. *Mayo Clin Proc* 52:641-649, 1977.

20. Bulkley BH, Roberts WC: Ankylosing spondylitis and aortic regurgitation. *Circulation* 48:1014-1027, 1973.

21. Bergfeldt L, Edhag O, Vedin L, Vallin H: Ankylosing spondylitis: An important cause of severe disturbances of the cardiac conduction system. Prevalence among 223 pacemaker-treated men. *Amer Jour Med* 73:187-191, 1982.

22. Russell ML, Gordon DA, Ogryzlo MA, McPhedran BS: The cauda equina syndrome of ankylosing spondylitis. *Ann Intern Med* 78:551-554, 1973.

23. Mason RM, Murray RS, Oates JK et al.: Prostatitis and ankylosing spondylitis. *Br Med Jour* 1:748-751, 1958.

24. Radford EP, Doll R, Smith PG: Mortality among patients with ankylosing spondylitis not given x-ray therapy. *N Engl J Med* 297:572-576, 1977.

25. Agudelo CA, Pisko EJ, Wall BA: Nephropathy in ankylosing spondylitis. *Arthritis Rheum* 26:930, 1983.

26. Marks SH, Barnett M, Calin A: Ankylosing spondylitis in women and men: A case-control study. *J Rheumatol* 10:624-628, 1983.

27. Resnick D, Dwosh IL, Goergen TG et al.: Clinical and radiographic abnormalities in ankylosing spondylitis: A comparison of men and women. *Radiology* 111:293-297, 1976.

28. Ostensen M, Romberg O, Husby G: Ankylosing spondylitis and motherhood. *Arthritis Rheum* 25:140-143, 1982.

29. Ansell B: Juvenile spondylitis and related disorders. In JMH Moll (ed.), *Ankylosing Spondylitis,* 1st Ed. London, Churchill Livingston, 1980, pp. 120-136.

30. Marks SH, Barnett M, Calin A: A case-control study of juvenile and adult-onset ankylosing spondylitis. *J Rheumatol* 9:739-741, 1982.

31. Rosenberg AM, Petty RE: A syndrome of seronegative enthesopathy and arthropathy in children. *Arthritis Rheum* 25:1041-1047, 1982.

32. Ball J: Pathology and pathogenesis. In JMH Moll, (ed.), *Ankylosing Spondylitis,* 1st Ed. London, Churchill Livingston, 1980, pp. 96-112.

33. Ryan LM, Carrera GF, Lightfoot RW et al.: The radiographic diagnosis of sacroiliitis. *Arthritis Rheum* 26:760-763, 1983.

34. Carette S, Graham D, Little H et al.: The natural history of ankylosing spondylitis. *Arthritis Rheum* 26:186-190, 1983.

35. Calin A, Marks S: Management of ankylosing spondylitis. *Bull Rheum Dis* 31:35-38, 1982.

36. Mintz G, Enriquez RD, Mercado U et al.: Intravenous methylprednisolone therapy in severe ankylosing spondylitis. *Arthritis Rheum* 24:734-736, 1981.

37. Resnick D, Dwosh IL, Goergen TG et al.: Clinical and radiographic "re-ankylosis" following hip surgery in ankylosing spondylitis. *Am Jour Roentgen* 126:1181-1188, 1976.

38. Reiter H: Ueber eine bisher unerkannte Spirochaeteninfektion (spirochaetosis arthritica). *Deut Med Wschr* 42:1535-1536, 1916.

39. Keat A: Reiter's syndrome and reactive arthritis in perspective. *N Engl J Med* 309:1606-1615, 1983.

40. Paronen I: Reiter's disease: A study of 344 cases observed in Finland. *Acta Med Scand* (suppl. 212) 131:1-112, 1948.

41. Calin A: Reiter's syndrome. In WN Kelley, ED Harris, S Ruddy, CB Sledge (eds.), *Textbook of Rheumatology,* 1st Ed. Philadelphia, W.B. Saunders, 1981, pp. 1033-1046.

42. Fox R, Calin A, Gerber RC, Gibson D: The chronicity of symptoms and disability in Reiter's syndrome: An analysis of 131 consecutive patients. *Ann Intern Med* 91:190-193, 1979.

43. Good AE, Kawanish H, Schultz JS: HLA-B27 in blacks with ankylosing spondylitis or Reiter's disease. *N Engl J Med* 294:166-167, 1976.

44. Calin A: The relationship between genetics and environment in the pathogenesis of rheumatic diseases. *West J Med* 131:205-218, 1979.

45. Willkens RF, Arnett FC, Bitter T et al.: Reiter's syndrome: Evaluation of preliminary criteria for definite diagnosis. *Bull Rheum Dis* 32:65-68, 1982.

46. McEwen C, DiTata D, Lingg C et al.: Ankylosing spondylitis and spondylitis accompanying ulcerative colitis, regional enteritis, psoriasis, and Reiter's disease. *Arthritis Rheum* 14:291-318, 1971.

47. Good AE: Reiter's disease: A review with special attention to cardio-vascular and neurologic sequelae. *Semin Arth Rheum* 3:253-286, 1974.

48. Ruppert GB, Lindsey J, Barth WF: Cardiac conduction abnormalities in Reiter's syndrome. *Amer J Med* 73:335-340, 1982.

49. Butler MJ, Russell AS, Percy JS, Lentle BC: A follow-up study of 48 patients with Reiter's syndrome. *Amer J Med* 67:808-810, 1979.

50. Moll JMH, Wright V: Familial occurrence of psoriatic arthritis. *Ann Rheum Dis* 32:181-201, 1973.

51. Wright V: Psoriatic arthritis. In WN Kelley, ED Harris, S Ruddy, CB Sledge (eds.), *Textbook of Rheumatology,* 1st Ed. Philadelphia, W.B. Saunders, 1981, pp. 1047-1062.

52. Brewerton DA, Caffrey M, Nicholls A et al.: HLA-B27 and arthropathies associated with ulcerative colitis and psoriasis. *Lancet* 1:956-958, 1974.

53. Armstrong RD, Panayi GS, Welsh KI: Histocompatibility antigens in psoriasis, psoriatic arthropathy, and ankylosing spondylitis. *Ann Rheum Dis* 42:142-146, 1983.

54. Bennett RM: Psoriatic arthritis. In DJ McCarty (ed.), *Arthritis and Allied Conditions,* 9th Ed. Philadelphia, Lea and Febiger, 1981, pp. 642-655.

55. Leonard DG, O'Duffy JD, Rogers RS: Prospective analysis of psoriatic arthritis in patients hospitalized for psoriasis. *Mayo Clin Proc* 53:511-518, 1978.

56. Roberts MET, Wright V, Hill AGS et al.: Psoriatic arthritis: A follow-up study. *Ann Rheum Dis* 35:206-212, 1976.

57. Lambert JR, Wright V: Psoriatic spondylitis: A clinical and radiologic description of the spine in psoriatic arthritis. *Quart J Med* 46:411-425, 1977.

58. Lambert JR, Wright V: Eye inflammation in psoriatic arthritis. *Ann Rheum Dis* 35:354-356, 1976.

59. Fallet GH, Arroyo J, Kischer TL: Sternoclavicular hyperostosis: Case report with a 31-year follow-up. *Arthritis Rheum* 26:784-790, 1983.

60. Rosner IA, Richter DE, Huettner TL et al.: Spondyloarthropathy associated with hidradenitis suppurative and acne conglobata. *Ann Intern Med* 97: 520-525, 1982.

61. Bauer W, Bennett GA, Zeller JW: Pathology of joint lesions in patients with psoriasis and arthritis. *Trans Assoc Am Phys* 56:349-352, 1941.

62. Black RL, O'Brien WM, Van Scott et al.: Methotrexate therapy in psoriatic arthritis. *JAMA* 189:743-747, 1964.

63. Dorwart B, Gall ED, Schumacher HR, Krauser RE: Chrysotherapy in psoriatic arthropathy. *Arthritis Rheum* 21:513-515, 1978.

64. Richter MB, Kinsella P, Corbett M: Gold in psoriatic arthropathy. *Ann Rheum Dis* 39:279-280, 1980.

65. Cornbleet T: Action of synthetic antimalarial drugs on psoriasis. *J Invest Derm* 26:435-436, 1956.

66. Perlman SG, Gerber LH, Robert RM et al.: Photochemotherapy and psoriatic arthritis. A prospective study. *Ann Intern Med* 91:717-722, 1979.

67. Palumbo PJ, Ward JE, Sauer WG, Scudamore HH: Musculoskeletal manifestations of inflammatory bowel disease: Ulcerative and granulomatous colitis and ulcerative proctitis. *Mayo Clin Proc* 48:411-416, 1973.

68. Greenstein AJ, Janowitz HD, Sachar DB: The extraintestinal complications of Crohn's disease and ulcerative colitis: A study of 700 patients. *Medicine* 55:401-412, 1976.

69. Bywaters EGL, Ansell BM: Arthritis associated with ulcerative colitis. *Ann Rheum Dis* 17:169-183, 1958.

70. Stein HB, Schlappner OLA, Boyko W et al.: The intestinal bypass arthritis-dermatitis syndrome. *Arthritis Rheum* 24:684-690, 1981.

71. Hodgson HJF, Potter PJ, Jewell DP: Immune complexes in ulcerative colitis and Crohn's disease. *Clin Exp Immunol* 29:187-196, 1977.

72. Dekker-Saeys BJ, Meuwissen SGM, van den Berg-Loonen WHD et al.: II. Prevalence of peripheral arthritis, sacroiliitis, and ankylosing spondylitis in patients suffering from inflammatory bowel disease. *Ann Rheum Dis* 37:33-35, 1978.

73. Good AE: Enteropathic arthritis. In WN Kelley, ED Harris, S Ruddy, CB Sledge (eds.), *Textbook of Rheumatology,* 1st Ed. Philadelphia, W.B. Saunders, 1981, pp. 1063-1078.

74. Fernandez-Herlihy L: Arthritis after jejunoileostomy for intractable obesity. *J Rheumatol* 4:135-138, 1977.

75. Dequeker J, Jamar R, Walravens M: HLA-B27, arthritis and *Yersinia enterocolitica* infection. *J Rheumatol* 7:706-710, 1980.

76. Short CD, Klouda DT, Smith L: *Campylobacter jejuni* enteritis and reactive arthritis. *Ann Rheum Dis* 41:287-288, 1982.

Chapter 11

CRYSTAL-INDUCED ARTHRITIS

Carlos A. Agudelo, M.D.

Certain crystals have been found to induce an acute synovitis in humans. Monosodium urate, calcium pyrophosphate dihydrate, hydroxyapatite, depot corticosteroid preparations, and possibly calcium oxalate are crystals associated with synovial inflammation.

The pathophysiology of crystal-induced synovitis is not completely understood and the presence of a particular crystal does not explain the events associated with such inflammatory reaction, since in some instances crystals may be found after all inflammation has subsided or in asymptomatic joints (1).

Acute arthritis is the most common form of synovitis induced by such crystals, but chronic joint disease may also occur. This acute arthritis has similar characteristics with a rapid onset, self-limited attacks, often monoarticular in the early stages, phagocytosis of the inducing crystal by polymorphonuclear leukocytes with subsequent release of lysosomal enzymes and other inflammatory mediators. Differences in crystal morphology and clinical presentation are helpful in diagnosis.

Gout

The term gout is traced to the Latin word "gutta" (a drop), and reflects the Hippocratic belief that the disease was caused by a poison, falling drop by drop into the joint, and signifies a heterogenous group of diseases in which characteristic manifestations include an increased plasma urate level, monosodium urate crystal deposits in or around joints and recurrent attacks of acute arthritis, usually self-limited in the early stages of the disease. In some patients, uric acid urolithiasis and/or renal disease involving glomerular, tubular, and interstitial tissues may occur.

Hippocrates in the fifth century B.C., referred to gout as podagra, cheiragra, or gonagra, depending on the joint involved (the big toe, the hand, or knee, respectively) (2). Some of his aphorisms are well known, including "eunuchs do not take the gout" and "a woman does not take the gout unless her menses have stopped." It was already recognized that a tendency towards the development of gout might be inherited. Galen (A.D. 131-200) first described the tophaceous deposits and the term "gout" is credited to Geoffros de Villehardouin, a French historian. Anthony Van Leeuwenhoek, a Dutch merchant, inventor of the microscope, first observed urate crystals in a gouty tophus in 1679. Their nature was unknown at the time. Thomas Sydenhan, who suffered from the disease for over 30 years, published a classic description of gout in 1683. In 1776, Scheele, a Swedish chemist, described uric acid in a kidney stone and Wollaston in 1797 demonstrated urate in a tophus. The association of hyperuricemia to gout, is credited to A. D. Garrod in 1848. A few years later, Garrod introduced his "thread test" to identify gouty individuals. In his books, he wrote that true gouty inflammation is always accompanied by deposition of urate of soda in the inflamed part, that the deposit is crystalline and that the deposit is the cause, not the effect, of the gouty inflammation. He pointed out as well the importance of kidney function in gout. Freudweiler and His in 1899 were able to induce an inflammatory reaction by the injection of urate crystals into subcutaneous tissues of experimental animals (2). These experiments and Garrod's writings went unnoticed until McCarty and Hollander in 1961 (3) described monosodium urate crystals in acutely inflamed joints from gouty individuals. They applied as well the polarizing microscope in the identification of such crystals.

Seegmiller, Rosenbloom, and Kelley (4) described the first specific enzymatic defect associated with gout, that of hypoxanthine-guanine-phosphoribosyl transferase deficiency present in children with the Lesch-Nyhan syndrome.

The history of colchicine parallels that of gout. Alexander of Tralles (A.D. 525-605) described the antiinflammatory effect of colchicine in patients with acute gout. Probenecid was introduced in 1950 (5-6) and allopurinol in 1963 (7).

Epidemiology

Hyperuricemia is a biochemical abnormality defined solely by the serum urate concentration. Uric acid is the final product in purine metabolism; humans lack the enzyme uricase which in other animals split uric acid into alantoin and CO_2 (as shown in Figure 11.1).

Hyperuricemia may be absolute or relative. Absolute hyperuricemia occurs when the limit of solubility of monosodium urate in serum has been exceeded (about 7 mg/100 ml). Relative hyperuricemia occurs when it exceeds the upper limit of an arbitrary normal range, usually defined as the central 95% of the distribution of urate values in the same sex and age group in the healthy population (9). At 37°C, the saturation value of urate in plasma is about 7.0 mg/100 ml. Using automated analyzers this value is higher and corresponds to a concentration of 7.5-8.0 mg/100 ml (10).

During childhood, serum urate values average 3.6 mg/100 ml in males and females (11). After puberty, these values rise but more so in males, averaging about 1 mg/100 ml higher for males until after the menopause when values in females rise further and approach or equal those in males (9). See Figure 11.2.

Hyperuricemia may be a result of increased uric acid production, as seen in enzyme defects, myeloproliferative diseases and other disorders of increased cell turnover, diminished uric acid excretion by the kidneys, or a combination of these mechanisms. Multiple conditions are associated with hyperuricemia (see Table 11.1).

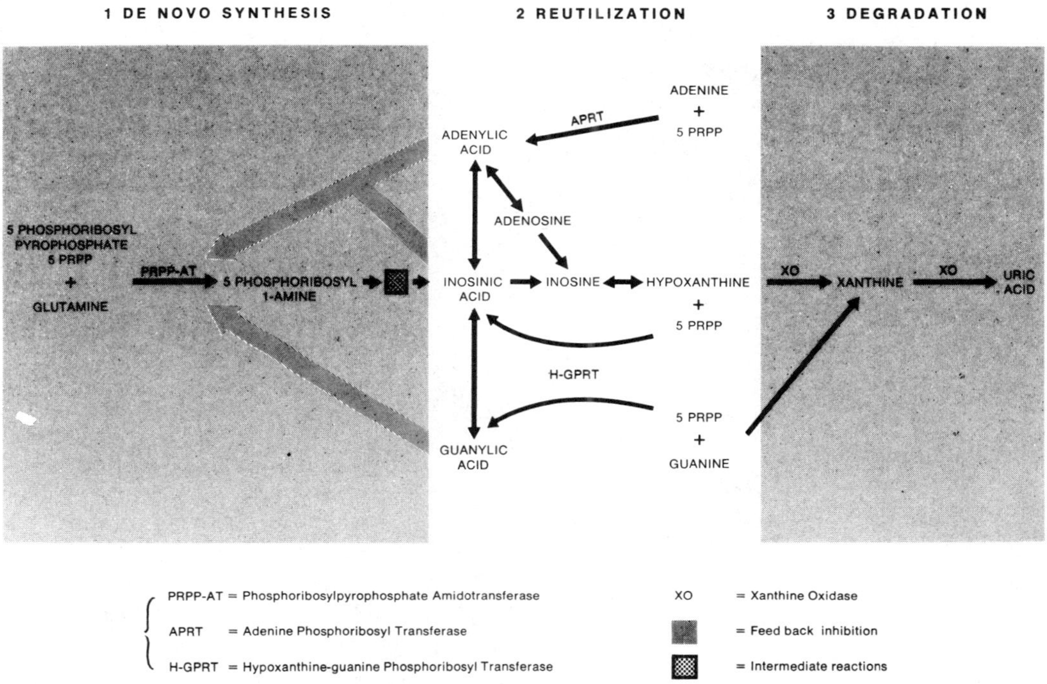

FIGURE 11.1 Purine metabolism and uric acid production (reproduced from *NEJM* (8) with permission).

Urate is almost completely filtered by the kidneys. At least 90% of filtered uric acid is reabsorbed, resulting in a relatively low clearance. It is thought that after filtration, subsequent steps of reabsorption-secretion-reabsorption-secretion occur at the tubules: 400–600 mg of uric acid/24 hr urine are excreted daily on a purine-free diet. About 25% of the urate is secreted into the gastrointestinal tract, where it is degraded by bacteria. This intestinal process does not influence plasma levels. Plasma solutions are saturated with urate at 6.4–6.8 mg/100 ml at 37°C, and at greater concentrations urate may precipitate as monosodium urate crystals. This precipitation is influenced by urate concentration, pH, and temperature. Not all factors involved in precipitation are known, since some individuals may tolerate high levels of plasma urate without ever demonstrating urate deposits and/or gouty attacks. Likewise not everybody with chronic hyperuricemia is at the same risk for the development of urate deposits or gouty attacks. What mechanism(s) may be involved in such predisposition is unknown.

Hyperuricemia, therefore, may occur as an isolated biochemical abnormality, often discovered by chance. The clinical management of these individuals is controversial, but there is no scientific evidence that the patient with asymptomatic hyperuricemia, if followed rather than treated, is in any real jeopardy (12).

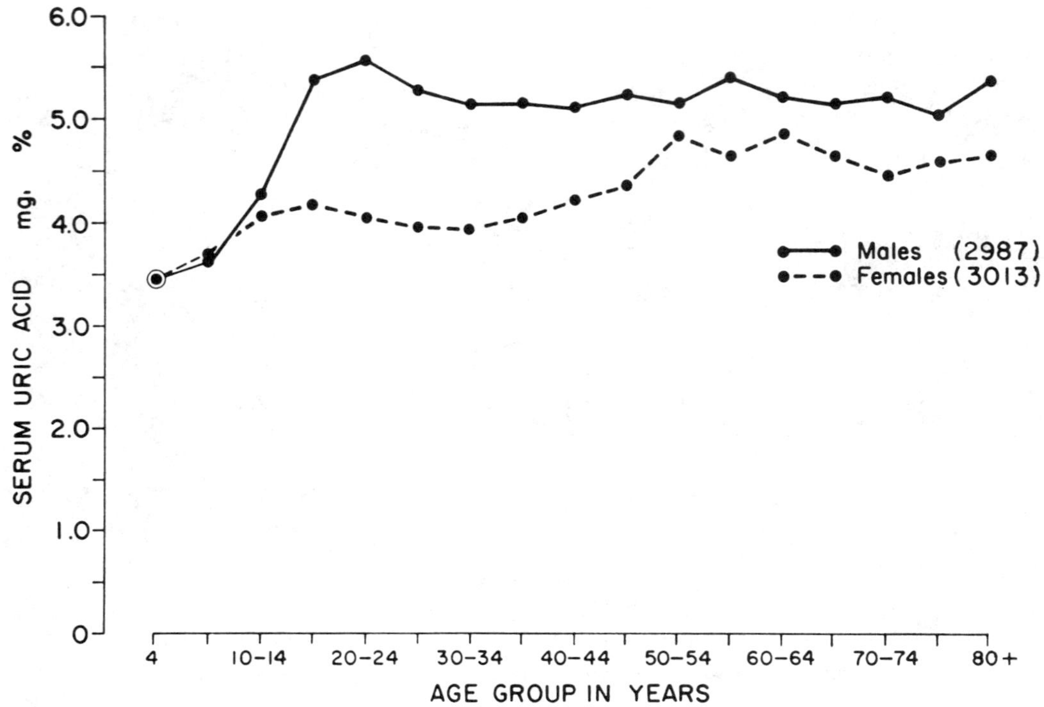

FIGURE 11.2 Sex-age-specific mean serum uric acid, Tecumseh, Michigan, 1959-60 (reproduced from *Amer Jour Med* (11) with permission of the journal and author).

Acute Gouty Arthritis

Acute gouty attacks are characterized by dramatic acute inflammation, usually monoarticular in the early stages of the disease and more frequently involving lower extremity joints. In about 60% of the patients, the first attack involves the first metatarsophalangeal joint, the classical podagra, with a sudden onset, often during the night, and within a few hours the affected joint becomes red, swollen, warm, and very tender with functional impairment. The acute attack resolves spontaneously or after medication in a few days and leaves no apparent sequelae. Fever and modest leukocytosis may occur. In some patients, the initial episodes may be polyarticular, usually in an asymmetric fashion. Bouts may be precipitated by trauma, surgery, and alcohol. Rarely tophaceous deposits may be found at the time of the first attack, as occasional patients have been described with tophaceous deposits who apparently had never had a gouty attack. Although hyperuricemia is characteristic of gout, normal serum urate values may be seen during the acute attack in 20-30% of patients. The reason for this is not completely clear but it appears that sudden changes in serum urate levels may precipitate gouty attacks.

TABLE 11.1 Conditions Associated with Hyperuricemia

Primary gout
Enzyme deficiencies (i.e., Lesch-Nyhan syndrome)
Myelolymphoproliferative diseases
Chronic hemolytic anemias
Sarcoidosis
Renal insufficiency
Drugs; diuretics, low dose salicylates; pyrazinamide, cytotoxic drugs, low dose uricosurics
Lead
Alcoholism
Ketoacidosis-increased lactate
Starvation
Obesity
Toxemia of pregnancy
Hypertension

As the disease evolves into a chronic state, if untreated, large tophi may develop, as in Figure 11.3, and the acute episodes may become polyarticular and more constant inflammation will be present, leading to a destructive type of arthritis with tophaceous deposits in joints and surrounding tissues. In this stage, confusion with rheumatoid arthritis is possible, as the physical findings may mimic a rheumatoid process in some patients. A high sedimentation rate and a positive rheumatoid factor, mostly in alcoholics with gout, have been described and these will add to the confusion. Gout occurs primarily in males over the age of 30; in females, it is more likely to occur after the menopause. Acute attacks involving the distal interphalangeal joint of the hand have been described.

McCarty and Hollander in 1961 (3) demonstrated monosodium urate crystals in synovial fluids of patients with acute gouty arthritis, thus gout became the first of the crystal-induced arthritides in which a specific crystal was identified in joint fluids. Since then, the presence of intracellular monosodium urate crystals in synovial fluids from acutely inflamed joints has been considered diagnostic of gout. Occasionally, the gouty attack may coincide with another process such as infection, pseudogout, or osteoarthritis. Even though rheumatoid arthritis is a common disease, the coexistence of both diseases, rheumatoid arthritis and gout, in the same individual, is very rare (14).

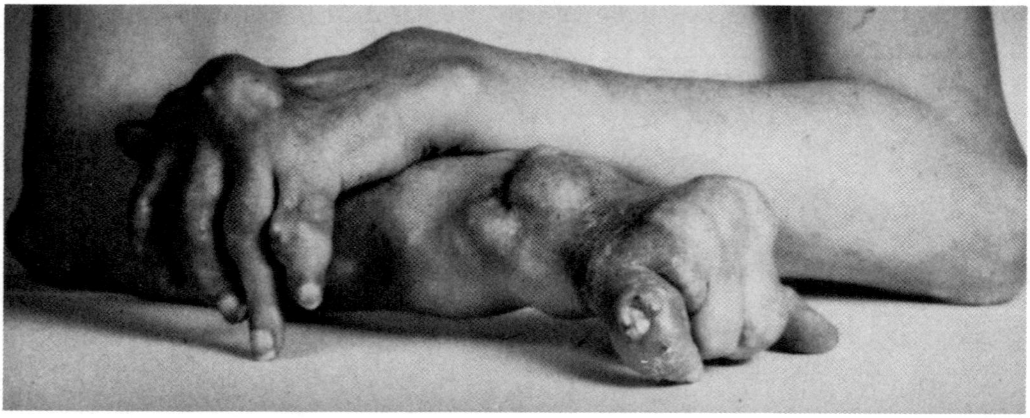

FIGURE 11.3 Multiple subcutaneous nodules (tophi) over elbows, arms, and hands in chronic tophaceous gout. (Reprint from the Revised Clinical Slide Collection of the Rheumatic Diseases, copyright 1981, used by permission of the Arthritis Foundation.)

Identification of urate crystals requires the use of a compensated polarizing microscope, but often times they may be seen under regular light microscopy as fine needle-like structures, either intra- or extracellular (see Figure 11.4). By compensated polarizing microscope, monosodium urate crystals are typically strongly negatively birefringent. Standard microscopes may be modified to identify crystals using two polarizing discs and a color compensator. Cellophane tape in association with polarizing discs can turn an ordinary light microscope into a polarizing one (13).

Monosodium urate (MSU) crystals are phlogistic and when injected into human knee joints or joints from experimental animals induce an inflammatory reaction, with pain, swelling, warmth, erythema, and functional impairment. This inflammatory reaction of intraarticular crystal injection peaks at about 4 hr. Synovial fluid aspiration reveals a high leukocyte count and phagocytosis of crystals by polymorphonuclear leukocytes (PMN). Under experimental conditions, acute inflammation does not occur in the absence of PMN. Phagocytic synovial lining cells may be important as well in the initial steps of the inflammatory reaction. Crystals are ingested by PMN, and are enveloped by a phagosomal vacuole. There is subsequent degranulation and release of lysosomal enzymes and other inflammatory mediators with rupture of the phagosomal membrane. Several other mechanisms and/or interactions may be important in triggering the acute inflammatory reaction, such as coating of the crystal with IgG, complement components, and clotting factors.

As the acute gouty attack subsides, the patient becomes asymptomatic until a new attack in the same or other joint occurs. This interval period, between attacks, is variable and may last from a few weeks to several years. During this asymptomatic period, the diagnosis of gout is based on the previous history of self-limited episodes of acute arthritis, the clinical response to colchicine, hyperuricemia, and the identification of monosodium urate crystals either by aspiration of visible tophaceous material or asymptomatic first metatarsophalangeal (1) or knee joints.

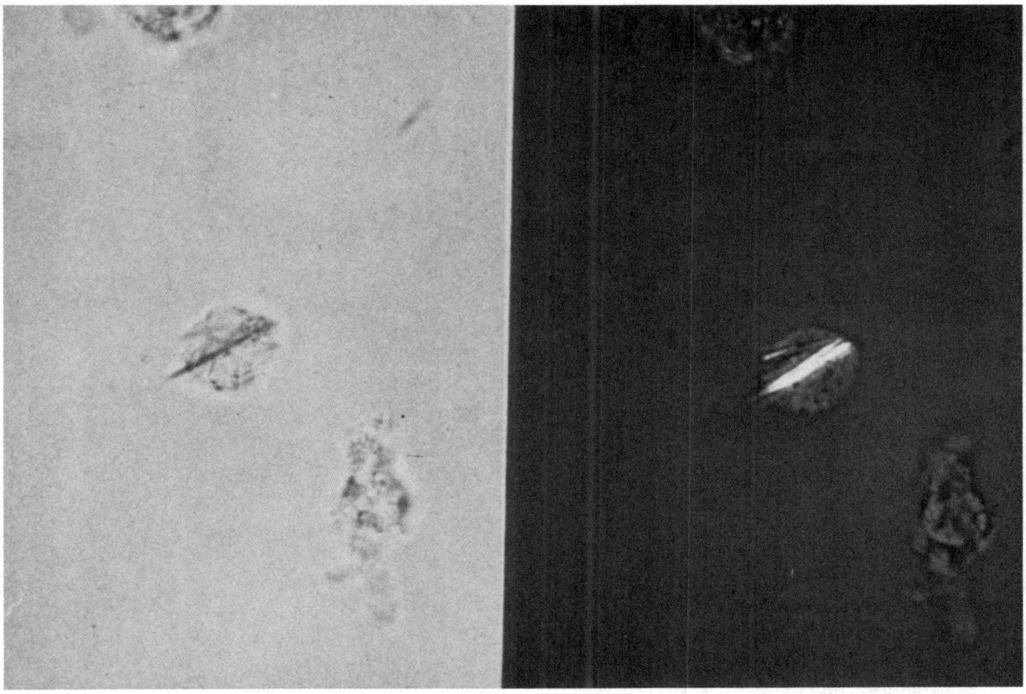

FIGURE 11.4 A needle-like monosodium urate (MSU) crystal within a leukocyte, viewed under regular and polarized light. (Reprinted from the Revised Clinical Slide Collection on the Rheumatic Diseases, copyright 1981, used by permission of the Arthritis Foundation.)

Tophaceous deposits may be seen on the helix of the ear, over extensor surfaces of the elbows as subcutaenous nodules or over joints (see Figure 11.3); these deposits are usually firm and when needled a white chalky material is obtained which will reveal multiple typical monosodium urate crystals under the compensated polarizing microscope.

Deposition of sodium urate crystals in the renal interstitial tissue and the resulting inflammatory reaction leads to parenchymal renal damage or urate nephropathy. Of interest is that apparently this type of renal involvement occurs only in patients with gout and not those with asymptomatic hyperuricemia. Chronic renal disease with progressive renal failure may occur. The use of uricosurics or xanthine-oxidase inhibitors may have prevented the development of the renal lesions in many patients. Hypertension is often found in the gouty population and contributes to the renal damage. Renal stones composed of uric acid are found in about 10-25% of gouty patients. However, most patients with uric acid stones do not have hyperuricemia or gout. Renal stones result from a persistently acid urine which favors precipitation or uric acid, and is only sometimes associated with an increased urinary uric acid concentration.

In patients with chronic gout, polyarticular attacks may be more frequent and occasionally a symmetric polyarthritis mimicking rheumatoid arthritis may occur. A history of initial self-limiting attacks with podagra, improvement after colchicine, hyperuricemia, and synovial fluid analysis will establish the diagnosis.

Classification

Hyperuricemia is a metabolic abnormality considered necessary for the development of gout. Hyperuricemia may result from an increase in the rate of uric acid production, a decrease in renal excretion, or most commonly a combination of both. Hyperuricemia may be primary or secondary. Most cases of hyperuricemia and gout may be classified as primary, where the molecular defect remains undefined. Many of these patients have underexcretion or overproduction of uric acid and the inheritance appears to be polygenic. A few cases are associated with specific enzyme defects such as that occurring in patients with partial deficiency of hypoxanthine-guanine-phosphoribosyl transferase, with x-linked inheritance. This is considered a primary form of hyperuricemia since the major clinical manifestations are a result of the hyperuricemia. These patients usually present at a young age with either renal stones or gouty arthritis, marked hyperuricemia, and high urinary excretion of uric acid (more than 800 mg/24 hr). A few cases of gout and hyperuricemia associated with an increased activity of PRPP synthetase have been described. In these patients, the defect has an x-linked inheritance leading to increased purine biosynthesis and increased production of uric acid.

The only other enzyme defect identified that leads to hyperuricemia is that of glucose 6-phosphatase (von Gierke's glycogen storage disease type 1), classified as a secondary form of hyperuricemia (15). There are other numerous causes of secondary hyperuricemia. In most cases, this results from a decrease in the renal excretion of uric acid, such as in patients with renal insufficiency. Patients with gout resulting from renal insufficiency have normal urate production and seldom have tophi (16). One of the most frequent causes of hyperuricemia is that associated with diuretics. Volume depletion and decreased secretion of uric acid may be mechanisms involved in diuretic-induced hyperuricemia.

Differential Diagnosis

The differential diagnosis of the patient presenting with acute arthritis, includes crystal-induced synovitis (gout, pseudogout, calcium apatite, and depocorticosteroid preparations), infection, trauma, Reiter's syndrome, Lyme arthritis, and palindromic rheumatism. The history, clinical presentation, and careful examination of the synovial fluid with crystal identification are necessary to establish the diagnosis.

Laboratory Features

Even though hyperuricemia is considered necessary for the development of gout, about 5% of the patients may have high normal serum urate values. During the acute attack 20-30% of the patients will demonstrate normal serum urate values. If repeated within a few days, most serum urates will be in the hyperuricemic range.

Synovial effusions in acute gout are typically inflammatory, with most fluids having 5000 to 40,000 WBC/mm^3, mostly polymorphonuclear leukocytes. Monosodium urate crystals can be readily identified in these fluids either intra- or extracellularly. In about 5-10% of these gouty effusions, calcium pyrophosphate dihydrate crystals also may be seen. In an occasional patient, infectious arthritis may coincide with the gouty attack. Complete synovial analysis including examination under compensating polarizing microscope, gram smear, and culture (based on clinical presentation) are of utmost importance in the management of the patient with acute arthritis. Acute gouty effusions without detectable crystals on initial examination have been reported, and such fluids may contain crystals visible only by electron microscopy. Careful reexamination of the fluid by experienced observers usually reveals crystals in such gouty fluids.

Tissues obtained from patients suspected of gout (synovial biopsy, subcutaneous nodules, tophus) should be fixed in absolute alcohol, as formalin fixatives contain water which dissolves urate crystals. During the acute attack the synovium reveals acute inflammation with fibrin, polymorphonuclear cell infiltration, and vascular congestion. Some dilated vessels may show margination of polymorphonuclear leukocytes. Microtophi may be seen even during the first attack. Urate crystals in the tophus are parallel to each other surrounded by an amorphous matrix when examined by electron microscopy. Under light microscopy, tophi are formed by radially arranged clusters of crystals within an amorphous matrix. In the synovial fluid, crystals may be seen in large mononuclear cells some of which are synovial linging cells as well as in PMN (17).

Radiologically, during the acute attack and early stages of the disease, only swelling of the soft tissue may be seen. In chronic gout, destructive lesions with a punched-out appearance are seen, most often in the subchondral bone at the bases or heads of phalanges. The most typical location of these punched-out lesions is at the medial aspect of the head of the first metatarsal-phalangeal joint and their edge may show a thin shell-like configuration continuous with adjacent bone contour, or the "overhanging margin" described by Martel (18). Osteoporosis is usually absent. These radiological abnormalities are a consequence of tophaceous deposits and asymmetric nodular masses may be seen. The joint space is usually preserved until late in the disease (19). (See Chapter 3 for further discussion of radiographic features.)

Prognosis and Management

Gout is one of the few rheumatological disorders where specific therapy aimed at correcting the metabolic disorder is available. Because of this, fewer cases of destructive, severe, tophaceous gouty arthritis are now seen. Once the diagnosis is confirmed, most patients are readily controlled on uricosurics or xanthine-oxidase inhibitors.

The treatment of gout involves several phases outlined below and in Chapter 4. Once the diagnosis of the acute attack is confirmed, treatment using appropriate rest of the inflamed joint(s) and antiinflammatory drugs is required. When the acute attack subsides, definitive therapy requires antiinflammatory prophylaxis and control of the hyperuricemia to prevent recurrent attacks, joint damage, and urate or uric acid nephropathy.

For the management of the acute attack, several drugs are available. Colchicine, if given early in the attack, has been considered quite specific; it can be used either by mouth or intravenously. Oral colchicine has been a classical agent in the treatment of the gouty attack; however, due to the frequency and severity of gastrointestinal side effects with nausea, vomiting, and diarrhea, the intravenous route is preferred by many clinicians. Orally, it is given as 0.5 or 0.6 mg tablets, 1 or 2, every 1-2 hours until either improvement or gastrointestinal side effects occur, or 12-14 tablets have been given. After a few hours of such treatment, significant relief is common and the dosage may be tapered to 1 tablet, 2 or 3 times daily. Intravenously, 2 mg of colchicine is given in 20 ml of normal saline. Another 1 mg dose may be given at 4-6 hour intervals up to a total of 4 mg/24 hr. Inadvertent extravenous infiltration may be very irritating. As the patient improves he/she can be switched to oral maintenance therapy. Intravenous colchicine is associated with little or no gastrointestinal toxicity and offers a rapid response. Rarely, in large doses, colchicine may produce bone marrow depression, leukopenia, and renal or hepatic toxicity. The mechanism of colchicine action in so specifically relieving crystal-induced inflammation is not completely understood, but may involve the inhibition of a chemotactic factor produced by phagocytizing leukocytes; this chemotactic factor may be a major mediator of the acute urate-induced synovitis. Other possible mechanisms include the interference with microtubular subunit protein aggregation in PMN, inhibiting lysosomal degranulation and release of lysosomal enzymes during phagocytosis of urate crystal, and suppression of leukotreine B_4 (LTB_4), a product of the lipooxigenase pathway of arachidonic acid metabolism.

Other useful medications in controlling the acute attack are the nonsteroidal antiinflammatory agents. Phenylbutazone is a very effective drug. However, potential serious side effects, including bone marrow suppression, fluid retention, gastric or duodenal ulceration limit its usefulness and most clinicians prefer other available nonsteroidals. Aspirin and other salicylates, though uricosuric at high doses, probably should not be used in the management of gouty arthritis, since lower doses induce hyperuricemia. Indomethacin in doses up to 200 mg/day in divided doses is very effective as well. At this large dose, the drug is often not well tolerated, particularly in the elderly, producing central nervous system, gastrointestinal, and metabolic side effects. Like phenylbutazone and other prostaglandin synthetase inhibitors, it leads to fluid retention. In some patients with mild, preexisting renal insufficiency, acute renal failure and hyperkalemia have been precipitated (hyporeninemic hypoaldosteronism). Other nonsteroidals may have the potential for inducing similar problems. Sulindac in doses of 200 mg twice daily may have the advantages of twice daily dosage, probably less gastrointestinal irritation, and less renal toxicity. Other nonsteroidals are being tested for their use and effectiveness in acute gout. In an occasional patient with an acute gouty attack of a large joint such as the knee, local intraarticular depot corticosteroid injection may be indicated.

Recurrence of acute gouty attacks can be prevented by controlling the hyperuricemia, which may take several months to achieve. Effective prophylaxis during this period is accomplished by adding small doses of colchicine, indomethacin, or other nonsteroidal antiinflammatory drug.

Effective control of hyperuricemia is achieved pharmacologically by increasing the renal excretion of uric acid, through the use of uricosurics, or by decreasing its synthesis. Uricosurics include probenecid and sulfinpyrazone, and are indicated if the patient excretes less than 600 mg of uric acid in 24 hours or if allergic to allopurinol. Probenecid is administered in dosages of 1.5 to 3.0 g daily. At lower doses, it may cause hyperuricemia. Possible side effects include dermatitis and gastrointestinal complaints. Probenecid inhibits the metabolic clearance of several nonsteroidal antiinflammatory drugs, including naproxen, indomethocin, and diflunisal, but not ibuprofen (20). It inhibits as well the renal excretion of many acidic drugs and markedly increases the plasma levels of methotrexate. Sulfinpyrazone is given in dosages from 200 to 400 mg/day in divided doses. It is chemically similar to the pyrazolones, and may lead as well to an increase in the plasma levels of warfarin, and inhibits the metabolic clearance of tolbutamide (20).

The only xanthine-oxidase inhibitor presently available is allopurinol. As seen in Figure 11.1, xanthine-oxidase catalyses the final two steps in the degradation pathway of purine metabolism ending in uric acid. In vivo, allopurinol is metabolized to oxipurinol which has a longer half-life, and both are strong xanthine-oxidase inhibitors. Allopurinol is administered in doses of 100-600 mg/

day in one dose; main indications for its use include patients who are overproducers and overexcretors (more than 600–800 mg of uric acid in 24 hours), in those with severe tophaceous gout, in patients with chronic renal insufficiency and in those allergic to uricosurics. Toxic reactions are usually related to skin rashes. Rarely, severe side effects such as vasculitis, toxic epidermal necrolysis, granulomatosus hepatitis, or agranulocytosis may occur. Many of these reactions occur early, after only a few weeks of therapy, and are frequently related to preexisting renal disease. In patients with preexisting renal disease or in the elderly, allopurinol therapy, when necessary, should be initiated at lower dosages, i.e., 50–100 mg/day with slow gradual increments until therapeutic control is achieved. Rarely oxipurinol nephrolithiasis may occur.

There is no uniform opinion regarding the management of asymptomatic hyperuricemia. It is best to avoid unnecessary medications. Studies of renal function, perhaps at 6-month intervals, may uncover those patients at high risk for the development of renal damage. Treatment of patients with renal uric acid calculi is directed at increasing urine production by increasing fluid intake, maintenance of alkaline urine, and the reduction of total uric acid excretion.

Many patients with hyperuricemia and gout are obese and consume large amounts of alcohol. Slow weight reduction and moderation in alcohol consumption may help in the control of the hyperuricemia.

Pseudogout

Synovial crystal deposition of calcium pyrophosphate dihydrate (CPPD) was first described by McCarty, Kohn, and Faires in 1962 (21). Because of the clinical similarities with gout, it was named pseudogout. This disease tends to involve large joints such as the knees, wrists, shoulders, but rarely it may involve the first metatarsal-phalangeal joint. Calcification, visible by x-ray, in cartilage or menisci, is often but not invariably present (chondrocalcinosis). Such calcifications were first described by Zitnan and Sitaj (22).

Even though no clinical data on prevalence exist, it has been estimated that there are about two to three patients with gout for every one with pseudogout. At autopsy about 5% of the adult population have CPPD crystals in their knee joints at the time of death (23) but values may be higher in the elderly.

The initial site of CPPD crystal deposition is probably the articular cartilage. Large tophus-like masses in degenerated cartilage have been described. Changes in the equilibrium of CA^{++}, phosphorus, and Mg^{++} may induce changes in the CPPD deposits, allowing some crystals to escape into the joint where they may in turn induce an inflammatory reaction in a similar manner to that seen with other phlogistic crystals.

Diagnosis

CPPD deposition disease may mimic different rheumatological syndromes. It may resemble infectious arthritis, gout, rheumatoid arthritis, osteoarthritis, traumatic arthritis, neuropathic joint disease, and ankylosing spondylitis.

McCarty has described five clinical patterns based on a clinical analysis of 80 cases (24):

Pseudogout. As the term implies, the attacks are similar to gout, usually lasting from one day to several weeks; several joints may be involved but the most common are the knees, wrists, and shoulders. Occasionally, the MTP joint may be affected. In old patients, fever may be present and the clinical presentation may mimic a septic arthritis. Infectious arthritis, gout, and osteoarthritis of the same joint may coincide with pseudogout. Diuretics, trauma, and severe illness may precipitate an attack. Joint aspiration and crystal identification are necessary for a proper diagnosis. About one-third of the patients may present with this pattern.

Pseudorheumatoid arthritis. Less than 10% of the patients have multiple joint involvement, mimicking rheumatoid arthritis, but usually from one to several joints are more inflamed than others and osteoporosis is unusual. Occasionally, however, the differential diagnosis may be difficult as both diseases may coexist in the same individual.

Pseudoosteoarthritis. This is the most common form. Women outnumber men. Symmetric involvement occurs with knees, wrists, shoulders, and MCP most commonly affected. Clinical and radiological findings are those of osteoarthritis, with superimposed chondrocalcinosis. Flexion contractures may be present, and are clinically useful when occurring in joints not usually affected by osteoarthritis, such as wrists and MCP. CPPD crystals may be found in roentgenographically negative joints, especially those with extensive degenerative changes.

Lanthanic. This form also is common, and includes patients with asymptomatic joints with chondrocalcinosis demonstrated by x-ray.

Pseudoneuropathic. In this form, Charcot-like arthropathy, in the absence of neurologic deficit, has been found. Some cases may occur in tabetic patients.

Hereditary forms of the disease have been described in Czechoslovakia, Chile, Spain, Holland, and Switzerland. Autosomal inheritance in some has been found. Usually there is a lack of association with metabolic conditions. True bony ankylosis has been described in familial cases and in some of these individuals spinal calcifications may be confused radiographically with ankylosing spondylitis.

Pseudogout has been associated with a number of degenerative and metabolic diseases including hyperparathyroidism, hemochromatosis, gout, hypothyroidism, ochronosis, and Wilson's disease.

Laboratory Features

The diagnosis of CPPD deposition disease is based on clinical presentation, x-ray findings, and demonstration of characteristic weakly positive birefringent rhomboid or rod-like crystals by compensated polarized light microscopy (see Figure 11.5). Crystals may be seen as well under regular light microscopy, either extra- or intracellularly. Synovial fluid may contain from only a few WBC to as many as 100,000 but white counts in most fluids range from 2000 to 20,000 WBC/mm^3. Recently, a simple, rapid screening method to detect calcium-containing crystals has been described using alizarin red stain and ordinary light microscopy. With this method, CPPD, calcium apatite, and calcium oxalate crystals may be identified even in cases where they have been missed by polarized light (25). Further studies to confirm this finding are needed.

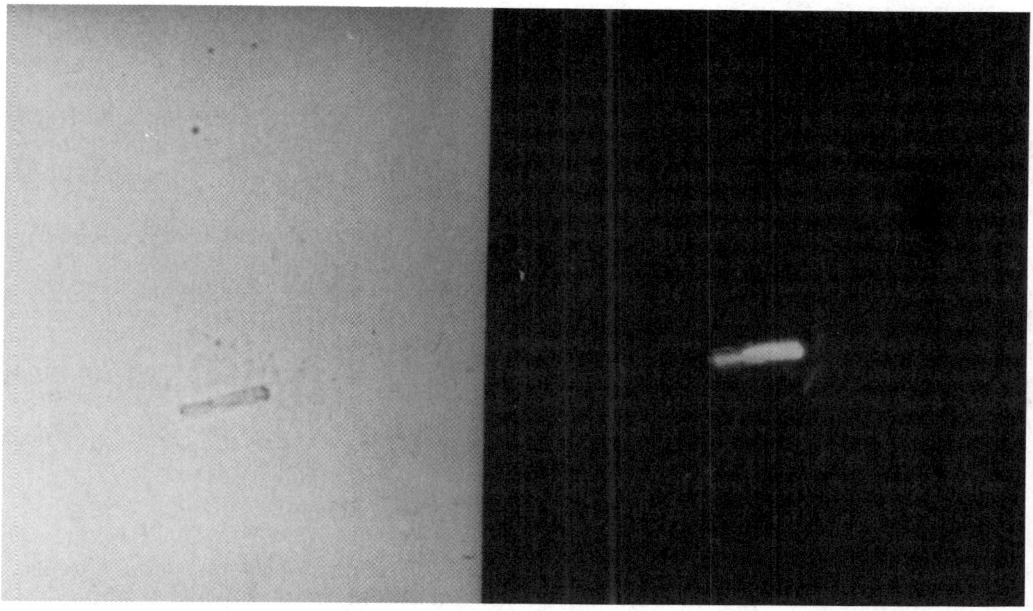

FIGURE 11.5 A calcium pyrophosphate dihydrate (CPPD) crystal, viewed under regular and polarized light. (Reprinted from the Revised Clinical Slide Collection on the Rheumatic Diseases, copyright 1981, used by permission of the Arthritis Foundation.)

The roentgenographic features of CPPD consist of linear and punctate calcification of fibrocartilage and hyaline cartilage of multiple joints, frequently bilateral and symmetrical (26), as discussed in Chapter 3.

Prognosis and Management

Acute attacks are usually self-limited and joint function is preserved. In those with other types, such as pseudorheumatoid, pseudoosteoarthritis, and pseudoneuropathic, more severe destructive changes may occur, leading to or accompanied by loss of joint function.

Intravenous colchicine, 2 mg (see treatment of acute gout), may be quite effective in the management of the acute attack. Nonsteroidal antiinflammatory agents are also useful in the management of the acute episode or for chronic inflammation. Patients with CPPD deposition disease should be screened for other possible associated metabolic diseases as previously discussed.

Hydroxyapatite Deposition Disease

Calcium apatite is present in bone and in certain pathologic calcifications, calcific tendonitis, and periarthritis. The calcium apatite crystals have been found to induce inflammation in a similar manner to those of monosodium urate and CPPD. Attacks may affect one or several joints and are usually self-limited (27).

McCarty et al. have described a chronic, painful degenerative condition of the shoulders, characterized by decreased mobility or stability, radiographic evidence of rotator cuff damage and microspheroids containing hydroxyapatite crystals in 12 of 13 synovial fluids. They named this condition the "Milwaukee shoulder" (28). Synovial fluid will reveal clumps of tiny apatite crystals, not birefringent. These clumps may be phagocytized by neutrophils. They may stain with alizarin red, or may be identified through electron microscopy or x-ray diffraction.

Patients undergoing chronic dialysis may present with a destructive arthropathy of the shoulders, highly inflammatory synovial fluid, and calcium apatite crystals. Similar crystals, as well as CPPD crystals have been demonstrated during attacks of acute arthritis and periarthritis in patients undergoing maintenance peritoneal dialysis (29). Apatite crystals may be seen as well in rheumatoid arthritis, gout, osteoarthritis, and CPPD deposition. Either colchicine or nonsteroidal antiinflammatory drugs may be helpful during acute attacks of calcium apatite-induced inflammation.

Other Crystal-Induced Arthropathies

Depot preparations of corticosteroids are microcrystalline and may induce acute inflammation when injected into joints or periarticular tissues. Only a small percentage of patients (3%) will develop this complication which is self-limited, beginning a few hours after injection, and subsiding within 1-2 days. Synovial fluid aspiration will reveal the crystal injected, many of them inside phagocytizing cells. This corticosteroid-induced attack must be differentiated from an infectious process, which would usually not begin so early after injection.

Calcium oxalate crystals have been identified in synovial fluids and cartilage from patients with chronic renal failure. Roentgenograms of affected joints may reveal chondrocalcinosis, secondary to calcium oxalate and not to CPPD (30).

Cholesterol crystals may occur in chronic effusions mostly from rheumatoid arthritis patients. They do not seem to be phlogistic.

References

1. Agudelo CA, Weinberger A, Schumacher HR, Turner R, Molina J: Definitive diagnosis of gout by identification of urate crystals in asymptomatic metatarsal-phalangeal joints. *Arthritis Rheum* 22:559-560, 1979.

2. Wyngaarden JB, Kelley WN: An abbreviated history of gout. In JB Wyngaarden, WN Kelley (eds.), *Gout and Hyperuricemia.* New York, Grune and Stratton, 1976, pp. 3-12.

3. McCarty DJ Jr, Hollander JL: Identification of urate crystals in gouty synovial fluids. *Ann Int Med* 54:452-460, 1961.

4. Seegmiller JE, Rosenbloom FM, Kelley WN: An enzyme defect associated with a sex-linked human neurological disorder and excessive purine synthesis. *Science* 155:1682-1684, 1967.

5. Talbott JH, Bishop C, Norcross BM et al.: Clinical and metabolic effects of benemid in patients with gout. *Trans Assoc Am Physicians* 64:372-377, 1951.

6. Goodman AB, Yu T-F: Benemid p-(di-N-propyl-sulfamyl) benzoic acid uricosuric agent in chronic gouty arthritis. *Trans Assoc Am Physicians* 64:279-288, 1951.

7. Rundles RW, Wyngaarden JB, Hitchingo GH et al.: Effects of a xanthine-oxidase inhibitor on thiopurine metabolism, hyperuricemia, and gout. *Trans Assoc Am Physicians* 76:126-140, 1963.

8. Rastegar A, Thier SO: The physiological approach to hyperuricemia. *N Engl J Med* 286:470-476, 1972.

9. Kelley WN: Approach to the patient with hyperuricemia. In WN Kelley, ED Harris, S Ruddy, CB Sledge (eds.), *Textbook of Rheumatology,* Philadelphia, W.B. Saunders, 1981, pp. 494-500.

10. Wyngaarden JB, Kelley WN: Epidemology of hyperuricemia and gout. In JB Wyngaarden, WN Kelley (eds.), *Gout and Hyperuricemia.* New York, Grune and Stratton, 1976, pp. 21-37.

11. Mikkelsen WM, Dodge HJ, Valkenburg H: The distribution of serum uric acid values in a population unselected as to gout or hyperuricemia. *Am J Med* 39:242-251, 1962.

12. Klinenberg JR: The management of asymptomatic hyperuricemia. *Clin Rheum Dis* 3:160-167, 1977.

13. Owen DS: A cheap and useful compensated polarizing microscope. *N Engl J Med* 285:1152, 1971.

14. Agudelo CA, Turner RA, Panetti M, Pisko E: Does hyperuricemia protect from rheumatoid inflammation? A clinical study. *Arthritis Rheum* 27: 443-448, 1984.

15. Kelley WN: Gout and related disorders of purine metabolism. In WN Kelley, ED Harris, S Ruddy, CB Sledge (eds.), *Textbook of Rheumatology.* Philadelphia, W.B. Saunders, 1981, pp. 1397-1437.

16. Sorenson LB: Gout secondary to chronic renal disease: Studies on urate metabolism. *Ann Rheum Dis* 39:424-430, 1980.

17. Agudelo CA, Schumacher HR: The synovitis of acute gouty arthritis. *Human Path* 4:265-278, 1973.

18. Martel W: The overhanging margin of bone: A roentgenologic manifestation of gout. *Radiology* 91:755, 1968.

19. Resnick D: Crystal-induced arthropathy: Gout and pseudogout. *JAMA* 242:2440-2442, 1979.

20. Day RO, Graham GG, Champion GD, Lee E: Clinically significant drug interactions with antirheumatic drugs. In EC Huskisson (ed.), *Anti-Rheumatic Drugs.* New York, Praeger, 1983, pp. 37-54.

21. McCarty DJ, Kohn NN, Faires JS: The significance of calcium phosphate crystals in the synovial fluid of arthritis patients: The "pseudogout syndrome" I. Clinical Aspects. *Ann Int Med* 56:711-737, 1962.

22. Zitnan D, Sitaj D: Chondrocalcinosis polyarticularis (familiaris). *Cesk Radiol.* 14:27, 1960.

23. Howell DS: Diseases due to deposition of calcium pyrophosphate and hydroxyapatite. In WN Kelley, ED Harris, S Ruddy, CB SLedge (eds.), *Textbook of Rheumatology*. Philadelphia, W.B. Saunders, 1981, pp. 1438-1454.

24. McCarty DJ: Pseudogout. Articular chondrocalcinosis. In J Hollander (ed.), *Arthritis and Allied Conditions,* 7th Ed. Philadelphia, Lea and Febiger, 1966, pp. 947-963.

25. Paul H, Reginato AJ, Schumacher HR: Alizarin red S staining as a screening test to detect calcium compounds in synovial fluids. *Arthritis Rheum* 26: 191-200, 1983.

26. Genant HK: Roentgenographic aspects of calcium pyrophosphate dihydrate crystal deposition disease (pseudogout). *Arthritis Rheum* 19:307-328, 1976.

27. Schumacher HR, Smolyo AB, Tse RL, Maurer K: Arthritis associated with apatite crystals. *Ann Int Med* 87:411-416, 1977.

28. McCarty DJ, Halverson PB, Carrera G, Brewer BJ, Kozin F: "Milwaukee Shoulder." Association of microspheroids containing hydroxiapatite crystals, active collagenase, and neutral protease with rotator cuff defects. I. Clinial Aspects. *Arthritis Rheum* 24:464-473, 1981.

29. Chalmers A, Reynolds W, Oreopoulos DG, Meema HE, Meinlock H, DeVeber GA: The arthropathy of maintenance intermittent peritoneal dialysis. *Can Med Assoc J* 123:635-638, 1980.

30. Hoffman GS, Schumacher HR, Paul H, Cherian V, Reed R, Ramsey AG, Franck WA: Calcium-oxalate microcrystalline-associated arthritis in end-stage renal disease. *Ann Int Med* 97:36-42, 1982.

Chapter 12

NONARTICULAR RHEUMATISM

Christopher M. Wise, M.D.

Many patients with musculoskeletal pain do not have definable arthritis, myositis, or bony abnormalities to explain their pain. Problems in periarticular structures and "pain amplification syndromes" frequently cause pain that may at first seem to be attributable to arthritis. A large number of syndromes have been described to account for this large area of rheumatology. In this chapter we will discuss these various nonarticular forms of rheumatism, the diagnosis of most of which must be based on a careful history and physical exam, but very few laboratory tests.

Table 12.1 lists the general categories of pathology that may cause non-articular musculoskeletal pain. Muscles, ligaments, tendons, and tendon sheaths may be irritated and stressed in such ways as to cause severe regional pain. The bursae of the body are numerous and are frequent sources of pain. Nerve entrapment syndromes, reflex sympathetic dystrophy, and referred pain syndromes may also give rise to regional pain that must be distinguished from intraarticular causes of pain. Fibrositis, or fibromyalgia, is a diffuse pain syndrome associated with multiple periarticular tender areas, but no specific pathology. Each of these entities will be discussed separately, and then specific regions of the body will be discussed in relation to nonarticular pain syndromes.

TABLE 12.1 General Causes of Nonarticular Musculoskeletal Pain

Muscle pain (spasm, strain, cramp)
Ligamentous strains and sprains
Tendonitis and tenosynovitis
Bursitis
Nerve entrapment syndromes
Reflex sympathetic dystrophy
Referred pain
Fibrositis (fibromyalgia)

General Causes of Nonarticular Rheumatic Pain

Muscle Pain

Injuries and abnormalities in muscle may cause pain. Muscle spasm represents prolonged excessive muscle unit acitivity and causes dull aching and tenderness. This results from irritation of nerves supplying blood vessels and local lactic acidosis. Blunt trauma to muscles can cause damage of fibers, rupture of blood vessels, and edema, and results in the same symptoms. Muscle strain results from overexertion, usually in a poorly conditioned muscle group, and causes sudden localized pain. On occasion, overuse of muscles may result in tearing of fascial planes and muscle sheaths, and results in herniation of muscle. Muscle cramp is a sudden localized contraction of muscle and usually results from fatigue, electrolyte or other metabolic imbalance (1). In most cases, there will be a history of recent overuse to which the localized muscle problem can be attributed. Common sense, rest, and application of cold, with progressive mobilization, local heat, and stretching exercises are usually required for rehabilitation of these usually minor problems. On occasion, muscle pain may result from inflammatory muscle diseases, which are discussed in Chapter 16.

Ligamentous Strains and Sprains

Ligaments are the tough, fibrous, connective tissue structures which connect and stabilize joints against stress. These are usually part of the joint capsule itself. A strain is usually a symptomatic condition in which pain is localized to the ligament and is associated with a stable joint. Treatment of strains is usually symptomatic. A sprain, on the other hand, may be painless, but is, by definition, associated with an unstable joint and ligamentous laxity. Treatment of this usually requires immobilization to allow the joint capsule and ligament to heal and stabilize the joint against further trauma.

Tendonitis and Tenosynovitis

Problems with tendons can occur anywhere along their course. When there is tenderness and irritation at the insertion of tendons into bone, this is referred to as an enthesopathy. Although this is seen in ankylosing spondylitis and other related syndromes, it may occur without any obvious etiology except possibly trauma or overuse. Many tendons also have an associated synovial-lined sheath and irritation here is referred to as tenosynovitis. This may occur as a localized condition as well as in systemic disease. Tendon function may be impaired by local trauma, systemic disease, inflammation, fibrosis, impaired blood supply, and atrophy or degeneration (2). A diagnosis of tendonitis is purely clinical and requires knowledge of local anatomy and a careful physical exam. On occasion, calcification may be seen within tendons on x-rays, but this is not usually the case.

Bursitis

A bursa is a synovial-lined space containing little or no fluid. Bursae are located outside of the joint space, usually between tendons, ligaments, bony structures, and other soft tissues. They serve to provide frictionless motion and lubrication between these various structures. They are located at various points around the body, and as many as 156 different bursae have been identified (3). There are many consistent locations for these bursae, but many are variable from one individual to another. Almost any disease process that affects joints may also affect bursae. Thus, bursitis may result from generalized inflammatory disease such as rheumatoid arthritis, infection, and crystal deposition. More frequently, bursitis results from localized trauma, mechanical irritation, or adjacent tendonitis. Many occupationally related bursitis syndromes have been given specific names, while most are unnamed. Evaluation of bursitis requires exclusion of other causes of pain in localized areas as well as a knowledge of frequently identified syndromes. On occasion, bursitis may be so severe as to cause a large collection of fluid, as in olecranon bursitis, and aspiration of the fluid should be part of the evaluation of any undiagnosed bursitis, especially to rule out crystal depostion or infection.

Nerve Entrapment Syndromes

Entrapment of peripheral nerves is a common cause of extremity pain, tingling, and sensory and motor dysfunction. The term entrapment indicates a mechanical irritation by which a specific peripheral nerve becomes locally injured in a vulnerable anatomic site (3). Nerve compression can occur at any point where a peripheral nerve passes through an opening in fibrous tissue or through an osseofibrous canal. Although symptoms referable to transient disturbances in peripheral nerves are a common experience in normal people, pathologic entrapment neuropathy results in persistent symptoms from focal nerve damage (4). The number of recognizable nerve entrapment syndromes has increased over the past several years with recognition of the frequency of focal damage of nerves and with the refinement of electrophysiologic techniques to confirm such damage. In the majority of entrapment neuropathies, there is no specific anatomic abnormality of the relationship of the nerve to the surrounding tissues, but in many cases, structural anomalies or traumatic abnormalities may be associated. In addition, certain primary peripheral nerve disorders may predispose nerves to damage at common sites of pressure or traction (3).

In addition to a careful neurologic examination, the evaluation of suspected entrapment neuropathy should include electromyography (EMG) and motor and sensory nerve conduction studies. Performance and interpretation of these tests require considerable expertise and experience and the clinician should be aware of the significance and limitations of each test. In general, motor and sensory nerve conduction studies are helpful in detecting slowing of conduction between two given points in the course of a nerve. Thus, most peripheral nerve entrapment syndromes can be detected by these studies. More proximal lesions, such as thoracic outlet syndrome or nerve root irritation at the level of the spine, will show EMG evidence of denervation and reinnervation with rest fibrillation, larger amplitudes, and less synchronous action potentials of longer duration. In proximal lesions, peripheral nerve conduction studies done distal to the lesion will be normal.

Reflex Sympathetic Dystrophy

The reflex sympathetic dystrophy syndrome (RSDS) is a syndrome of pain and tenderness which may involve one or more of the extremities. It is characterized by intense burning pain and is associated with vasomotor instability, trophic skin changes, and swelling (5,6). Radiographic evidence of patchy bone demineralization occurs when the condition is long-standing. Radionuclide bone scanning may show abnormalities on flow studies and static images in up to 80% of patients. An example of this is shown in Figure 12.1, which demonstrates increased uptake of tracer in the affected extremity.

A majority of patients with RSDS have a history of a precipitating event, with the most common being soft tissue injury, fracture, surgery, myocardial infarction, or stroke. There is also a significant association with emotional disturbance at the time of onset. Although this syndrome usually involves one upper extremity, some studies indicate that the condition may be bilateral in a majority of patients. The lower extremities may be involved as well, and in these cases, diagnosis is particularly difficult. Because of this and because of many of its clinical features, this syndrome has been known by many other names over the years, including causalgia, shoulder-hand syndrome, reflex neurovascular dystrophy, acute atrophy of bone, and Sudeck's atrophy.

Referred Pain

Pain which seems to have a musculoskeletal origin may be due to deeper visceral structures. This is particularly true for pain syndromes involving the shoulders, chest wall, low back, and hips. Shoulder pain, in particular, may be a manifestation a large variety of visceral lesions, including pulmonary neoplasm, myocardial or pericardial disease, diaphragmatic disorders, and subdiaphragmatic processes involving the gallbladder, liver, stomach, or pancreas. Chest wall and thoracic spine pain may be mistaken for cardiac, pulmonary, or esophageal lesions. Pain in the low back, pelvic girdle, and leg may represent referred pain from diseased abdominal or pelvic structures. A careful history and complete physical examination are mandatory parts of the investigation of nonspecific pain syndromes. In general, when pain is referred from a visceral structure, joint motion is normal and does not produce pain and tender points are relatively minimal or nonexistent.

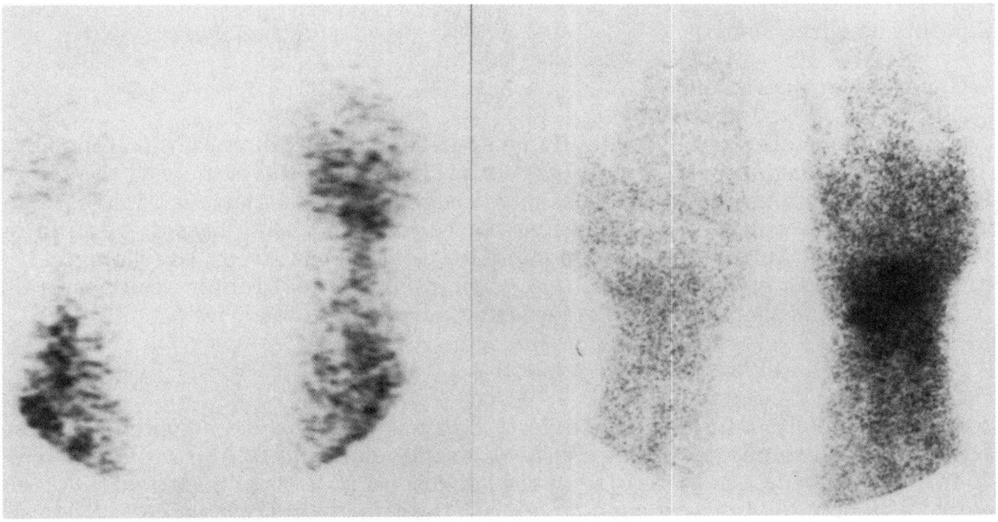

FIGURE 12.1 Radionuclide bone scan of a patient with reflex sympathetic dystrophy of the left upper extremity, demonstrating increased uptake on both dynamic (A) and static (B) images.

Fibrositis

General Features

The term fibrositis is used to describe a syndrome of widespread musculoskeletal pain and aching in the trunk and limbs, accompanied by multiple local tender points, but few, if any other objective physical or laboratory findings (7,8,9). Historical aspects of this still poorly defined disorder are discussed by Bennett (9). The term was first coined in 1904 to describe lumbago and arm pain and has since been used by various authors to describe various types of nonspecific musculoskeletal pain. Other terms which have been used to describe this syndrome, some of which are based on theories of etiopathogenesis, include fibromyositis, fibromyalgia, muscular rheumatism, nonrestorative sleep syndrome, pain amplification syndrome, and universal musculoskeletal pain enhancement syndrome. Primary fibrositis refers to patients with this syndrome who have no other underlying disease. Secondary fibrositis is used to distinguish the patient in which there is an associated disease state in which the same mechanisms as present in primary fibrositis are important in amplification of pain.

Fibrositis is thought to be much more common among women, with some studies showing only about 15% of cases occurring in men (10). It is primarily a disease of middle age, being most often seen in the 20-50 year-old group, although it can occur in juveniles and in older patients. The overall incidence and prevalence of this condition are undetermined, but it may represent as much as 16% of what is seen in a private rheumatology practice (11).

Etiopathogenesis

General Considerations

Fibrositis is characterized by virtually no specific changes in muscle or tendon histology, electromyography, blood tests or radiographs. Nevertheless, the clinical picture and associated complaints have suggested many avenues of investigation. Currently, most investigators consider fibrositis to be the result of an interaction of several factors, including personality, emotional stress, psychological disturbance, and sleep disturbance. In addition, mechanical factors and posture may play a role in triggering or exacerbating symptomatology.

Personality and Psychological Aspects

The "fibrositic personality" has been described by many authors. Typically, these patients are said to be demanding, perfectionist type patients who set high standards for themselves. They are often very successful in their occupations. Various types of psychological disturbance have been described, and one recent study using MMPI scales found that patients with fibrositis scored significantly higher on many scales when compared with patients with rheumatoid arthritis or other pain syndromes. The scales for measuring hypochondriasis and hysteria were particularly high, but the wide variety of changes suggest that patients with fibrositis form a heterogenous group with a higher frequency of psychological disturbance in general, but without specific types of psychological disturbances (12).

Mechanical Factors

The neck and low back region are among the most symptomatic of the painful areas in fibrositis syndrome. The cervical spine is particularly subject to stresses during sleep (8). The skull and thorax are supported during sleep, but the neck is more subject to sagging and compressive forces. Exaggeration of the forces from position of sleep may cause pain, interfere with sleep, and help perpetuate the cycle of pain and sleep disturbance. Mechanical factors in the low back are similarly thought to play a role in perpetuating the pain syndrome.

Sleep Disturbance

A great deal of evidence has implicated sleep disturbance as a key pathogenetic factor in the initiation and perpetuation of the fibrositis syndrome. In addition to a high frequency of complaints of disturbed sleep and generalized exhaustion, recent studies have shown abnormalities in sleep in patients with fibrositis (7,8). Patients with fibrositis have decreases in stage III and stage IV slow-wave sleep with frequent intrusions of alpha rhythm. In addition, a pain syndrome indistinguishable from fibrositis has been reproduced in normal subjects by intentional deprivation of stage IV non-REM sleep by use of a buzzer or other arousal. This study, performed in healthy college students, resulted in multiple tender points, tiredness, arthralgias, and pain similar to that seen in typical patients with fibrositis. In addition, it was found that subjects in better physical condition were less likely to develop fibrositic syndromes. Finally, another study has shown that fit persons tend to have higher levels of non-REM sleep than unfit subjects (13). The interactions between sleep, pain sensitivity, personality, and psychological stress and underlying neurochemical abnormalities remain to be specifically delineated.

Although a generally diminished pain threshold has been thought to be an important mechanism, a recent study suggests that only the specific trigger points are more pain-sensitive (14).

Clinical Features

Historical Aspects

The pain of fibrositis is a widespread, poorly localized and often deep aching pain. Pain is often referrable to muscle, areas of ligament attachment, or bony prominences rather than the joints themselves. When fibrositic pain is peripheral, it may have a swelling or numbing character. Stiffness, which is often felt with activity, is different from that felt in rheumatoid arthritis or other inflammatory arthropathies. There is no true morning stiffness, but sometimes a few minutes of aching and lethargy on arising. Pain is often made worse by cold or humid weather and often is worse during times of anxiety and stress. Local heat and massage often relieve symptoms but may paradoxically make symptoms worse.

Associated Features

Extreme exhaustion, with or without sleep disturbance, is a common complaint. Many patients may not notice specific sleep disturbance, but have a history of being light sleepers for many years. Patients will often notice sleep disturbance which tends to correspond to times of psychological stress. Fatigue and exhaustion may be even more disabling than the pain itself. Classically, extreme fatigue in the morning will be present, will improve within the first few hours of the day, and then become worse late in the afternoon and in the evening. Symptoms of depression, such as decreased energy, loss of sexual interest, reduced appetite, constipation, or even suicidal ideas may be seen. A wide variety of other functional symptoms may coexist in patients with fibrositis. Patients often may have been evaluated by cardiologists for noncardiac chest pain, by gastroenterologists for irritable bowel syndrome; other symptoms such as headache and urinary frequency may be present.

Examination and Trigger Points

The patient with fibrositis will have a remarkably normal physical examination, particularly in light of the severity of symptoms. During the examination, the patient typically seems very uncomfortable and apprehensive and seems to have difficulty relaxing. All joints should have normal range of motion, although sometimes full range is achieved only after gentle persistence. Muscle strength should be normal, but sometimes is inconsistent and poorly sustained (8). Tenderness without evidence of other pathology is the hallmark of the physical examination in fibrositis. Some patients will be diffusely tender, demonstrating a "touch me not" quality. Several specific and reproducible areas of tenderness have been proposed and investigated by several authors. In general, these involve muscle, bone, fibrous tissue, and musculotendinous junctions, and no histologic abnormalities can be demonstrated in these areas. Smythe has proposed a list of 14 specific tender points (see Figure 12.2 and Table 12.2) (7,8). In addition, several other sites are frequently tender, and the total number of tender points may range as high as 25 (9). Skin fold tenderness and reactive hyperemia, most prominent particularly in the upper scapular and trapezius area, are seen in most patients with fibrositis, and may provide some clue to the pathogenesis of the disorder.

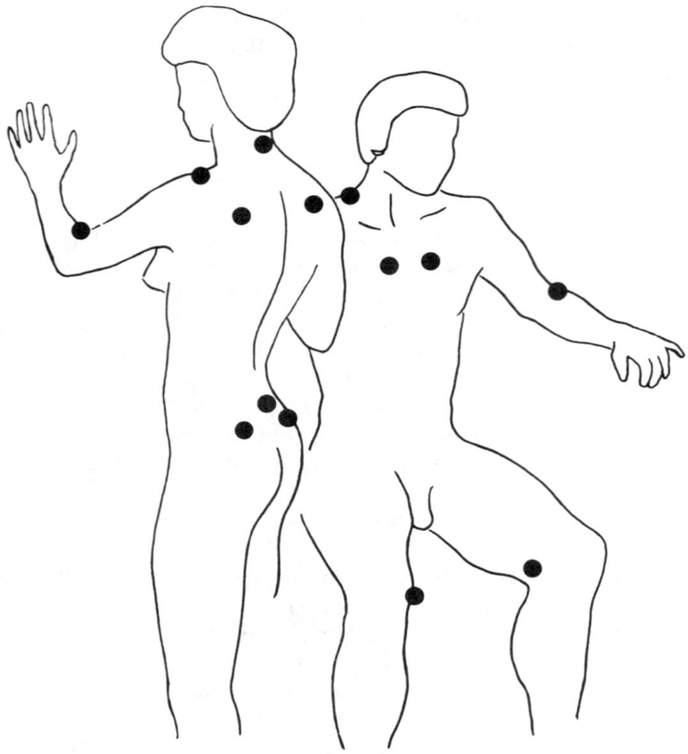

FIGURE 12.2 The 14 trigger points of fibrositis. (Reprinted from the Bulletin on Rheumatic Diseases, copyright 1977. Used by permission of the Arthritis Foundation.) (See Table 12.2 and text.)

Several sets of criteria for the diagnosis of fibrositis have been set forth. Probably the best known and most frequently followed are those suggested by Smythe (8) (see Table 12.3). A prerequisite for the use of these criteria would be a physical examination that shows no evidence of joint swelling or limitation of motion, and no abnormalities of erythrocyte sedimentation rate, liver enzymes, rheumatoid factor, antinuclear antibody, muscle enzymes, or sacroiliac films. Other authors have suggested that the above criteria are too strict, and suggest altering the second item to "local tenderness at 10 of the 25 specified sites" (9). The diagnosis of fibrositis is still a diagnosis of exclusion, and should be considered only after inflammatory or degenerative arthropathies or other possible causes of diffuse musculoskeletal pain are eliminated by history, physical examination, and appropriate laboratory testing.

Differential Diagnosis of Fibrositis

The differential diagnosis of fibrositis is essentially that of other entities that cause diffuse, widespread arthralgias (see Table 12.4). The term secondary fibrositis refers to the syndrome when it occurs in a patient with an underlying musculoskeletal syndrome. Patients with rheumatoid arthritis, for example, may have their synovitis under good control, but pain, sleep disturbance, and other

TABLE 12.2 Tender Points in the Fibrositis Syndrome

The typical 14 points (7,8): (See Figure 12.2)	Lateral epicondyles (elbows) (right and left) Second costochondral junctions (right and left) Trapezius skinfolds (right and left) Supraspinatus origin (near medial scapula) (right and left) Lower cervical spine (midline) Lower lumbar spine (midline) Gluteus medius (upper outer buttocks) (right and left) Medial fat pad (anserine bursae-knees) (right and left)
Other nonspecific points (9): (All bilateral)	Occipital insertion-nuchal muscles Intertransverse ligaments (C4-6) Medial aspects rhomboid Gluteal muscles, SI area Muscle-Achilles tendon junction Heel pad Medial epicondyle (elbows) Greater trochanter (hips)

TABLE 12.3 Diagnostic Criteria for Fibrositis (8)

Diffuse nonspecific aching for more than 3 months

Local tenderness at 12 of 14 trigger points

Tenderness over upper scapular or trapezius skin roll

Sleep disturbance and/or morning fatigue

factors may interact to reproduce the entire fibrositis syndrome without an apparent worsening in the degree of synovitis or other indicators of disease activity. Similarly, patients with osteoarthritis or any other musculoskeletal syndrome may have fibrositis superimposed on their underlying disease. Psychogenic rheumatism is a term used to describe bizzare musculoskeletal complaints without any obvious anatomical explanation and usually with some sort of underlying psychiatric disturbance (15). In most of these syndromes, such as hysteria, malingering, or conversion reactions, the pain is not only out of proportion to the findings, but specific tender points and skin fold tenderness are not present. Well-defined arthropathies, such as rheumatoid arthritis, seronegative spondyloarthropathies, or osteoarthritis, usually do not present significant diagnostic problems, but early in these conditions, laboratory studies and x-ray findings may be normal

TABLE 12.4 Differential Diagnosis of Fibrositis - Other Causes of Diffuse Musculoskeletal Pain

Secondary fibrositis (fibrositis superimposed on preexisting disease)
Psychogenic rheumatism
Rheumatoid arthritis
Seronegative spondyloarthropathies
Osteoarthritis
Polymyalgia rheumatica
Hypothyroidism
Connective tissue syndromes (SLE, polymyositis, scleroderma, Sjögren's syndrome)
Malignancy

or negative and only careful follow-up establishes one of these alterntive explanations for pain. In elderly patients with new onset of diffuse aching and stiffness, polymyalgia rheumatica should be a top consideration. Physical findings in this syndrome are often minimal, but the sedimentation rate should be elevated, usually markedly so, and is very helpful in establishing a diagnosis. Hypothyroidism is frequently complicated by diffuse myalgias, stiffness, and myopathy. Usually other more specific symptoms and signs are present, such as weight gain, cold sensitivity, and myxedema, but this should be suspected, particularly in elderly patients and is easily ruled out by appropriate laboratory testing. Diffuse connective tissue syndromes, such as SLE, polymyositis, scleroderma or Sjögren's syndrome, may initially present with diffuse nonspecific symptoms and few specific clinical findings. Appropriate initial laboratory testing and careful history and physical with close follow-up is necessary to establish these diagnoses. Finally, underlying malignancy should be suspected in patients who are at a high risk for developing malignancy, such as elderly patients, heavy smokers, or any one with weight loss or other systemic symptoms. Various mechanisms may account for such musculoskeletal pain, including hypertrophic osteoarthropathy, carcinoma polyarthritis, or bony metastasis.

Laboratory Findings

As noted previously, normal laboratory studies are essential for the diagnosis of fibrositis, and helpful in excluding other syndromes that may closely mimic this. Laboratory evaluation should be complete, and usually includes normal sed rate, muscle and liver enzymes, rheumatoid factor, and antinuclear antibodies. X-rays of painful areas, particularly when there are any suggestions of abnormalities on examination of the joints, should be undertaken at some point during the evaluation, particularly when symptoms persist in one area out of proportion to others.

Prognosis and Management

Natural History and General Principles of Therapy

The natural history of this condition is poorly documented, probably reflecting its relatively recent recognition. Overall, fibrositis tends to be a very difficult condition to treat effectively. Patients often feel that their complaints are not taken seriously and that the lack of hard findings on examination or laboratory testing have labeled them as "quitters" or "fakers." The physician's lack of experience in dealing with this syndrome and undue reliance on medication and inadequate time for explanations often contribute to this (9). Patients with fibrositis often become disenchanted and skeptical of their medical therapy, and "doctor shopping" is frequently seen.

After thorough evaluation, a careful explanation of the nature of this condition should be the first priority. The following should be explained:

1. This is not a crippling illness.
2. Mechanical stresses, particularly in the neck and lower back, often serve to aggravate the condition.
3. Sleep disturbance plays a role.
4. Exercise and conditioning are important in rehabilitation.
5. Emotional and psychologic stresses may contribute.

After careful explanation, therapy should be directed toward medical management of pain and sleep disturbance, physical modalities to alleviate mechanical factors and improve conditioning, and psychological support, as summarized in Table 12.5.

TABLE 12.5 Management of Fibrositis - General Principles

Continued observation and investigation for other possible causes of pain

Explanation and education

Medical therapy:
- analgesia - nonsteroidal antiinflammatories in small doses,
- sleep disturbance - tricyclic or other antidepressants, muscle relaxants

Physical modalities and exercises:
- Muscle strengthening and stretching
- General conditioning
- Local measures (heat, ice, massage, trigger point injection)
- Correction of mechanical problems

Psychological intervention:
- Education
- Stress reduction (behavior modification, biofeedback, support groups)

Medical Therapy

Any of the nonsteroidal antiinflammatory medications may be used, usually in small analgesic doses, as part of the management of fibrositis. Although these are frequently effective and may be sufficient for pain control and allow return to functional activity, these should not be relied upon exclusively. Medications directed at restoring normal sleep patterns have been used. Chlorpromazine and benzodiazipines are occasionally helpful, but usually not for sustained periods. Tricyclic antidepressants, such as amytriptiline and doxapin, have been suggested. In general, patients with fibrositis tend to be more subject to intolerable side effects from these medications, as opposed to those in whom these medications are used strictly for depression (7,8). Morning drowsiness is a particular problem in many, and for this reason, very small doses should be tried initially, and the dose should be gradually increased afterwards. Newer antidepresants such as trazadone, and muscle relaxants, such as cyclobenzaprine, have been suggested by a few authors.

In general though, too much reliance on medical therapy without careful explanation of the syndrome and attention to physical and psychological factors is to be discouraged.

Physical Modalities

Various physical modalities, often initially taught by a physical therapist and continued at home are often helpful to relieve muscle tightness and spasm and reduce the hypersensitivity of trigger points. Stretching exercises, local heat, ice, ultrasound, and transcutaneous electrical nerve stimulation have been used with variable success. Correction of mechanical problems in the cervical and lumbar spine may be particularly helpful. The use of a cervical ruff to support the neck at night, exercises to strengthen lumbar and abdominal musculature, and postural training to avoid lumbar hyperextension should be considered where appropriate. A careful evaluation of the level of physical activity and encouragement of gradually increased general exercise should be undertaken, particularly since muscle conditioning is helpful in reducing pain thresholds and enhancing sleep.

Psychological Management

Although it is often difficult to change the work and living habits of the typical hypersensitive and perfectionist patient with fibrositis, specific advice about holidays away from responsibilities and cares may be helpful (8). Careful discussion with the patient about the relationship of pain and fatigue to emotional stresses both at home and on the job is useful in identifying situations that contribute to worsening. Often the realization of these relationships allows the patient to make changes in responsibility and the response to them. The encouragement of recreational release, and getting out from under self-imposed loads can be helpful as well. Behavioral modification, biofeedback, and psychological support groups, or participation in a pain clinic for psychological support is often very successful (see Chapter 5).

Clinical Features of Specific Regional Pain Syndromes

Head and Neck

Temporomandibular Joint Dysfunction

Pain related to dysfunction of the temporomandibular joint is relatively common. Several systemic disease processes can involve this joint, the most common being rheumatoid arthritis and ankylosing spondylitis. Psoriatic arthritis, gout, infectious arthritis, and tumors may also involve the joint and degenerative joint disease may be found here as well, although x-ray changes correlate poorly with symptoms (16,17). In the absence of obvious articular pathology, several terms have been used to describe this syndrome of poorly understood facial pain, including TMJ syndrome, myofascial pain-dysfunction syndrome, and atypical facial neuralgia. This syndrome is seen more commonly in young to middle-aged females who present with chronic pain in the jaw occasionally radiating to the ear and neck. These are often associated with TMJ noises, irregular and limited jaw motion, and a sensation of pressure in the ear or tinnitus. Grinding of the teeth (bruxism) during sleep is often seen and pain is usually made worse by chewing or talking. Although malocclusion of the teeth is often associated with this syndrome, there is considerable doubt about the role it plays, since correction of these malocclusions has not uniformly alleviated the symptoms. A careful examination of the oral pharynx, palpation of the joint from inside the mouth and anterior to the ear, and x-ray of the TMJ are important in excluding organic causes for the symptoms. Several forms of therapy have been used with variable success. The use of a joint spacer or bite plate during sleep, and instructions for proper sleep with neck support are helpful in selected individuals. Isometric jaw exercises, local corticosteroid injection, biofeedback training, and tricyclic antidepressants are recommended in refractory cases (16).

Vascular Syndromes

Carotidynia is a syndrome of facial pain which is intermittent or persistent, localized over the temporomandibular area and sometimes radiating to the temple and ear. This has been described in young to middle-aged patients with a high incidence of past history or family history of migraine headaches (18). There may be associated tenderness and sometimes palpable swelling of the external carotid artery, and there are usually trigger points within the trapezius and posterior neck muscles. All laboratory and pathologic studies are normal. Most authors believe this represents a "migraine equivalent," although there are no visual or other associated symptoms. Treatment recommendations include local trigger point injection, tricyclic antidepressants, and occasionally ergot preparations and other medications used in migraine. Exercises, such as active resistance shoulder shrugging and neck-erector strengthening, may also be useful (16).

Cervical Fibrositis and Strain

Pain in the muscles of the posterior neck is a common complaint. The syndrome of pain and spasm often occurs after trauma, and may have its onset several weeks after the trauma. On physical examination, active motion may be markedly limited and although passive motion may ultimately be normal, guarding and spasm may make this maneuver extremely difficult. The head is often held in a rigid position, and sometimes spasm will cause rotation and tilting of the head (torticollis). In the typical cervical syndrome, pain is usually worse with sitting or upon arising in the morning and improves with motion. Radiographic evaluation is mandatory in most cases to exclude cervical spine disease, although degenerative changes are so common in older age groups that there may be no relationship between the pain syndrome and radiographic changes. Management inclused avoidance of prolonged motionless periods, correct sleeping posture, and sometimes injection of trigger points in the trapezius and paraspinous muscles. Exercises to mobilize and stretch muscles are helpful and cervical traction of 8-20 lb may often be necessary. Muscle relaxants, antiinflammatory and analgesic medication, and occasionally tricyclic antidepressants are advocated. Careful observation and follow-up are important, with particular attention being paid to development of possible cervical nerve root impingement syndromes.

Cervical Nerve Root Syndromes

Neck pain associated with pain radiating to the shoulders or further down the arms suggests nerve root impingement. This may be due to disc degeneration, root sleeve injury, trauma, or osteophyte encroachment on the neural foramina. Dull aching in the shoulder suggests C5 nerve root irritation. A positive Spurling maneuver and decreased vibratory and pin prick sensation over the deltoid region are also strongly suggestive. Radiographs of the cervical spine should include oblique views to demonstrate the neural foramina. Electrodiagnostic studies may be normal early, but should show abnormalities on EMG (16). Treatment principles are much the same as for cervical strain. The use of a neck collar or neck pillow for sleeping sometimes helps relieve spasm. Local heat, trigger point injection, and muscle strengthening exercises as well as home cervical traction and muscle relaxants are usually successful in reversing the syndrome. Refractory cases may require further studies and consideration of surgery. Occipital neuralgia is a similar syndrome occurring as a result of irritation of the sensory root of the second cervical nerve. This may occur as a result of trauma or in association with degenerative disease. Any evaluation for possible cervical nerve root irritation requires a functional knowledge of anatomy with special reference to sensory dermatomes, as shown in Figure 12.3. The evaluation of muscle groups for strength and reflexes is also an essential part of this evaluation.

Shoulder Girdle

Rotator Cuff Lesions

The rotator cuff is a group of four muscles which form a common tendon group which blends with the joint capsule and inserts on the humerus (as shown in Figure 12.4). The subscapularis is the main medial rotator, the supraspinatus works with the deltoid as an abductor, and the teres minor and infraspinatus are external rotators. Degenerative and inflammatory lesions within this rotator cuff are probably the most common cause of shoulder pain (4). Although controversy exists about exact etiologic and pathogenetic mechanisms, most authors believe that the initial pathologic event in the rotator cuff occurs in the supraspinatus tendon, which is particularly prone to thinning, humeral impingement against the coracoacromial arch, and traumatic inflammation. Problems here occur most commonly in patients over the age of 45 in whom occupational or leisure activities involve shoulder stress. The pain is usually of a dull nature, is localized to the lateral deltoid region, and is worse with certain movements, particularly abduction.

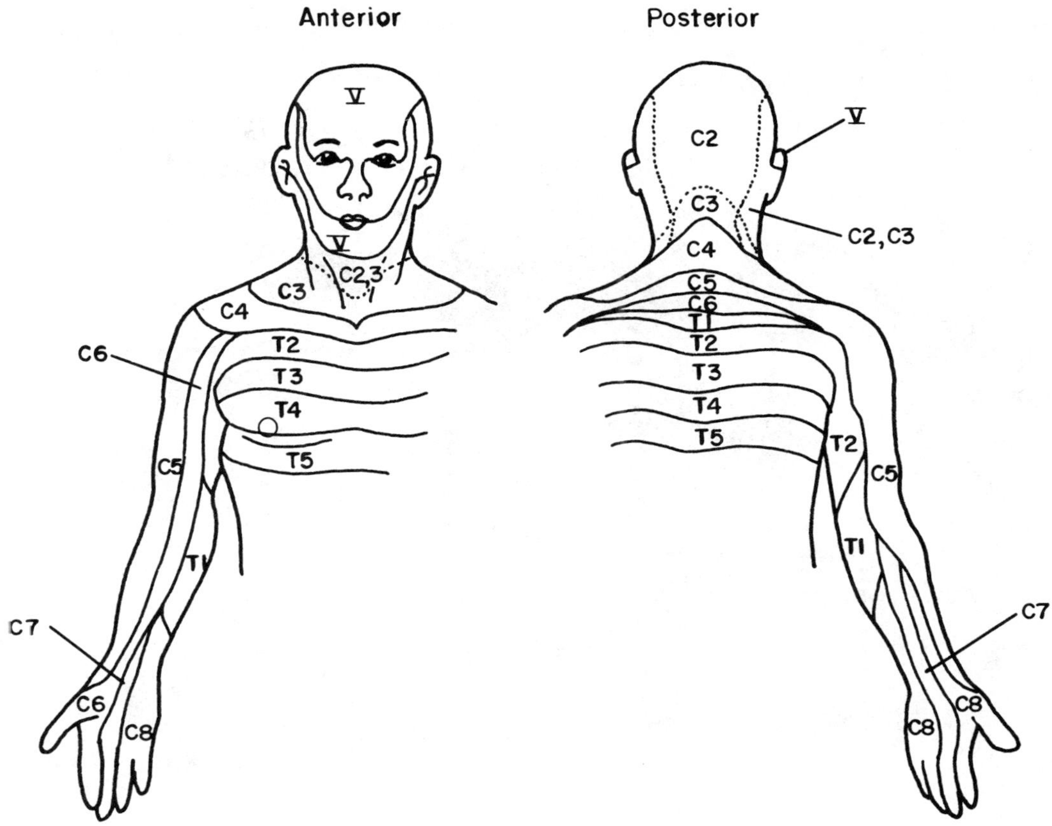

FIGURE 12.3 The sensory dermatomes of the upper extremity, demonstrating regions of pain and paresthesia related to specific cervical nerve root involvement.

Night pain is a very common characteristic, and examination reveals diffuse, poorly localized tenderness, with pain exacerbated by resisted movement involving the affected portion of the rotator cuff. Passive range of motion is normal, but active range of motion may reveal loss of normal scapulohumeral rhythm. X-rays are usually normal in uncomplicated rotator cuff tendonitis, although calcific densities may be seen in chronic processes. This condition is best managed with a combination of local heat or cold, range of motion exercises, antiinflammatory medications, and local steroid injection to enable a more vigorous exercise program.

In younger patients, calcific tendonitis may be seen more commonly. Hydroxyapatite crystals have been identified in these deposits and the clinical presentation is similar to that of acute, crystal-induced periarthritis, with abrupt onset of severe pain which affects sleep and any movement of the shoulder. Temporary rest with gradual mobilization, antiinflammatory drugs, and local injection with anesthetic agent or steroid preparations are usually successful.

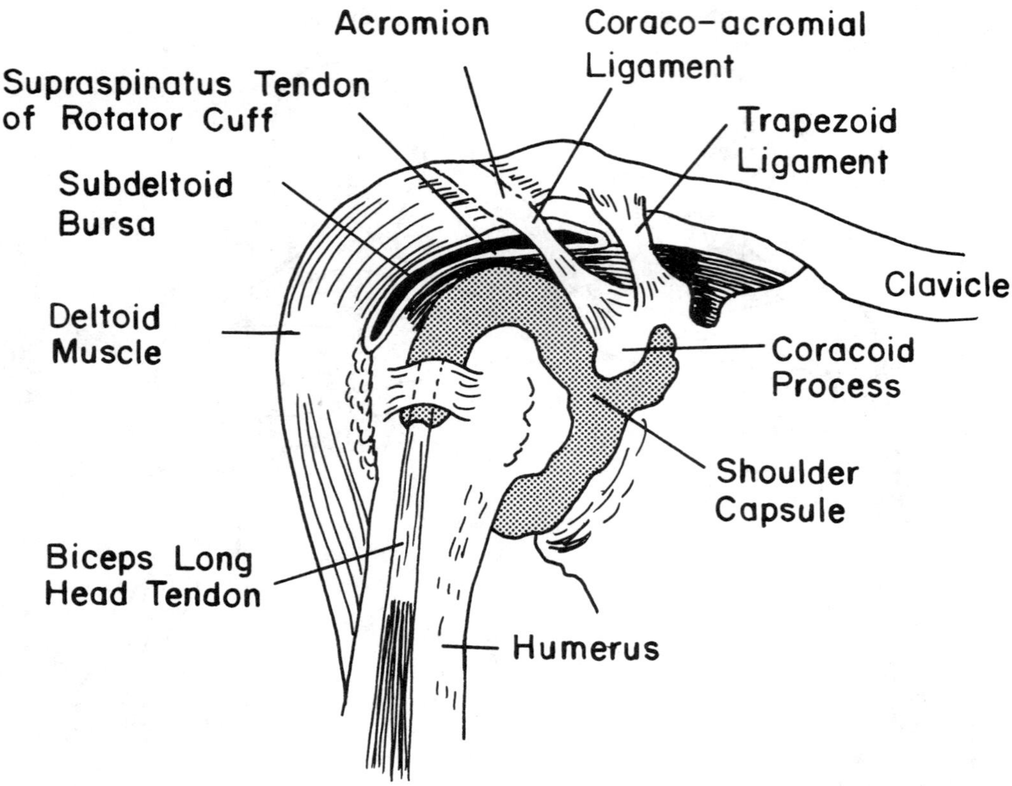

FIGURE 12.4 Anterior view of the functional anatomical structures of the shoulder.

Rotator cuff tears occur usually as a result of a degenerative process, and almost always in patients over the age of 50. This occurs most commonly in the supraspinatus portion of the rotator cuff. There will often be an abrupt painful episode, followed by relative comfort and subsequent severe pain and immobility. Abduction is the movement most commonly affected and passive movement is usually normal, but the patient will display a "drop arm" sign, where the patient is unable to maintain the arm in a horizontal position. X-rays of the shoulders will usually show elevation of the humeral head in relation to its usual location in the glenoid fossa. As the condition becomes chronic, rotator cuff atrophy occurs and the arm is held in a position close to the body. Arthrography may be necessary to confirm the diagnosis, with extravasation of dye from the glenoid fossa into the subacromial bursa being apparent. Complete rotator cuff ruptures, when they occur acutely, should be surgically repaired, while partial tears are chronic problems and usually require aggressive conservative management as with the other rotator cuff syndromes.

Bicipital Syndromes

The long head of the biceps originates at the superior aspect of the glenoid fossa and arches over the humeral head anteriorly through the bicipital groove (see Figure 12.4). Much of its course is intraarticular, and thus the biceps tendon can become involved in any intraarticular process. Tendonitis and tenosynovitis in the biceps tendon are characterized by chronic anterolateral pain which sometimes radiates to the arm and forearm. Pain is usually worse with repetitive activities, especially over the head. Examination will reveal anterior tenderness with extreme pain as the tendon is rolled under the fingers. A positive Yergason sign is elicited by forced supination of the forearm causing pain in the anterior shoulder. This syndrome is also managed conservatively with analgesic and antiinflammatory medication and local heat. Corticosteroid injection into the tendon sheath, or into the joint capsule itself often gives dramatic pain relief and allows the patient to maintain range of motion and help prevent a more diffuse process and adhesive capsulitis.

Other bicipital syndromes include tendon elongation, tendon dislocation, and rupture of the long head of the biceps. All of these conditions may cause pain and, in the case of rupture, a lump may be seen in the biceps muscle. Unless these occur acutely in a young patient, conservative management is usually preferable and very little function is lost by rupture of the long head of the biceps.

Bursitis

Bursitis as a primary event is actually relatively uncommon. Virtually all cases of subacromial bursitis are preceded by tendonitis in the rotator cuff, biceps tendon, or an inflammatory process in the shoulder joint with secondary spread to the overlying bursa (4).

Adhesive Capsulitis (Frozen Shoulder)

Chronic pain in the shoulders associated with gradual progressive restriction of all joint movement is known by various terms. The term frozen shoulder is a medical colloquialism rather than a diagnosis (19). Other terms which are more descriptive and carry more pathogenic implications include periarthritis, pericapsulitis, adhesive capsulitis, and obliterative bursitis. This condition occurs almost exclusively in patients over the age of 40 and may occur in association with a number of conditions, not all of which are primarily shoulder, but Chronic rotator cuff tendonitis is a very common cause of frozen shoulder but myocardial infarction, cerebral vascular accident, local trauma, intrapulmonary processes, thyroid disease, and diabetes have all been associated with this condition. Pain is usually diffuse, interferes with sleep, and is associated with a gradual loss of movement. The classically described natural history of this condition is that of a cycle of freezing, frozen, and thawing (4). The first phase typically lasts 10-36 weeks and is characterized by gradual stiffening. The second phase lasts from 4 to 12 months with less severe pain, but maximally restricted shoulder movement. The third phase is characterized by gradual recovery over a 5 to 26 month period. Although eventual recovery of functional shoulder movement is the rule, several studies have suggested that most patients are left with at least some residual loss of motion (19). The pathogenesis of this poorly understood syndrome is complex, but several theories have been put forth to describe what is pathologically a gradual contraction of the shoulder capsule. Trauma and internal derangement, immobilization, localized compression neuropathy, autonomic neuropathy, certain immunological mechanisms, and psychogenic factors are all believed to play a role in the development of this syndrome. Several studies have shown an association between diabetes and frozen shoulder with one series reporting an incidence of 10.8% of diabetics having frozen shoulders (20). The aims of treatment are to relieve pain and restore shoulder motion and function. There is general agreement that preventive measures to encourage range of motion in high-risk individuals is helpful. Management of pain, antiinflammatory medications, local heat, corticosteroid injection, and even local injection of the shoulder joint under pressure have all been used in selected cases (4,19, 21,22). Manipulation under general anesthesia has also been utilized as a last resort (22).

Articular Abnormalities

The shoulder joint functionally consists of four separate joints: the sternoclavicular, acromioclavicular, scapulothoracic, and glenohumeral. The sternoclavicular joint can be involved in a large number of diseases, most frequently rheumatoid arthritis, ankylosing spondylitis, various types of infectious arthritis, and sometimes in the other spondyloarthropathies. Disease here is easily detected by swelling, warmth, and tenderness in this area. The glenohumeral joint can be involved in several disease processes, most commonly rheumatoid arthritis, ankylosing spondylitis and related syndromes, gout, and pseudogout. In addition, previous trauma and specific occupations, such as truck driving, may predispose to osteoarthritis of the shoulder. In general, though, osteoarthritis is an infrequent cause of shoulder pain. Internal derangements of the acromioclavicular joint may occur in rheumatoid arthritis, secondary osteoarthritis, or after trauma. When this joint is diseased, pain will be localized to the superior aspect of the shoulder and there will be marked tenderness at the joint itself. Pain is particularly severe with motions of throwing and with adduction of the arm across the chest in a horizontal plane. X-rays will often show joint space narrowing and osteophyte formation. Treatment of this syndrome is usually successful with nonsteroidal antiinflammatory drugs, along with physical therapy and exercises, although local corticosteroid injection or even resection of the distal clavicle may be necessary for symptomatic relief (4).

Milwaukee Shoulder

Recently, a group of elderly women with painful shoulders, decreased mobility, and instability has been described. Radiographic features include evidence of complete rotator cuff tear and degenerative changes in the glenohumeral joint. Synovial fluid analysis has revealed a relatively low number of white cells, and careful analysis for crystals has shown microspheroids containing hydroxyapatite crystals (23). Synovial tissue has shown extensive osteochondromatosis with calcific foci and microvilli (24). Although pathogenesis of this syndrome is unclear, the authors hypothesize that hydroxyapatite deposition is the initiating event, followed by release into the synovial fluid, engulfment by macrophages, and release of enzymes which damage the rotator cuff.

Shoulder-Hand Syndrome (Reflex Sympathetic Dystrophy)

This poorly understood symptom complex classically is characterized by a painful stiff shoulder followed by dystrophic changes in the ipsilateral hand and fingers (5,6). The clinical course often consists of three stages. The first is characterized by should pain with redness and edema of the extremity. The skin is hot, dry, and usually very tender to the touch and the pain is often of a burning quality (causalgia). Radiographically, patchy osteoporosis may occur rapidly, even as early as a few days after onset. In the second stage of disease, shoulder movement increases, hand edema lessens, and muscle, skin, and subcutaneous atrophy occur. In the third stage, dystrophic changes are the most severe with marked atrophy of skin and subcutaneous tissues and brittle ridged nails. Pigmentary changes can also occur. Treatment of this syndrome involves early recognition and measures to reduce pain and inflammation in the shoulder and prevent contracture with progressive physical therapy. As noted previously, radionuclide scanning will show increased tracer uptake in the affected extremity in about 80% of patients, and is a useful tool in early diagnosis. Kozin et al. (6) have reported that a short course of tapering systemic corticosteroids may be highly effective if utilized early in the disease, and those with abnormal radionuclide scans appear to be more likely to respond. Others have reported efficacy with stellate ganglion blockade, but this appears to be less successful than was previously thought.

Thoracic Outlet Syndrome

Compression of the neural and vascular structures that supply the upper extremity may lead to a wide variety of clinical syndromes. Paresthesias, pain, and loss of motor function as well as swelling and vascular instability are prominent symptoms, and sensory deficit, cool skin, weakness, and muscle atrophy may be detected. In addition, certain maneuvers, such as the Adson maneuver, or manipulation of the shoulder and arm to reproduce or alleviate symptoms may be useful diagnostically. Anatomic structures which often cause these problems include cervical ribs, anomalous thoracic ribs, scalene muscle abnormalities, and compression between the rib and clavicle. In addition, certain unusual positions, such as prolonged hyperabduction, may also cause symptoms of neurovascular compression. Although conservative management with education, exercise, and physical therapy are successful in most patients, surgical intervention may be necessary.

Elbow

Figure 12.5 demonstrates various structures about the elbow that may give rise to pain.

Epicondylitis

Pain and tenderness at the bony prominences on the medial and lateral aspects of the elbow may result from strain or low-grade tear at the insertion of the forearm musculature here (25,26). Irritation at the attachment of the extensor muscles at the lateral epicondyle is often referred to as lateral epicondylitis or tennis elbow. The flexor muscles insert in the medial epicondyle region, and problems here are often referred to as medial epicondylitis or golfer's elbow. Tennis elbow is most frequently seen in the 40-60 year age group, and oftens results from overuse or incorrectly performed activities, such as in playing tennis. Pain may be acute or chronic and is usually worse with grasping or supination of the wrist.

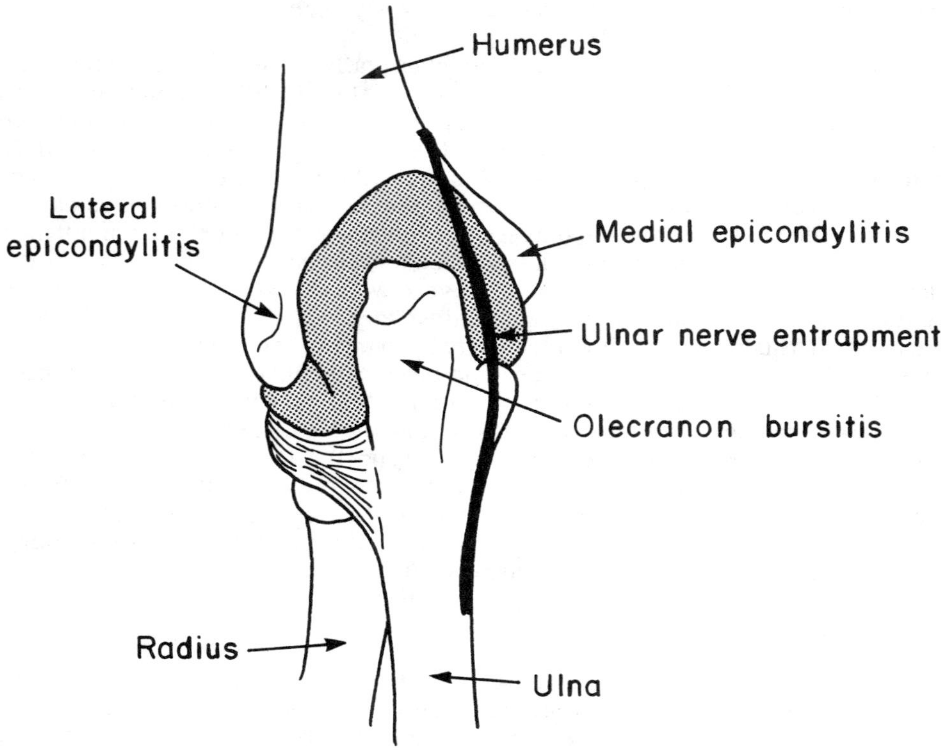

FIGURE 12.5 Posterior view of the elbow, demonstrating common causes of nonarticular pain.

Examination usually reveals obvious tenderness over the involved area. All laboratory studies should be normal in this condition, and movement of the elbow joint itself should be entirely normal. A conservative approach results in successful resolution of the problem in over 90% of the patients. The use of a tennis elbow band to provide forearm stability is advocated during activities. In addition, mild analgesic or antiinflammatory medications are often helpful. Local corticosteroid injections are successful in a majority of patients (27). A series of exercises to stretch and strengthen the forearm musculature is recommended as well (25).

Bursitis

The largest and most commonly diseased bursa about the elbow is the posteriorly placed olecranon bursa. Inflammation here may result from systemic inflammatory diseases, such as gout, rheumatoid arthritis, or infectious processes. Trauma may also cause a bursitis here, and activities that require prolonged pressure over this area are often implicated in the pathogenesis of this syndrome. An acute or subacute bursitis usually requires investigation to rule out a septic process. Analysis of the bursal fluid with white cell count, glucose determination, gram stain and culture should be performed in most cases. Even in the absence of fever or an obvious site of inoculation, septic bursitis should be suspected. Most patients with septic bursitis have low glucose levels in bursal fluid and the white cell count is almost always above 1000 (28). Infectious bursitis should be managed with repeated aspiration and appropriate antibiotics. Inflammatory conditions often respond well to local steroid injection. Posttraumatic bursitis should respond to a combination of aspiration, avoidance of pressure on the area, and local steroids if the fluid recurs. Other types of bursitis described around the elbow include a bursitis near the biceps insertion at the head of the radius in the antecubital fossa, and bursitis at the triceps insertion on the olecranon process, but these entities are rare.

Nerve Entrapment Syndromes

Poorly defined pain in the elbow and forearm in the absence of other abnormality should suggest a nerve entrapment syndrome at the elbow. Symptoms may be reproduced by placing a tourniquet over the elbow, but peripheral nerve conduction tests are often necessary to clearly define this. A radial tunnel syndrome has been described in which the radial nerve is compressed in the region of lateral epicondyle. In this syndrome, pain is reproduced with passive stretching or resisted extension of the middle finger. The pronator syndrome is a median nerve entrapment by the pronator muscles. In this syndrome, pain is reproduced by resistance to pronation in flexion of the wrist. Ulnar nerve entrapment behind the medial epicondyle can result from repeated minor trauma or pressure. On occasion, retrograde paresthesia from a carpal tunnel syndrome at the wrist may cause forearm and elbow pain.

Hand and Wrist

Ligamentous Injuries

A painful hand or wrist following a sports injury, trauma, or falling on the outstretched wrist should suggest a lesion of the tendons, ligaments, articular discs, or fracture to the bone itself. A fractured scaphoid bone may not be obvious on initial x-rays, and these should be repeated 2 weeks after the injury if pain persists. Sprain of the radioulnar joint may result in hypermobility and a "piano key" sign of the distal ulna. Sprain of the trapezium-first metacarpal joint usually results in pain at the base of the thumb and limitation of pinch grasping. Pisiform-triquetral injury results in pain on flexion or ulnar deviation, and tenderness over the hypothenar aspect of the palm. Immobilization and reconstructive surgery are usually indicated for these if instability persists.

Hypermobility

Generalized joint hypermobility may occur as a result of heritable systemic diseases, such as Marfan's syndrome and Ehlers-Danlos syndrome, but also may occur in 5-10% of normal individuals (29). Hand pain without swelling and instability may be complaints, particularly in children or young adults. Although premature osteoarthritis of the carpal-metacarpal joint may occur, there is some disagreement as to whether hypermobility predisposes to degenerative changes (30). Muscle strengthening exercises, avoidance of hyperextension, and supportive devices are suggested in patients with hypermobility and complaints referable to this.

DeQuervain's Tenosynovitis

Pain at the base of the thumb and into the radial aspect of wrist associated with grasping or wrist movement should suggest this diagnosis. This entity is seen commonly, particularly in young women, and is usually associated with chronic trauma, overuse, or repetitive activity. Tenderness is usually maximal in the lower part of the "snuffbox area" along the tendons of the abductor pollicis longus and extensor pollicis brevis. Thickening may also be obvious here. A positive Finklestein maneuver, shown in Figure 12.6, should confirm the diagnosis (see Chapter 1). Treatment of this syndrome begins with avoidance or modification of repetitive thumb movement or pinch grasping that may have initiated the pathologic sequence of events. Splinting of the thumb and wrist with local steroid injection into the tendon sheath is usually effective although surgical release of the tendons is necessary in occasional refractory cases (31).

Flexor Tenosynovitis

Tenosynovitis in a flexor tendon of any of the fingers, with nodular expansion of the tendon may result from low-grade trauma, overuse, or may be associated with systemic inflammatory disease. When this occurs in the thumb, it usually occurs in the flexor pollicis longus tendon, while in the other fingers, the flexor sublimis tendons are involved. The patient will complain of snapping, intermittent locking of the digit in flexion, or triggering. Examination will reveal triggering on active

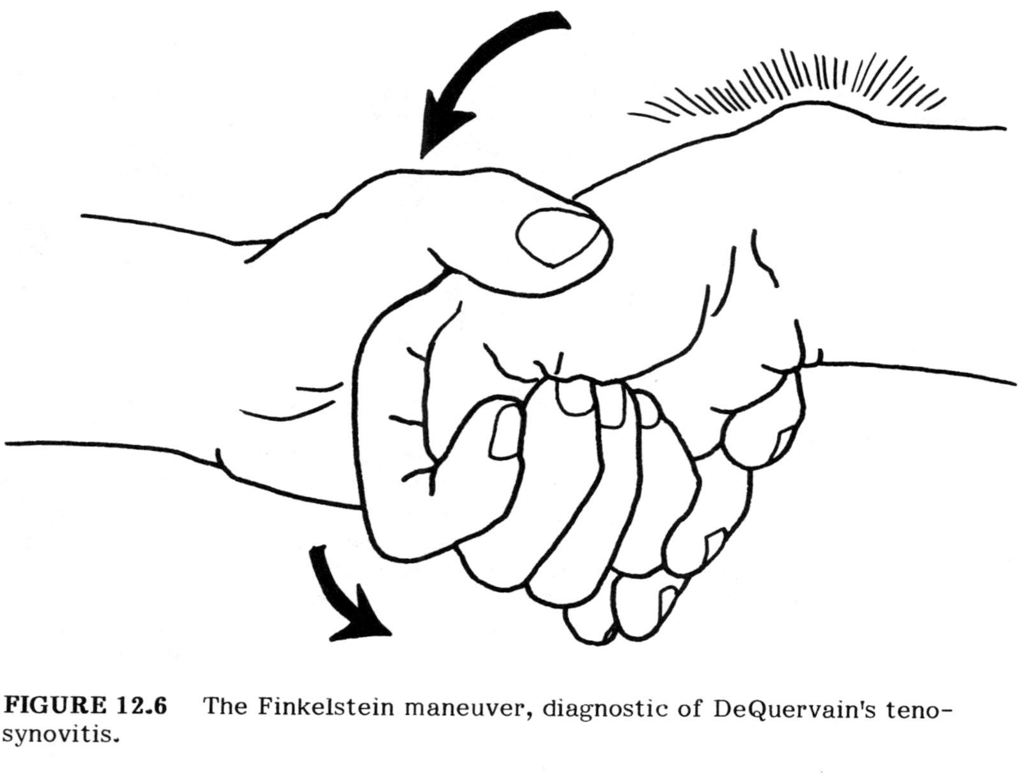

FIGURE 12.6 The Finkelstein maneuver, diagnostic of DeQuervain's tenosynovitis.

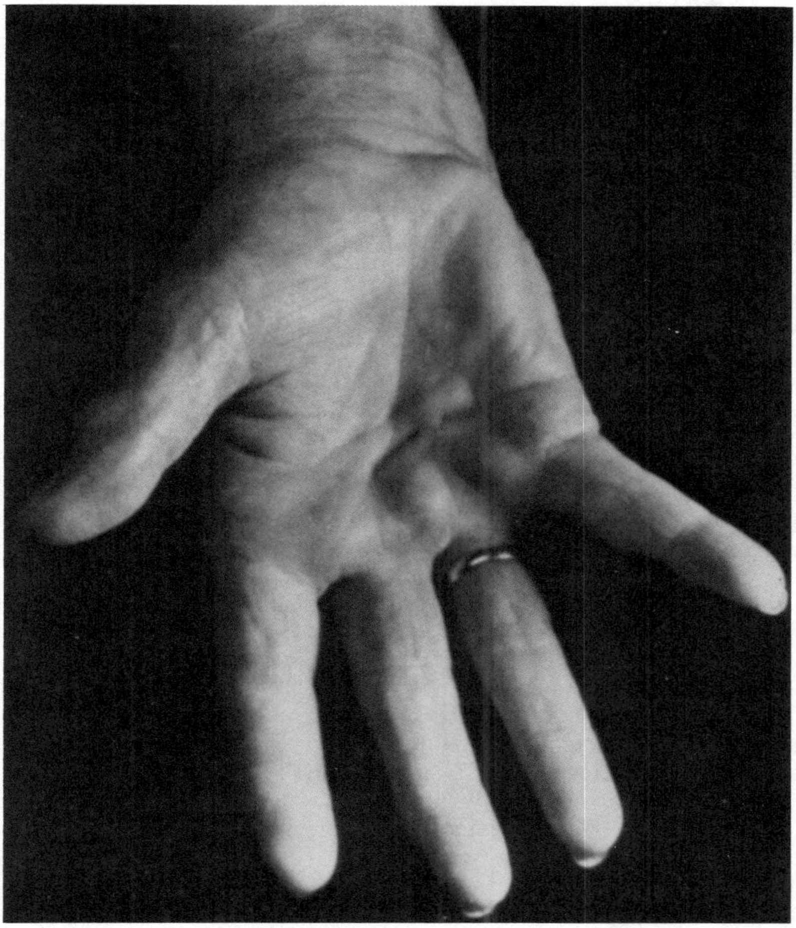

FIGURE 12.7 Dupuytren's contractures of the palmar fascia (see text). (From Sheon RD, Moskowitz RW, Goldberg VM: *Soft Tissue Rheumatic Pain: Recognition, Management, Prevention.* Philadelphia, Lea and Febiger, 1982.)

and passive movement with tenderness along the tendon sheath in the palmar aspect, usually at the level of the MCP joint. Often a nodule on the tendon may be palpated as it moves during flexion and extension. Treatment includes avoiding pressure and repetitive movement, splinting of the involved digit, or local injection of steroid and anesthetic into the tendon sheath. If this is unsuccessful, surgical release is indicated.

Dupuytren's Contractures (Figure 12.7)

Painless, nodular fibrosing lesions of the palmar fascia progressing to fibrosis and and contracture were first described by Dupuytren in 1834. This occurs most commonly in the palmar fascia and radiates to the fourth or fifth fingers, but may involve the other fingers as well. The flexor tendons themselves are not involved, but the inflammatory and fibrotic process surrounds the tendons. This syndrome occurs in 1-3% of Caucasian males and occurs about 10 times more frequently in men than women. There is a high frequency of familial involvement, suggesting a genetic predisposition. The condition may be associated with a large number of other localized systemic scleroses, including Garrod's knuckle pads, Peyronie's disease, sclerosing cholangitis, and Riedel's thyroiditis. Some studies have also suggested an association with cirrhosis of the liver and epilepsy (32). Histologically, fibrosis, giant cells and vascular hyperplasia have been noted. Treatment of this condition is unsatisfactory in most patients. Passive stretching and local corticosteroid injections are advocated by some, while surgery should be considered only if functional impairment or progressive deformity develops. There is a high rate of recurrence, and most patients should be advised to adapt to the disorder.

Carpal Tunnel Syndrome

Symptoms of pain, numbness, and tingling in the distribution of the median nerve in the hand should suggest entrapment of this nerve in the carpal tunnel area. Typically, patients with this disorder have pain that is worse at night, or on awaking in the morning. Occasionally, symptoms of motor impairment may predominate with difficulty pinching or holding objects. Symptoms may also worsen after use of the hands in certain tasks such as knitting, grasping objects, or driving (33). Weakness and atrophy of the thenar muscles occur when the condition is chronic. Examination of the joints of the hands should be normal and wrist movement may be essentially normal, although there may be tenderness and swelling in the volar aspect of the wrist, especially in the flexor tendon sheaths here. Positive Tinel's and Phalen's maneuvers are usually present (see Chapter 1). Electrodiagnostic testing will show abnormal conduction of the median nerve across the wrist in over 90% of patients. Carpal tunnel syndrome may occur as a result of repetitive activities requiring the flexors of the wrist, or may result from direct trauma with resulting edema in the area. Any inflammatory disease which can cause tenosynovitis may result in a carpal tunnel syndrome, and this is most typically seen in rheumatoid arthritis, but it may also occur in gout or pseudogout. Other associated conditions include osteoarthritis, pregnancy, diabetes, hypothyroidism, acromegaly, and amyloidosis. Most patients with carpal tunnel syndrome do not have one of these underlying processes, but complete physical examination and appropriate laboratory testing should be performed with these associated conditions in mind. When symptoms are early and have not resulted in any thenar atrophy, conservative measures may be attempted. Splinting of the wrist, particularly at night, may result in gratifying improvement in the symptoms. Local steroid injection in the flexor tendons at the wrist may also be very helpful but should be carried out with great care using a very small bore (25-27-gauge needle). If these measures fail or if thenar atrophy is present, surgical release should be undertaken.

Ganglia (Figure 12.8)

Cystic swellings over the dorsal aspects of the hands and wrists are frequently caused by ganglia. These represent thin-walled cysts near joint capsules or tendon sheaths, but do not usually contain synovial lining cells. They may be unilocular or multilocular and usually contain a noninflammatory jelly-like fluid. They may occur spontaneously or as a result of trauma or may be associated with underlying arthritis. Ganglia are usually not painful unless strategically located on or near tendon sheaths and infrequently cause functional impairment. Therapy is usually not indicated, since spontaneous disappearance may occur. Local pressure and

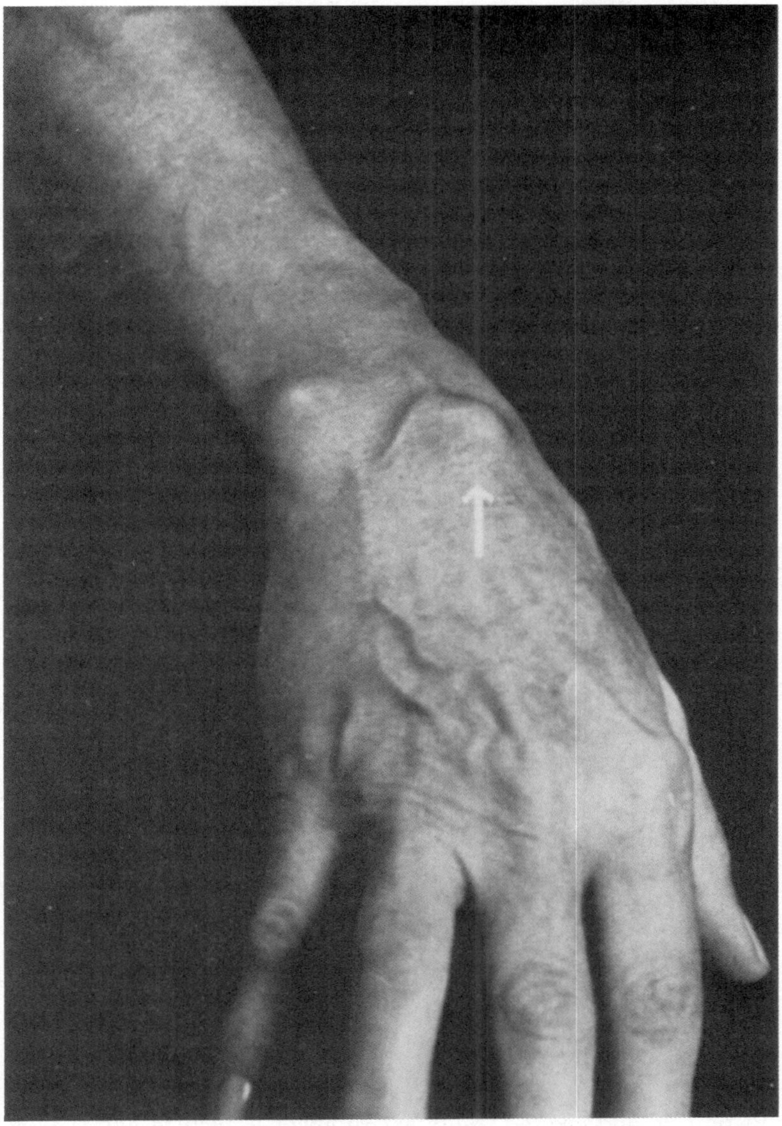

FIGURE 12.8 Dorsal ganglia of the wrist (see text). (From Sheon RD, Moskowitz RW, Goldberg VM: *Soft Tissue Rheumatic Pain: Recognition, Management Prevention.* Philadelphia, Lea and Febiger, 1982.)

intentional rupture of ganglia is successful in some, as is aspiration and injection of local steroid. Surgical removal is rarely indicated (26,31).

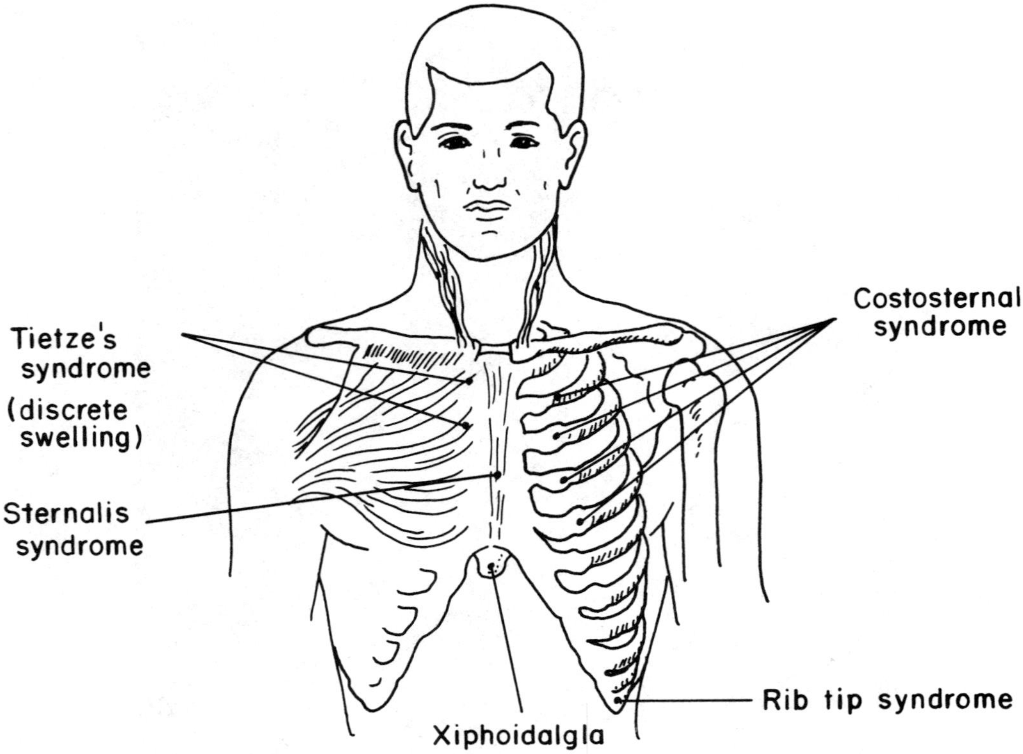

FIGURE 12.9 Anterior view of the chest, demonstrating various myofascial syndromes causing chest wall pain.

Chest Wall

Figure 12.9 demonstrates a wide variety of structures of the chest wall that may cause musculoskeletal chest pain.

Myofascial Chest Wall Syndromes

Evaluation of pain in and around the chest requires a careful and thorough examination of the entire patient. Disturbances arising in the head, neck, or cervical spine as well as subdiaphragmatic causes need to be excluded before attributing chest pain to the thoracic wall. In addition, exclusion of cardiac and pulmonary causes is essential and, in particular, exclusion of coronary disease in patients at high risk for developing this should be the physician's first priority. Several conditions have been described in which chest pain can be attributed to tenderness of chest wall structures in the absence of discrete swelling or bony abnormalities of the ribs themselves. Although the terms diffuse costochondritis and the chest wall pain syndrome are used to describe these syndromes as a group, several distinct clinical entities have been described (34). The costosternal syndrome describes conditions where pain is limited to the anterior part of the chest wall. This may radiate to the whole chest and may be accentuated by deep breathing, but is usually intermittent over several days but sometimes for months or years.

There is tenderness and reproducible pain at one or more costosternal junctions and pain may be reproduced by horizontal traction on the arm flexed across the chest (35). The sternalis syndrome is characterized by pain directly over the center of the sternum, probably at the sternal synchondrosis or in the sternalis muscle itself. The pain in this syndrome is generally less severe and less intermittent than with the costosternal syndrome. Xiphoidalgia is a syndrome characterized by spontaneous anterior chest pain associated with discomfort and tenderness of the xiphoid process at the lower end of the sternum. Pain in this syndrome is usually intermittent and may be aggravated by eating, lifting, or certain movements. This syndrome tends to be self-limited. The rib-tip syndrome is associated with severe sharp pain associated with hypermobility of the anterior end of the costal cartilage of one of the lower ribs. Pressure over the involved area may produce painful clicking, and pain may be aggravated by abduction of the arm. The "hooking maneuver" where the examiner's fingers are hooked under the ribs and the ribs are pulled forward, should reproduce the snap and pain. Etiology of these chest wall syndromes is unclear, but muscular strain, misuse, or poor posture have been implicated. All laboratory studies should be normal in these syndromes, but sedimentation rate, chest x-ray and special views of the ribs, as well as electrocardiogram and other investigation for cardiac disease, should be performed to exclude other causes of chest pain. Management should generally be conservative, since many of these syndromes are self-limited and spontaneously disappear. Exclusion of organic disease, explanation, and reassurance may go a long way in relieving the patient's anxiety. Elimination of aggravating factors and poor posture as well as certain exercises have been advocated (34). The "cornering" exercise or the standing pushup in a corner is suggested to allow strengthening and stretching of the pectoralis and other chest wall muscles. This is performed with the patient facing the corner with his feet positioned about 2 feet away and each arm on an adjacent wall at shoulder height with the fingers pointed toward the corner. Mild analgesics, nonsteroidal antiinflammatory medications, and local injection of steroids and local anesthetics into localized trigger points may be helpful.

Tietze's Syndrome

This disorder is characterized by pain, tenderness, and enlargement at the costochondral junctions. It may be acute, intermittent or chronic and is usually localized to one or two costochondral junctions (38). Histologically, only mild increased vascularity and cartilage proliferation is seen. The etiology of this condition is unknown, but x-rays and other laboratory studies are routinely negative. Spontaneous remission may occur, but antiinflammatory medications or local corticosteroid injections may be necessary, as well as local application of heat or cold.

Thoracic Spine Syndromes

Various lesions of the thoracic vertebrae or intervertebral discs may cause pain in the chest wall. Juvenile kyphosis with epiphysitis (Scheuermann's disease) occurs mainly in adolescents and is characterized by vertebral end-plate irregularity and herniation into the vertebral body with some anterior wedging of the vertebra. Osteoporosis and osteomalacia may result in compression fractures that cause back and chest pain. Herniated dorsal intervertebral discs are unusual but may cause severe back and chest wall pain. Ankylosing spondylitis and other related conditions may cause inflammation at the costovertebral junctions and result in back and chest wall pain as well as pain on inspiration.

Low Back

It has been estimated that 70-80% of the general population will experience low back pain at some point during adult life (37,38,39). The impact of this on our society from the standpoint of inconvenience, loss of work, and disability cannot be underestimated. It is estimated that up to half of all loss of work due to rheumatic complaints is due to back pain and that back pain is the chief complaint of nearly 20% of the patients seen in rheumatologic practice and nearly 40% in general orthopedic and neurosurgical practice. The vast majority of back pain is caused by disease localized to the back, and seldom represents an emergency requiring immediate intervention (37,39). Nevertheless, certain elements of the history and physical should alert the clinician to nonarticular causes of back pain or elements that warrant acute intervention. Older patients with continuous progressive back pain that is worse in a recumbent position should be carefully examined with occult malignancy or other systemic diseases in mind. Careful attention to the breast, prostate, thyroid, pelvis, and lymphatics, as well as a chest x-ray, evaluation for anemia, hypercalcemia, or liver or bone enzyme abnormalities should be undertaken. The association of back pain and fever warrants a more aggressive diagnostic evaluation for osteomyelitis, meningitis, or septic discitis. In younger patients with back pain associated with prominent morning stiffness, ankylosing spondylitis should be a consideration. Symptoms of bowel or bladder dysfunction, weakness of ankle dorsiflexion, the presence of ankle clonus, or color changes in an extremity should also suggest something other than a simple mechanical problem as a cause of low back pain.

Lumbosacral Strain

Probably the majority of patients with musculoskeletal low back pain do not have sufficient findings to suggest a herniated disc as the cause of the symptoms. A large number of terms are used to describe this syndrome, including low back derangement, lumbosacral strain, the posterior joint syndrome, or the facet syndrome. This condition may be either acute, subacute, or chronic. Most patients will describe pain after tasks that involve movement or lifting and a sensation of "catching" that may lead to immobilization in a slightly bent forward position. The syndrome is often self-limited, lasting for about 4 days in most cases. Chronic recurring pain may develop, which is usually aggravated by activity and improved with rest. Physical examination may reveal degrees of tenderness in the musculature and in the sacroiliac region. Motion causes pain and is therefore limited. The site of pathology in this syndrome is unclear, but various authors have implicated facet joint subluxation, transient disc prolapse, partial ligament tear, muscle insertion tear, or muscle hemorrhage. Mechanical back pain of this type occurs usually in middle age. Radiographs of the low back area are usually normal, and disc space narrowing and osteophytes are often incidental findings unrelated to the acute pain syndrome. Several contributing factors have been implicated in low back syndromes, including postural deficits, improper work habits, or weakness of supporting muscles.

Treatment of lumbosacral strain varies with the acuteness and duration of the problem. Bed rest in a semi-Fowler position (supine, hips flexed, legs elevated) is suggested initially in acute cases. This will allow muscle spasm to subside. Drug therapy with mild analgesics, muscle relaxants, and nonsteroidal antiinflammatory agents may be helpful. Although controlled data for the use of these types of drugs are sparse, most clinicians employ some combination of the above. As pain and muscle spasm subside after acute episodes, gradual mobilization and gentle flexion exercises are suggested. The use of local heat and other physical modalities, manipulation, corsets, braces, traction, local injection therapy, and acupuncture have all been advocated, but most of these modalities are controversial and controlled data are either lacking or show no benefit (37,38,39,40). Probably most important for the prevention of recurrence in both acute and chronic cases is education about the mechanics of the low back in order to avoid aggravating stresses (see Table 12.6). Therapeutic exercises are another cornerstone of management of the painful low back (39). The most frequently prescribed exercises, the Williams' flexion exercises (41), are designed to strengthen both lumbar and abdominal muscles and increase the support of the spine, as well as reduce pain by relaxing muscles in spasm. Several variations on these exercises have been suggested by various authors (see Figure 12.10). The general principles of muscle strengthening remain the same, although several modifications have been made because of the belief that some of the Williams' exercises actually increase intradiscal pressure.

Disc Herniation

Over 90% of all lumbar herniations occur at the L4-L5 or L5-S1 levels (38). Classic presentation is that of severe back and leg pain, spasm, limitation of spinal movement and restriction of straight leg raising. Specific neurologic findings should be present. In L3-L4 disc herniation (L4 nerve root), there will be a sensory loss over the anteromedial leg, quadriceps weakness, and diminished knee reflex. In L4-L5 disc herniation (L5 nerve root), senosry loss is more often over the distal lateral leg and dorsal foot with weakness in the toe dorsiflexors, particularly the extensor hallucis longus. In L5-S1 disc herniation (S1 nerve root), sensory loss will be over the posterior calf, lateral heel and lateral three toes. Weakness in the gluteal muscles, hamstrings, and calf may be present and the ankle reflex is frequently diminished or absent. Routine radiographic evaluation for lumbar disc disease may be normal, although in long-standing cases there may be significant disc space narrowing. Electromyography may be valuable in localizing a lesion, demonstrating findings of denervation. CT scanning may also demonstrate a herniated disc. Myelography is the definitive laboratory study, but

TABLE 12.6 Principles of Education for Patients with Low Back Pain Syndromes

Avoid hyperextension of the low back
Suitable night support (firm mattress or board)
Support low back when sitting
Use of armrests while sitting
Avoid prolonged forward flexion (as in vacuuming, washing, bed making)
Lift objects with back in a neutral position (flex knees, hold objects close to body)

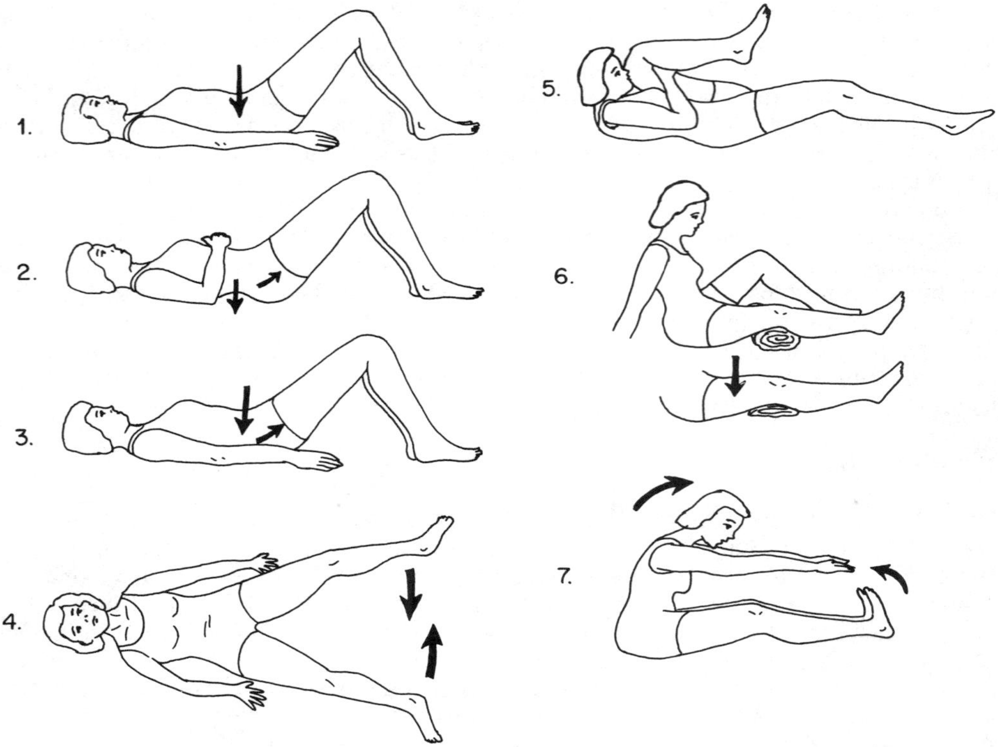

FIGURE 12.10 Typical flexion exercises used in rehabilitation following lumbar strain. These should begin with a few repetitions of each, increasing gradually up to 10 minutes, 3 times daily: 1) contract abdominal muscles as hard as possible, 2) contract the gluteal muscles, 3) contract abdominal and gluteal muscles together (pelvic tilt), 4) contract hep adductors and pelvic floor, 5) knee-chest exercise, 6) quadriceps strengthening (isometric), 7) achilles and hamstring stretching.

should be reserved for those in whom surgery is being considered. Treatment varies with the age of the patient, severity and duration of symptoms, and degree of nerve root entrapment. Conservative management with rest and analgesics, and other measures used for strain may be successful but laminectomy of the involved segment and removal of the disc is recommended in those that do not respond to conservative measures or in those with severe neurologic deficit. Chemonucleolysis (injection of chymopapain) has recently been approved for use in this country as an alternative to surgery in selected cases, but is associated with a relatively high incidence of allergic and sometimes life-threatening reactions (42).

Spondylolisthesis

This term refers to slipping and dislocation of one vertebral body in relationship to that below, leaving the posterior elements attached. This occurs as a result of spondylolysis, usually a congenital bony abnormality of the pars intraarticularis of the pedicle of the vertebrae. Pain in this syndrome often radiates into the buttocks or lower extremities and is aggravated by forward bending. Physical findings include abnormal straight-leg raising and, on occasion, neurologic findings as with a herniated disc. X-rays will usually reveal an abnormality, although many patients will have spondylolisthesis without symptoms. Therapy should be conservative at first, and flexion type exercises have been shown to be more successful than those involving extension (43). Bracing and restriction of activities are often necessary, and surgical intervention with arthrodesis, resection of loose posterior elements, or bilateral posterior fusion has been advocated (38).

Vertebral Abnormalities

Compression fractures of the vertebral end plate, multiple myeloma or metastatic carcinoma, Paget's disease, or other metabolic abnormalities involving bone all may cause back pain, and for this reason x-rays of the back are important at some point to rule out these abnormalities.

Sciatica and Other Nerve Entrapment Syndromes

Sciatica is a symptom complex which can result from many entities affecting the low back. Symptoms include pain as well as numbness, tingling, and burning and these latter neuritic features may occur at some distance from the area of pain. Activities that increase intraabdominal pressure such as lifting, pushing, coughing, or sneezing usually aggravate this sort of pain. A herniated lumbar disc is a frequent cause of sciatica, but several other entities should be suspected if neurologic findings are absent. Entrapment neuropathy of the sciatic nerve may occur from direct injury from sitting on a hard surface, and rarely may be caused by spasm of the piriformis muscle in the buttock. The sciatic nerve may also become entrapped in the posterior thigh between myofascial bands, but this is very rare. Spinal stenosis may result from degenerative changes in the lumbar spine, or any other entity that may narrow the spinal canal (developmental abnormalities, Paget's disease, arachnoiditis). Characteristic symptoms include nerve root irritation and worsening of pain and paresthesias with walking (pseudoclaudication). Night pain may occur in the upper thighs. Symptoms in spinal stenosis are intermittent at first but frequently become progressive, constant, and bilateral. Physical examination will usually reveal bilateral findings of nerve root compression. Electromyographic studies are almost always abnormal. Computerized axial tomography or myleography is required to confirm the diagnosis and also quantitate the degree of stenosis (44). Surgery for this condition can be fairly extensive, and is not uniformly successful. For this reason, conservative measures are usually employed first, particularly in elderly individuals, although wide decompression may be necessary to relieve symptoms (36).

Myofascial Back Pain

This condition has variably been referred to as fibrositis of the low back or tension myositis, and may well represent a variation of what is referred to as lumbosacral strain (39). In this syndrome, pain seems to be more localized to the gluteal-fascia or specific muscle groups or bursae, such as the iliocostalis, sacrospinalis, or interspinous bursa. Pain is dull and aching, is worse with working or sitting and improves with heat, walking, or bed rest. When subacute or chronic, these occur most frequently in the third to fifth decades of life and are rarely associated with a definite injury or acute pain. These may be seen in association with degenerative disc disease or other local problems and are therefore sometimes very difficult to distinguish. By definition, these syndromes are associated with definite trigger points which cause accentuation of pain when palpated. Episacroiliac fibrofatty nodules (lipomas) may coexist. Injection of trigger points, local heat, exercises, and various analgesics, antiinflammatory, and muscle relaxing medicines may be helpful. In addition, antidepressants may help improve the pain-sleep disturbance cycle that makes this syndrome quite similar to that seen in generalized fibrositis (39).

Pelvic Girdle

A wide variety of syndromes may cause nonarticular pelvic girdle pain. Figures 12.11 (anterior view) and 12.12 (posterior) demonstrate various structures that may give rise to these syndromes.

Osteitis Condensans Ilii

Sclerosing densities on the iliac side of the pelvic bone may sometimes mimic sacroiliitis radiographically, but careful examination reveals a normal sacroiliac joint space and no changes on the sacral side. This condition is most commonly seen in women of child-bearing years, and may be related to stress during pregnancy, labor, and delivery. It is also seen in males who have been exposed to trauma or contact sports (26). Although this entity may be asymptomatic, diffuse pelvic pain and symptoms of sciatica may be present.

Osteitis Pubis

This condition is characterized radiographically by erosion, sclerosis, and widening of the symphysis pubis. A majority of patients with this disorder are middle-aged women who complain of pain in the low anterior pelvis radiating into the thighs. There may be a waddling gait, and tenderness is reproduced by pressure over the area. This condition may be seen in ankylosing spondylitis, chondrocalcinosis, and sometimes may represent regional spread of infection after prostate or bladder surgery (39). The condition is frequently self-limited, but may respond to antiinflammatory agents or local corticosteroid injection. Progressive worsening or radiographic progression of the condition suggests an infectious process and warrants further investigation with biopsy of the lesion.

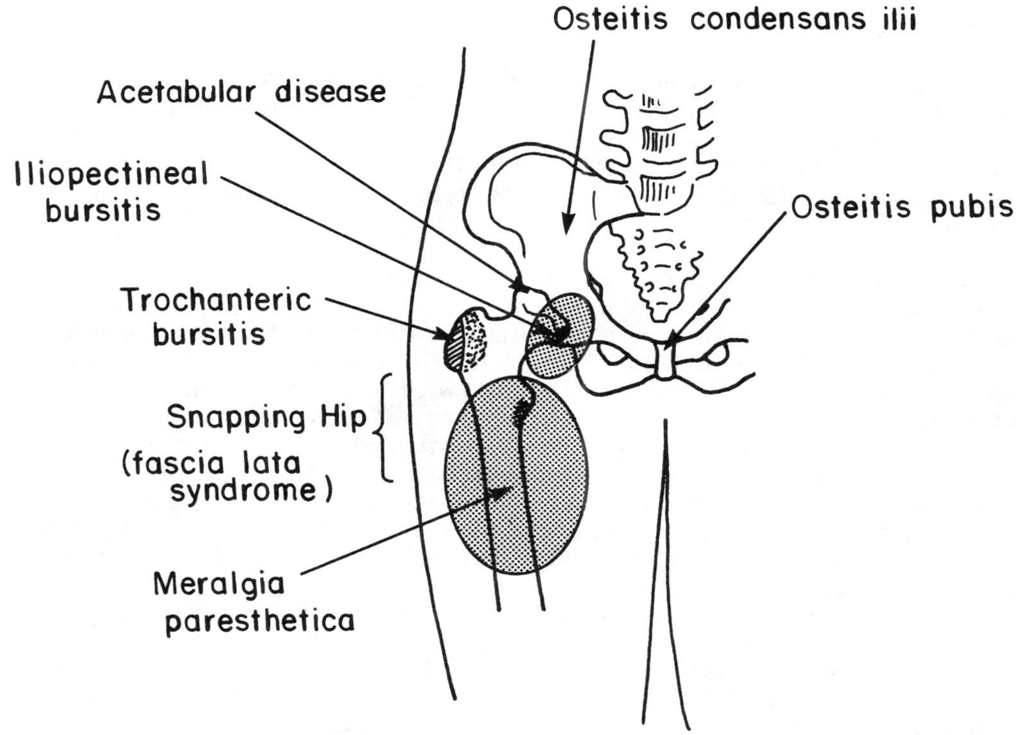

FIGURE 12.11 Anterior view of the pelvis, showing common causes of anterior hip girdle pain (see text).

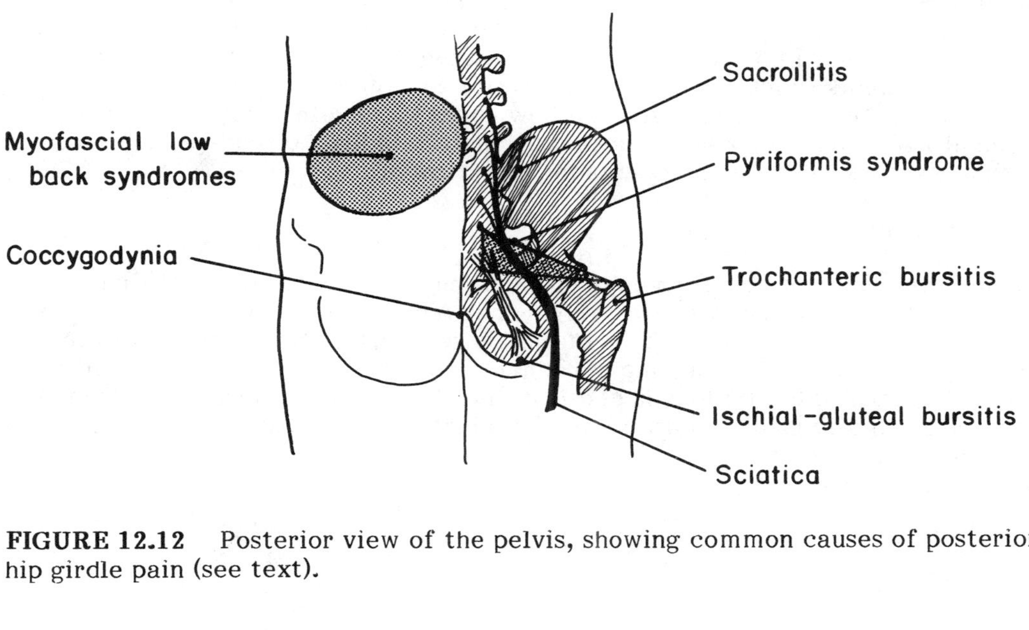

FIGURE 12.12 Posterior view of the pelvis, showing common causes of posterior hip girdle pain (see text).

Coccygodynia

Pain over the coccyx may represent referred pain from the lower lumbar region, visceral structures in the pelvis or rectum, or may represent a local inflammatory or posttraumatic condition involving the coccyx itself. Local treatment includes the use of a thick foam rubber cushion with the center cut out and, on occasion, local anesthetic or steroid injection in the area. Surgical resection is rarely indicated.

Snapping Hip and Fascia Lata Syndrome

The fascial plane extending down the lateral aspect of the thigh may be a source of a snapping sensation in this area which may or may not be associated with pain. The painless snapping hip may be associated with subtle leg length discrepancy, affecting the longer leg (26). This snapping may be reproduced on examination, most easily brought out by flexion from a position of adduction and extension. Inflammation or tightness of the fascia lata may result from overuse or disuse. Vague pain on arising, partially relieved by walking, and later aggravated by further prolonged walking are characteristic (46). Pain is most easily reproduced with the patient on the table with the involved hip uppermost, and downward pressure is placed on the straight leg held over the edge of the table. Pain should be reproduced along the area of fascia lata, and tenderness may also be detected here. Dimpling along the fascia has also been described, and is thought to result from adhesions. Local injection of steroids with anesthetic into symptomatic locations is often helpful. In addition, exercises designed to stretch the fascia should be performed by the patient with weight applied to the ankle (3-10 lb) as the leg is held extended over the edge of a table, as in the examination noted above.

Trochanteric Bursitis

The bursa lying between the laterally placed trochanter of the femur and the overlying tendon of the gluteus maximus is particularly prone to acute and chronic irritation and subsequent low-grade inflammation. Probably one of the most common causes of pain in and around the hip, this disorder is characteristically associated with pain which is more severe at night, but may get worse with certain movements which require gluteal strain. Symptoms may improve with local heat application or sleeping with a pillow under the involved buttock to keep body weight lifted off the bursa, but local anesthetic-corticosteroid injection is usually dramatically successful and results in prompt relief.

Iliopectineal Bursitis

Pain in the anterior pelvis, groin, and thigh sometimes radiating to the knee may be caused by irritation of the bursa lying between the iliopsoas muscle and the iliopectineal eminence. This type of pain is very difficult to distinguish from that of true hip joint disease, and hip movement and x-rays of the joint space itself should be normal before this diagnosis is entertained. Local heat, antiinflammatory or analgesic medications, or careful injection of the bursa with corticosteroid are often successful.

Ischial-Gluteal Bursitis

Exquisite pain over the ischial prominence, made worse with sitting or lying, may result from irritation of the bursa over the ischial prominence, and has been referred to as "weaver's bottom," "tailor's bottom," or "back pocket wallet syndrome," often being caused by repetitive trauma in this area. Point tenderness over the ischial tuberosity, reproducing the painful syndrome is helpful in making this diagnosis, but intrinsic hip disease and sciatica should be ruled out, since the latter conditions may coexist (47). Careful injection of the area with anesthetic and corticosteroid may be undertaken but care should be taken to avoid injection of the sciatic nerve.

Entrapment Neuropathies

Intermittent numbness and tingling in the hips and thighs should suggest an entrapment neuropathy. The abdominal cutaneous nerve can occasionally be irritated at the margin of the rectus muscle, and result in burning pain across the lower abdomen. The obturator nerve may be irritated following a pelvic fracture, osteitis pubis, or in association with an obturator hernia, and result in pain in the groin traveling down the inner thigh. Probably the most common of the entrapment neuropathies involves the lateral femoral cutaneous nerve, and is known as meralgia paresthetica. This syndrome is characterized by paresthesia and pain over the upper anterolateral thigh. This entrapment occurs at the anterior superior iliac spine, and may result from a leg length discrepancy, prolonged sitting with crossed legs, or as a result of marked abdominal obesity or use of a tight corset or belt. Local steroid injections are recommended as are avoidance of contact pressure or weight loss for relief of symptoms (46).

Pyriformis Syndrome

The pyriformis muscle may cause sciatic nerve irritation or may itself become irritated due to strain and cause pain and tenderness in the buttock between the ischium and the greater trochanter. This syndrome is sometimes seen in joggers, and usually responds to a combination of local ice or heat, rest, and toe-touching exercises with the legs crossed.

Knee

As shown in Figure 12.13, the knee is a very complex structure, and pain may be caused by stress or irritation of any of several areas.

Patellofemoral Pain Syndromes

Pain and crepitation in the area of the patella which is worse during activities that require knee flexion under stress suggests one of the patellofemoral pain syndromes. Chondromalacia of the patella is commonly part of this syndrome and probably results from a variety of mechanical problems, including malalignment of the quadriceps with lateral displacement of the patella, abnormal medial patellar facet or hypermobility (48,49). In this syndrome, pain is reproduced when the examiner presses the patella during knee motion. Radiological evaluation will show loss of cartilage, irregularity of the patella facets, and deviation of the patella. Tangential views of the patella (skyline view) are necessary to demonstrate these abnormalities. A similar type of pain may be caused by tendonitis

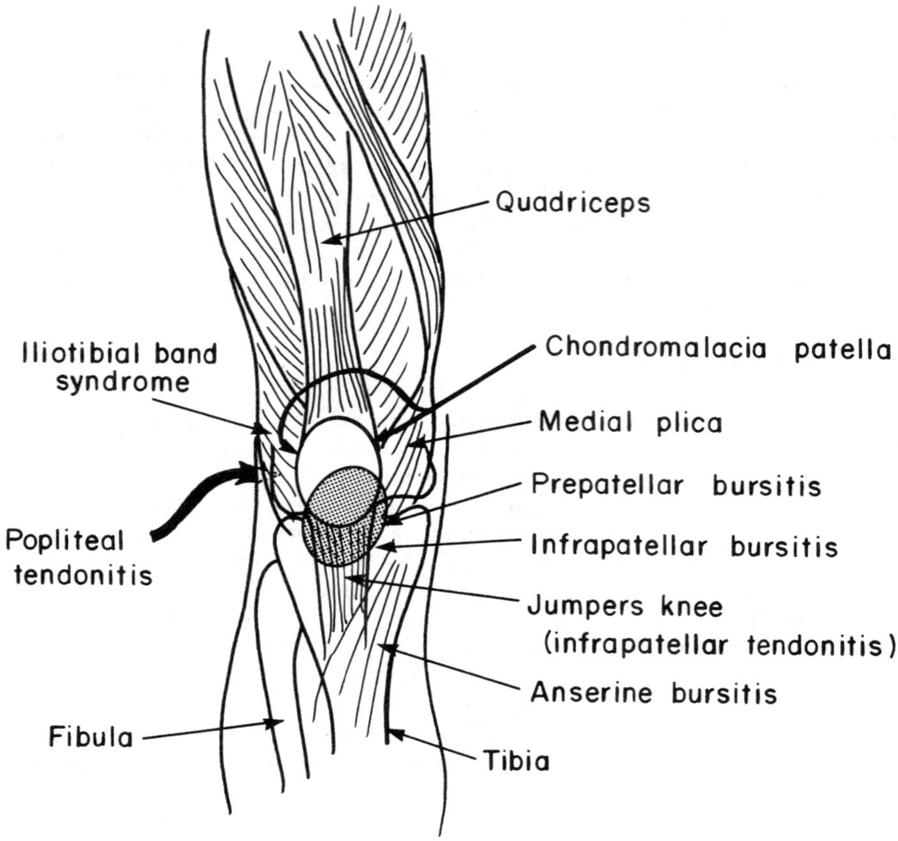

FIGURE 12.13 Common causes of nonarticular knee pain (see text).

of the infrapatella tendon which often results from jumping in athletic endeavors (jumper's knee). Patellofemoral pain syndromes are managed initially by conservative measures, such as antiinflammatory drugs, restriction of activity, and quadriceps strengthening exercises. These exercises are designed to maintain muscle tone and may serve to correct patellar alignment. Where conservative measures fail, surgical correction of the abnormality or patellar shaving may be necessary.

Bursitis

There are at least 12 bursa located in the knee region. Among the better known anteriorly are the suprapatellar, prepatellar, and infrapatellar bursae. Posteriorly are located the gastrocnemius and semimembranous bursae between the muscle groups. Medially are located the sartorius and anserine bursae. Any of these bursae may become inflamed either as a result of local trauma or systemic inflammatory disease. Pain, swelling, and point tenderness over the involved area are characteristic. Anserine bursitis is characterized by medial knee pain, very often in the fat pad, and is seen more often in obese females. Pain at night is a characteristic feature or anserine bursitis. Swelling and fluctuance should suggest infection, and aspiration should be undertaken as with other forms of bursitis. Aspiration of fluid with or without injection of local steroids is often therapeutic, but avoidance of the repetitive initial trauma is a necessary part of the management as well.

Popliteal Tendinitis

Pain and tenderness in the posterior or posterior-lateral aspect of the knee should suggest this diagnosis. Straight-leg raising is painful, and local corticosteroid injection in the tender points often provides dramatic relief (50).

Pellegrini Stieda Syndrome

Trauma or soft tissue injury to the medial or lateral collateral ligament about the knee may result in swelling, transient localized synovitis, restriction of knee flexion and calcification in the area of the ligament. This syndrome occurs most often in adult males, and calcification appears 3-4 weeks after an injury. Calcification may be seen without symptoms, but the syndrome is usually painful, and gradually resolves over several months (51).

Iliotibial Band Syndrome

The lower end of the fascia lata inserts over the lateral tibial condyle. Vigorous running, hiking, or other exercise may result in pain in the lateral knee secondary to friction and inflammation of this tendon as it courses over the lateral femoral condyle. Pain is particularly severe when the knee is held at 30-40° while supporting weight. Effusion or instability does not occur, and the syndrome usually responds to rest, antiinflammatory medication, or local steroid injection.

Plica Syndrome

As the knee joint and suprapatellar pouch develop, they eventually join, leaving behind several folds or shelves of synovium at their junction, known as plica (52, 53). The medial suprapatellar plica is the most common of these, and may become irritated by blunt trauma or twisting. Pain over the medial aspect, locking, and giving way are common symptoms. Physical examination will reveal a palpable snap over the medial femoral condyle. Diagnosis must be confirmed by arthoscopy, and excision of the offending plica can be accomplished during this procedure. Conservative treatment with hamstring stretching, rest, and antiinflammatory medications are helpful in some patients.

Lower Leg

Shin Splints

This term is used to describe syndromes of pain and discomfort in the lower leg that occur after repetitive overuse such as in jogging, running, or excessive walking. Pain is usually felt along the lower half of the medial border of the tibia. A dull aching sensation usually occurs at first with exertion and is relieved by rest, but later may become continuous. The syndrome is usually related to overuse of underdeveloped, untrained muscles, and probably results from increased pressure in the posterior tibial muscles (the posterior compartment just behind the interosseous membrane (54,55). Stress fracture or musculotendinous tears should be considered in the differential diagnoses and should be ruled out. The initial step in management is rest and avoidance of running on hard surfaces. Exercises to stretch and strengthen the posterior tibial muscles and use of proper supportive footwear are essential to prevent recurrence.

Anterior Compartment Syndrome

The anterior compartment is much more prone to increased pressure with resulting ischemia. Symptoms may be similar to that of shin splints, but usually begin 10-12 hours after unaccustomed exercise or after serious trauma (54). Increased pain in the anterior compartment after passive toe flexion is an early sign of the syndrome, and may be followed by pallor and extreme tenderness over the area. When severe, the syndrome requires measurement of compartment pressure to confirm the diagnosis, and surgical decompression by fasciotomy.

Osgood-Schlatter Disease

This syndrome results from avulsion of the tibial tubercle at the insertion of the patellar tendon usually after trauma or extreme overuse, and occurs almost exclusively in adolescent boys. Pain in this syndrome will occur when climbing stairs, kneeling, or in other activities requiring quadriceps movement. Radiographic evaluation may be unremarkable, but fragmentation or avulsion may be evident. Management of this generally benign syndrome usually includes casting for several weeks, temporary avoidance of contact sports, and quadriceps strengthening exercises.

Leg Cramps

Cramps in the lower leg, often occurring at night, occur in people of all ages, but are more common in elderly individuals. These should be differentiated from the cramp of intermittent claudication, which should occur during use and be relieved by rest. Cramps may be seen in normal individuals, but may also be seen after usually heavy exertion, during pregnancy, as a result of intrinsic muscle disease or motor neuron disease, or as a result of sodium or potassium depletion. In addition, certain medications, especially phenothiazines, terbutaline, and morphine have been associated with cramps (1). Medications commonly used for this condition include quinine and diphenhydramine. In addition, phenytoin, procainamide or dantrolene have been used in refractory cases. Exercises to stretch the calf muscle before retiring have been used with some success (56). The patient is instructed to stand 2-3 feet from the wall, place the hands on the wall and climb up the wall with the hands with the heels kept flat on the floor.

Restless Leg Syndrome

Vague pain, often exquisite and associated with a restless sensation and continuous leg movement, has been described in a number of patients. Although considered to be of psychogenic or hysterical origin by many, others have implicated overuse of caffeine in this poorly described syndrome (57). Leg stretching exercises and low doses of tricyclic antidepressants have been used with some success (54).

Reflex Sympathetic Dystrophy

Throbbing, burning pain in the leg, often following minor trauma, associated with signs of vascular instability and later atrophy of the skin and osteoporosis can be seen in the lower extremity. Physical findings and laboratory studies are similar to that seen in the upper extremity, where it is much more common and easily recognized (see above). Analgesic medication, vigorous physical therapy, and a short course of oral prednisone may be beneficial.

Ankle and Foot

Pain in the ankle and foot may result from simple sprains or one of several other entities, illustrated in Figure 12.14.

Ankle Sprain

Ankle sprains probably represent the most common soft tissue problem in the ankle. Sprains are classified in three grades: grade 1 involves mild ligamentous stretching, grade 2 implies a partial disruption of ligaments, and grade 3 represents complete ligament disruption (58). The collateral ligaments on either side of the ankle

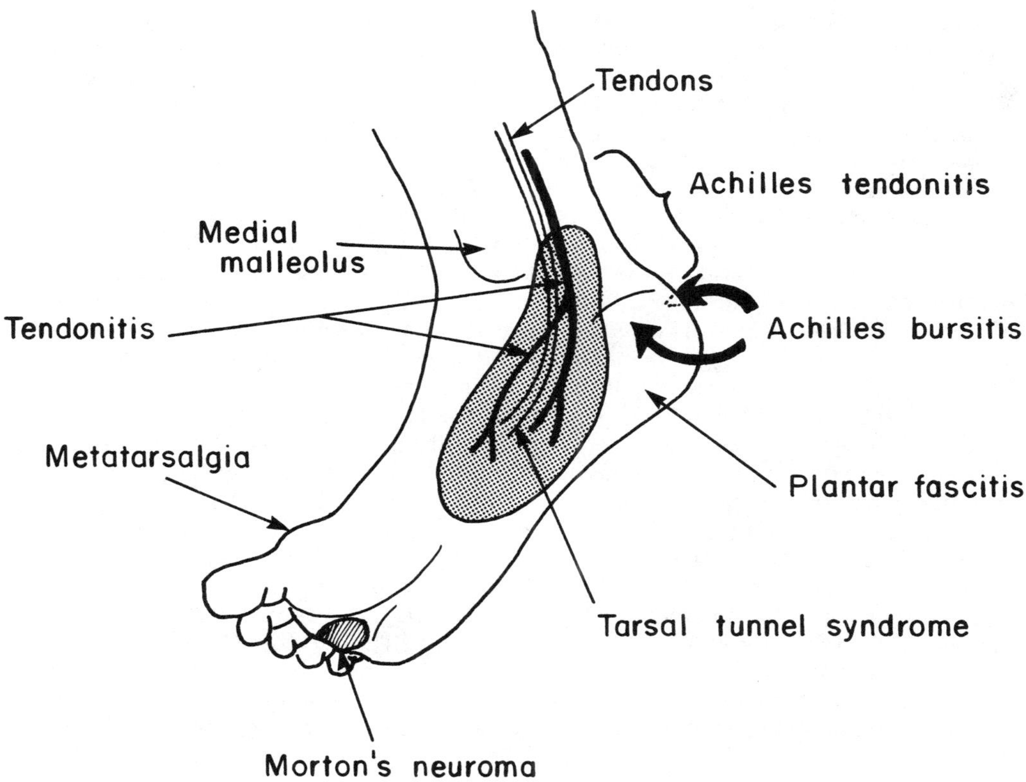

FIGURE 12.14 Common causes of foot pain (see text).

may be injured but this usually occurs in the lateral ligaments and is associated with inversion of the ankle. On examination, pain will be increased on forced inversion, and there will be tenderness in one or more of the three components of the lateral collateral ligaments, below the lateral malleolus. The medial collateral ligament may also be strained, and findings here are similar. Management of ankle sprain depends on the severity of the injury. Grade 1 sprains can be managed with local cold, elevation, and rest for the first 24-48 hours. Radiographic examination to exclude avulsion fracture or other bony abnormality should be undertaken in most cases, and when instability is present, stress radiographs are often obtained to document this. More extensive injury may require casting. Gradual remobilization, ankle strapping and elastic support, and supportive shoes should be used during the recovery. Lack of rapid response and any question of ligamentous instability are indications for early orthopedic referral, since seemingly trivial injuries may result in significant impairment of future athletic endeavors.

Tendonitis

Pain in the ankle region associated with local areas of tenderness and low-grade inflammation should suggest tendonitis of one of the many tendon sheaths crossing the ankle joint. Overuse syndromes or systemic inflammatory disease may involve the tibialis anterior, tibialis posterior, extensor digitorum longus or peroneal tendons. In these situations, tenderness should be localized over the affected area. These syndromes usually respond to immobilization, physical therapy to maintain range of motion, and antiinflammatory medications or local tendon sheath injections. Peroneal tendon dislocation is relatively common and is often associated with a snapping sensation and feeling of ankle instability, but little pain. Occasionally, dislocation can be detected by careful inspection of the area of the lateral malleolus. This dislocation may spontaneously reduce, but often requires cast immobilization or surgery. Achilles tendonitis causes pain in the heel, often radiating up into the calf and is worsened by dorsiflexion. There is often marked tenderness, swelling, and warmth over the achilles tendon, particularly near its insertion at the calcaneous, and bursitis in the superficial and deep bursa near the insertion may coexist. This syndrome may be seen in any of the spondyloarthropathies, but is most often due to overuse, particularly in joggers or in those using improperly fitting shoes (58). Complete rupture of the Achilles tendon may be seen, particularly as a sports-related injury in an untrained individual. This is usually associated with an audible snap during strenuous activity. On examination, an abnormal Thompson test will be seen. In this test the patient kneels on a chair and the examiner squeezes the calf muscle. A lack of plantar flexion of the foot represents a positive test. Achilles tendonitis is best managed by rest, local application of ice (acutely) and heat (chronically), and gradual remobilization. The use of an orthotic device to elevate the heel during walking or jogging is helpful, and stretching exercises designed to stretch the heel cord (as described above for leg cramps) are important during the rehabilitation period. Aspirin and other nonsteroidal antiinflammatories are helpful during this phase as well. Because of the risk of Achilles tendon rupture, local injection of corticosteroid is contraindicated in most cases. Complete Achilles tendon rupture necessitates early orthopedic consultation for immobilization or surgical repair.

Heel Pain

Pain in the heel may result from a wide variety of conditions, including bursitis, tendonitis, periostitis, fasciitis, or spurs. Nodular lesions over the lower Achilles region, referred to as "pump bumps," often result from poorly fitting shoes and may be associated with bursitis (59). Bursitis over the lateral aspect of the heel is often referred to as "last bursitis" and also results from poorly fitting shoes (60). Pain at the base of the heel often results from subcalcaneal bursitis or plantar fasciitis.

Plantar Fasciitis

The plantar fascia is a thick deep ligamentous structure that courses from its attachment on the tuberosity of the calcaneous distally into five slips, one attaching at each toe. Strain of this fascia may result from jumping, prolonged standing, and may be seen in association with rheumatoid arthritis, gout, or ankylosing spondylitis (61). In addition, an association with obesity and flat feet has been noted. Although this syndrome is often associated with radiographic evidence of plantar heel spurs, the relationship between spurs and fasciitis is somewhat unclear. Plantar fasciitis is characterized by plantar foot pain which is made worse with walking. There should be reproducible tenderness along the fascia, sometimes with localized point tenderness, made worse by forced dorsiflexion of the foot. Management of underlying problems, such as obesity, correction of flat feet, or treatment of underlying systemic disease should be undertaken first. The use of arch supports (either rigid or foam rubber) may be helpful, and often must be gradually introduced over a period of several weeks. Local injection of tender points with steroids and anesthetic with a very small gauge needle is useful. Nonsteroidal antiinflammatory medications are helpful as well. In addition, in those patients who must walk on concrete floors, the use of crepe-soled shoes is helpful (59).

Metatarsalgia

Pain acorss the ball of the foot (MTP joints) can result from a variety of conditions, including pes cavus, shortened Achilles tendon, Morton's neuroma, or inflammatory arthritis of the MTP joints themselves (62). Deformities of the first metatarsal may result in abnormal mechanics of weight-bearing for the rest of the metatarsal arch and result in ligamentous and muscular strain causing pain across the arch. The second metatarsal is relatively immobile, and the region under the head of this bone is particularly subject to aggravation by poorly fitting shoes. Painful bunions associated with hallux valgus deformity or corns and calluses, associated with irritation by confining shoes are common causes of metatarsalgia. Careful evaluation for underlying articular abnormalities should be undertaken in evaluation of these syndromes. Properly fitting shoes with a broad toe box are often helpful. A metatarsal bar, placed behind the metatarsal heads, will often result in tremendous symptomatic relief by reducing stress across the metatarsal heads. Self-molding inserts and other types of shoe inserts that provide cushioning and support for the entire foot are helpful as well. Weight reduction and proper shoes are the most important aspects of management. In athletes or other very active patients, stress fractures of the metatarsals should be suspected. When localized pain is palpated over one of the metatarsals, x-rays will often be normal during the first few weeks, and follow-up radiographs or bone scan may be necessary to demonstrate the abnormality. The second and third metatarsal shafts are the most commonly fractured. Most stress fractures will respond to immobilization, but casting may be necessary in patients who will not restrict their activities, as with compulsive long-distance runners.

Flat Feet

The loss of the normal longitudinal arch of the midfoot (pes planus) may be congenital or may result from faulty posture, obesity, trauma, or underlying rheumatic disease (59,62). Various types of flat feet are described, including spastic, rigid, or flexible, the latter being the most common and most important type. Many patients with flat feet have no symptoms. A flexible flat foot will appear normal, but the arch flattens with weight-bearing. When symptomatic, this will result in muscular fatigue and aching which is worse with prolonged walking or standing. Change in work habits or other foot injuries that result in abnormal gait may cause previously asymptomatic flat feet to become symptomatic. Treatment with orthotics and adjustment of shoes are designed to move the center of gravity to the outside of the foot and remove pressure from symptomatic areas (59). This usually involves a shoe with a tight instep, firm heel support, and a low heel. Exercises to strengthen intrinsic foot muscles may be helpful.

Disorders of the Toe

Hallux valgus deformity is often associated with a painful bursitis over the medial aspect. In addition to inflammatory arthritis, this condition may result from a congenital medial rotation of the metatarsal, and is exacerbated by overuse of ill-fitting shoes or high-heeled shoes. Prolonged hallux valgus deformity may result in loss of motion of the great toe, termed hallux rigidus. Treatment of disorders of the great toe begins with the use of shoes having an enlarged toe box and felt or other pads to reduce irritation of overlying bursa. The use of rigid sole support is also helpful. Local corticosteroid injection may provide temporary symptomatic relief, but surgical intervention is often necessary. The hammer toe deformity may result from lateral pressure from a hallux valgus or from tight shoes. The second toe is most frequently involved, with the toe being forced upward, resulting in forced flexion of the PIP and pointing of the tip of the toe downward. Painful callous formation over the dorsal aspect often results, and unless shoe modifications can be made to accommodate the toe, surgical intervention and correction of the deformity may be necessary.

Entrapment Neuropathies

The tarsal tunnel syndrome and interdigital nerve entrapment are the most common entrapment neuropathies in the foot. The tarsal tunnel syndrome results from entrapment of the posterior tibial nerve as it passes through the tunnel beneath the medial malleolus at the ankle (63). This syndrome is characterized by aching, burning, and tingling in the plantar and distal foot and toes. Sometimes pain will radiate to the calf. Symptoms are often worse at night or after prolonged standing. Physical examination reveals minimal abnormality in the joints, and no neurologic deficit. A Tinel's test may be performed by tapping over the area posterior and inferior to the medial malleolus, and symptoms should be reproduced by this maneuver. Tarsal tunnel syndrome may be seen in rheumatoid arthritis or other inflammatory conditions, or may result from local mechanical problems, such as trauma, fracture, or dislocation in the ankle area. Diagnosis may be confirmed by nerve conduction studies across the affected area, but normal values do not entirely exclude the syndrome. The syndrome often responds to local injection of a corticosteroid-anesthetic mixture, although surgical decompression may be necessary. Entrapment neuropathy of interdigital nerves may occur on the plantar surface of the foot between the heads of the metatarsals, most commonly between the third and fourth toes. This may or may not be associated with a neuroma in the region, often referred to as Morton's neuroma. Pain in the area of the metatarsal heads, radiating into the toes, and tingling and burning in nature should suggest this syndrome. Symptoms may be aggravated by walking on hard surfaces or wearing tight or high heeled shoes (59). Physical examination shows tenderness in the plantar aspect over the third and fourth metatarsals, and compression of the area will reproduce the symptoms. Direct pressure over the plantar aspect of this area, especially when associated with distal paresthesia, is even more specific. Management begins with conservative measures, most often designed to decrease pressure over the metatarsal heads and increase plantar flexion by the use of metatarsal supports or bars. Broad-toed shoes may allow more room for metatarsal heads and decrease compression on the nerve, and local corticosteroids may be helpful. Surgical removal of the neuroma and the nerve may be required, but often leaves an area of numbness.

References

1. Joekes AM: Cramp. *Clin Rheum Dis* 5:873-881, 1979.

2. Bywaters EGL: Lesions of bursae, tendons, and tendon sheaths. *Clin Rheum Dis* 5:883-926, 1979.

3. Nakano K: Entrapment neuropathies. In WN Kelley, ED Harris, S Ruddy, CB Sledge (eds.), *Textbook of Rheumatology,* 1st Ed. Philadelphia, W.B. Saunders, 1981, pp. 1829-1846.

4. Wakefield G: The entrapment neuropathies. *Clin Rheum Dis* 5:942-955, 1979.

5. Bland JH, Merrit JA, Boushey DR: The painful shoulder. *Semin Arthritis Rheum* 7:21-47, 1977.

6. Kozin F, Ryan LM, Carerra GF et al.: The reflex sympathetic dystrophy syndrome (RSDS) II. Scintigraphic studies, further evidence for the therapeutic efficacy of systemic corticosteroids, and proposed diagnostic criteria. *Am Jour Med* 70:23-30, 1981.

7. Smythe HA, Moldofsky H: Two contributions to understanding the "fibrositis syndrome." *Bull Rheum Dis* 28:928-931, 1978.

8. Smythe HA: Fibrositis and other diffuse musculoskeletal syndromes. In WN Kelley, ED Harris, S Ruddy, CB Sledge (eds.), *Textbook of Rheumatology,* 1st Ed. Philadelphia, W.B. Saunders, 1981, pp. 485-493.

9. Bennett RM: Fibrositis - Misnomer for a common rheumatic disorder. *West J Med* 134:405-413, 1981.

10. Yunus MB, Masi AT, Calabro JJ et al.: Primary fibromyalgia (fibrositis): Clinical study of 50 patients with matched normal controls. *Semin Arth Rheum* 11:151-171, 1981.

11. Mazanec DJ: First year of a rheumatologist in private practice. *Arthritis Rheum* 25:718-719, 1982.

12. Payne TC, Leavitt F, Garron PC et al.: Fibrositis and psychologic disturbance. *Arthritis Rheum* 25:213-217, 1982.

13. Griffin SJ, Trinder J: Physical fitness, exercise and human sleep. *Psychophysiology* 15:447-450, 1978.

14. Campbell SH, Clark S, Tindall EA, Forehand ME, Bennett RM: Clinical characteristics of fibrositis. I. A "blinded" controlled study of symptoms and tender points. *Arthritis Rheum* 26:817-824, 1983.

15. Rotes-Querol J: The syndromes of psychogenic rheumatism. *Clin Rheum Dis* 5:797-805, 1979.

16. Sheon RP, Moskowitz RW, Goldberg VM: The head and neck. *Soft Tissue Rheumatic Pain: Recognition, Management, Prevention,* 1st Ed. Philadelphia, Lea and Febiger, 1982, pp. 13-32.

17. Marbach JJ: Arthritis of the temporomandibular joints and facial pain. *Bull Rheum Dis* 27:918-921, 1977.

18. Loushin LL: Carotidynia. *Headache* 17:192-195, 1977.

19. Rizk TE, Pinals RS: Frozen shoulder. *Semin Arth Rheum* 11:440-452, 1982.

20. Bridgman JF: Periarthritis of the shoulder and diabetes mellitus. *Ann Rheum Dis* 31:69-71, 1972.

21. Cogen L, Anderson LG, Phelps P: Medical management of the painful shoulder. *Bull Rheum Dis* 32:88-92, 1982.

22. Kozin F: Painful shoulder and the reflex sympathetic dystrophy syndrome. In DJ McCarty (ed.), *Arthritis and Allied Conditions,* 9th Ed. Philadelphia, Lea and Febiger, 1979, pp. 1091-1120.

23. McCarty DJ, Halverson PB, Carrera GF, Brewer BJ, Kozin F: "Milwaukee shoulder" - Association of microspheroids containing hydroxyapatite crystals, active collagenase, and neutral protease with rotator cuff defects. I. Clinical Aspects. *Arthritis Rheum* 24:464-473, 1981.

24. Garancis JC, Cheung HS, Halverson PB, McCarty DJ: "Milwaukee shoulder" - Association of microspheroids containing hydroxyapatite crystals, active collagenase, and neutral protease with rotator cuff defects. III. Morphologic and biochemical studies of an excised synovium showing chondromatosis. *Arthritis Rheum* 24:484-491, 1981.

25. Sheon RP, Moskowitz RW, Goldberg VM: The Elbow. *Soft Tissue Rheumatic Pain: Recognition, Management, Prevention.* Philadelphia, Lea and Febiger, 1982, pp. 81-92.

26. Hazelman BL, Laurin CA, Tremblay GR: The injured joint with a "normal" x-ray. In WN Kelley, ED Harris, S Ruddv, CB Sledge (eds.), *Textbook of Rheumatology,* 1st Ed., W.B. Saunders, 1981, pp. 1809-1828.

27. Nevellos, AB: The treatment of tennis elbow with triamcinolone acetonide. *Curr Med Res Opin* 6:507-509, 1980.

28. Ho G, Tice AD, Kaplan SR: Septic bursitis in the prepatellar and olecranon bursae. *Ann Intern Med* 89:21-27, 1978.

29. Kirk JA, Ansell BM, Bywaters EGL: The hypermobility syndrome: Musculoskeletal complaints associated with generalized joint hypermobility. *Ann Rheum Dis* 26:419-425, 1967.

30. Jessee EF, Owen DS, Sagar KB: The benign hypermobile joint syndrome. *Arthritis Rheum* 23:1053-1056, 1980.

31. Sheon RP, Moskowitz RW, Goldberg VM: The wrist and hand. *Soft Tissue Rheumatic Pain: Recognition, Management, Prevention,* 1st Ed. Philadelphia, Lea and Febiger, 1982, pp. 93-114.

32. Graham JR: Localized systemic scleroses. In WN Kelley, ED Harris, S Ruddy, CB Sledge (eds.), *Textbook of Rheumatology,* 1st Ed. Philadelphia, W.B. Saunders, 1981, pp. 1235-1250.

33. Gelberman RH, Aronson D, Weisman NH: Carpal tunnel syndrome. *J Bone Joint Surg* 62A:1181-1184, 1980.

34. Sheon RP, Moskowitz RW, Goldberg VM: The thoracic cage and dorsal spine region. *Soft Tissue Rheumatic Pain: Recognition, Management, Prevention,* 1st Ed. Philadelphia, Lea and Febiger, 1982, pp. 115-134.

35. Epstein SE, Gerber LH, Borer JS: Chest wall syndrome. A common cause of unexplained cardiac pain. *JAMA* 241:2793-2797, 1979.

36. Calabro JJ: Costochondritis. *N Engl J Med* 296:946-947, 1977.

37. Quinet RJ, Hadler NM: Diagnosis and treatment of backache. *Semin Arthritis Rheum* 8:261-287, 1979.

38. Grabis SL, Mankin HJ: Pain in the lower back. *Bull Rheum Dis* 30:1040-1045, 1980.

39. Sheon RP, Moskowitz RW, Goldberg VM: The low back and pelvis. *Soft Tissue Rheumatic Pain: Recognition, Management, Prevention,* 1st Ed. Philadelphia, Lea and Febiger, 1982, pp. 135-171.

40. Mendelson G, Selwood TS, Kranz H, Loh TS, Kidson MA, Scott DS: Acupuncture treatment of chronic low back pain. A double-blind placebo-controlled trial. *Amer Jour Med* 74:49-55, 1983.

41. Wagner CJ: Williams' flexion regime in the treatment of low back pain. *J Int Coll Surg* 18:69-76, 1952.

42. Onofrio BM: Chemonucleolysis - Past and Present (Editorial), *Mayo Clin Proc* 58:207-208, 1983.

43. Gramse RR, Sinaki M, Ilstrup DM: Lumbar spondylolisthesis. A rational approach to conservative treatment. *Mayo Clin Proc* 55:681-686, 1980.

44. Jacoby RK, Sims-Williams H, Jayson MIV, Baddeley H: Radiographic stereoplotting - A new technique and its application to the study of the spine. *Ann Rheum Dis* 35:168-170, 1976.

45. Rodnan GP, Schumacher HR: Disorders of the lower back. *Primer on the Rheumatic Diseases,* 8th Ed. Atlanta, Arthritis Foundation, 1983, pp. 147-149.

46. Sheon RP, Moskowitz RW, Goldberg VM: The pelvis and thigh region. *Soft Tissue Rheumatic Pain: Recognition, Management, Prevention,* 1st Ed. Philadelphia, Lea and Febiger, 1982, pp. 172-184.

47. Swartout R, Compere EL: Ishiogluteal bursitis. *JAMA* 227:551-552, 1974.

48. Abernathy PJ, Townsend PR, Rose RM, Radin EL: Is chondromalacia patellae a separate clinical entity? *J Bone Joint Surg* 608:205-210, 1978.

49. Insall J: Current concepts review, patellar pain. *J Bone Joint Surg* 64A: 147-152, 1982.

50. Sheon RP, Moskowitz RW, Goldberg VM: The knee. *Soft Tissue Rheumatic Pain: Recognition, Management, Prevention,* 1st Ed. Philadelphia, Lea and Febiger, 1982, pp. 185-205.

51. Peterson HA: Leg aches. *Pediatr Clin North Am* 24:731-736, 1977.

52. Hardaker WT, Whipple TL, Bassett FH: Diagnosis and treatment of the plica syndrome of the knee. *J Bone Joint Surg* 62A:221-225, 1980.

53. Reid GD, Glasgow M, Gordon DA et al.: Pathologic plicae of the knee mistaken for arthritis. *J Rheumatol* 7:573-576, 1980.

54. Sheon RP, Moskowitz RW, Goldberg VM: The foreleg region. *Soft Tissue Rheumatic Pain: Recognition, Management, Prevention,* 1st Ed. Philadelphia, Lea and Febiger, 1982, pp. 206-212.

55. D'Ambrosia RD et al.: Interstitial pressure measurements in the anterior and posterior compartment in athletes with shin splints. *Am J Sports Med* 5:127-131, 1977.

56. Daniell HW: Simple cure for nocturnal leg cramps. *N Engl J Med* 301:216, 1979.

57. Lutz EG: Restless legs, anxiety, and caffeinism. *J Clin Psych* 39:693-695, 1978.

58. Jones SJ, Bates BT, Osteriing LR: Injuries to runners. *Am Jour Sports Med* 6:40-50, 1978.

59. Sheon RP, Moskowitz RW, Goldberg VM: The ankle and foot. *Soft Tissue Rheumatic Pain: Recognition, Management, Prevention,* 1st Ed. Philadelphia, Lea and Febiger, 1982, pp. 213-241.

60. Layfer LF: "Last" bursitis - A cause of ankle pain. *Arthritis Rheum* 23: 261, 1980.

61. Furey JG: Plantar fasciitis: The painful heel syndrome. *J Bone Joint Surg* 57A:672-673, 1975.

62. Rodnan GP, Schumacher HR: The foot. *Primer on the Rheumatic Diseases,* 8th Ed. Atlanta, Arthritis Foundation, 1983, pp. 162-163.

63. Goodgold J, Kopell HP, Spielholz NI: The tarsal-tunnel syndrome. *N Engl J Med* 273:742-745, 1965.

Chapter 13

SYSTEMIC LUPUS ERYTHEMATOSUS

Carlos A. Agudelo, M.D.

General

Systemic lupus erythematosus is a chronic, systemic, immunologically mediated disease of unknown etiology, affecting primarily young females and characterized by the presence of multiple autoantibodies and a variable clinical course (1).

The term lupus, a Latin derivative (lupus - wolf), has been used for several centuries to describe cutaneous conditions. The first recognition of systemic lupus erythematosus (SLE) is credited to Kaposi in 1872. Hebra in 1845 had described the "butterfly" appearance of the facial rash. Between 1895 and 1903 William Osler emphasized the systemic nature of the disease with polymorphic skin lesions, arthritis not progressing to crippling deformity, visceral manifestations (including gastrointestinal crisis), endocarditis, pericarditis, nephritis, and central nervous system involvement. In 1924 Emanuel Libman and Benjamin Sacks (2) described "a hitherto undescribed form of valvular and mural endocarditis." In this article they described four young patients with fever, endocarditis, pericarditis, pleuritis, arthritis, dermatitis, and nephritis, fulfilling current criteria for the diagnosis of SLE. They described as well the onion skin lesion of the splenic arteries. In 1922 Keith and Rowntree reported four patients with SLE and nephritis and stressed that nephritis was a common complication of SLE. Another important contribution to our understanding of SLE was that of Baehr, Klemperer, and Schiffrin with the description of the "wire loop" appearance of glomeruli in kidney biopsies in 1935. Klemperer, Pollack, and Baehr in 1941 introduced the term "diffuse connective tissue disorders." In 1948, Hargraves, Richmond, and Morton described the LE cell seen frequently in the bone marrow in patients with SLE and this soon became a useful diagnostic test. Immunofluorescence was introduced by Coons in 1951 and Friou described its application to blood and tissues of SLE patients in 1957 (1). In 1971, preliminary criteria for the classification of SLE were proposed (3), and in 1982 changes were made and a new revised criteria emerged (4).

Incidence and Prevalence

SLE occurs more frequently in young women between the ages of 15 and 40, but children and older individuals are often affected. Females are affected 7-10 times more commonly than males. Even though this condition occurs in all races, it appears to be more common in blacks and Chinese. A prevalence of 1 in 245 black women aged 15-64 has been reported, and overall prevalence of SLE in the United States is about 1 in 1000 women. An increased incidence of SLE, other connective tissue diseases, and serologic abnormalities has been reported in relatives of patients with SLE.

Etiopathogenesis

Animal Models for SLE

The New Zealand Black (NZB) and NZB/NZWF1 hybrid mouse and two new strains of mice (MRL/1 and BXSB) and the canine lupus model have significantly contributed to the understanding of pathogenetic mechanisms involved in SLE (5). Multiple factors may play a role in the development of SLE, including genetic, immunologic, environmental, hormonal, and viral influences. The studies in animal models suggest that diverse genetic backgrounds are consistent with the development of SLE. Early in their development there is a polyclonal B-cell hyperactivity which persists throughout the life of the animal with no demonstrable T-cell regulatory abnormality. The predilection to disease in the female NZB/WF1 appears related to the female sex hormone environment. Hormonal manipulation with testosterone suppresses proteinuria, reduces autoantibodies, and prolongs survival, while castration of the male increases disease expression. Studies on both mice and humans have failed to demonstrate a viral etiology.

In humans, genetic influences may be important in the development of SLE (6). HLA typing studies have described associations with the HLA-D region, mostly HLA-DRW2 and HLA-DRW3. A higher incidence of SLE and other immunological abnormalities such as positive ANA and false-positive STS have been described in relatives of patients with SLE. Several deficiencies of the complement system have been described in association with SLE and other connective tissue diseases.

Hormonal factors may play a role and may partially explain the predominance of SLE in women of child-bearing age, the association with Klinefelter syndrome, and the possible influence of contraceptive pills. Certain drugs and ultraviolet light are environmental factors that may precipitate the disease in some predisposed individuals.

There is no solid proof that immune complexes are central in the pathogenesis of SLE, but they are thought to mediate tissue damage found in many organs and tissues of SLE patients. Complexes of various nuclear antigens and antibodies will fix complement and lead to such tissue damage. Other antibodies directed against cell membrane antigens may cause tissue damage as well (6).

Clinical Features

The clinical presentation of SLE may be quite protean. The disease may have a sudden onset, sometimes after sun or drug exposure, with high fever, multisystem involvement, polyserositis, CNS manifestations, or may run a chronic course with remissions and exacerbations. SLE may be a relatively benign condition with minimal arthralgias, arthritis, and immunologic abnormalities. Most SLE patients will first seek medical attention because of musculoskeletal or dermatological manifestations.

Musculoskeletal Manifestations

Polyarthralgias and/or polyarthritis are the most common manifestations, and arthritis occurs in 80–90% of patients. The small joints of the hands, wrists, and knees are most commonly involved, and the disease is usually symmetrical. Multiple joints may be involved at any one time, mimicking rheumatoid arthritis, or there may be only involvement of a few joints. In many patients arthritis is not only the most common but the major manifestation of the disease. Tendonitis may also occur. The arthritis of SLE is typically nondeforming and erosions are not usually seen; a few patients (5%) may develop ulnar deviation and swan neck deformities secondary to chronic inflammatory changes in the soft tissues of the joint. Morning stiffness is a frequent complaint, usually lasting less than one hour, and joint symptoms may be severe. Clinical findings may be quite mild and often do not correlate with symptomatology. Joint function is usually preserved. SLE should always be suspected in patients presenting with a chronic nondeforming polyarthritis. In most patients, synovial fluid shows less than 3000 cells/mm^3 with a good to fair mucin clot and viscosity; LE cells may be present (7). Occasionally, higher white counts in the synovial fluid are found, and in cases of monoarticular presentation, infectious arthritis should be considered.

Aseptic necrosis of the bones may occur in the absence of corticosteroid therapy, but in most cases is associated with its long-term use. Younger females may be at higher risk for the development of this complication and the hips, knees, and shoulders are most frequently affected.

An inflammatory myopathy, manifested by pain and tenderness of muscle and proximal weakness may occur. The diagnosis is confirmed by elevated enzymes, EMG, and biopsy findings. It should be differentiated from a steroid-induced myopathy which usually does not cause elevation of muscle enzymes and lacks inflammatory components on biopsy.

Cutaneous Manifestations

The dermatologic manifestations of SLE are numerous and some type of rash is noted in about 80% of patients. (See Table 13.1.)

These cutaneous lesions may be highly specific, such as discoid lupus, or nonspecific such as urticaria, purpura, and vasculitis. The malar rash, shown in Figure 13.1, frequently adopting a butterfly distribution and sparing the nasolabial folds, is quite common and characteristic of lupus. This lesion usually leaves no scarring and is different from the discoid lesions characterized by erythema with follicular plugging, telangiectasia, and atrophy. Discoid lesions, as seen in Figure 13.2, may occur as a localized process (discoid lupus) with no other clinical or serological evidence of SLE or as manifestation of SLE and in both settings the lesions are histologically undistinguishable. About 30% of the patients give a history of photosensitivity. A seasonal relationship to the onset of SLE has been

TABLE 13.1 SLE. Mucocutaneous Manifestations

Butterfly rash
Malar rash
Discoid lesions
Photosensitivity
Urticaria
Vasculitis - microinfarcts
Raynaud's phenomenon
Oral ulcerations
Nail changes
Alopecia
Maculopapular eruption
Purpura
Bullous lesions

described, with more patients noting the onset of SLE during the summer months in the southeast. In patients with established disease, sun exposure may lead to exacerbations or additional manifestations.

Maculopapular eruptions resembling drug reactions, erythema multiformlike eruptions, urticaria, periungual erythema, and nail changes with pitting, ridging, and onycholysis may occur. Vasculitic skin lesions occur in about 30% of SLE patients and frequently are associated with other signs or symptoms of active disease. Often these lesions occur in hands and feet, on the palms and soles and on the tips of the fingers and toes, and they may be tender. Microinfarcts may develop and an occasional patient may develop digital arteritis; livedo reticularis is another vascular manifestation occasionally occurring in patients with SLE. When sitting or standing patients may develop a dusky discoloration in the feet (8).

Bullous lesions have been described and a recent association with dermatitis herpetiformis has been reported. Oral mucosal ulcerations have been identified in about 30% of patients. These ulcerative lesions are usually painless, occurring in the hard or soft palate, and are often associated with active disease. Since they are asymptomatic it is important to look for them. Nasal ulcerations may lead to septum perforation. Histologically, mucosal lesions show nonspecific mononuclear cell infiltrates with immunoglobulins and complement deposits in vessel walls and along epithelial borders.

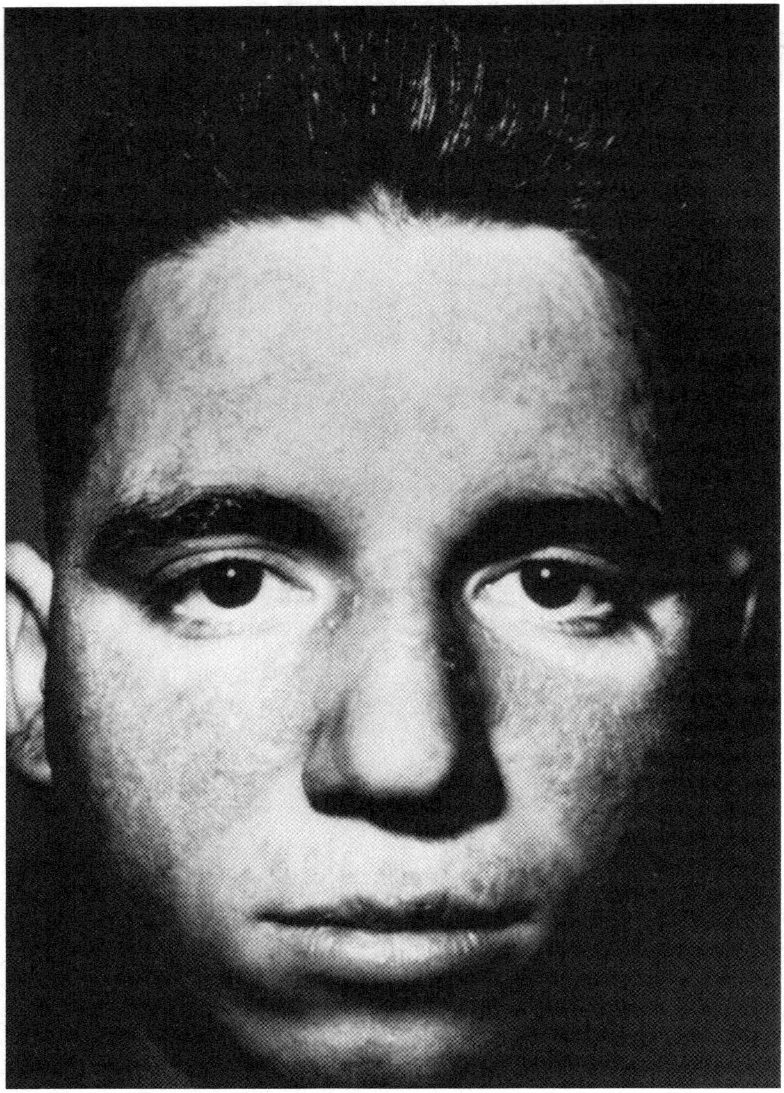

FIGURE 13.1 Typical butterfly malar rash of SLE. Often related to sun exposure, this rash will usually heal without scarring. (Reprinted from the Revised Clinical Slide Collection on the Rheumatic Diseases, copyright 1981. Used by permission of the Arthritis Foundation.)

Recently a subset of SLE patients has been identified as ANA-negative lupus and characterized by photosensitivity and polycyclic, annular, cutaneous lesions; these patients frequently have antibodies directed against cytoplasmic RNA macromolecules, anti-RO (SSA) (9).

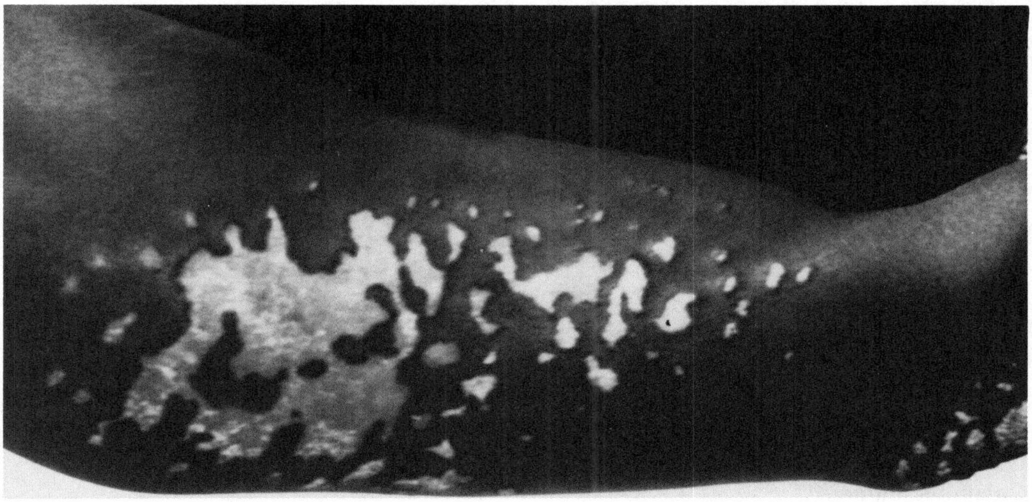

FIGURE 13.2 Rash of discoid lupus, which may occur with or without evidence of systemic disease. These lesions may be located on the face, scalp, trunk, or any extremity. They often begin as keratotic erythematous plaques, and heal with thinning and hyper- or hypopigmentation.

Rheumatoid-like subcutaneous nodules have been noted in a small percentage of patients. They are usually smaller than the nodules in rheumatoid arthritis and are often of short duration. Raynaud's phenomenon is found in up to 20% of the patients with SLE; it may be the first sign of the disease, persisting for several years before other manifestations occur. Even though it has been excluded from the 1982 criteria, it continues to be a useful clue to the disease.

Alopecia is quite common and an important manifestation occurring in up to 65% of patients. The distribution may be patchy or total, and new hair growth may alternate with alopecia. Most often the patients complain about diffuse hair loss which may occur at initial presentation or later on during disease flares. Documentation of hair loss initially can be made by gently pulling a small amount of hair. Hair usually will regrow with control of the disease. Discoid lesions in the scalp heal with scarring and atrophy and leave areas of alopecia and hypo- or hyperpigmentation. As with Raynaud's phenomenon, alopecia has been excluded from the recent criteria; however, it continues to be useful in the diagnosis and management of the disease.

Serositis

Pleural effusions are common in SLE and occur in about 35% of the patients. They are usually small to moderate and can be bilateral. Pleuritic pain without definite pleural effusion is common as well. Most often the pleural fluid is clear exudate with a high protein content, normal sugar and during acute exacerbations polymorphonuclear cells predominate; LE cells may be present and complement levels are low. Pleural tissue shows mild inflammatory infiltrate mainly composed of lymphocytes, macrophages, mononuclear cells, and neutrophils. Perivascular accumulation of such cells may be noted.

Pericarditis is the most common cardiac manifestation of SLE and occurs in about 30% of the patients. Typically, patients present with substernal chest pain which is aggravated by motion and pericardial or pleural rubs may be heard. There may be other signs or symptoms of active disease. The electrocardiogram is often helpful, but echocardiography is the most sensitive method of confirming the diagnosis. Pericardial thickening may be found and rarely pericardial tamponade or calcific deposits with constrictive signs occur. Pericardial fluid is an exudate with low complement levels. Pathologically, immunoglobulin and complement deposits are found with foci of fibrinoid degeneration and inflammatory cell infiltration (10).

Abdominal pain is a frequent complaint in SLE patients and in some it may be due to aseptic peritonitis. Persisting abdominal pain or localizing findings on physical examination should be viewed as an emergency as it may represent infarction, bowel perforation, vasculitis, or some other abdominal catastrophe. Ascites has been described in about 4% of SLE patients and peritoneal involvement was found in 60% of patients at postmortem examination in one study.

Cardiovascular

Pericarditis is the most common cardiac manifestation as previously discussed. Other manifestations listed in Table 13.2, include myocarditis, endocarditis, coronary artery disease, arrhythmias, and congenital heart block (10).

Evidence of myocarditis is found in 25-50% of autopsy studies. Earlier studies, perhaps reflecting more severe, untreated cases, found a higher incidence of myocarditis, while more recent studies have found a lower incidence. Myocarditis may be manifest clinically by unexplained tachycardia, enlarged heart, gallop rhythm, or new murmurs. Even though reduction in left ventricular function by echocardiography has been detected, lupus myocarditis usually does not lead to cardiac insufficiency. Although subepicardial and myocardial fat is increased in SLE patients at autopsy, this may be related to chronic corticosteroid therapy, rather than the disease process itself.

TABLE 13.2 Cardiac Manifestations of SLE

Pericarditis
Myocarditis
Endocarditis
Coronary artery disease
Arrhythmias
Congenital heart block

Nonbacterial endocarditis in SLE was described by Libman and Sacks in 1924 (2). Although this is not a clinical diagnosis, it is frequently a postmorten finding. Systolic murmurs are common in patients with SLE but they do not correlate with endocarditis at autopsy. Mitral and aortic valve disease leading to aortic insufficiency has rarely been reported. Pathologically, the vegetations are small, 1-4 mm in diameter, occurring near the edge of the ventricular side of the valve, on chordae tendinae, papillary muscles, or mural endocardium. There might be necrosis of valve tissue with lymphocytes and plasmacytic infiltrates occasionally leading to calcific deposits; IgG and complement deposits have been detected by immunofluorescent studies and a preponderance of left-sided lesions has been reported.

Coronary artery disease as the result of vasculitic involvement or secondary to atherosclerosis may occur. There have been several reports of young SLE patients, without familial predisposing factors to ischemic heart disease, dying of myocardial infarction proven to be atherosclerotic in origin at autopsy. High-dose chronic corticosteroid therapy may have played a role in the induction of these early atherosclerotic lesions in lupus.

Conduction abnormalities and congenital heart block may occur, although high grade heart block and life-threatening arrhythmias are very uncommon in SLE. Pathological study of conduction tissue has noted foci of inflammatory cells as well as fibrosis along the course of this specialized tissue.

Blant and Stephen first described the phenomenon of congenital heart block in the offspring of a lupus patient (11). Since that time about 100 cases of neonatal lupus have been reported and the syndrome has been characterized by congenital heart block, transient cutaneous lesions, or both; occasionally hepatic or hematological abnormalities have been noted. It has been estimated that one-third of children born with congenital heart block, will have mothers who have or will develop SLE, Sjögren's syndrome, rheumatoid arthritis, or some other connective tissue disease. It is thought that a maternal antibody, anti-SSA/Ro passes across the placenta to the fetus where it induces tissue damage. The skin lesions resolve and the heart lesion heals but leaves permanent sequelae with endomyocardial fibrosis or fibroelastosis. This prevents the atrial-ventricular node from connecting with the His bundle, leading to permanent complete heart block. The autoantibody is only a transient phenomenon in the infant, disappearing within 6 months, but is a permanent serological abnormality in the mother. The syndrome may recur in successive pregnancies and affected children may be at risk for developing SLE later in life. A recent association with the HLA-DR3, HLA-MB2, HLA-MD2, and HLA-B8 in the mothers but not in the infants has been noted (12, 13).

Pulmonary Manifestations

Even though multiple pulmonary manifestations have been described, pulmonary involvement in SLE has been less well studied and characterized (14). Radiographic evidence of pleural involvement is present in about one-third of the patients at some time during the course of the disease but pleuritic pain and dyspnea are more common. Pleuritis may be unilateral or bilateral and it may occur in association with pericarditis. Small pleural effusions are the rule and the pleural fluid is normally clear but hemorrhagic effusions have been reported. The fluid is an exudate and glucose levels are normal. WBC count in the pleural fluid is usually less than 5000 cells, pH is normal, and LDH is less than 500 units. LE cells may be present and antinuclear antibodies may be positive. Low C3 and C4 have been reported. Pleural histology shows a cellular infiltrate consisting mainly of lymphocytes and plasma cells. (See Serositis.)

The frequency of pulmonary parenchymal lesions due to SLE ranges from 9 to 98% in different studies, reflecting the specialized interest of various authors. Haubt, Moore, and Hutchens recently reviewed the clinical and pathologic features of 120 patients with SLE described in autopsy records (14). Interstitial pneumonitis, interstitial fibrosis, pulmonary vasculitis and pulmonary hematoxylin bodies were attributable to SLE. Alveolar hemorrhage, wall necrosis, edema, and hyaline membranes, previously attributed to SLE were found in many cases to be secondary to intercurrent infection, congestive heart failure, renal failure, aspiration, increased intracranial pressure, and oxygen toxicity.

Acute pneumonitis in SLE may present with fever, dyspnea, pleuritic chest pain, and cough. Gross hemoptysis has been noted in a few patients. Chest x-ray will demonstrate bibasilar infiltrates. Episodes may be self-limited or the patients may go on to develop chronic infiltrates. Those patients developing dyspnea on exertion usually are found to have diffuse interstitial lung disease and the diagnosis is based on the radiographic findings of persistent, diffuse interstitial infiltrates. Pulmonary function tests reveal a restrictive pattern. Pathology is nonspecific with some thickening of the alveolar walls noted and moderate plasma cell infiltration. Immunofluorescence has showed immune complex deposits in the alveolar walls. In those patients with SLE presenting with pulmonary manifestations, drug toxicity (immunosuppressives) and infection have to be excluded.

Renal Manifestations

The incidence of clinically serious renal involvement in SLE is about 50%. Virtually all patients with systemic lupus erythematosus whose renal tissue is studied by light microscopy, immunofluorescence, and electron microscopy prove to have some evidence of involvement. Nephritis is a prominent feature of the disease and a major cause of morbidity and mortality. Renal disease in lupus occurs early, is more frequent in women, and the first clue to its presence is an abnormal urinalysis with proteinuria, hematuria, and cellular casts often in combination (see Table 13.3). Occasionally significant renal involvement is found despite a normal urinalysis. Most patients with active renal disease show evidence of multisystem involvement and a number of immunological abnormalities (8,15).

Proteinuria is the most common urinary abnormality and it may be minimal, moderate, or severe as in the nephrotic syndrome. Often, there is hematuria and cell casts. Red cell casts are found in those patients with glomerulitis and correlate with more severe involvement such as diffuse proliferative glomerulonephritis. Hypertension is unusual in the absence of corticosteroid therapy except in patients with severe renal involvement.

The classification of renal disease in SLE is based on renal biopsy findings obtained by light microscopy (LM), electron microscopy (EM), and immunofluorescence (IF), as seen in Table 13.4.

The incidence of the various forms of lupus nephritis is difficult to assess since renal biopsies are not obtained on all SLE patients and the value of biopsies has been questioned. Completely normal renal biopsies are unusual in SLE and most patients will show some type of abnormality. Patients with mesangial or minimal lupus glomerulonephritis will have normal-appearing glomeruli or may show some increase in mesangial cells and matrix on light microscopy. Immunofluorescence will reveal IgG and C3 deposits in the mesangium and electron dense deposits by EM. Mild proteinuria and hematuria may be noted and in general these patients have a good prognosis. Occasionally, however, there will be progression to a more serious form of involvement such as diffuse proliferative glomerulonephritis.

TABLE 13.3 Renal Abnormalities at Diagnosis and During the Course of SLE

	Within 6 Months of Diagnosis %	At Diagnosis or During Course of Disease %
Proteinuria (any)	54	78
Persistent trace	6	4
1+	13	11
2+	5	11
3+	9	13
4+	19	27
Hematuria	35	42
WBC	30	42
Casts	23	30
Fixed specific gravity	6	8
Serum albumin <3 g	26	31
Serum creatinine >1.5 mg	20	31
BUN <21	67	59
21-35	13	19
36-50	6	6
51-70	3	4
>70	3	10
Cholesterol 280	28	41

Modified from Rothfield N (8).

TABLE 13.4 Classification of Renal Involvement in SLE

Normal with no immune deposits
Normal by LM with immune deposits
Mesangial lupus nephritis
Mild (focal) glomerulonephritis
Diffuse proliferative glomerulonephritis
Membranous glomerulonephritis
Interstitial and tubular nephritis

Patients with focal proliferative glomerulonephritis will show increased mesangial matrix and hypercellularity with segmental proliferation, necrosis and leukocytic infiltration in less than 50% of the glomeruli. Subendothelial electron dense deposits by EM and immunoglobulins, and C3 by IF will be evident. Some deposits may be noted as well in the subepithelial and intramembrane areas. The prognosis in these patients is usually good and urinary abnormalities include a mild proteinuria and hematuria. Nephrotic syndrome is uncommon and renal function is usually normal.

Diffuse proliferative glomerulonephritis (DPGN) is the most serious form of renal involvement in lupus. Virtually all glomeruli are involved with hypercellularity; sclerotic changes may be present and may be a sign of poor prognosis. IF and EM show extensive mesangial, subendothelial, and subepithelial deposits with uneven distribution. This type of nephritis carries the worst prognosis, with approximately 70-80% 5-year survival. Moderate to heavy proteinuria is common and, during periods of exacerbation, hematuria and RBC casts are noted. During active disease and at times antedating changes in renal function, antibodies to native DNA and low serum complement levels are often seen. Renal insufficiency is more common in DPGN. Thus, elevation in serum creatinine and serum uric acid levels early in the course of the disease might be a clue to this form of nephritis, if a renal biopsy is not done.

Membranous lupus nephritis is characterized by diffuse thickening of glomerular capillary walls with no proliferation. Immunofluorescence reveals deposits of immunoglobulins and complement along the basement membranes and this involvement leads more frequently to nephrotic syndrome. A few RBC's may be noted in the urine but this is not a frequent finding and DNA antibodies are usually negative. Despite control of the disease, most of the patients continue to have persistent proteinuria and may develop mild renal insufficiency. Their prognosis is usually good.

In other patients, interstitial and tubular renal disease is noted. These may occur in combination with glomerulonephritis and the histological findings are of focal or diffuse infiltrates with inflammatory cells and immune deposits. Some patients may develop a very severe type of renal involvement with rapidly progressing glomerulonephritis, hypertension, and necrotizing vasculitis with fibrinoid necrosis; they have a very poor prognosis and these may be a subset of patients with diffuse proliferative glomerulonephritis.

Nervous System Involvement

A wide variety of neurological and psychiatric manifestations have been described in SLE and involvement of the nervous system is now recognized in 25-75% of patients (16). The recognition and treatment of nervous system manifestations of SLE are difficult and prognosis is variable. The clinical variability and the lack of specific diagnostic laboratory criteria may complicate distinction from the neurological sequelae of secondary metabolic disturbance, drug treatment, or incidental illness (17). Bresnihan has proposed a clinical classification of CNS lupus, as seen in Tables 13.5 and 13.6 (16).

Psychiatric manifestations are very common. Mild mood changes to overt psychosis occur. Some patient may develop an organic psychosis with hallucinations, delirium, etc., or functional changes with anxiety and depression. Psychiatric problems may be due to the disease itself, coinciding with periods of activity, or may be a reaction to the disease or medications. Occasionally, psychotic features may coincide with the introduction of high-dose corticosteroid therapy and, if due to the medication, usually clear on reduction of the dose. CNS involement

TABLE 13.5 Classification of CNS Lupus

Primary	Neurological Psychiatric Mixed neuropsychiatric
Secondary	Uremia Hypertension Infection Coagulopathy Corticosteroids

Reproduced from Bresnihan (16), *Clinics in Rheumatic Disease,* W.B. Saunders, 1982.

TABLE 13.6 Neurological Manifestations of Primary CNS Lupus

Anatomical	Pathophysiological	Clinical
Meningeal	Aseptic meningitis	Meningism, headache
Cerebral	Cortical atrophy	Loss of higher function, dementia
	Vascular episodes	Strokes, subarachnoid hemorrhage, migraine
	Seizure disorders	Grand mal, petit mal, Jacksonian, temporal lobe
	Movement disorders	Chorea
	Extrapyramidal disorders	Rigidity, tremor
	Pseudotumour cerebri	Headaches
	Hypothalamic-pituitary disorders	Inappropriate ADH secretion
Cerebellar		Ataxia
Spinal	Transverse myelitis, apparent demyelination	Paraparesis, multiple sclerosis-like disorder
Peripheral nerves (cranial, spinal)	Basal meningitis, neuritis, neuromuscular junction disorder	Cranial and peripheral sensory and motor neuropathies, mononeuritis multiplex, myasthenia gravis, Guillain-Barré syndrome

Reproduced from Bresnihan (16), *Clinics in Rheumatic Disease,* W.B. Saunders, 1982.

correlates with highly active severe disease and worse prognosis. Neurological features may occasionally be the initial manifestation of the disease. Grand mal seizures occur in about 20% of patients and may be severe. Petit mal seizures, Jacksonian fits, and temporal lobe epilepsy also occur. Some patients may present with a clinical picture resembling multiple sclerosis. Peripheral neuropathy is seen in about 5% of patients. Aseptic meningitis occurs but is a diagnosis of exclusion.

There is no characteristic pathological lesion of CNS lupus. Microscopic infarcts are common, but in other patients gross hemorrhagic lesions may be seen. Occasionally immune complex deposits have been seen in choroidal vessels, but true vasculitis is rare.

Gastrointestinal Manifestations

Abdominal pain is a frequent complaint of patients with SLE and may represent a mild serositis. In other patients the pain may be more severe, such as that seen associated with pancreatitis. Vasculitis with mesenteric arteritis and perforation of the colon may occur. As with any other patient, other causes of abdominal pain, such as appendicitis, must be considered; thus, early surgical consultation is important in the evaluation of patients with abdominal pain.

In other patients, GI symptoms may be secondary to drug therapy, such as GI irritation caused by nonsteroidal antiinflammatory agents, high-dose corticosteroid therapy, or immunosuppressives. In association with other signs of active disease, mild abnormalities of liver function may be noted. In most patients, however, such abnormalities may be secondary to aspirin or other medications. Hepatosplenomegaly may occur.

Ocular Manifestations

Probably the most frequent ocular manifestation in SLE is that due to keratoconjunctivitis sicca (Sjögren's syndrome). The patients may complain of dry eyes or may have been using artificial tears. Conjunctivitis, episcleritis, and papilledema have also been reported. Retinal lesions in the form of small, white exudates in the absence of hypertension or diabetes are usually a manifestation of retinal vasculitis (cytoid bodies). They are seen in about 10% of SLE patients and their presence is highly suggestive of systemic lupus erythematosus. Blindness secondary to vasculitis has been reported. Subcapsular cataracts in corticosteroid-treated patients may be seen.

Sjögren's syndrome is probably underdiagnosed in SLE patients. Due to the multisystem nature of both entities, SLE and primary Sjögren's syndrome, it may be difficult at times to differentiate these conditions from each other.

Pregnancy in SLE

Menstrual abnormalities with periods of amenorrhea are seen in patients with SLE and tend to coincide with periods of severe active disease. Flares may occur during pregnancy or immediately after delivery or abortion. Many patients with mild lupus go through pregnancy without developing particular problems; however, they have to be followed closely and treated vigorously with corticosteroids should signs of active disease develop. Patients with a previous history of lupus nephritis, those with active disease at the beginning of pregnancy, or those who develop the disease while pregnant are at high risk of developing severe flares during pregnancy or in the period following delivery (18). Close interaction among rheumatologist, obstetrician, and pediatrician during this period is of utmost importance.

Except for transient immunological abnormalities, mild malar rash, and the occurrence of congenital heart block, no other abnormalities are usually noted in children born to SLE mothers.

Diagnosis

In 1971, the American Rheumatism Association proposed preliminary criteria for the diagnosis of SLE (3). These criteria were revised and updated to incorporate new immunologic knowledge and improve disease classification in 1982 (4). At least four of the 11 criteria listed in Table 13.7 must be present serially or simultaneously during any interval of observation for the purpose of identifying patients with SLE. It appears that not all 11 criteria have equal diagnostic value, and it has been suggested that malar rash, discoid rash, photosensitivity, renal, neurologic, or immunological disorder have better discriminating ability (19).

These new 1982 criteria excluded Raynaud's phenomenon and alopecia, which had been included in the 1971 criteria. These findings were excluded because of low sensitivity and specificity, but they continue to be useful in some patients.

Clinical Variants

There may be many clinical similarities between SLE, mixed connective tissue disease, and primary Sjögren's syndrome. Patients with SLE may have high titers of RNP antibodies, a hallmark for mixed connective tissue disease. In other patients an overlap syndrome may exist with characteristics of other connective tissue diseases such as dermatomyositis, polymyositis, or rheumatoid arthritis.

Over 90% of patients with active SLE have antinuclear antibodies. Therefore, less than 10% of patients with active disease will fulfill criteria for the diagnosis but have a negative ANA test and are thus called ANA negative lupus. Some of these patients may have anticytoplasmic and anti-Ro antibodies. These ANA-negative patients have a high incidence of dermatitis and photosensitivity and a lower incidence of renal and neurological manifestations. A similar clinical presentation may occur in patients with complement deficiencies, usually in those with C2 deficiency.

Several inherited deficiencies of the complement system have been associated with connective tissue diseases (mostly SLE) and infections (see Table 13.8). Homozygous or heterozygous deficiencies of C2 are the most common deficiencies and many of these patients develop a connective tissue disorder of which SLE is the most frequently found. Dermatomyositis, vasculitis, discoid lupus erythematosus, and juvenile rheumatoid arthritis have also been described. Dermatological manifestations are common (20).

Drug-Induced SLE

A number of medications are able to induce a clinical syndrome resembling systemic lupus erythematosus (see Tables 13.9, 13.10) (21,22). Clinical differentiation from idiopathic SLE is made on the basis of exposure to the offending drug, improvement of the symptoms following discontinuation of the drug (although immunological abnormalities may persist for a long time), normal serum complement levels and a low frequency of renal involvement and absence of anti-DNA antibodies. ANA antibodies in drug-induced SLE are usually antihistone antibodies. Lupus-like syndromes were first described after hydralazine therapy in 1954. In 1962, procainamide-induced lupus was described. Prolonged therapy with hydralazine leads to positive ANA in approximately one-third of the patients. Only a few

TABLE 13.7 Diagnostic Criteria for SLE (8)

Criterion	Definition
Malar rash	Fixed erythema, flat or raised, over the malar eminences, tending to spare the nasolabial folds
Discoid rash	Erythematous raised patches with adherent keratotic scaling and follicular plugging; atrophic scarring may occur in older lesions
Photosensitivity	Skin rash as a result of unusual reaction to sunlight, by patient history or physician observation
Oral ulcers	Oral or nasopharyngeal ulceration, usually painless, observed by a physician
Arthritis	Nonerosive arthritis involving 2 or more peripheral joints, characterized by tenderness, swelling, or effusion
Serositis	Pleuritis - convincing history of pleuritic pain or rub heard by a physician or evidence of pleural effusion OR Pericarditis - documented by ECG or rub or evidence of pericardial effusion
Renal	Persistent proteinuria greater than 0.5 g/day or greater than 3+ if quantitation not performed OR Cellular casts - may be red cell, hemoglobin, granular, tubular or mixed
Neurologic	Seizures - in the absence of offending drugs or known metabolic derangements; e.g., uremia, keto-acidosis, or electrolyte imbalance OR Psychosis - in the absence of offending drugs or known metabolic derangement, e.g., uremia, keto-acidosis, or electrolyte imbalance
Hematologic	Hemolytic anemia with reticulocytosis OR Leukopenia - less than 4000/mm^3 total on 2 or more occasions OR Lymphopenia - less than 1500/mm^3 in the absence of offending drugs OR Thrombocytopenia - less than 100,000/mm^3 in the absence of offending drugs

Immunologic	Positive LE cell preparation OR Anti-DNA: antibody to native DNA in abnormal titer OR Anti-Sm: presence of antibody to Sm nuclear antigen OR False-positive serologic test for syphilis known to be positive for at least 6 months and confirmed by *Treponema pallidum* immobilization or fluorescent treponemal antibody absorption test
Antinuclear antibody	An abnormal titer of antinuclear antibody by immunofluorescence or an equivalent assay at any point in time and in the absence of drugs known to be associated with drug-induced lupus syndrome

TABLE 13.8 Inherited Complement Deficiencies and Associated Diseases

Component	Associated Diseases			Other
	SLE	Infection	Renal	
Classical Pathway				
C1q	+++	+	+	
C1r	+++	+	+	
C1s	+	0	0	
C2	+++	++	++	Vasculitis, asthma
C4	+++	+	+	
Alternative Pathway				
P (properdin)	0	+	0	
B	(none reported)			
D	(none reported)			
C3	0	+++	+	
Terminal Sequence (C3)				
C5	+	+++	0	
C6	+	+++	0	
C7	+	+++	+	
C8	++	+++	0	
C9	+	+++	0	

TABLE 13.8 (Cont'd)

Component	Associated Diseases SLE	Infection	Renal	Other
Control Proteins				
CHNH (C1 inhibitor)	++	0	0	Hereditary angioedema
1 (C3b/C4b inactivator)	0	+++	0	
H (β1H)	(none reported)			
C (C4 binding protein)	(none reported)			

0 = none reported.
+ = low or only one patient reported.
++ = occurs more often than expected.
+++ = number of patients reported indicates strong association with component deficiency.
Modified from Rynes (20).

TABLE 13.9 Drugs Capable of Activating Lupus Through Probable Pharmacological Properties (Group 1)

Hydralazine
Procainamide
Anticonvulsants
Mephenytoin
Dyphenylhydantoin
Primidone
Trimethadione
Ethosuximide
Carbamazepine
Phenylethylacetylurea
Isoniazid
Chlorpromazine

Reproduced from Alarcon-Segovia (22), *Clinics in Rheumatic Disease*, W.B. Saunders, 1975.

TABLE 13.10 Other Drugs Implicated in the Causation of Systemic Lupus Erythematosus and/or Antinuclear Antibodies (Group 2)

Animosalveilic acid	Oxyphenisatin
Chlorthalidone	Penicillin
D-penicillamine	Phenylbutazone
Griseofulvin	Practolol
Guanoxan	Propylthiouracil
Isoquinazepon	Quinidine
L-dopa	Reserpine
Methyldopa	Streptomycin
Methysergide	Sulphonamides
Methylthiouracil	Tetracycline
Oral contraceptives	Tolazamide

Reproduced from Alarcon-Segovia (22), *Clinics in Rheumatic Disease*, W.B. Saunders, 1975.

patients so treated will develop drug-induced lupus. It has been found that slow acetylators are more likely to develop a lupus-like syndrome after hydralazine, procainamide, and isoniazid therapy. After 6 months of therapy with procainamide most patients will develop positive ANA's but only about 10% may go on to develop drug-induced lupus. Symptoms such as fever, malaise, weakness, and weight loss occur. As in the case of idiopathic lupus, arthralgias are frequent and a nondeforming arthritis occurs. Pleuropulmonary involvement is common, particularly after procainamide therapy, with pleuritis reported in over one-third of the patients. Pericardial tamponade and constrictive pericarditis have been described. In distinction to idiopathic SLE, dermatitis occurs in less than one-third of the patients.

Possible mechanisms by which different medications induce antinuclear antibodies and drug-induced lupus include a predisposition such as that occurring in slow acetylators or some other genetic markers, a cross-reactivity of drugs with nuclear antigens, or perhaps interaction of the medications with lymphocytes (21). Once the diagnosis of drug-induced lupus is established or suspected, the offending drug should be stopped. In many patients the symptoms will resolve within a few days or weeks. However, in some others, the symptoms may persist for longer periods of time, particularly in SLE induced by hydralazine. In those patients with severe drug-induced lupus, corticosteroids may be required.

Laboratory

General

Hematological abnormalities are very common in patients with SLE (23). Anemia occurs in most patients during active disease and it may be of immune or non-immune origin. Most often the patients will have a normocytic and normochromic anemia with normal bone marrow iron stores and a low serum iron. This is called anemia of chronic disease. This anemia is usually mild and treatment is directed to the control of the systemic disorder. In some patients the anemia may be complicated by chronic blood loss, renal disease, or be drug-induced. Even though a positive Coombs test may be present in about 20% of the patients with SLE, significant autoimmune hemolytic anemia occurs in less than 10% of the patients. Some patients may have a mild chronic hemolytic process for which the bone marrow is able to compensate and in some others the hemolytic anemia may be quite severe with hemoglobin values dropping to 4-5 g%. This type of anemia usually responds to corticosteroid therapy. A few cases or pure red-cell aplasia have been described. Bone marrow depression may be present and may be either secondary to the disease itself or drug-induced, such as that occurring with cytotoxic therapy.

Leukopenia occurs in about 30-50% of the patients at some time in the course of their disease. Depression of circulating granulocytes is common and it may be due to peripheral destruction secondary to antigranulocyte antibodies or to decreased marrow production. Circulating lymphocytes also may be reduced and in some cases correlate with severe disease. The lymphopenia may be secondary to cytotoxic antibodies (23).

Mild thrombocytopenia with counts between 100,000 and 150,000 is common. Severe thrombocytopenia, usually secondary to peripheral destruction, occurs in about 5% of the patients. Evans syndrome (hemolytic anemia and idiopathic thrombocytopenic purpura) may be the first manifestation of the disease. Defects in granulocytes and platelet function have been described.

Generalized lymphadenopathy occurs in about 20% of the patients and it may be an early manifestation. Pseudolymphoma and lymphoma usually of the non-Hodgkins class have been described.

Coagulation abnormalities have been described, and are mostly due to the presence of an inhibitor of clotting factors or the so-called lupus anticoagulant. This inhibitor affects both the intrinsic and extrinsic pathways of the coagulation system by interfering with the binding of phospholipid to form prothrombin activator. It may be present as well in other conditions and is not limited to SLE. In some patients, this anticoagulant may be associated with a tendency for thrombotic events and its presence has been correlated with the false-positive serologic test for syphilis. The lupus anticoagulant can be identified by the presence of a marked prolongation of the partial thromboplastin time. These patients are not more prone to bleeding. Specific inhibitors of factors VIII, IX, and XII also have been described and their identification is important since they may lead to bleeding episodes.

False-positive serologic test for syphilis occurs in about 20% of the patients and it may be the first manifestation of the disease. Its recognition is very important to avoid unnecessary concern to the patients or their families. Occasionally, positive treponemal antibodies have been described with the FTA or MHAT tests.

A characteristic feature of SLE is the presence of numerous serologic abnormalities. Hypergammaglobulinemia is common. The sedimentation rate is elevated and may remain high in clinically apparent remissions. Increases in serum C-reactive protein may correlate with active disease or infection.

Multiple antibodies directed against nuclear and cytoplasmic constituents have been found, including antibodies against native (double-stranded) and single-stranded DNA, DNA-histone, and nuclear-RNA proteins. The LE cell was first described in 1948 by Hargraves et al. It is present in about 70% of the patients with active disease. However, ANA testing, which is positive in over 90% of the patients, is preferred by most clinicians and laboratories. The presence of antinuclear antibodies lacks diagnostic specificity and must be correlated with clinical findings. Testing by immunofluorescence may reveal several patterns: 1) homogenous or diffuse pattern; 2) a peripheral, rim, or shaggy pattern which is present in about 20% of the patients and is quite specific for SLE; 3) speckled pattern which correlates best with anti-SM or anti-RNP antibodies (ribonucleoprotein); and 4) nucleolar. High titers of RNP and antinucleolar antibodies are more frequently seen in mixed connective tissue disease and scleroderma respectively. Anti-Sm antibodies may be present in about 25% of the patients, but they are highly specific for SLE. Antibodies against native (double-stranded) DNA are present in about 25-70% of the patients depending on the test used for their detection. Their presence at high levels correlates well with serious, active renal disease. Ro and La antibodies (SSA-SSB) may be present in a small percentage of patients, mostly in those with secondary Sjögren's. A positive rheumatoid factor occurs in about 30% of the patients with SLE. Immune complexes are commonly found (see Chapter 2).

Activation of the complement system either through the classic or the alternate pathway occurs often in SLE. Low complement levels, CH5O, C3, and C4 correlate best with active renal disease. Inherited deficiencies of component of the complement system have been described and these patients may be more susceptible to connective tissue diseases.

Other Laboratory Abnormalities

Mild cerebrospinal fluid abnormalities may be present during episodes of CNS disease. Modest elevations in CSF protein and cell count with a normal fluid pressure may correlate with organic disease. Lowered CSF fluid C_4 levels have been associated with active CNS lupus, and antineuronal antibodies have been described. EEG and brain-scan are not considered useful tests in the diagnosis or management of CNS lupus. CT scans may uncover vascular abnormalities, cerebral infarcts, and atrophy, and they may prove to be more useful in CNS lupus.

Pathological abnormalities have been described in each of the different organ systems. The place of renal biopsy in the diagnosis and management of lupus nephritis has been questioned and its role remains controversial. Even though renal biopsy abnormalities will be demonstrated in most patients with SLE, the identification of those patients with more severe forms of the disease as well as those with milder forms is important. We advocate use of renal biopsy early in the course of the disease since early identification of diffuse proliferative glomerulonephritis may allow the institution of prompt and vigorous therapy before significant renal damage occurs.

Immunofluorescence of the skin using antibodies to immunoglobulins and complement reveals immunoglobulin and complement deposits at the dermal-epidermal junction (the lupus band test) in about 50% of uninvolved skin and in almost 100% of patients with skin lesions. Even though it may be positive in patients with inactive disease, it is most often positive in those with severe active disease and appears to correlate with anti-DNA antibodies and renal disease. The test is not specific for lupus since it can be positive in other diseases. Recently, a possible subset of SLE patients has been described and characterized by renal involvement, positive ANA, and positive lupus band test of the skin as the only manifestations of the disease.

Prognosis and Management

Prior to the description of LE cells and antinuclear antibodies most diagnosed cases of SLE were of patients with severe disease fulfilling six or more of today's criteria. Because of this, the prognosis was considered quite poor and the 5-year survival was less than 30-40%. Since that time the prognosis has progressively improved with 5-year survival approaching 90% in recent series, as we have learned more about the disease and milder cases are being diagnosed. Most patients will experience at some time in the course of their disease generalized symptoms such as arthralgias, myalgias, easy fatigability, and fever.

Proper management of the disease depends on an appreciation of the enormous variability of the potential course of the illness in any one patient (24). The onset of the disease and subsequent exacerbations may be related to precipitating factors such as infections, sun sensitivity, drugs (such as oral contraceptives, penicillin, and sulfonamides), operations, pregnancy, and emotional stress. General measures include education of the patient and his or her family regarding the disease, proper rest during periods of active disease, avoidance of drugs such as those previously mentioned or the ones the patient may have reacted to in the past, and avoidance of excessive sunlight, particularly those with photosensitivity. There are a number of sunscreen products available for protection. These should be applied to areas vulnerable to sunburn 30-60 minutes before going out in the sun.

Improved criteria for the diagnosis and increased awareness of the disease by physicians and the public have led to early recognition in many patients, and milder forms are being diagnosed. Many patients have a benign, mild form of the disease requiring only observation. Many of these patients have arthralgias, occasionaly episodes of arthritis, mild dermatitis, mild hematological abnormalities, and a positive ANA requiring no specific medication. The continued improvement in the survival rates of SLE patients observed during the last 30 years may be due to multiple factors, including improvement in our knowledge of the natural course of the disease, early diagnosis, diagnosis of milder forms and of possible complications, early detection of infection, corticosteroids and better antibiotics.

In some patients, however, arthritis can be more severe with signs of chronic active disease and a symmetric polyarthritis mimicking rheumatoid arthritis early on. The nondeforming appearance, good functional status, low WBC in the synovial fluid, and the positive ANA help differentiate the arthritis of SLE from rheumatoid arthritis. Aspirin, other salicylates, or other nonsteroidal antiinflammatory agents and hydroxychloroquine may be required. Some SLE patients may be more sensitive to toxicity from ibuprofen and serious side effects may occur. In those patients with a history of renal involvement nonsteroidals should be avoided since they may induce further renal damage. In a few patients aspirin can induce hepatic toxicity that improves after discontinuation of the drug. For those patients with articular and dermatological manifestations significant enough to require treatment, hydroxychloroquine, 200-400 mg daily, may be effective. Its usefulness is limited due to retinal toxicity with potential blindness and the patients require ophthalmological evaluations at baseline and every 4-6 months. Occasional flares occur during spring and summer months and antimalarials might be used during this period. As the patient improves the dosage may be reduced to 200 mg daily and in some patients the drug may be stopped for several months. Retinal toxicity appears to correlate with higher cumulative doses, and after a total dose of 400 g has been reached, the medication should be stopped to avoid ocular toxicity.

Corticosteroid therapy has a clearly beneficial effect on the severity of many clinical features of systemic lupus erythematosus and improves survival in high-risk patients (24). Indications for the use of corticosteroids include severe multisystem involvement, severe autoimmune hemolytic anemia, or thrombocytopenic purpura. Starting dosages range from 60 to 80 mg daily in divided doses (every 6-8 hours) and, as the patient improves, the medication is switched to once a day therapy. With further improvement, slow tapering should be continued and in some patients control may be achieved with alternate day therapy.

In some patients with multisystem organ involvement and fever, control may be achieved with lower doses of prednisone therapy, starting at 20-30 mg daily in divided doses. As control is achieved, the medication is slowly tapered. As a guideline, once the disease is under control, we suggest tapering from 60 mg daily, decreasing the dose by 5-10 mg every week and trying to control the patient on alternate day corticosteroid therapy. The patient may be tapered from 60 mg daily to 60 alternating with 50 for 1 week, 60 alternating with 40 for another week, 60 alternating with 30 for another week, and 60-25 for another week. Thereafter, the lower dosage is tapered more slowly, eventually reaching a dosage of 60 mg every other day. This alternate day dose then may be gradully tapered further. If, during this period, disease activity flares, adjustments in medication made be made. Occasionally, on days off the prednisone, the patients may have mild arthralgias not requiring therapy. For those with more severe articular symptoms, salicylate therapy might be of benefit. In many patients, active disease may be controlled on very low doses of corticosteroid therapy, in the range of 10 mg every other day. At this low dose, few side effects are noted and further decreases in the dose may bring about flares of the disease requiring daily therapy.

The management of lupus nephritis and severe CNS disease is more controversial (24-28). Even though most of these patients are treated with high-dose corticosteroid therapy, the value of such therapy remains unproven in well-controlled studies. Those patients with mesangial, focal, or membranous glomerulonephropathy, carry a better prognosis, and may require less vigorous therapy, thus avoiding the side effects associated with long-term high-dose corticosteroid therapy. For those patients with diffuse proliferative glomerulonephritis, many medications have been advocated, including high-dose corticosteroid therapy, pulse methyl-prednisolone therapy, combination with other immunosuppressive medications (cyclophosphamide, azathioprine, chlorambucil), and plasmapheresis. These multiple therapies reflect the lack of evidence that any particular one is better than any other in the treatment of lupus nephritis. The protean nature of the disease with many different clinical presentations makes the selection of therapy even more difficult for the clinician. Those patients with diffuse proliferative glomerulonephritis and persistently elevated anti-DNA antibodies and persistently low C3 have a worse prognosis and warrant aggressive therapy. Acute deterioration of renal function due to active disease also may respond to corticosteroid or immunosuppressive therapy. Vigorous therapy for patients with advanced renal disease may produce more toxicity than benefit and in these patients a program of chronic hemodialysis and/or renal transplantation may be more suitable. Many of the patients at this stage of the disease are only mildly symptomatic if at all and most of the immunological abnormalities disappear. The results of renal transplantation have been good even though an occasional patient may have a flare of the disease, perhaps as a consequence of normalization of renal function or decreases in the immunosuppressive therapy.

The treatment and prognosis of nervous system involvement in systemic lupus erythematosus are difficult to assess. This is due to the clinical variability, lack of specific diagnostic laboratory criteria, and other complicating factors such as metabolic disturbance, medication, or incidental illness such as infection or hypertension. Therapy should be individualized and every attempt should be made to exclude other causes for CNS symptoms such as CNS infections, hypertensive crisis, uremia or other metabolic disturbance, and steroid-induced psychosis. Often, patients may develop psychological symptoms which are secondary to the knowledge of having a chronic disease that may be fatal. Symptoms from active disease, weight gain, and changes in appearance from steroid therapy may also be significant contributing factors. For those patients with more severe symptoms such as psychosis or for those who become suicidal, psychiatric care will be necessary. Headaches are being recognized more frequently in patients with SLE. These may be secondary to hypertension, infection, or active disease.

Aseptic meningitis occurs and occasionally may be seen in patients treated with ibuprofen. Different types of movement disorders are described, including epileptic seizures and chorea. In patients with seizures it is very important to exclude other possible causes, such as hypertension or infection. The seizures may be due to active disease and control attained by corticosteroid therapy and antiepileptic medication. Status epilepticus has a worse prognosis and IV corticosteroid therapy in high doses together with antiepileptic measures and medications may be beneficial in some patients.

Several immunosuppressives, including azathioprine, cyclophosphamide, and chlorambucil, and plasmapheresis have been used to treat patients with severe SLE. Severe side effects including bone marrow depression, hemorrhagic cystitis, infection, and the possibility of increased risk for the development of neoplastic disorders in the case of immunosuppressives, limit their potential usefulness.

Patients with SLE may receive the influenza vaccination. It is suggested that immunization be performed when the patient is not taking large doses of corticosteroids or immunosuppressives.

References

1. Talbott JH: Historical background of discoid and systemic lupus erythematosus. In EL Dubois (ed.), *Lupus Erythematosus,* 2nd Ed. Los Angeles, University of Southern California Press, 1974, pp. 1-11.

2. Libman F, Sacks B: A hitherto undescribed form of valvular and mural endocarditis. *Arch Int Med* 33:701-737, 1924.

3. Cohen AS, Reynolds WE, Franklin EC, Kulka JP, Ropes MW, Shulman LE, Wallace SL: Preliminary criteria for the classification of systemic lupus erythematosus. *Bull Rheum Dis* 21:643-648, 1971.

4. Tan EM, Cohen AS, Fries JF, Masi AT, McShane DJ, Rothfield NF, Schaller JG, Talal N, Winchester RJ: The 1982 revised criteria for the classification of systemic lupus erythematosus. *Arthritis Rheum* 25:1271-1277, 1982.

5. Dixon FJ: Murine lupus. An overview. *Arthritis Rheum* 25:721-725, 1982.

6. Zvaifler NJ: Etiology and pathogenesis of systemic lupus erythematosus. In WN Kelley, ED Harris, S Ruddy, CB Sledge (eds.), *Textbook of Rheumatology,* 1st Ed. Philadelphia, W.B. Saunders, 1981, pp. 1079-1105.

7. Labowitz R, Schumacher HR: Articular manifestations of systemic lupus erythematosus. *Ann Int Med* 74:911, 1971.

8. Rothfield N: Clinical features of systemic lupus erythematosus. In WN Kelley, ED Harris, S Ruddy, CB Sledge (eds.), *Textbook of Rheumatology,* 1st Ed. Philadelphia, W.B. Saunders, 1981, pp. 1106-1132.

9. Maddison PJ, Provost TT, Reichlin M: Serological findings in patients with ANA-negative systemic lupus erythematosus. *Medicine* 60:87-94, 1981.

10. Chang RW: Cardiac manifestations of SLE. *Clin Rheum Dis* 8:197-206, 1982.

11. Blant RK, Stephen RA: Complete A-V block in a fetus: Case report. *Am Heart J* 30:615-618, 1945.

12. Lee LA, Bias WB, Arnett FC, Huff JC, Norris DA, Harmon C, Provost TT, Weston WL: Immunogenerics of the neonatal lupus syndrome. *Ann Int Med* 99:592-596, 1983.

13. Abruzzo J: The neonatal lupus syndrome, autoantibodies and connective tissue disease. Editorial. *Ann Int Med* 99:716, 1983.

14. Haupt HM, Moore GW, Hutchins GM: The lung in systemic lupus erythematosus. *Am J Med* 71:791-798, 1981.

15. Adu D, Cameron JS: Lupus nephritis. *Clin Rheum Dis* 9:153-182, 1982.

16. Bresnihan B: CNS lupus. *Clin Rheum Dis* 8:183-195, 1982.

17. Gibson T, Myers A: Nervous systemic involvement in systemic lupus erythematosus. *Ann Rheum Dis* 35:398-406, 1976.

18. Jungers P, Dougados M, Pelissier C, Kutten F, Tron F, Lesavre PL, Bach JF: Lupus nephropathy and pregnancy. *Arch Int Med* 142:771-776, 1982.

19. Manu P: Serial probability analysis of the 1982 revised criteria for the classification of systemic lupus erythematosus. *N Engl J Med* 23:1460, 1983.

20. Rynes RI: Inherited complement deficiency states and SLE. *Clin Rheum Dis* 8:29-47, 1982.

21. Harmon C, Portanova J: Drug-induced lupus: Clinical and serologic studies. *Clin Rheum Dis* 8:121-135, 1982.

22. Alarcon-Segovia D: Drug-induced systemic lupus erythematosus and related syndromes. *Clin Rheum Dis* 1:573-582, 1975.

23. Budman DR, Steinberg AD: Hematologic aspects of systemic lupus erythematosus. *Ann Int Med* 86:220-229, 1977.

24. Steinberg AD: Management of systemic lupus erythematosus. In WN Kelley, ED Harris, S. Ruddy, CB Sledge (eds.), *Textbook of Rheumatology,* 1st Ed. Philadelphia, W.B. Saunders, 1981, pp. 1133-1150.

25. Albert DA, Hadler NM, Ropes MW: Does corticosteroid therapy affect the survival of patients with systemic lupus erythematosus? *Arthritis Rheum* 22:965-969 , 1979.

26. Kaplan D: Treatment of systemic lupus erythematosus. *Arthritis Rheum* 20: S 175-179, 1977.

27. Friedman EA: Lupus nephritis: What to do until the data arrives. Editorial. *Nephron* 19:190-192, 1977.

28. Sergent JS, Lockshin MD, Klempner MS, Lipsky BA: Central nervous system disease in systemic lupus erythematosus. *Amer J Med* 58:644-654, 1975.

Chapter 14

PROGRESSIVE SYSTEMIC SCLEROSIS (SCLERODERMA)

Edward J. Pisko, M.D.

Introduction

General Comments

Progressive systemic sclerosis (PSS, scleroderma) is a multisystem disorder which results in degenerative fibrotic changes of numerous organs including the skin, esophagus, lungs, heart, small bowel, and kidney (1,2,3). The presence of target organ lymphocytic infiltration (4) suggests that cellular autoimmune mechanisms (5,6) may be in part responsible for the chronic, inflammatory changes. PSS is relatively unique among the autoimmune connective tissue diseases because one major target of the autoimmune inflammatory process is the small artery and arteriole (7,8). This results in narrowing and occlusion of these vessels which can lead to tissue ischemia and tissue fibrosis. Life-threatening disease often results when the renal or pulmonary vessels become narrowed.

A large variety of diseases may be associated with scleroderma, which literally means hardening of the skin. A classification of these diseases is shown in Table 14.1. It is obvious that PSS is only one of many diseases that may give rise to scleroderma. PSS can be grouped with mixed connective tissue disease, morphea, and other forms of localized scleroderma, eosinophillic fasciitis and graft vs host disease as the scleroderma syndromes.

In general, the scleroderma syndromes are grouped together because of their clinical and histological features, as well as their probable autoimmune etiology. The scleroderma-like disorders which make up the rest of Table 14.1 sometimes have a better defined etiology.

TABLE 14.1 Classification of Scleroderma*

Progressive Systemic Sclerosis

- PSS with diffuse scleroderma: symmetric, diffuse involvement of the skin (scleroderma) affecting trunk, face, proximal and distal portions of the extremities; relatively early appearance of disease of the esophagus, intestine, heart, lung, and kidney.
- CREST syndrome: relatively limited involvement of the skin, often confined to the fingers and face; prominence of calcinosis, Raynaud's phenomenon, esophageal dysfunction, sclerodactyly, telangiectasia, and prolonged delay in appearance of distinctive internal manifestations (including severe pulmonary arterial hypertension and biliary cirrhosis).
- Overlap syndromes, including sclerodermatomyositis and mixed connective tissue disease.

Eosinophilic Fasciitis

Congenital Fascial Dystrophy

Localized (Focal) Forms of Scleroderma
- Morphea
  - Plaque-like
  - Guttate
  - Generalized
  - Less typical forms: subcutaneous morphea, keloid morphea
  - Possibly superficial primary atrophic morphea (atrophoderma Pasini-Pierini)
- Linear scleroderma, with or without melorheostosis
- Scleroderma *en coup de sabre*, with or without facial hemiatrophy

Chemically-Induced Scleroderma-like Conditions
- Vinylchloride disease
- Pentazocine-induced fibrosis
- Bleomycin-induced fibrosis
- Possibly trichloroethylene-induced fibrosis
- Scleroderma-like illness after use of L-5-hydroxytryptophan and carbidopa

Digital Sclerosis and Joint Contractures Associated with Juvenile-Onset Diabetes Mellitus

Diseases with Skin Changes Resembling Scleroderma (Pseudoscleroderma)
- Edematous
  - Scleredema adultorum of Büschke
  - Scleredema related to diabetes mellitus
  - Scleromyxedema (papular mucinosis)

Indurative and/or atrophic
- Lichen sclerosus et atrophicus
- Porphyria cutanea tarda
- Acromegaly
- Myeloma-associated and primary amyloidosis
- Skin thickening associated with plasma cell neoplasia with peripheral polyneuropathy
- Phenylketonuria
- Carcinoid syndrome
- Localized lipoatrophy, including Gower's panatrophy, lipoatrophy of ankles, orbicular lipoatrophy
- Congenital poikiloderma, including Rothmund's syndrome, Rothmund-Thompson syndrome
- Werner's syndrome
- Progeria
- Acrodermatitis chronica atrophicans

---

*From the *Primer on the Rheumatic Diseases,* 8th Ed. Atlanta, GA, Arthritis Foundation, p. 59 (used with permission).

The numerous terms used in discussing the diseases characterized by scleroderma can cause confusion. These terms have been defined (Table 14.2) by the American Rheumatism Association (ARA) Committee which provided criteria for the diagnosis of PSS (9) (Table 14.3).

PSS has been divided into two major groups: generalized diffuse disease and CREST syndrome (1). The characteristics of these two forms of PSS are summarized in Table 14.4. CREST syndrome refers to the clinical constellation of calcinosis, Raynaud's phenomenon, esophageal dysmotility, and telangiectasia. These patients often will have had Raynaud's phenomenon for many years prior to diagnosis and they often live for several decades. They may succumb to such disease complications as late onset primary pulmonary hypertension (10). The concept of CREST syndrome is clinically useful although patients will sometimes be difficult to categorize. The localized scleroderma syndromes have an excellent prognosis as does eosinophilic fasciitis which is a fascinating newly recognized illness that responds to corticosteroids (11,12). Mixed connective tissue disease (13) (MCTD, Chapter 17) is an overlap syndrome with features of systemic lupus erythematosus, polymyositis, and PSS. Many of these patients closely resemble PSS patients with time and MCTD is therefore included as a scleroderma syndrome. Human graft vs host disease is a iatrogenic disease which gives rise to a syndrome with features of PSS and Sjögren's syndrome (14). The association of PSS with the autoimmune diseases, MCTD, Sjögren's syndrome, primary biliary cirrhosis, Hashimoto's thyroiditis, and graft vs host disease provides further evidence for an autoimmune etiology for PSS. Figure 14.1 pictorially shows the interrelationships between PSS and several of the other autoimmune diseases.

Historical Aspects

The historical aspects of PSS have been reviewed by Rodnan et al. (3). Patients with scleroderma were described during the eighteenth century. However, some of these patients most likely did not have true scleroderma, but another illness called scleredema. Scleredema is a rare, usually self-limited disorder in which there is postinfectious skin induration over the neck, trunks, and flanks. Unlike

TABLE 14.2 Glossary of Clinical Terms Used in Description or Classification of Systemic Sclerosis*

1. Typical sclerodermatous skin changes: tightness, thickening, and nonpitting induration, excluding the localized forms of scleroderma (morphea or linear scleroderma)
   a) Sclerodactyly: above-indicated changes limited (to fingers and toes)
   b) Proximal scleroderma: above-indicated changes proximal to the metacarpophalangeal or metatarsophalangeal joints, affecting other parts of the extremities, face, neck, or trunk (thorax or abdomen); usually bilateral, symmetrical, and almost always including sclerodactyly

2. Other skin manifestations attributable to systemic sclerosis or comparable disorders
   a) Digital pitting scars or loss of substance from the finger pad: depressed areas at tips of digits or loss of digital pad tissue as a result of digital ischemia rather than trauma or exogenous causes
   b) Bilateral finger or hand edema: firm but pitting edema, especially involving fingers (includes puffy, sausage-like swelling of fingers) or the dorsal aspect of the hands
   c) Abnormal skin pigmentation: hyperpigmentation often containing areas of punctate or patchy hypopigmentation or depigmentation ("pepper and salt")
   d) Telangiectasia: visible macular dilatation of superficial blood vessels which collapse upon pressure and fill slowly when pressure is released; distinguished from rapidly filling spider angioma with central arteriole and from dilated linear superficial vessels
   e) Raynaud's phenomenon: at least a two-phase color change in fingers and often toes consisting of pallor, cyanosis, and/or reactive hyperemia in response to cold exposure or emotion, as determined by patient's history or physician's observation

3. Visceral manifestations
   a) Bibasilar pulmonary fibrosis: bilateral reticular pattern of linear or lineonodular densities which are most pronounced in basilar portions of the lungs on standard chest roentgenogram; may assume appearance of diffuse mottling or honeycomb lung, and should not be attributable to primary lung disease
   b) Lower (distal) esophageal dysphagia: substernal discomfort on swallowing or sensation of food holdup in the retrosternal location
   c) Lower (distal) esophageal dysmotility: hypoperistalsis or aperistalsis, as demonstrated by either cineesophagram or fluoroscopy or by manometric study, often accompanied by evidence of decrease in lower esophageal sphincter tone with reflux of gastric contents into the esophagus
   d) Colonic sacculations: wide-mouthed diverticula of colon located along the antimesenteric border; found on barium enema examination; these sacculations may also occur in ileum and jejunum

*From *Arthritis Rheum* 23:583, 1980 (used with permission).

TABLE 14.3 ARA Scleroderma Criteria Cooperative Study (SCCS): Preliminary Clinical Criteria for Systemic Sclerosis*

Proximal scleroderma is the single major criterion; sensitivity was 91% and specificity was over 99%.

Sclerodactyly, digital pitting scars of fingertips or loss of substance of the distal finger pad, and bibasilar pulmonary fibrosis contribute further as minor criteria in the absence of proximal scleroderma.

One major or two or more minor criteria were found in 97% of definite systemic sclerosis patients, but only in 2% of the comparison patients with systemic lupus erythematosus, polymyositis/dermatomyositis, or Raynaud's phenomenon.

*Excludes localized scleroderma and pseudosclerodermatous disorders. From *Arthritis Rheum* 23:587, 1980 (used with permission).

TABLE 14.4 Significant Difference Between 555 PSS Patients with Diffuse Scleroderma and CREST Syndrome Seen at the University of Pittsburgh, 1972 to 1983*

	Diffuse (N = 248)	CREST (N = 307)
Mean age at onset (years)	45	41
Mean disease duration, onset to diagnosis (years)	1.7	8.0
Raynaud's phenomenon as initial symptom	36%	78%
Arthralgias/arthritis	75%	50%
Tendon friction rubs	67%	3%
Myositis	19%	8%
Esophageal stricture	17%	8%
Pulmonary hypertension	rare	10%
Cardiac involvement	27%	5%
Renal involvement	25%	rare
Anticentromere antibodies	3%	50%
Cumulative survival at 5 years from diagnosis (%)	58%	74%
Calcinosis of digits	7%	43%
Telgangiectasia of digits	32%	82%
Calcified granuloma on chest radiograph	14%	67%
Rib notching on chest radiograph	16%	0%

*From Medsger TA Jr: *Orth Rev* 13:268, 1984 (with permission).

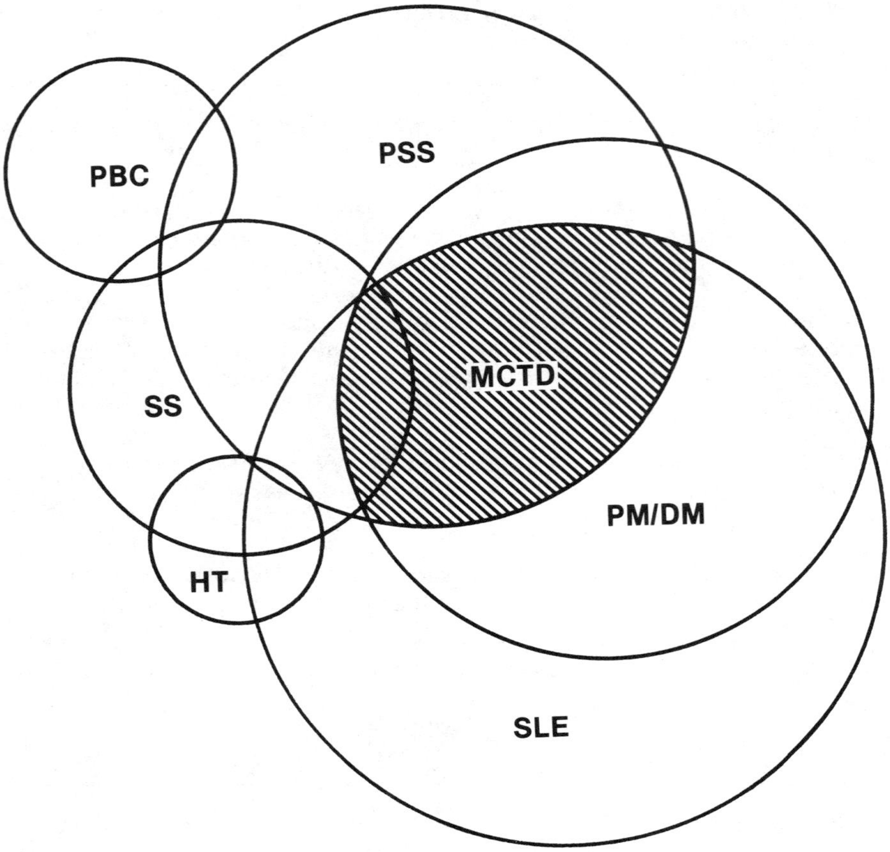

FIGURE 14.1 The relationships between progressive systemic sclerosis (PSS) and several of the other autoimmune diseases. Overlaps between PSS and other autoimmune diseases are common, but only mixed connective tissue disease (hatched bars) with features of polymyositis/dermatomyositis, PSS, and systemic lupus erythematosus is considered a separate entity. [Progressive systemic sclerosis (PSS), systemic lupus erythematosus (SLE), mixed connective tissue disease (MCTD), Hashimoto's thyroiditis (HT), Sjögren's syndrome (SS), primary biliary cirrhosis (PBC)].

PSS, scleredema spares the hands and is not associated with Raynaud's phenomenon or internal organ system involvement. Internal organ systemic involvement with scleroderma was described during the nineteenth century, and the twentieth century saw increasing awareness that scleroderma encompassed a multisystem disorder with prominent skin changes and marked changes in the internal organs. The term progressive systemic sclerosis was first used by Goetz in 1945 (15) in order to emphasize that what was then known as scleroderma was a multisystem disorder with degenerative and fibrotic changes, not only in the skin, but in numerous internal organ systems. There is a trend towards changing the name of this illness from PSS to systemic sclerosis because the word progressive is frightening to patients and implies a worse prognosis than is often the case.

Although they were not the first to describe calcinosis associated with scleroderma, Thiebierge and Weissenbach emphasized this association. O'Leary and Waisman introduced the term acrosclerosis to describe the simultaneous occurrence of Raynaud's phenomenon with sclerodactyly and sclerodermatous changes of the face. The concept of CRST syndrome (16) and, with the recognition of prominent gastrointestinal involvement, CREST syndrome, gradually evolved from these descriptions to describe a subset of patients with a more favorable prognosis who might have had Raynaud's phenomenon for a decade or longer before diagnosis. These patients were also more likely to develop primary pulmonary hypertension as a late manifestation of their disease (10). Primary biliary cirrhosis is also seen more commonly in CREST patients (17). CREST patients may also have relatively unique autoantibodies such as those to the chromosome centromere complex (18).

Mixed connective tissue disease (MCTD) was first described by Sharp et al. in 1972 (13). Although overlap syndromes between the connective diseases had been known, Sharp emphasized the relatively unique serological findings of this disease. Subsequent reports have emphasized the finding that with time many MCTD patients are clinically indistinguishable from patients with PSS.

Shulman described eosinophilic fasciitis in 1977 (11). This illness is characterized by acute painful swelling and induration of the skin of the extremities. Full-thickness skin biopsies show round cell infiltration with eosinophils that predominates in the fascia but which is also seen in the skin, subcutis, and muscle.

Epidemiology

The incidence of PSS has been described as being between 4.5 and 12 cases per million per year (1,2). It is a disease of women (female to male ratio of approximately 4 to 1) between the ages of 30 and 50. The disease rarely occurs in childhood, although all ages have been affected. Patients are fairly evenly divided between generalized diffuse PSS and CREST syndrome. There are no apparent geographic or racial factors which affect the incidence of this disease. Familial occurrence has rarely been described and inheritance may be linked to HLAD or HLADR histocompatibility antigens, although further work will be necessary to better define the HLA specificities in this disease.

Silica dust may predispose individuals to the development of PSS. Workers exposed to polyvinyl chloride may develop a scleroderma-like illness characterized by distal osteoloysis of the digits, Raynaud's-like syndrome and hepatic and pulmonary fibrosis (19). Patients given bleomycin may develop typical sclerodermatous skin changes, particularly of the hands (20).

Etiopathogenesis

Introduction

Progressive systemic sclerosis is a disease of unknown etiology, but an autoimmune etiology is suspected (1,5,6). The possible factors underlying the autoimmune phenomena have not been addressed with the exception of studies suggesting possible genetic linkages which may have important implications for the autoimmune nature of this disease. The issue of an infectious process underlying the autoimmunity in PSS has not been addressed. Although humoral abnormalities are found in PSS, cellular immune mechanisms are probably of more importance. In this sense, PSS more closely resembles dermatomyositis/polymyositis. PSS is also characterized by prominent microvascular abnormalities and tremendous changes in collagen metabolism leading to fibrosis (1,2,5-8). The relationship between the autoimmune abnormalities and the vascular and fibrotic abnormalities in PSS is an important area of study.

PSS as an Autoimmune Disease

The immune abnormalities in PSS which are outlined in Table 14.5 can be divided into humoral, cellular, and mediator (lymphokine/monokine) abnormalities. Figure 14.2 depicts the possible interrelationship between these multiple abnormalities.

Humoral Abnormalities

PSS is frequently associated with antinuclear antibodies (18,21), immune complexes (21,22) and hyperglobulinemia. However, there is less evidence that these autoantibodies are pathogenic than in systemic lupus erythematosus, where autoantibody-containing immune complexes are likely causes of renal disease. Deposits of immunoglobulin and complement have been found in kidney biopsies of PSS patients (23), but the role of these deposits, which are usually intraarterial, is unknown. The presence of these deposits in the arterial wall leads to the speculation that they may be playing a role in precipitating the severe vasoconstriction which is pathogenic in scleroderma renal disease. However, inflammation is not a prominent finding when kidney biopsies are performed on patients with PSS renal disease,

Cellular Immune Abnormalities

Perhaps the most important evidence implicating cellular mechanisms in the pathogenesis of PSS is the finding of lymphocytic infiltrations in the skin, gastrointestinal tract, muscle, synovium, and other organs. These lymphocytes are predominantly T cells. Generally, it has been found that PSS patients have fewer peripheral T cells, and this finding often correlates with more severe organ system involvement. It is not known whether the decrease in peripheral blood T cells is simply related to increased tissue deposition or is due to other mechanisms, such as antibody and complement-mediated destruction of the lymphocytes. B-lymphocyte numbers are normal in the peripheral blood of PSS patients. The ratio of helper (OKT4) to suppressor/cytotoxic (OKT8) lymphocytes as measured by monoclonal antibodies is generally increased in PSS although not all studies have confirmed this. This increased ratio of helper:suppressor lymphocytes could be, in part, responsible for some of the autoantibody formation in this disease. It is important to note that both peripheral blood and tissue lymphocyte populations may vary with disease stage. In addition, reactivity of PSS lymphocytes to concanavalin A, pokeweed mitogen, and phytohemagglutination is generally decreased, and this abnormality may also correlate with internal organ system involvement. Delayed hypersensitivity by skin testing is apparently normal in PSS patients despite the other abnormalities of cellular immunity.

TABLE 14.5 Immunologic Abnormalities in Progressive Systemic Sclerosis*

B-Cell Activity

- Serologic abnormalities
  - Rheumatoid factor
  - Antinuclear antibodies
  - Immune complexes
- Serum proteins - increase, usually mild, in serum IgG concentration
- Deposition of immunoglobulin (IgM) and complement components (including C3) in kidney

Cellular Immune (T-Cell) Reactivity

- Peripheral lymphopenia, affecting T lymphocytes
- Presence of T-lymphocyte infiltrates in dermis and other tissues
- Disturbance in immunoregulation
- Stimulation of peripheral blood lymphocytes by cutaneous antigen(s) and collagen
- Lymphokine stimulation of collagen production by dermal fibroblasts

Occurrence of PSS- and Sjögren's Syndrome-like Disease in Individuals with Graft-Versus-Host Reaction after Bone Marrow Transplantation

Association of PSS with Sjögren's Syndrome and Hashimoto's Thyroiditis

*From the *Primer on the Rheumatic Diseases,* 8th Ed. Atlanta, GA, Arthritis Foundation, p. 63 (used with permission).

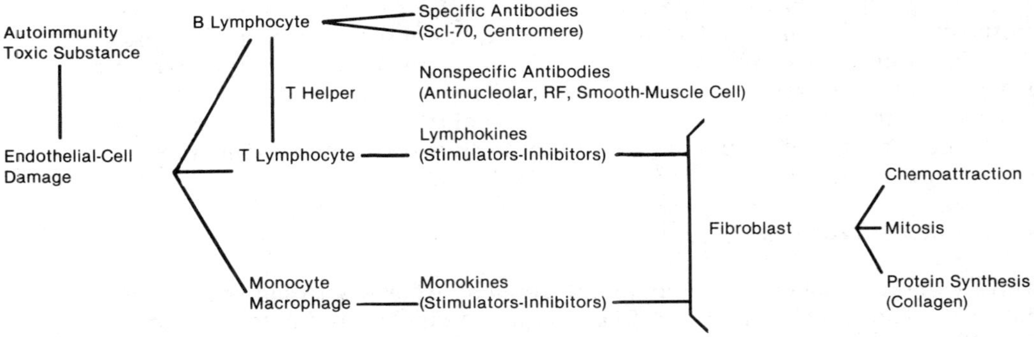

FIGURE 14.2 The complex factors that may be important in the pathogenesis of PSS are pictured in this figure. From Fleischmejer, *Arch Dermatol* 119:960, 1983 (used with permission).

Abnormal Lymphokine/Monokine Production

As previously noted, skin biopsies from patients with early PSS reveal infiltrates in the lower dermis consisting of lymphocytes and monocytes/macrophages (4). There is also an increase in the number of fibroblasts which are presumably responsible for the increased collagen production that is commonly seen. A variety of lymphokines and monokines (6) have been described which can either increase or decrease fibroblast proliferation, chemotaxis, or the production of collagen and glycosoaminoglycans. It is postulated that the lymphocytes and monocytes found in the PSS skin may have stimulatory or inhibitory effects on dermal fibroblasts. Presumably an imbalance between such stimulating factors and other suppressor factors may be responsible for the increased fibroblast activity in PSS. T-helper activity in PSS may also be increased giving rise to the increased B-cell reactivity. The specific T-cell factors controlling fibroblast function have not been elucidated with the exception of gamma interferon which may be playing an inhibitory role. Blood vessel type IV collagen, exposed after endothelial cell damage, may be an important antigen in stimulating soluble mediator release.

PSS as a Disease of the Microvasculature

The microvascular abnormalities in PSS may be of preeminent importance in the pathogenesis of this disease. The evidence for disturbances in the microcirculation comes from nailfold capillaroscopy studies (24) and electron microscopic studies (8). The former studies reveal a substantial loss of capillaries with dilation of remaining capillaries, and the latter studies have revealed distinctive morphological changes consisting of reduplication of the basement membrane, degenerative and necrotic changes of the endothelial cells, and marked adventitial fibrosis sometimes associated with perivascular round cell infiltrates. Serum factors may be responsible for the endothelial damage (25). Antibodies to type IV (basement membrane) collagen or immune complexes may also be important. Endothelial cells produce factor VIII and the finding of increased levels of factor VIII as well as von Willebrand antigen, plasma B-thromboglobulin, and platelet aggregates provides further evidence of sustained vascular injury in PSS (26,27).

PSS as a Disease of Disordered Fibroblast Activity

Increased numbers of fibroblasts are found in PSS skin and the available evidence suggests that they have increased metabolic activity, manifested by increased synthesis of collagen and glycosaminoglycan, particularly hyaluronic acid (6,28, 29). These activated fibroblasts are more likely to occur in the deeper layers (reticular and subcutaneous) of the skin. It is possible, but unlikely, that PSS is a disease caused by a primary defect of fibroblasts leading to overactivity. It is more likely that soluble immune mediators are responsible for this increased activity which also takes place in the vessel wall.

Animal Models for PSS

White leghorn chickens develop an autoimmune illness with many features of PSS (30). The tight skin mouse (31) and bleomycin-treated rats (32) may provide us with new insights into the pathogenesis of PSS.

Clinical Features

General

The typical PSS patient presents as a woman in her thirties or forties who often will have experienced Raynaud's phenomenon for several years. She now notes swelling of her hands and, to a lesser extent, her face. Further questioning may reveal dysphagia, polyarthralgias, and myalgias. Occasional patients present with widespread diffuse edematous swelling of their extremities, face, and trunk. These patients may be less aware of their Raynaud's phenomenon and are more likely to have dysphagia, polyarthralgias and polymyalgias, palpitations, and dyspnea. Crampy abdominal pain with constipation or diarrhea may be somewhat more likely to be present in the patients presenting with long-standing Raynaud's phenomenon. Occasional patients with PSS may present with features suggestive of an inflammatory arthritis resembling rheumatoid arthritis. PSS patients may also appear to have primary polymyositis when they first present. Rare patients develop esophageal, large intestine, or pulmonary manifestations of PSS before cutaneous involvement is manifest. Features suggestive of systemic inflammation such as fever, fatigue, and morning stiffness are not particularly common in PSS. However, patients with major organ system involvement may experience malaise and fatigue.

Raynaud's Phenomenon

Raynaud's phenomenon (33,34) consists of vasospasm with episodic blood flow changes of peripheral areas such as the hands, feet, and also occasionally the tip of the nose, tongue, and ears. Over 95% of PSS patients will have Raynaud's phenomenon. Raynaud's phenomenon consists of three classic phases: pallor with diminished blood flow, cyanosis in which there is relative tissue ischemia, and finally erythema in which there is a reactive hyperemia as blood flow is restored. Raynaud's phenomenon may be accompanied by paresthesias (burning and tingling) and/or pain. A large variety of illnesses may be associated with Raynaud's phenomenon (Table 14.6). A careful history, physical examination, and appropriate laboratory tests will eliminate most of the possibilities. Debate exists about the significance of idiopathic Raynaud's phenomenon, but most patients without an apparent associated condition are referred to as having Raynaud's disease. Most patients seen by a rheumatologist for Raynaud's phenomenon have or develop a connective tissue disease, usually PSS or MCTD.

When Raynaud's phenomenon is present for many years prior to the development of the PSS skin lesions, the patients usually fall into the CREST variant category of PSS. With generalized diffuse PSS, Raynaud's phenomenon may occur several months prior to or contemporaneously with the onset of skin symptoms. Because of the sometimes dramatic onset of diffuse generalized PSS, patients may overlook the Raynaud's symptoms. If a patient is presumed to have PSS without Raynaud's phenomenon, the possibility that the patient has another scleroderma-like illness should be sought. Scleredema, in particular, may be responsible for diffuse induration of the skin without Raynaud's phenomenon and should be considered.

TABLE 14.6 Disorders Associated with Raynaud's Phenomenon

Neurovascular Compression

- Thoracic outlet syndromes (e.g., cervical rib, scalenus anticus syndrome)
- Crutch pressure
- Carpal tunnel syndrome

Arterial Diseases

- Thromboangiitis obliterans
- Thromboembolism
- Arteriosclerosis

Blood Abnormalities

- Cryoglobulinemia
- Cryofibrinogenemia
- Cold hemagglutinins
- Monoclonal gammopathy
- Polycythemia

Occupational

- Percussion and vibratory tool workers (e.g., chain saw)
- Traumatic-occlusive arterial disease
- Vinylchloride workers

Drugs and Toxins

- Ergot
- Methylsergide
- β Adrenergic blocking drugs
- Chemotherapy

Connective Tissue Diseases

- Systemic sclerosis
- Systemic lupus erythematosus
- Mixed connective tissue disease
- Rheumatoid arthritis
- Dermatomyositis/polymyositis

Miscellaneous

- Reflex sympathetic dystrophy
- Hypothyroidism
- Pheochromocytoma
- Neoplasm
- Primary pulmonary hypertension
- Variant angina

*From Spencer-Green, G. *Bull Rheum Dis* 33:3, 1983 (used with permission).

Skin Involvement

PSS skin involvement occurs in virtually all patients and the presence of the typical cutaneous features is the most important diagnostic feature in PSS (Table 14.3). There are three phases of skin involvement in PSS. The first phase (Figure 14.3) is the early edematous phase in which the skin of the hands and feet can be dramatically swollen with sausage-like swelling of the digits. Pitting edema can occur, but the swelling is characteristically nonpitting. This phase may persist in some patients with the CREST syndrome variant of the disease and MCTD; patients may also persist at this stage for many years.

During the second or indurative phase of PSS skin disease (Figure 14.4), one finds the classic PSS skin findings. The skin becomes tight and taut with the development of contractures, particularly of the fingers. In patients with diffuse generalized PSS, the skin changes occur not only over the hands and feet but over the face, trunk, and upper arms and thighs. These changes are often accompanied by dramatic hyperpigmentation which can be interspersed with areas of hypopigmentation. Telangiectasias occur over involved areas.

Some patients will enter into a third phase of PSS skin involvement in which there is skin softening. This phase has also been called the atrophic phase. Skin wrinkling which is lost during the second or classic disease phase may return during this phase although the normal appearance of the skin is not restored. Despite skin thinning and softening, there is not a return to histologically normal skin. The presence of this phase is responsible for the enthusiasm for so many PSS treatments, and it is important to realize that PSS patients' skin may soften spontaneously in the absence of treatment.

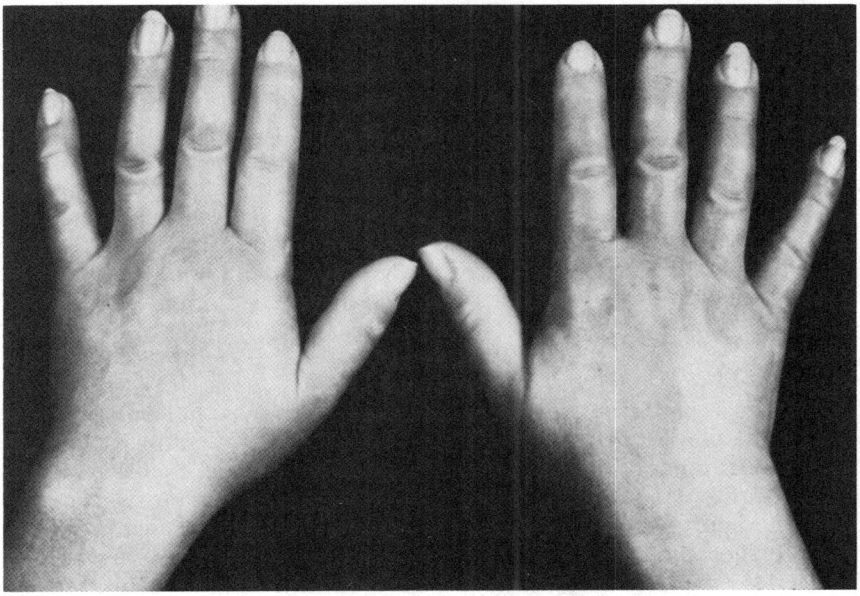

FIGURE 14.3 Early edematous (puffy) changes in a patient with PSS. (From the *Revised Clinical Slide Collection on the Rheuamtic Diseases*. Copyright 1981. Used by permission of the Arthritis Foundation.)

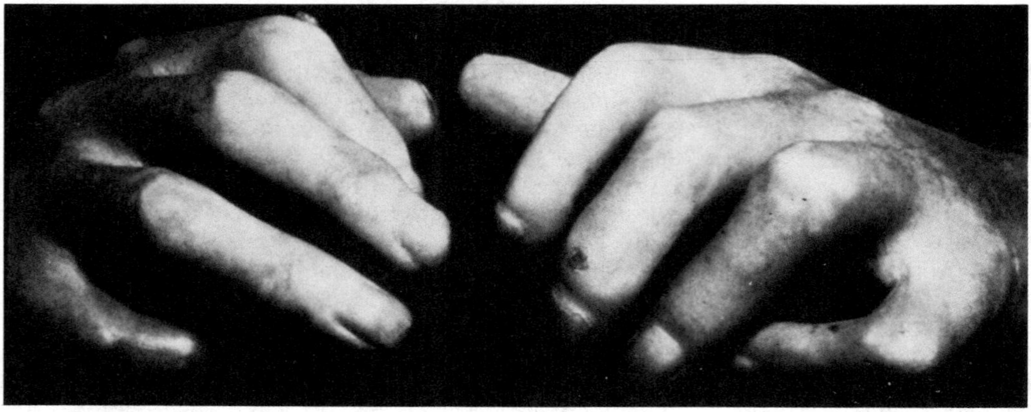

FIGURE 14.4 Typical PSS skin changes during the indurative phase of the disease. The skin has become quite tight causing flexion contractures. There are also areas of hyperpigmentation and hypopigmentation. Distal digit resorption has also occurred. (From the *Revised Clinical Slide Collection on the Rheumatic Diseases*. Copyright 1981. Used by permission of the Arthritis Foundation.)

Scarring of the digital pulp may occur at any phase and is generally present with PSS skin disease. With advanced disease there may be resorption of the distal digits. Digital pulp scars may antedate PSS skin changes in the presence of Raynaud's phenomenon. Dilated nailfold capillary loops or telangiectasias are often seen with the unaided eye in PSS or with long-standing Raynaud's phenomenon. Soft tissue subcutaneous calcification consisting of calcium apatite can occur, particularly over the volar aspect of the distal digits. Large conglomerates of calcium apatite are sometimes found over the forearms and the knee or elbow bursae.

During the second or classic phase of PSS, ulcerations can occur over the small joints of the hands and over bony prominences. These ulcers are notoriously difficult to treat, and they may become secondarily infected. Gangrene of the distal fingertips can occur at any stage of PSS skin involvement and may be associated with Raynaud's alone without skin involvement.

Esophagus

Esophageal disease is present in over 90% of PSS patients, but only about half of these patients display significant symptoms. Postprandial fullness or burning may occur as an initial complaint, but with more severe disease, frank dysphagia may occur with patients complaining of solid foods getting stuck on swallowing. Some patients develop quite severe reflux esophagitis with rather constant pain requiring aggressive therapy. Esophageal perforation and hemorrhage are fortunately rare. The distal two-thirds of the esophagus generally becomes dilated, but esophageal stricture can also occur.

A cineesophagram is the most useful test utilized to evaluate PSS patients for esophageal involvement. In addition to revealing the decreased motility, it can also reveal an associated hiatal hernia and perhaps reflux esophagitis as well as stricture. A conventional barium swallow is not as useful as a cineesophagram. Manometrics are the most sensitive method of evaluating esophageal disease revealing poor secondary and tertiary waves as well as the decreased lower esophageal sphincter tone that allows reflux esophagitis to occur. Once the diagnosis of PSS esophageal disease is made, some gastroenterologists prefer to perform endoscopies to evaluate recurrent symptoms. Esophagitis can be directly visualized and strictures, if found, can be readily dilated. Esophageal disease can become a major clinical problem when severe symptoms result in a decrease in oral intake. The subsequent weight loss must be distinguished from malabsorption which can occur with PSS small bowel involvement.

Lung

Over 90% of PSS patients will have pulmonary involvement. Most patients will not experience severe disability from lung disease, but pulmonary disease can lead to severe debility and follows kidney disease as a cause of death in PSS. Lung involvement in PSS can be divided into three general areas: pleural, interstitial, and vascular (35). Pleural disease can be found in 60-100% of patients at autopsy with primarily fibrotic changes being present. Pleural effusion can occur but symptomatic pleural disease is rare. Patients with severe interstitial pulmonary disease and severe pulmonary hypertension secondary to primary vessel disease belong to two separate groups. One group often has the CREST variant of PSS and develops pulmonary hypertension as a late manifestation of their disease without developing significant interstitial disease (10). The typical patient with diffuse generalized PSS insidiously develops interstitial disease which can lead to cor pulmonale.

Interstitial pulmonary involvement in PSS can be detected by roentgenographic, spirometric, or diffusion studies. Roentgenograms are not a particularly sensitive means of detecting PSS lung disease and are open to variability in interpretation. The typical picture is that of interstitial or a nodular-interstitial pattern involving the lower two-thirds of the lungs. Small cystic areas occur but the cysts are generally less than 1.5 cm. Diffusion studies such as the single-breath carbon monoxide diffusion study are a sensitive way to detect pulmonary involvement in PSS. About 33-90% of patients may have a low carbon monoxide diffusion capacity. This wide variability in the prevalence of low carbon monoxide diffusion may be related to technique and/or the case mix between diffuse and CREST patients. The carbon monoxide diffusion capacity primarily measures abnormalities in the ventilation:perfusion ratio, and reflects alveolar damage or fibrosis leading to lung areas that are perfused without adequate gas exchange.

Spirometry is abnormal in 80-100% of PSS patients. PSS lung disease is classically thought to be restrictive, but obstructive disease occurs about as frequently as restrictive disease. Small airway disease is frequently present and accounts for most of the remaining patients without frank restrictive or obstructive disease. The classic patient with restrictive disease has a decreased vital capacity, residual volume, and total lung capacity presumably on the basis of pulmonary fibrosis and poor compliance (35). Small airway disease is frequently found in PSS and can be detected by measuring maximal, midexpiratory flow, or closing volume. Small airway disease is a likely precursor to obstructive pulmonary disease. The relationship between small airway disease and subsequent restrictive disease is less clear but the strict categorization of patients with restrictive and obstructive disease is probably not justified as the fibrotic process in the lung is quite diffuse.

Recently, gallium scans have been utilized to evaluate PSS patients for inflammatory lung disease (36). Changes on gallium scan may correlate with the presence of inflammatory cells by bronchoalveolar lavage. Studies such as these, which may be indicative of a more acute inflammatory process, may be utilized in the future as a guide to therapy. At the present time, PSS lung disease is generally not recognized until fibrosis has occurred.

As mentioned, CREST patients who have little in the way of interstitial pulmonary disease, may develop quite severe primary pulmonary hypertension. The mechanisms responsible for precipitating this dreaded occurrence are not clear at the present time. This is a principal cause of late mortality in this subset of PSS patients.

Heart

Cardiac disease in PSS can take many forms (Table 14.7). The primary involvement with the PSS disease process may lead to pericardial, myocardial (37), and conduction system abnormalities (38). In addition, pulmonary and renal disease can secondarily affect the cardiac status and, as noted, primary pulmonary hypertension can be a devastating late manifestation of PSS. Cardiac disease follows lung and kidney disease as a cause of death in PSS.

Pericardial disease consisting primarily of fibrosis occurs in one-third to two-thirds of patients with PSS at autopsy. Pericardial disease can result in tamponade but, in most instances, pericardial disease is asymptomatic, and there is little evidence of diminished cardiac function secondary to its presence.

Myocardial disease is present in about one-half of PSS patients at autopsy and myocardial fibrosis occurs in a patchy manner that does not correspond to a single large vessel. The finding of contraction band necrosis in PSS myocardium (37) gives a clue to the etiology of PSS heart disease. This histological picture is seen when coronary blood flow is temporarily interrupted and then reperfusion is allowed to occur. The coronary vessels are patent, and it is thought that small vessel coronary spasm is the cause of the histological changes and subsequent fibrosis.

TABLE 14.7 Cardiac Manifestations of PSS

Pericardial disease (usually fibrous)
Myocardial involvement (fibrosis probably secondary to small vessel disease with ischemia and reperfusion leading to contraction band necrosis)
Congestive heart failure secondary to scleroderma kidney disease with severe hypertension
Cor pulmonale secondary to respiratory failure with interstitial lung disease
Cor pulmonale secondary to primary pulmonary hypertension, i.e., with little or no pulmonary fibrosis.

Fibrosis also occurs in the conducting system possibly related to the interruption of the blood supply and the subsequent arrythmias are quite common in PSS patients. Sudden death, presumably on the basis of arrythmia, is a not uncommon occurence with PSS. Congestive heart failure can be a sequela of cardiac fibrosis but may also be associated with PSS renal disease with its severe hypertension. Cor pulmonale occurs in patients with interstitial lung disease and respiratory failure. Cor pulmonale is most severe when associated with primary pulmonary hypertension in CREST patients.

Small Bowel

Involvement of the small bowel occurs in about 10% of PSS patients clinically but may be present in one-half of the patients at autopsy. It is usually associated with esophageal disease and occasionally occurs without cutaneous PSS. CREST patients may be more susceptible to symptomatic small bowel disease. The tremendous weight loss seen in one autopsy series of PSS patients (47) may be secondary to relatively asymptomatic small bowel disease with malabsorption.

The pathologic process consists of atrophy of the muscularis with fibrosis leading to decreased motility. Roentgenographic studies may reveal dilated areas of bowel, particularly the second or third segments of the duodenum and the jejunum. Malabsorption results from bacterial overgrowth in the hypomotile bowel. Bile salts may be depleted leading to a malabsorption of fats and fat-soluble vitamins. Seventy-two hour stool for fat studies and D-xylose absorption studies may be valuable in documenting malabsorption. Malabsorption usually responds to institution of broad spectrum antibiotics such as tetracycline or neomycin. Antibiotics may need to be rotated as resistant organisms occur. Although the malabsorption may be treatable, these patients' overall condition may deteriorate as the PSS disease process progresses.

Abdominal pain, cramping, diarrhea, and constipation may also occur with small bowel disease in the absence of malabsorption. The symptoms are difficult to treat but the judicious use of bulking agents and laxatives may be of some benefit. Intestinal pseudoobstruction occurs with PSS and this may lead to unnecessary surgery.

Large Bowel

Large-bowel large-mouth sacculations occur in the colon, but they are usually an incidental asymptomatic finding. Pneumatosis intestinalis may also occur. The condition, in which air from the lumen enters the bowel wall, can lead to pneumoperitoneum.

Kidney

PSS renal disease (39–41) is a leading cause of death in PSS. The recognition of renal impairment and the institution of appropriate therapy is of extreme importance in order to help prevent the uniformly rapidly fatal course that patients with PSS renal failure had in the past. Renal disease is not confined to PSS patients with long-standing disease. The patients can present with renal disease or not uncommonly develop it in the first years of their illness. Although severe hypertension is usual in PSS renal disease, it is important to monitor the urine findings and renal function studies in order to detect more subtle abnormalities. Volume depletion may precipitate PSS renal disease and every effort should be made to prevent its occurrence.

The exact incidence of renal disease is unknown but, at autopsy, up to 90% of patients may have typical renal histological changes consistent with PSS. Similarly, a careful search for abnormalities of renal blood flow may result in a high percentage of patients with abnormalities. A much smaller number of patients develop azotemia, malignant hypertension, and proteinuria leading to renal failure. Proteinuria, which is usually mild, is the most common manifestation of PSS renal disease, and this may be present in up to one-third of patients. An active urinary sediment with cells and casts is not usually seen in PSS but is occasionally reported. Proteinuria, even without azotemia or hypertension, implies a worse prognosis for survival in PSS. Up to one-half of PSS patients may have hypertension. Three-quarters of these patients have a very benign course with mild to moderate hypertension. The remaining one-quarter of patients have malignant hypertension. These patients develop concomitant azotemia and renal failure, often associated with hypertensive encephalopathy and congestive heart failure as well as a microangiopathic hemolytic anemia. The outlook for these patients, while improving, remains poor. Azotemia can occur without hypertension, and these patients do not do appreciably better than hypertensive patients with azotemia.

Xenon-133 washout studies and angiographic data support the hypotheses that a diminution of cortical blood flow is a major abnormality in the PSS kidney. This can lead to diminished renal plasma flow in the face of a normal glomerular filtration rate. These effects are probably secondary to changes in the renin-aldosterone system with increased renins usually being found in patients with PSS renal disease. An elevated plasma renin may be a predictor of severe PSS renal disease. In some studies, plasma renin correlates with PSS histological changes and cold pressor testing elevates the renin levels in these patients. Figure 14.5 summarizes the complex interactions that can lead to renal failure in PSS. Decreased renal perfusion may be caused by hypovolemia secondary to blood loss or diuretic therapy. Congestive heart failure or pericardial disease may also lead to decreased renal perfusion. If recognized early and vigorously treated, renal failure may be avoided in these conditions. The role of steroidal and nonsteroidal antiinflammatory agents in diminishing renal blood flow in PSS has not been studied, but caution should be exercised when using these drugs which generally have little or no effect on the PSS disease process.

Muscle

Muscle may be involved in up to 80% of PSS patients although involvement is usually indolent and overshadowed by the other more dramatic manifestations of the disease. However, a frank myopathy with EMG, muscle enzyme, and biopsy changes may occur. These patients have marked proximal muscle weakness on examination with corresponding symptoms. Some of these patients with frank myopathy who were described in the past undoubtedly had mixed connective tissue disease (MCTD). However, PSS and polymyositis/dermatomyositis occur in some patients without serological evidence of MCTD. It is important to document such an inflammatory myopathy since treatment with corticosteroids is indicated. However, the majority of patients with PSS have normal or only mild increases in the creatine phosphokinase (CPK) and aldolase with a corresponding increase in urine creatine. These patients rarely complain of weakness, although proximal muscle weakness may be found on examination. In addition, proximal muscle atrophy can be found, perhaps related to the myopathy. Distal atrophy may also be present. This is probably related to the fibrosis and contractures present secondary to skin involvement. Only mild, noninflammatory changes may be found on biopsy in

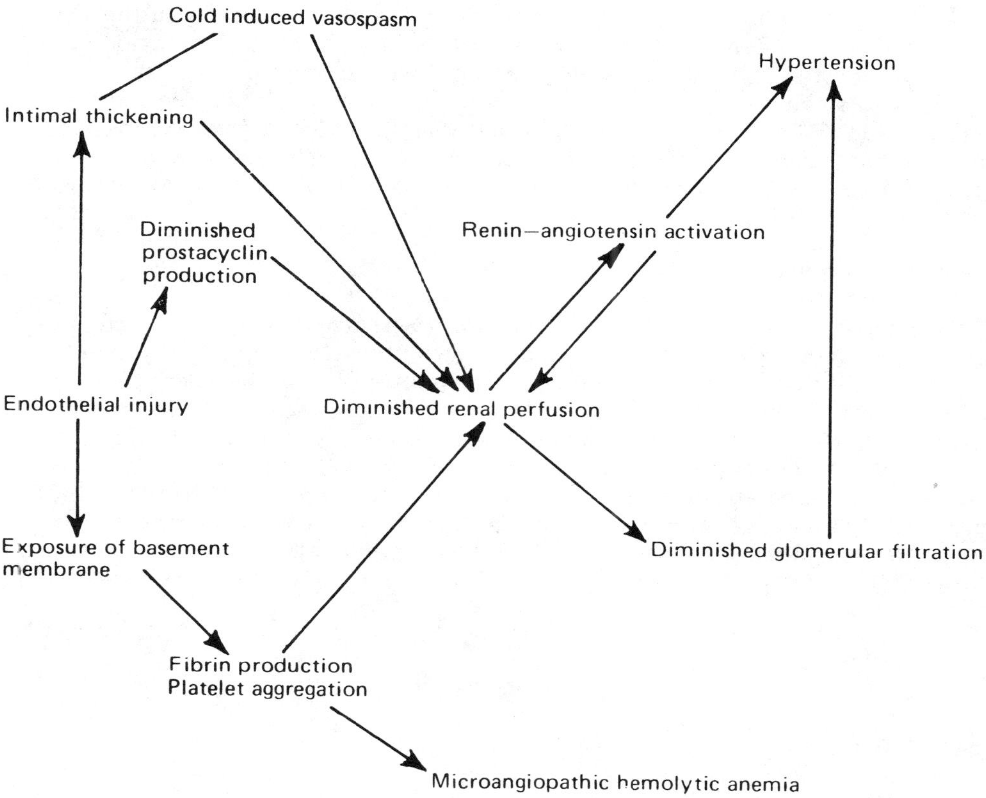

FIGURE 14.5 Proposed mechanisms for the pathogenesis of the renal disease found in PSS. From Nussbaum and Leroy. Renal involvement in scleroderma (systemic sclerosis), p. 293, in Bacon and Hadler (eds.), *The Kidney and Rheumatic Disease.* Butterworth Scientific, 1982 (used with permission).

these patients. The EMG is similarly undramatic. It is important to recognize that PSS patients often may have an indolent, noninflammatory myopathy in order to avoid potentially harmful treatment with corticosteroids which will benefit only those patients with myopathy resembling that seen in polymyositis.

Joints

Articular involvement in PSS is rarely a major manifestation of the disease but up to two-thirds of patients may have symptoms and signs of arthritis. Occasional patients may present with an inflammatory arthritis resembling rheumatoid arthritis. These patients gradually develop PSS over the next 2 years. The joints involved are similar to those involved in rheumatoid arthritis, but there is also a tendency for the development of erosive disease of the distal interphalangeal joints of the hand. This may be related to limited motion in these joints secondary to sclerodermatous skin changes with decreased motion. Joint erosions in PSS are usually localized. In general, the roentgenographic picture is much milder than that seen in rheumatoid arthritis. There is no true pannus in PSS and the synovial membrane, which may be infiltrated with lymphocytes early in the course of the disease, eventually becomes fibrotic. This leads to limitation of motion of the joints and tendons, as well as a leathery-like crepitus of the involved areas. Patients may complain of creakiness in their joints. The joint fluid contains less than 2000 white cells, usually mononuclear. Hydroxyapatite crystals may be found in the joint fluid of patients with soft tissue calcinosis associated with their PSS. Calcinosis may occur more frequently in patients with DIP disease.

Miscellaneous Organs

Sjögren's syndrome occurs in up to two-thirds of patients with PSS. Glandular fibrosis is more likely to occur in PSS than in patients with idiopathic Sjögren's or Sjögren's syndrome associated with other connective tissue disorders (42). Neurologic involvement with the PSS disease process is rare except for cranial neuropathies, particularly a sensory trigeminal neuropathy. Primary biliary cirrhosis is associated with the CREST variant of PSS (17) and PSS patients are more likely to develop autoimmune thyroid disease (Hashimoto's thyroiditis) (43). Patients with PSS may develop the anemia of chronic disease with extensive organ involvement. Malabsorption and/or blood loss may contribute to the anemia. Microangiopathic hemolytic anemia is an ominous complication of PSS renal disease.

Laboratory Tests

Serological Tests

Antinuclear Antibodies

Fluorescent antinuclear antibodies (FANA) may be positive in up to 96% of patients with PSS (18); however, a negative FANA should never be used to rule out the possibility of PSS in a patient. The likelihood of the FANA being positive in PSS is related to the technique utilized and is particularly related to the tissue substrate used in the test. When tissue culture substrates are used, a larger variety of patterns can be seen with the most common pattern being speckled. With some diligence, these speckles can be distinguished into two groups, coarse and fine-speckled. PSS patients with fine speckles may also have antibodies to a saline extractable nuclear antigen (Scl-70) on immunodiffusion. Only a small number of PSS patients have antibody to Scl-70, although this may be related to the relative insensitivity of immunodiffusion as a technique for detecting antibodies. When present, antibody to Scl-70 is relatively specific for the diffuse form of PSS. Coarse-speckled staining also occurs in PSS, but the nature of the antigen causing this pattern is unknown. Antinucleolar antibodies are also frequently found in diffuse PSS but are also seen in the CREST variant and occasionally in other diseases. The specificity of the nucleolar pattern for PSS increases with an increasing titer. In recent years, a new staining pattern has emerged in which antibodies are detected to the centromere portion of the chromosome. Like nucleolar staining, centromere staining may be difficult to distinguish from speckled-staining on tissue section substrates, but it is easier to detect on tissue culture slides. Antibody to the centromere occurs in the majority of PSS patients with the CREST variant but may also be present in diffuse PSS. Antibodies to nuclear RNP and SM are rarely detected in PSS patients when performed by immunodiffusion. Antibodies to nuclear RNP may be present in up to 20% of PSS patients using hemagglutination assays. This reflects the sensitive nature of these assays for antibodies to nuclear RNP. The diagnosis of mixed connective tissue disease should not be entertained unless titers of antibodies to nuclear RNP are quite high and in general antinuclear RNP antibodies should be detected by immunodiffusion. Antibodies to native DNA are rarely found in PSS.

Other Immunological Studies

Rheumatoid factors may be present in up to one-third of PSS patients (21) and hyperglobulinemia and circulating immune complexes may be detected in up to one-half of patients (21,22). However, complement levels are generally within normal limits, suggesting that immune complexes are not responsible for extensive complement-mediated injury in this disease. In one study, patients with immune complexes were more likely to have echocardiographic abnormalities (21). In general, however, the presence of immune complexes has not correlated well with disease severity. The Westergren erythrocyte sedimentation rate may be elevated in approximately one-half of the patients. It has not been shown to correlate with organ system involvement or disease activity.

Other Laboratory Tests

As will be mentioned in the section on differential diagnosis, the detection of antinuclear antibodies, skin biopsy, and nailfold capillaroscopy are often valuable adjuncts to making the diagnosis of progressive systemic sclerosis. Once the diagnosis is established, the search for internal organ system involvement should be made in order to best treat the patient and also be in a better position to establish a prognosis. PSS patients should have a cineesophagram or manometric studies in order to establish the presence of esophageal involvement with this disease. Pulmonary involvement is actually as common as esophageal involvement, and all patients should have a spirometry with carbon monoxide diffusion capacity (35). A gallium lung scan (36) and/or a lung biopsy may help to establish the presence of inflammatory lung disease. However, at the present time there is no definite treatment for this entity, and these tests may not be justified. The role of treatment in preventing pulmonary fibrosis in this illness may become clearer over the next decade. An echocardiogram should be performed on PSS patients in order to evaluate the patient for pericardial disease as well as myocardial contraction abnormalities (21,44). Valvular abnormalities are occasionally seen, but the relationship between these abnormalities and the PSS disease process is not yet clear. An EKG should be performed on all patients and a 24-hour Holter monitor recording may be necessary to establish the presence of arrythmias which are not uncommon in PSS. The latter should be performed in the presence of signs or symptoms consistent with an arrythmia. The presence of renal disease should continually be monitored by performing blood pressure determinations. Frequent urinalyses, BUN's, and creatinines, as well as creatinine clearances, will help establish early renal disease in the absence of hypertension. The serum renin may be a sensitive indicator of PSS renal disease. However, the sample must be obtained under careful conditions and controlled fluid load. Renal biopsy or renal angiography are generally not performed because the presence and severity of renal disease can be established on the basis of clinical and laboratory parameters.

Roentgenograms of the hands can show erosive changes as well as distal osteolysis with associated calcinosis. These findings are rare in patients with early PSS, and hand roentgenograms are not usually of diagnostic importance.

Muscle enzymes such as the CPK and aldolase do not need to be performed routinely in the absence of symptoms or signs of a myopathy. If there are only minimal symptoms and mild elevations in the CPK and aldolase, careful clinical follow-up and repeat testing is indicated. With severe symptoms or signs of myopathy and, in particular, with marked elevation in the muscle enzymes, an EMG and muscle biopsy should be performed.

A small bowel roentgenogram may reveal involvement of the intestine with the scleroderma disease process. There may be dilation of the second and third portions of the duodenum as well as the jejunum with hypomotility being present. Small bowel biopsy will often be positive but is generally not needed to diagnose small bowel involvement with the PSS process. Seventy-two hour stool for fat determinations and a D-xylose absorption test may also be performed to evaluate the patient for malabsorption. Neither roentgenograms nor other studies need to be performed in the absence of symptoms or signs of malabsorption. B12 and iron levels may need to be performed in the presence of malabsorption as a guide to supplemental therapy.

Pathology

Histological examination of the digital arteries reveals intimal proliferation often leading to occlusion and adventitial fibrosis which can be severe. Reduplication and fraying of the internal elastic lamina and subendothelial fibrosis can also occur. Skin biopsies classically reveal thinning of the epidermis with loss of rete pegs. There is loss of dermal appendages and an increase in dermal collagen. Only homogenization of collagen may be seen in early disease. Large accumulations of lymphocytes (T cells) may occasionally be seen in the dermis and subcutis, particularly with early disease (4). Increased subepidermal melanin may also be seen. Skin biopsy specimens in PSS are thicker than control biopsies and weigh considerably more than normal biopsy specimens (45). Electron microscopy of PSS skin reveals increased amounts of immature collagen.

Synovial histology reveals infiltration of the synovium with lymphocytes and plasma cells. The synovium may become covered by a dense network of fibrin, and synovial fibrosis is a late finding. Muscle biopsy may reveal atrophy and necrosis of muscle fibers with extensive perimysial and epimysial fibrosis. Lymphocytic and plasma cell infiltration of muscle may occur in a manner similar to that seen in polymyositis.

Abnormal esophageal histologic changes are generally confined to the lower two-thirds of the organ. Mucosal thinning may occur with ulceration. The submucosa can be infiltrated with increased amounts of collagen, and submucosal round cell intiltrates also occur. The muscularis may be atrophied and replaced by dense fibrotic tissue.

Lung histology (46) consists of extensive fibrosis leading to thickening of alveolar walls. Septal degeneration or rupture leads to areas of bullous emphysema. Peribronchial and interstitial fibrosis also occur. Sclerosis of the pulmonary artery leading to pulmonary hypertension may occur in the absence of extensive pulmonary changes, particularly in those patients with the CREST form of PSS. Alveolar and bronchiolar carcinoma are found with an increased frequency in PSS and they may arise in areas of chronic inflammation with scarring.

Examination of the heart reveals extensive fibrosis which can also be found in the conducting system. Narrowed vessels and round cell infiltration may also be seen. As previously noted, the presence of contraction band necrosis suggests that there is intermittent spasm in the coronary vessels with reperfusion.

Kidney histopathology is remarkably similar to that found in malignant nephrosclerosis with the exception of the finding of intense arterial adventitial fibrosis. The surface of the kidney may contain cortical infarcts. Microscopic examination can reveal marked intimal hyperplasia of medium and small arteries. There is deposition of acid mucopolysaccharides in the vessel wall and fibrinoid necrosis of the vessel walls including those of the glomerular tufts.

The histopathology of the small bowel reveals changes similar to those seen in the esophagus with submucosal infiltration of collagen and atrophy of the muscularis often associated with severe fibrosis. Atrophy at the muscularis layer of the large bowel may result in the large-mouth sacculations in the colon which are relatively specific for PSS.

Differential Diagnosis and Diagnostic Criteria

The preliminary criteria for the classification of progressive systemic sclerosis were established in 1980 by a subcommittee of the American Rheumatism Association (9). These criteria which were shown in Table 14.3 were established as a means of setting definite criteria that would allow general agreement on the diagnosis of PSS in order to facilitate clinical trials and clinical research in the area of PSS. These criteria were not developed as an aid to diagnosing early disease. Patients with overlap syndromes were excluded from the final analysis of this study and the final criteria refer only to PSS patients. As can be seen, the single major criterion is proximal scleroderma. This is quite sensitive and specific for PSS. The minor criteria of sclerodactyly, digital pitting scars of the fingertips, and bibasilar pulmonary fibrosis also contribute to the diagnosis. The major difficulty for patients with early disease is making the diagnosis of proximal scleroderma.

As previously mentioned, the typical PSS patient will present with a long history of Raynaud's phenomenon and puffiness or swelling of the hands. The diseases associated with Raynaud's phenomenon are numerous (Table 14.6), but most can be ruled out with a careful history and physical examination. If the Raynaud's phenomenon occurs with physical signs of swelling and induration of the skin, then the patient most likely has an autoimmune connective tissue disorder such as PSS or mixed connective tissue disease. Most of the other diseases associated with scleroderma (Table 14.1) are not usually associated with Raynaud's phenomenon. Bleomyocin toxicity and vinyl chloride exposure may occasionally be associated with Raynaud's-like symptoms, but in these instances, the exposure history will help to distinguish these patients from PSS.

When no obvious cause for scleroderma skin changes is found, there are three general tests which are beneficial in establishing a diagnosis of early scleroderma. Recent advances in the detection of fluorescent antinuclear antibodies in PSS have enabled clinicians to use these tests more readily to establish the diagnosis (18). If the patient has an antibody to the centromere portion of the chromosome, then the diagnosis of the CREST variant of progressive systemic sclerosis is likely. Antibodies to nucleoli, especially in high titer, are relatively specific for the diffuse form of PSS. Detection of antibodies to the Scl-70 antigen by immunodiffusion is yet another test which is reasonably specific for diffuse PSS. If the fluorescent antinuclear antibody test is positive in a speckled pattern, the diagnosis of MCTD should be entertained. If antibodies to RNP are present by immunodiffusion, then the patient most likely has mixed connective tissue disease. These patients may eventually develop a disease which closely resembles PSS, but the clinical course is different enough from PSS to classify this illness as a separate entity. As mentioned, PSS patients may have low titers of antibodies to RNP by hemagglutination techniques. A positive ANA can also be indicative of SLE; however, the diagnostic criteria for SLE will usually enable one to distinguish SLE patients from those with PSS.

A skin biopsy may also be useful in diagnosing early PSS. The classic findings of generalized thickening secondary to accumulation of increased amount of collagenous connective tissue, loss of dermal appendages, and thinning of the epidermis may not all be present. However, the marked increase in dermal collagen with homogenization which occurs during the early stages of this illness can lend a great deal of support to the diagnosis of PSS. In addition, there may be large collections of lymphocytes in the dermis and subcutis, especially in early disease.

Nailfold capillaroscopy (24) with a dissecting microscope may help make the diagnosis of early PSS. The small blood vessels are markedly abnormal in PSS. The orientation of the capillaries in the nailfolds is such that one can get a good view of them on their long axis. The large dilated capillary loops that are seen in scleroderma may also be seen in dermatomyositis. However, these findings are not usually found in SLE or rheumatoid arthritis. Their presence, therefore, helps to establish the diagnosis of PSS.

There are several other scleroderma syndromes which need to be distinguished from PSS. As previously mentioned, the clinical picture and the specific serology of MCTD enables one to readily distinguish it from PSS, although some authors believe MCTD should be a subset of PSS.

Localized scleroderma can take several forms including morphea and linear scleroderma. Morphea consist of plaque-like areas with scleroderma skin changes. The skin is generally thickened with a waxy-shiny surface that becomes sclerotic, although the skin may appear more inflammatory early in the course of these lesions. Early sclerotic lesions are generally surrounded by a violaceous erythematous area of inflammation. The biopsy can closely resemble that seen in PSS although there tends to be more of a mononuclear inflammatory infiltrate. These skin areas tend to soften and involute with time, sometimes leaving areas of hyper- or hypopigmentation. Morphea is generally not associated with internal organ disease, and therefore is not a major problem although it can be a cosmetic problem, particularly on the face.

Linear scleroderma is generally a disease of childhood in which there is a linear streak of sclerotic skin on the upper or lower extremities. One side of the face may also be involved especially over the forehead and scalp, and this has been referred to as the *en coup de sabre* malady. These lesions can be associated with hemiatrophy, particularly of the face, but also of the extremities. Joint contractures can occur secondary to linear scleroderma. Melorheostosis refers to a linear fibrotic hyperostosis of bone that may coexist with linear scleroderma. Patients with localized scleroderma may have serological evidence of autoantibodies and rheumatoid factors suggesting that localized forms of scleroderma may be etiologically linked to PSS.

Eosinophilic fasciitis is a scleroderma syndrome which has only recently been described (11,12). The typical patient is a young or middle-aged adult who develops painful induration of the extremities after vigorous exercise. The disease can also appear in the absence of vigorous exercise and all ages may be affected. A striking eosinophilia and hyperglobulinemia may be found in the early stages of this disease, and they serve as a guide to the diagnosis. Histologic evidence is necessary to make the diagnosis, and a deep biopsy including skin, subcutis, fascia, and muscle should be obtained. The diagnostic finding is thickening and inflammation in the fascia with a marked infiltration of mononuclear cells as well as eosinophils. Increased fibrosis and inflammation may be found in other areas of the biopsy. Both the muscularis and subcutis are often infiltrated with inflammatory cells. This disease often resolves spontaneously, although treatment with low-dose corticosteroids is usually used with good relief of the painful induration of the skin. Both the peripheral eosinophilia and the eosinophilia on biopsy may have resolved by the time a biopsy is performed and the absence of eosinophilia does not preclude the diagnosis. The finding of aplastic anemia in a few patients with eosinophilic fasciitis points to its probable autoimmune etiology and is a cause of concern. This disease is potentially not as benign as was originally expected. Eosinophilic fasciitis patients usually do not have antinuclear antibodies, Raynaud's phenomenon, or internal system involvement consistent with PSS.

Graft vs host disease is an interesting illness that occurs in recipients of bone marrow transplants (14). These patients have features of PSS and Sjögren's syndrome. This illness, in which donor lymphocytes are capable of inducing autoimmune disease in recipients, is of interest for the light that it may shed on the pathogenesis of PSS.

Scleredema, also known as scleredema adultorum of Buschke, is an illness that can occasionally be confused as scleroderma. This illness often follows acute infection of the upper respiratory tract or ear. Children are more often affected and the illness tends to be self-limited with resolution over 6-12 months, although scleredema can become chronic. This illness, which can also be associated with diabetes mellitus, is characterized by painless swelling and induration of the skin over the trunk, flanks, face, and possibly lower extremities. Sparing of the hands and feet helps to distinguish this illness from scleroderma, and Raynaud's phenomenon usually does not occur. Histologically, there are swollen collagen bundles, but there is preservation of the rete pegs and accessory glands.

Amyloid disease can be associated with cutaneous papules consisting of amyloid protein. Occasionally, the skin infiltration becomes diffuse and there can be widespread edema and hardening of the skin.

Scleromyxedema (lichen myxedematosus papular mucinosis) is an illness in which there may be thickening of the skin associated with widespread lichenoid eruption of soft papules. Abnormal serum immunoglobulins are occasionally detected in these patients who have deposits of acid mucopolysaccharide in the upper portion of the dermis.

Porphyria cutanea tarda may be associated with induration of skin similar to that seen in scleroderma. The skin changes have a predilection for occurring on sun-exposed skin.

Vinylchloride workers develop an illness characterized by Raynaud's phenomenon, soreness and tenderness of the finger tips, nodular induration of the skin, the hands, and forearms, associated with synovial thickening of the proximal interphalangeal joints (19). Roentgenograms may reveal osteolysis of the distal phalanges. Hepatic and pleural fibrosis, pulmonary fibrosis, and splenomegaly have all been described in this syndrome.

Bleomycin therapy for malignancy may lead to pulmonary fibrosis and scleroderma-like skin changes associated with Raynaud's phenomenon (20). Histological changes in the skin resemble those seen in scleroderma, and bleomycin has been administered to experimental animals as a model for scleroderma and pulmonary fibrosis (32).

Course and Prognosis

PSS is a disease with an extremely variable clinical course. In one large study the mean survival rate in PSS was 45% at 7 years (48). As previously mentioned, patients with the CREST syndrome generally have a better prognosis than patients with diffuse scleroderma. Figure 14.6 depicts the mean survival in a recent study in which patients were separated into diffuse PSS and CREST groups (49). Survival is related to organ system involvement (48), and renal involvement remains an extremely poor prognostic finding with a mean survival measured in months despite advances in therapy. Patients with cardiac involvement have a worse prognosis than those with pulmonary disease. In general, patients without any internal organ involvement do quite well.

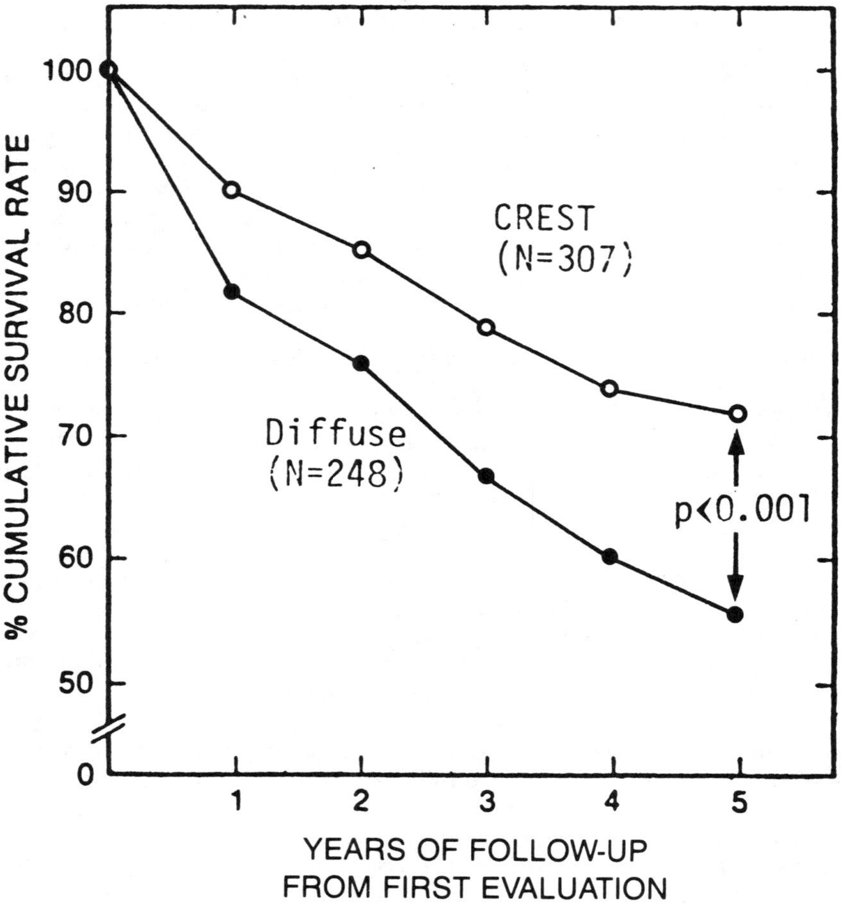

FIGURE 14.6 Cumulative survival rate from time of first University of Pittsburgh evaluation for patients with PSS and either CREST syndrome or the diffuse form of the disease. From Medsger, *Ortho Rev* 13:267, 1984 (used with permission).

The clinical course of the skin disease often goes through the edematous, indurative and thickened, and atrophic stages. However, the skin can soften and appear normal at any stage of disease although this tends to be a late finding. True remissions do occur with PSS. Internal organ system involvement also may stabilize for many years, suggesting that the term progressive may be an unnecessary burden for patients to bear. Unfortunately, the disease does tend to be progressive despite occasional long intervals of relative disease inactivity.

Treatment

It is quite difficult to make an adequate assessment of therapeutic improvement in a disease such as PSS. Despite these difficulties, it is becoming increasingly apparent that therapeutic intervention can be beneficial in many patients (49,50). For purposes of clinical trials and when treating individual patients, it is important to decide whether the patient has CREST syndrome or generalized diffuse PSS. It is also important to distinguish between early and late disease. CREST patients are primarily troubled by Raynaud's phenomenon, gastrointestinal motility problems, and the late occurrence of pulmonary hypertension. Generalized diffuse PSS patients have more difficulty with cutaneous, pulmonary, cardiac, renal, muscular, and joint involvement. These patients may also have symptomatic gastrointestinal disease. The patterns of cutaneous disease differ between CREST and generalized diffuse PSS. With generalized diffuse PSS there is a tendency towards gradual thinning of the skin as the early edematous and indurative phases give rise to a more atrophic stage of disease. There may also be spontaneous softening of the skin. In contrast, while skin involvement in CREST syndrome is relatively milder, there is a trend toward greater skin thickening with time. Any benefits attributable to the treatment of skin disease in PSS, must be analyzed against this background. In addition, in clinical trials and with individual patients one must keep in mind disease duration. Given these difficulties it is not surprising that there are few double-blind controlled treatment trials in PSS. The small numbers of patients at most medical centers and the expense of large multicentered trials are also a major factor in limiting these studies. Despite these difficulties, there has been a great deal more enthusiasm about the treatment of PSS over the last decade.

Vascular System

Warm socks and mittens, avoidance of cold, and the maintenance of an adequate core body temperature with clothing such as sweaters is of extreme importance in preventing vasospasm in PSS. These measures can often control the vasospasm leading to Raynaud's phenomenon and they may prevent renal and cardiac reflex vasospasm.

Vasoactive drugs (51) are used in three separate situations to treat PSS. These drugs are used to treat Raynaud's phenomenon, PSS renal disease, and pulmonary hypertension. In addition, some individuals believe that these drugs should be tried empirically because of the belief that the vascular abnormalities in PSS are of primary importance in the pathogenesis of the disease. In keeping with this philosphy, low-dose aspirin and dipyridamole have been used to treat PSS patients. There are known platelet and clotting abnormalities in PSS which may be contributing to the vascular abnormalities and in order to correct these abnormalities and to possibly influence the course of the disease, these relatively benign medications may be given.

TABLE 14.8 Vasoactive Drugs Used in the Treatment of PSS*

Drug	Organ System or Symptom Being Treated: Raynaud's Phenomenon	Hypertension/ Renal Disease	Pulmonary Hypertension
Guanethidine	+	+	
Alphamethyldopa	+	+	
Reserpine	+		
Phentolamine	+		+
Phenoxybenzamine	+		
Hydralazine	+	++	+
Prazosin	++	+++	+
Tolazoline	+		
Nitrates	+	++	+
Nifedipine	++	+	++
Captopril	++	++++	++
Minoxidil	+	+++	
Metoprolol		+++	

*Relative efficacy of drugs for specific situations, ranging from occasionally (+), to usually (++++) effective.

Table 14.8 shows the large number of presynaptic sympathetic blockers, postsynaptic alpha blockers, and vascular smooth muscle dilators which have been used to treat Raynaud's phenomenon. More recently, the calcium channel blockers have been utilized with some success. Captopril, an angiotensin-converting enzyme inhibitor, is also effective in treating Raynaud's, but its toxicities preclude its usage for uncomplicated Raynaud's phenomenon. The beta blockers are generally contraindicated in Raynaud's phenomenon as they may exacerbate the problem causing more reflex alpha spasm. Nifedipine and prazosin seem to be most effective in treating Raynaud's phenomenon. Local application of nitropaste may also be effective in treating secondary digital ulcerations. Raynaud's phenomenon may become refractory to any of the agents listed after an initial response.

Hypertension which is unassociated with proteinuria, azotemia, or decreased renal function may respond to prazosin or hydralazine. The presence of elevated renins and/or the presence of azotemia, decreased renal function, or proteinuria may call for the utilization of a drug that blocks renin release such as captopril, which is the most effective drug in treating PSS renal disease (52). It has major side effects such as nephrotic syndrome and leukopenia and should be used with caution. Captopril is not always an effective treatment for PSS renal disease and may need to be combined with other drugs such as prazosin for effective treatment. Diuretics such as furosemide may be necessary when fluid retention or congestive heart failure is a problem or when there is failure to get a satisfactory antihypertensive response. In general, diuretics should be used with caution because they may cause vascular depletion and further renin release.

Metoprolol is a beta blocker which inhibits renin release and therefore may provide effective therapy for PSS renal disease. It may exacerbate Raynaud's phenomenon or asthma and should be used cautiously. Both prazosin and minoxodil may be used concomitantly with metoprolol for control of PSS hypertension. A nitroprusside drip occasionally controls hypertension when other agents have failed. Nephrectomy often allows for much easier blood pressure control. The combination of antihypertensive therapy and dialysis has led to increased survival in PSS patients who previously would all have died with a mean 6-month survival after developing renal disease.

The treatment of pulmonary hypertension which occurs as a late complication of CREST syndrome is quite difficult. Nifedipine, hydralazine, prazosin, captropril, and nitrates can be tried either empirically or their hemodynamic effects can be measured at the time of heart catheterization. Patients may quickly become refractory to vasodilator therapy in this condition.

Gastrointestinal Disease

Esophageal Disease

Reflux esophagitis can be managed using the usual measures of antacids, elevating the head of the bed on blocks, and avoiding food before retiring. The histamine antagonists such as cimetidine and ranitidine may be necessary to control symptoms. Esophageal dilation may be necessary when stricture occurs.

Malabsorption

Malabsorption can be treated with antibiotics such as tetracycline and neomycin. Hypomotility, which underlies the malabsorption is occasionally amenable to metaclopramide. Vitamin supplementation with B_{12}, iron, and other vitamins may be necessary in the face of malabsorption. Dietary supplements may be necessary including those containing medium chain triglycerides. Hyperalimentation may be required in severe cases. Constipation is occasionally the major complaint and may be managed with appropriate bulking agents and laxatives.

Heart Disease

Arrhythmias, congestive heart failure, and pericardial disease should be managed using standard measures. Acute symptomatic pericardial disease may occasionally respond to moderate-dose corticosteroids. There is no definite role for the use of vasodilating agents in the prevention of myocardial fibrosis despite evidence that the cardiac lesion may be due to intermittent cardiac vasospasm. Hopefully, future studies will answer this question.

Lung Disease

There is no known therapy for the interstitial disease that occurs in PSS. Studies looking at gallium scans, pulmonary lavage studies, and biopsies may help identify patients with early active disease who could benefit from therapy before fibrosis occurs.

Muscle Disease

Corticosteroids should only be given to PSS patients with a definite myopathy diagnosed by the physical examintion, biopsy, EMG, and muscle enzymes. Prednisone in dosages between 20 and 60 mg may be given. Many patients will have a mild myopathy with slight elevations in their CPK and atrophy on biopsy. Because of the hazards of corticosteroids, these patients should not receive treatment.

Joint Disease

Nonsteroidal antiinflammatory agents can be utilized at moderate dosages such as those used to treat osteoarthritis. Nonacetylated salicylates have the advantage of having less gastrointestinal toxicity and less effect on renal blood flow. There is no evidence that the nonsteroidal antiinflammatory agents will have other than analgesic effects in this disease.

Skin Disease

D-penicillamine is now widely utilized to treat PSS skin disease, but it has not been definitely shown to be effective. In a large retrospective study (53), PSS patients had increased survival, less new organ system involvement, and more improvement of their skin than control patients who did not receive D-penicillamine. It is important to note that the patients that were part of this retrospective study did not have CREST syndrome, but had generalized diffuse PSS. These patients also had disease of only 3 years duration. It is not clear that D-penicillamine would benefit CREST patients or those patients with long-standing disease. It currently is quite difficult to perform a double-blind controlled study of D-penicillamine therapy in PSS because so many patients are treated with the drug and an expensive large multicentered study would be necessary to evaluate this therapy. In the absence of these double-blind controlled studies, one should keep in mind that D-penicillamine is a potentially quite toxic drug which should be administered with caution and informed consent.

Potassium P-aminobenzoate has been used for many years to treat PSS. Occasional patients seem to do well on this drug and note an exacerbation of their symptoms when they discontinue it. Skin rash and bone marrow depression may sometimes occur with this drug, which is not now commonly used.

Skin emollients help the dry skin found in PSS and should be applied frequently to be beneficial. PSS skin may be more susceptible to sun exposure, and sun screens may be necessary to avoid sun-exposed damage.

Miscellaneous Measures

Sjögren's syndrome and Hashimoto's thyroiditis leading to hypothyroidism may require appropriate supportive measures.

References

1. Rodnan GP: Progressive systemic sclerosis (scleroderma). In DJ McCarty Jr (ed.), *Arthritis and Allied Conditions,* 9th Ed. Philadelphia, Lea and Febiger, 1979, pp. 762-809.

2. LeRoy EC: Scleroderma (systemic sclerosis). In WN Kelley, ED Harris Jr, S Ruddy, CB Sledge (eds.), *Textbook of Rheumatology,* Philadelphia, W.B. Saunders, 1981, pp. 1211-1230.

3. Rodnan GP, Jablonska S, Medsger TA: Classification and nomenclature of progressive systemic sclerosis (scleroderma). *Clin Rheum Dis* 5:5-14, 1979.

4. Fleischmajer R, Perlish JS, Reeves JRT: Cellular infiltrates in scleroderma skin. *Arthritis Rheum* 20:975-984, 1977.

5. Haynes DC, Gershwin ME: The immunopathology of progressive systemic sclerosis (PSS). *Semin Arthritis Rheum* 11:331-351, 1982.

6. Fleischmajer R, Perlish JS, Duncan M: Scleroderma: A model for fibrosis. *Arch Derm* 119:957-962, 1983.

7. Campbell PM, LeRoy EC: Pathogenesis of systemic sclerosis: A vascular hypothesis. *Semin Arthritis Rheum* 4:351-368, 1975.

8. Fleischmajer R, Perlish JS, Shaw KV, Pirozzi DJ: Skin capillary changes in early systemic scleroderma. Electron microscopy and in vitro autoradiography with tritiated thymidine. *Arch Dermatol* 112:1553-1557, 1976.

9. Subcommittee for Scleroderma Criteria of the American Rheumatism Association Diagnostic and Therapeutic Criteria Committee. Preliminary criteria for the classification of systemic sclerosis (scleroderma). *Arthritis Rheum* 23:581-590, 1980.

10. Salerni R, Rodnan GP, Leon DF, Shaver JA: Pulmonary hypertension in the CREST syndrome variant of progressive systemic sclerosis (scleroderma). *Ann Intern Med* 86:394-399, 1977.

11. Shulman LE: Diffuse fasciitis with eosinophilia: A new syndrome? *Trans Assoc Am Physicians* 88:70-86, 1975.

12. Bennett RM, Herron A, Keogh L: Eosinophilic fasciitis. Case report and review of the literature. *Ann Rheum Dis* 36:354-359, 1977.

13. Sharp GC, Irvin WS, Tan EM, Gould RG, Holman HR: Mixed connective tissue - An apparently distinct rheumatic disease syndrome associated with a specific antibody to an extractable nuclear antigen (ENA). *Am J Med* 52:148-159, 1972.

14. Shulman HM, Sullivan KM, Weiden PL, McDonald GB, Striker GE, Sale GE, Hackman R, Tsoi M-S, Storb R, Thomas ED: Chronic graft-versus-host syndrome in man: A long-term clinicopathologic study of 20 Seattle patients. *Am J Med* 69:204-217, 1980.

15. Goetz RH: The pathology of progressive systemic sclerosis (generalized scleroderma) with special reference to changes in the viscera. *Clin Proc* (Capetown) 4:337-392, 1945.

16. Winterbauer RH: Multiple telangiectasia, Raynaud's phenomenon, sclerodactyly and subcutaneous calcinosis: A syndrome mimicking hereditary hemorrhagic telangiectasia. *Bull Johns Hopkins Hosp* 114:361-383, 1964.

17. Reynolds TB, Denison EK, Frankl HD, Lieberman FL, Peters RL: Primary biliary cirrhosis with scleroderma, Raynaud's phenomenon and telangiectasia. *Amer J Med* 50:302-312, 1971.

18. Tan EM, Rodnan GP, Garcia I, Moroi Y, Fritzler MJ, Peebles C: Diversity of antinuclear antibodies in progressive systemic sclerosis. Anticentromere antibody and its relationship to CREST syndrome. *Arthritis Rheum* 23:617-625, 1980.

19. Ward AM, Vdoon S, Watkins J, Walker AE, Darke CS: Immunological mechanisms in the pathogenesis of vinyl chloride disease. *Br Med J*:i:936-938, 1976.

20. Finch WR, Rodnan GP, Buckingham RB, Prince RK, Winkelstein A: Bleomycin-induced scleroderma. *J Rheum* 7:651-659, 1980.

21. Pisko E, Gallup K, Turner R, Parker M, Nomeir A-M, Box J, Davis J, Box P, Rothberger H: Cardiopulmonary manifestations of progressive systemic sclerosis: Associations with circulating immune complexes and fluorescent antinuclear antibodies. *Arthritis Rheum* 22:518-523, 1979.

22. Seibold JR, Medsger TA, Winkelstein A, Kelly RA, Rodnan GP: Immune complexes in progressive systemic sclerosis (scleroderma). *Arthritis Rheum* 25:1167-1173, 1982.

23. McCoy RC, Tisher CC, Pepe PF , Cleveland LA: The kidney in progressive systemic sclerosis. Immunohistochemical and antibody elution studies. *Lab Invest* 35:124-131, 1976.

24. Maricq HR, LeRoy EC Jr, D'Angelo WA, Medsger TA Jr, Rodnan GP, Sharp GC, Wolfe JF: Diagnostic potential of in vivo capillary microscopy in scleroderma and related disorders. *Arthritis Rheum* 23:183-189, 1980.

25. Kahaleh MB, Sherer GK, LeRoy EC: Endothelial injury in scleroderma. *J Exp Med* 149:1326-1335, 1979.

26. Kahaleh MB, Osborn I, LeRoy EC: Increased factor VIII/von Willebrand factor antigen and von Willebrand factor activity in scleroderma and Raynaud's phenomenon. *Ann Int Med* 94:482-484, 1981.

27. Kahaleh MB, Osborn I, LeRoy EC: Elevated levels of circulating platelet aggregates and beta-thromboglobulin in scleroderma. *Ann Int Med* 96: 610-613, 1982.

28. Buckingham RB, Prince R, Rodnan GP, Taylor F: Increased collagen accumulation in dermal fibroblast cultures from patients with progressive systemic sclerosis (scleroderma). *J Lab Clin Med* 92:5-21, 1978.

29. Rodnan GP, Lipinski E, Luksick J: Skin thickness and collagen content in progressive systemic sclerosis and localized scleroderma. *Arthritis Rheum* 22:130-140, 1979.

30. Gershwin ME, Abplanalp H, Castles JJ, Ikeda RM, vanderWater J, Eklund J, Haynes D: Characterization of a spontaneous disease of white leghorn chickens resembling progressive systemic sclerosis (scleroderma). *J Exp Med* 153:1640-1659, 1981.

31. Jimenez SA, Millan A, Bashey RI: Scleroderma-like alterations in collagen metabolism occurring in the TSK (tight skin) mouse. *Arthritis Rheum* 27:180-185, 1984.

32. Mountz JD, Downs Minor MB, Turner R, Thomas MB, Richards F, Pisko E: Bleomycin-induced cutaneous toxicity in the rat: Analysis of histopathology and ultrastructure compared with progressive systemic sclerosis (scleroderma). *Br J Derm* 108:679-686, 1983.

33. Spencer-Green G: Raynaud phenomenon. *Bull Rheum Dis* 33:1-8, 1983.

34. Blunt RJ, Porter JM: Raynaud syndrome. *Semin Arthritis Rheum* 10:282-308, 1981.

35. Guttadauria M, Ellman H, Emmanuel G, Kaplan D, Diamond H: Pulmonary function in scleroderma. *Arthritis Rheum* 20:1071-1079, 1977.

36. Baron M, Feiglin D, Hyland R, Urowitz MB, Shiff B: ^{67}Gallium lung scans in progressive systemic sclerosis. *Arthritis Rheum* 26:969-974, 1983.

37. Bulkley BH, Ridolfi RL, Salyer WR, Hutchins GM: Myocardial lesions of progressive systemic sclerosis. A cause of cardiac dysfunction. *Circulation* 53:483-490, 1976.

38. Clements PJ, Furst DE, Cabeen W, Tashkin D, Paulus HE, Roberts N: The relationship of arrhythmias and conduction disturbances to other manifestations of cardiopulmonary disease in progressive systemic sclerosis (PSS). *Am J Med* 71:38-46, 1981.

39. Nussbaum AI, LeRoy EC: Renal involvement in scleroderma (systemic sclerosis). In PA Bacon, NM Hadler (eds.), *The Kidney and Rheumatic Disease*. London, Butterworth Scientific, 1982, pp. 282-296.

40. Sommers SC, LeRoy EC: The relationship of hypertension and renal failure in scleroderma (progressive systemic sclerosis) to structural and functional abnormalities of the renal cortical circulation. *Medicine* 53:1-46, 1974.

41. Kovalchik MT, Guggenheim SJ, Silverman MH, Robertson JS, Steigerwald JC: The kidney in progressive systemic sclerosis: A prospective study. *Ann Intern Med* 89:881-887, 1978.

42. Cipoletti JF, Buckingham RB, Barnes EL, Peel RL, Mahmood K, Cignetti FE, Pierce JM, Rabin BS, Rodnan GP: Sjögren's syndrome in progressive systemic sclerosis (scleroderma). *Ann Intern Med* 87:535-541, 1977.

43. Medsger TA Jr: Thyroid disease in progressive systemic sclerosis: Increased frequency of glandular fibrosis and hypothyroidism. *Ann Intern Med* 95: 431-435, 1981.

44. Smith JW, Clements PJ, Levisman J, Furst D, Ross M: Echocardiographic features of progressive systemic sclerosis: Correlation with hemodynamic and postmortem studies. *Am J Med* 66:28-33 1979.

45. Rodnan GP, Lipinski E, Luksick J: Skin thickness and collagen content in progressive systemic sclerosis and localized scleroderma. *Arthritis Rheum* 22:130-140, 1979.

46. Young RH, Mark GJ: Pulmonary vascular changes in scleroderma. *Am J Med* 64:998-1004, 1978.

47. D'Angelo WA, Fries JF, Masi AT, Shulman LE: Pathologic observations in systemic sclerosis (scleroderma). *Am J Med* 46:428-440, 1969.

48. Medsger TA Jr, Masi AT, Rodnan GP, Benedek TG, Robinson H: Survival with systemic sclerosis (scleroderma): A life-table analysis of 309 patients. *Ann Intern Med* 75:369-376, 1971.

49. Medsger TA: Scleroderma: Recent advances in the treatment of progressive systemic sclerosis. *Orth Rev* 13:267-278, 1984.

50. Medsger TA Jr: Clinical trials in progressive systemic sclerosis. *Clin Rheum Dis* 9:655-670, 1983.

51. Coffman JD: Vasodilator drugs in peripheral vascular disease. *N Engl J Med* 300:713-717, 1979.

52. Whitman HH III, Case DB, Laragh JH, Christian CL, Botstein G, Maricq H, LeRoy EC: Variable response to oral angiotensin-coverting-enzyme blockade in hypertensive scleroderma patients. *Arthritis Rheum* 25:241-248, 1982.

53. Steen VD, Medsger TA Jr, Rodnan GP: D-penicillamine therapy in progressive systemic sclerosis (scleroderma). *Ann Int Med* 97:652-658, 1982.

Chapter 15

SJÖGREN'S SYNDROME

Christopher M. Wise, M.D., and
Elliott L. Semble, M.D.

Sjögren's syndrome is a chronic inflammatory disorder characterized by diminished lacrimal and salivary gland secretion (1). The primary clinical manifestations are dry eyes (xerophthalmia) and dry mouth (xerostomia), which result from lymphocytic and plasma cell infiltration of the lacrimal and salivary glands. In the late nineteenth and early twentieth centuries, several authors described some of the components of the syndrome (2). Leber first described keratitis, while Haden first described xerostomia. Mikulicz described a syndrome of lacrimal and salivary gland enlargement in 1892, which is pathologically identical to what we now know as Sjögren's syndrome (3). The first association between dry eyes, dry mouth, and arthritis was made by Dr. Henrik Sjögren, a Swedish ophthalmologist, in 1933. Since that time a great deal of information has been learned about this syndrome, and it has evolved from a medical curiosity to a relatively frequently diagnosed autoimmune disease.

Although there is no absolute definition of Sjögren's syndrome, the classic triad of dry eyes, dry mouth, and the presence of a connective tissue disease (usually rheumatoid arthritis) is usually sufficient. Several other clinical and laboratory diagnostic parameters have been introduced in recent years to help in the recognition of this disorder. Sjögren's syndrome may occur without any association disorder (the primary form), or it may occur in association with a variety of connective tissue diseases (the secondary form). Rheumatoid arthritis is the most commonly associated disease, but in recent years the syndrome has been increasingly recognized in association with systemic lupus erythematosus, progressive systemic sclerosis, mixed connective tissue disease, and polymyositis.

Sjögren's syndrome occurs most often in middle-aged and elderly females. Females constitute more than 90% of all patients with the diagnosis of Sjögren's syndrome, with a mean age of onset of 50 (1,2). The incidence of sicca syndrome (dry eyes and mouth) in elderly patients may range as high as 3%, but most of these patients probably have senile atrophy of the secretory apparatus rather than immunologic injury (3). The exact prevalence of the condition in the general population is difficult to determine, but autopsy studies suggest that the syndrome occurs in somewhat less than 1% of the population.

Etiopathogenesis

General Aspects

Genetic factors undoubtedly play a role in the development of Sjögren's syndrome. In addition to several reports of familial occurrence, other studies have shown a relatively high frequency of clinical and serologic abnormalities in younger relatives of patients with Sjögren's syndrome (3). Several studies have shown an increased incidence of the histocompatibility markers HLA-B8 and HLA-DW3 in patients with Sjögren's syndrome (4,5). Approximately 75% of patients with primary Sjögren's syndrome are positive for HLA-DW3, compared to 24% of controls. However, this HLA association is not seen in those patients with Sjögren's syndrome associated with rheumatoid arthritis. HLA-DW3 is also associated with several other autoimmune diseases, including celiac disease, dermatitis herpetiformis, myasthenia gravis, Grave's disease, chronic active hepatitis, Addison's disease, and insulin-dependent diabetes mellitus, in addition to systemic lupus erythematosus.

Infectious Agents

Several studies have attempted to implicate various infectious agents in the initiation of the immunologic process that characterizes Sjögren's syndrome. To date, attempts have been made to culture viruses from saliva, or demonstrate changes in antibody titers to specific viruses. However, these efforts have been unsuccessful, as have attempts to isolate a virus from salivary gland tissue. Particles resembling viruses have been demonstrated in renal tubular cells, major and minor salivary glands, vascular endothelium, and lymphocytes. Further studies have shown that these probably represent ultrastructural alterations in normal subcellular components rather than viral structures (3).

Immunologic Abnormalities

Sjögren's syndrome is characterized by numerous manifestations of hyperactivity of B lymphocytes. Hyperglobulinemia is seen in over 50% of patients, and autoantibodies and circulating immune complexes are often detected. Within the lymphoid infiltrates in the salivary glands, local synthesis of immunoglobulin has been described. Circulating immune complexes are detectable in a high proportion of patients, but their role in pathogenesis is unclear.

The B-cell hyperactivity and excess helper T-cell function seen in Sjögren's syndrome has been implicated in the tissue damage seen in this condition (6). However, a decrease in suppressor T cells has also been found in peripheral blood and salivary tissue of patients with this disorder and the importance of these lymphocyte abnormalities is unclear at this time.

Animal Models

The development of an inbred animal model of human SLE, the New Zealand black/white F1 hybrid mouse, has also greatly aided investigation of many aspects of Sjögren's syndrome (2). Lymphocytic infiltration in many organ systems is seen in this mouse, particularly in the salivary glands. In addition, lymphatic neoplasms may develop spontaneously later in the course of the disease, as sometimes occurs in humans with Sjögren's syndrome. Thus, this animal may serve as a model for Sjögren's syndrome, in addition to SLE, and may be a useful tool for investigating etiopathogenetic mechanisms in both diseases.

Clinical Features

Ocular Manifestations

Inflammation of the lacrimal glands results in decreased tear production and symptoms of dry eyes (keratoconjunctivitis sicca). In most series, 85-95% of patients complain of dry eyes, but as many as one-third to one-half of patients in other studies fail to have significant symptoms (2,7). A foreign body sensation, grittiness, or accumulation of thick, ropey secretions may be noted. In addition, patients may complain of erythema, photosensitivity, eye fatigue, or decreased visual acuity. Chronic dryness may result in disruption of the corneal epithelium which predisposes the eye to bacterial or viral infection.

The Schirmer's test is a screening procedure designed to detect the presence of dry eyes by measuring tear production. This is performed by using a strip of filter paper folded and placed over the lower lid near the middle to outer third (as shown in Figure 15.1). In normal individuals, the paper will demonstrate wetting of at least 15 mm after 5 minutes. Less than 5 mm is considered abnormal, although many older individuals without Sjögren's syndrome will demonstrate decreased wetting. Some authors advocate a second stage to the Schirmer's test, in which maximum tear production is stimulated with ammonia. Staining of the cornea with rose bengal dye and observation through slitlamp examination may demonstrate evidence of filamentary and punctate keratitis.

Oral Manifestations

Inflammatory changes in the salivary glands result in decreased production of saliva and symptoms of dryness of the mouth (xerostomia). Although not usually a presenting complaint, this symptom is present in a vast majority of patients at some point. Other manifestations of xerostomia include difficulty in swallowing, cracking and fissuring of the tongue and lips, loss of taste, and polydypsia. Lack of normal lubrication also predisposes to accelerated dental caries, particularly along the borders of the teeth adjacent to the gingiva.

Xerostomia is not a specific symptom of Sjögren's syndrome, and may also be seen in heavy smokers, mouth breathers, as a complication of certain drug therapy (particularly tricyclic antidepressants), and after irradiation of the salivary glands. Xerostomia may also be seen in states of dehydration, but should be accompanied by other signs. The earliest objective sign on physical examination is the absence of pooling of saliva in the floor of the mouth. There is not a single, simple objective test for the assessment of xerostomia. However, objective laboratory assessment of parotid and salivary gland involvement may be accomplished by sialography, assessment of parotid saliva flow, scintigraphy, or by labial biopsy.

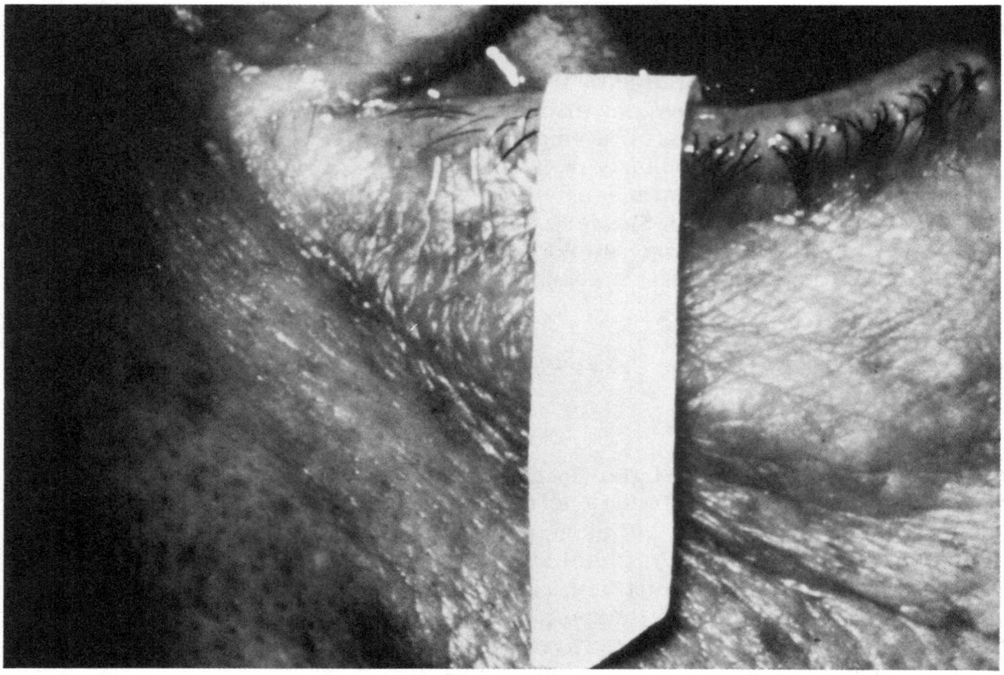

FIGURE 15.1 The Schirmer's test assesses tear production. It is performed by placing a strip of filter paper over the lower lid. Wetting is measured after 5 minutes (normally over 15-mm wetting). Reprinted from the Revised Clinical Slide Collection on the Rheumatic Diseases, copyright, 1981. Used by permission of the Arthritis Foundation.

Dryness of other mucosal membranes, including the nasal mucosa, upper respiratory tract, and vagina, may result in symptoms in these areas. Submandibular and parotid gland enlargement occurs in many patients, and may be either unilateral or bilateral (7).

Articular Manifestations

A mild, relapsing, nonerosive polyarthritis is common in Sjögren's syndrome (3). Approximately one-half of patients have articular symptoms which precede the onset of dry eyes and dry mouth. Arthralgias are even more common than true arthritis (8). The MCP's, PIP's, wrists, and knees are most often affected. Radiographic changes are usually minimal, but destructive changes may be seen.

Pulmonary Manifestations

Lung involvement in Sjögren's syndrome may take many forms, and occurs in 10-15% of patients (3,7). Chronic inflammatory changes around the bronchial glands may result in chronic bronchitis and obstructive changes. Recurrent pneumonitis and pleurisy have been described in a small number of patients. Chronic interstitial fibrosis of varying degree has also been described. In addition, many patients with normal radiographs may have evidence of restrictive disease and diminished gas transfer on pulmonary function testing.

Gastrointestinal and Hepatic Disease

Gastrointestinal involvement may be seen in Sjögren's syndrome. Antibodies to parietal cells may occur in 25-30% of patients and may be associated with atrophic gastritis. However, the overall incidence of overt pernicious anemia in one series was only 3.5% (9). Clinical pancreatitis may be seen, and extensive testing has detected subclinical abnormalities in pancreatic function in large numbers of patients.

Liver enlargement has been described in about 20% of patients, although liver enzyme abnormalities and biopsy-proven disease is relatively unusual. Primary biliary cirrhosis may be associated with Sjögren's syndrome. Antimitochondrial antibodies may be seen in about 10% of patients, and this is usually associated with histologic evidence of lymphocytic infiltrates in liver biopsy specimens. Chronic active hepatitis has also been described in a small number of patients with Sjögren's syndrome. In addition, features of Sjögren's syndrome have been found frequently in patients with chronic active hepatitis, and in a majority of patients with primary biliary cirrhosis (10).

Renal Disease

Renal tubular dysfunction resulting from lymphocytic interstitial infiltrates may occur in Sjögren's syndrome. Up to one-third of patients may demonstrate concentrating defects and inability to excrete an acid load. Nephrogenic diabetes insipidus and renal tubular acidosis may be seen as well as aminoaciduria, hypouricemia, and glycosuria (11). In addition to interstitial nephritis, glomerulonephritis has been described in a few patients (12).

Cutaneous Manifestations

Skin dryness is a common complaint of patients with Sjögren's syndrome and may be related to chronic inflammation of the sweat and sebaceous glands. Ulcerations of the lip and skin, angular stomatitis, purpura, and livedo reticularis may also occur.

Endocrine Abnormalities

Although Sjögren's syndrome typically involves the exocrine glands, several abnormalities of the endocrine system have been described. Thyroid disease may be seen in association with this syndrome. Antithyroglobulin and antithyroid microsomal antibodies may be detected in about 40% of patients, some of whom have histologic evidence of Hashimoto's thyroiditis (9,13).

Neuromuscular Manifestations

Neuromuscular features of Sjögren's syndrome include facial nerve palsy, trigeminal neuropathy, and other isolated cranial nerve abnormalities. Peripheral neuropathy, either a sensory or sensory-motor type, has also been described (9). A recent series described several central nervous system complications of Sjögren's syndrome, including hemiparesis, meningoencephalitis, cerebellar ataxia, subarachnoid hemorrhage, seizures, and myelopathy (14). Sjögren's syndrome was diagnosed prior to the onset of CNS disease in only 3 of the 16 patients in this series. Polymyositis, myasthenia gravis, and focal myositis may also be associated with Sjögren's syndrome.

Raynaud's Phenomenon and Vasculitis

Raynaud's phenomenon occurs frequently in patients with Sjögren's syndrome, probably in about 20–35% of patients (7). Vasculitic lesions occur in about 35% of patients (15). Vasculitis may involve the skin, nervous sytem, or visceral organs. Vasculitis has been associated with hyperglobulinemia, antibodies to SSA (see discussion of laboratory findings), and other autoantibodies, as well as anemia, leukopenia, or thrombocytopenia.

Disease Associations (Secondary Sjögren's Syndrome)

In the secondary form of Sjögren's syndrome, a variety of connective tissue diseases (e.g., rheumatoid arthritis, systemic lupus erythematosus, scleroderma) may be found.

Rheumatoid Arthritis

Sjögren's syndrome occurs in 10–20% of patients with rheumatoid arthritis, although with more extensive testing, the prevalence may be closer to 30% (2). Overall, 30–55% of all patients with Sjögren's syndrome have rheumatoid arthritis. Rheumatoid arthritis patients with or without Sjögren's syndrome have similar laboratory and genetic features. In the majority of patients, rheumatoid arthritis precedes the appearance of dry eyes and dry mouth by many years (16).

Systemic Lupus Erythematosus

The coexistence of Sjögren's syndrome and systemic lupus erythematosus is well known, but the exact frequency with which this occurs is uncertain. One early study found abnormalities of parotid glands by sialography, scintigraphy, or labial biopsy in almost all patients with SLE, but using more strict criteria, probably only about 30% of patients had Sjögren's syndrome (17). A more recent study found labial biopsy abnormalities compatible with Sjögren's syndrome in about 50% of SLE patients. In this study, symptoms of dry eyes or dry mouth did not always correlate with the histopathologic abnormalities, and abnormal Schirmer's tests were found in only about 20% of patients (18).

Scleroderma

Although previously thought to be relatively uncommon in scleroderma, the findings of Sjögren's syndrome are present in a significant percentage of patients with this disorder. One early study found evidence of keratoconjunctivitis in 40%, labial biopsy abnormalities in 50%, and sialographic or scintigraphic abnormalities in virtually all scleroderma patients (19). More recently however, only about 17% of patients were felt to fulfill criteria for Sjögren's syndrome by clinical features and labial biopsy (20). In the latter study, a large number of patients were found to have sclerosis and fibrosis on labial biopsy, but few of these patients had inflammatory changes or symptoms of Sjögren's syndrome.

Other Disease Associations

Sjögren's syndrome has also been associated with various other autoimmune diseases, including mixed connective tissue disease and polymyositis. It is also found in graft-vs-host disease (21), seen after bone marrow transplantation. Sjögren's syndrome has also been rarely associated with autoimmune hemolytic anemia (22). As previously discussed, there also exists a clinical overlap with autoimmune hepatic diseases, such as chronic active hepatitis and primary biliary cirrhosis.

Lymphoproliferation, Pseudolymphoma, and Lymphoma

A wide spectrum of lymphoproliferation, ranging from benign infiltration to malignant degeneration, occurs in Sjögren's syndrome (3,23). In the early stages of benign proliferation within exocrine glands, infiltration is limited to the periductal region. Diffuse involvement may occur with advancing disease resulting in destruction of the acini.

Progressive lymphocytic infiltration is termed pseudolymphoma. Massive salivary gland enlargement, lymphadenopathy, and pulmonary infiltrates may be found. Histopathologic findings in pseudolymphoma include loss of normal lymph node architecture, but malignant changes within the cells are not present. Pseudolymphoma is often associated with elevated levels of serum gammaglobulins.

Patients with Sjögren's syndrome are at increased risk for development of malignant lymphoreticular neoplasms, with a frequency of lymphoma as high as 5% in some centers (3). It may often be difficult to distinguish pseudolymphoma from true lymphoma either clinically or pathologically. A wide variety of lymphoid malignancies are seen, including Hodgkin's disease, non-Hodgkin's lymphoma, thymoma, and Waldenstrom's macroglobulinemia. Lymphoma is more likely to occur in patients with more severe extraglandular complications of Sjögren's syndrome.

Diagnosis

Dry eyes and dry mouth are not specific for Sjögren's syndrome, but may be seen in a number of other diseases, including hyperlipoproteinemia, hemochromatosis, sarcoidosis, and amyloidosis (1). Drugs with anticholinergic activity may cause xerostomia, and many normal elderly individuals may have diminished tear production.

The diagnosis of Sjögren's syndrome may be very difficult on the basis of clinical findings alone. Listed in Table 15.1 are several tests which have been developed to assess the presence and degree of lacrimal and salivary gland involvement. Schirmer's test, previously described, is an objective test used to quantitate tear production. Rose bengal staining may detect corneal abnormalities, as noted earlier. Salivary gland function may be studies by measuring parotid flow after lemon juice stimulation or by radionuclide scanning. Unfortunately, these tests are nonspecific, and abnormalities may be seen in other disease states.

Parotid sialography may show dilation, narrowing and atrophy of salivary ducts in Sjögren's syndrome, but may be abnormal as well in other conditions involving inflammation of these glands, including sarcoidosis.

The most sensitive and specific procedure for diagnosing Sjögren's syndrome is biopsy of one of the minor salivary glands in the labial region. The number of mononuclear cell aggregations in the tissue specimen is counted and scored. The most frequently used system was described by Greenspan in 1974 (24). Using this

TABLE 15.1 Diagnostic Tests in Sjögren's Syndrome

Schirmer's test
Rose bengal staining
Salivary gland function: Parotid flow rates, scintigraphy, sialography
Minor salivary gland biopsy

scoring system, aggregates of 50 or more mononuclear cells within salivary gland tissue constitute a focus of cells. The presence of greater than one focus for every 4 mm^2 of tissue is considered abnormal and characteristic of Sjögren's syndrome (24,25). An example of a typical positive minor salivary gland biopsy is seen in Figure 15.2.

There are no uniformly accepted criteria for the diagnosis of Sjögren's syndrome. However, most investigators would require a history of dry eyes or dry mouth, with abnormal Schirmer's test and/or rose bengal staining, and confirmation by minor salivary gland biopsy.

Laboratory Features

Normochromic normocytic anemia is a common finding in Sjögren's syndrome. Other hematologic abnormalities, such as leukopenia, eosinophilia, and thrombocytopenia have been occasionally reported. Hyperglobulinemia is frequently present and rarely cryoglobulinemia and hyperviscosity may occur. Levels of serum IgG, IgA, and IgM are elevated in most patients. The sedimentation rate is increased in the majority of patients, although correlation with disease activity is often poor.

Several studies have shown elevated levels of salivary immunoglobulins. Other authors have reported elevated levels of beta 2 microglobulin and lysozyme in saliva (3,26).

Autoantibodies

A wide variety of autoantibodies are seen in both primary and secondary Sjögren's syndrome, including antibodies directed against gastric parietal cells, thyroid microsomes and thyroglobulin, mitochondria, smooth muscle, and salivary duct antigens. Rheumatoid factors occur in a majority of patients, and are almost always seen in those with associated rheumatoid arthritis. Antinuclear antibodies occur in most patients as well, although the exact frequency is variable.

In 1975, a separate antigen-antibody system (SSA, anti-SSA and SSB, anti-SSB) was described. Initially anti-SSA and anti-SSB were felt to be highly specific for primary Sjögren's syndrome (27). Subsequent studies by the same authors and others have suggested that these autoantibodies may not be specific for primary Sjögren's syndrome, but may also be detected in Sjögren's syndrome associated with rheumatoid arthritis or other connective tissue diseases (28,29). Anti-SSA and SSB are also relatively common in SLE, even without evidence of coexistent Sjögren's syndrome.

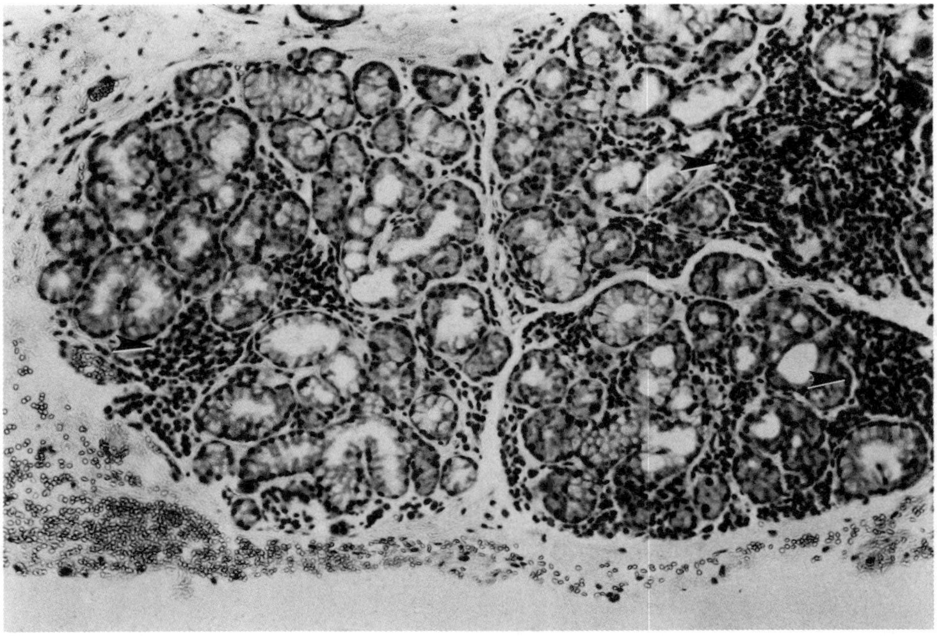

FIGURE 15.2 Photomicrograph of a minor salivary gland biopsy in a patient with Sjögren's syndrome. Arrowheads show three foci of lymphocytes, each of which has more than 50 cells. Mag X 330. (Courtesy of Dr. V.R. Challa, Department of Pathology, Bowman Gray School of Medicine.)

Pathology and Radiology

Pathologic changes may be seen in the major and minor salivary glands as well as the lacrimal glands. Biopsy of the major salivary gland is seldom recommended, unless there is some suggestion of a parotid malignancy. Biopsy of the minor salivary glands of the lip has become a relatively simple and useful procedure for diagnosing Sjögren's syndrome (25).

Characteristic histological finding of the salivary glands include lymphocytic and plasma cell infiltration. A sytem for quantitating the amount of inflammation has been devised as noted previously (24). A focal area of 50 or more inflammatory cells counts as a focus. A grade 0 biopsy shows no infiltration, while grade 1 indicates slight infiltration. Grade 2 biopsies show moderate infiltration, or less than 1 focus/4 mm^2. A grade 3 biopsy indicates 1 focus, and a grade 4 more than 1 focus/4 mm^2. A focus score of greater than 1 (grade 4) is considered diagnostic for the salivary component of Sjögren's syndrome (25).

Other pathologic abnormalities noted in the salivary glands of patients with Sjögren's syndrome include ductal dilation and epithelial cell hypertrophy. The growth of epithelial cells may result in the formation of epimyoepithelial islands that may cause ductal occlusion. These are rarely seen in minor salivary gland tissue, but are occasionally found in major salivary glands. These islands have been considered by some to be very specific for Sjögren's syndrome, but may also be seen in malignant lymphoid salivary tumors.

TABLE 15.2 Sjögren's Syndrome: General Principles of Management

Keratoconjunctivitis sicca: artificial tears and lubricants, nasolacrimal duct occlusion, mucolytic agents, ophthalmologic follow-up
Xerostomia: frequent fluids, oral lubricants, aggressive dental care
Major organ system disease (renal, neurologic, pulmonary, vasculitis, myositis): ? corticosteroids, ? cytotoxic/immunosuppressive drugs
Arthritis: nonsteroidal antiinflammatory drugs
Malignant transformation: observation for serologic, clinical changes

Radionuclide scanning with technetium pertechnetate may be useful diagnostically in Sjögren's syndrome, and usually shows increased uptake in involved glands. Sialography of the parotid glands is abnormal in most patients. However, the findings are nonspecific and may be confused with other disease entities, including infectious parotitis or sarcoidosis (30).

Prognosis and Management

Sjögren's syndrome is a relatively benign disorder. Patients may complain of only dry eyes and dry mouth for years, but occasionally extraglandular manifestations may cause serious morbidity. The development of lymphoma is potentially the most serious complication, particularly since these malignancies tend to be resistant to therapeutic intervention.

The treatment of Sjögren's syndrome involves a combination of measures to control keratoconjunctivitis sicca as well as recognizing and managing underlying organ system involvement. The general principles of therapy are summarized in Table 15.2.

Ocular dryness may be relieved by using methylcellulose eye drops during the day and ointments at night. Occasionally, occlusion of the nasolacrimal duct is useful in allowing accumulation of residual tears. Mucolytic agents may be necessary if large amounts of dry mucus collect about the eye. The most important aspect of treatment of ocular disease is careful ophthalmologic follow-up and treatment of secondary infection. Topical steroids should be avoided in most cases, because of the potential for corneal thinning. Drugs that decrease secretions, such as diuretics and tricyclic antidepressants, should be avoided.

The treatment of xerostomia may be particularly difficult. Most patients maintain oral moisture by drinking fluids frequently. Careful dental care is extremely important, as caries is a major problem. Avoidance of sugar intake and vigorous control of plaque should be encouraged. Early recognition and treatment of oral candidiasis may also be helpful. Various oral lubricants have been formulated and marketed, most of which contain glycerin. Dryness of other mucous membranes and skin is best treated by local moisturizers and lubricants.

The therapy of major organ system disease in Sjögren's syndrome remains largely empirical. Renal tubular acidosis should be treated appropriately with alkali. Corticosteroids and cytotoxic drugs may be of benefit in selected cases where vasculitis, neurologic complications, or renal disease cause severe illness, although overall efficacy of these agents has not been proven. Articular manifestations may be controlled in most cases with nonsteroidal antiinflammatory drugs.

Transformation into pseudolymphoma or lymphoma may sometimes be suspected by serologic changes. Laboratory features suggesting malignant transformation of Sjögren's syndrome include the appearance in the serum of a monoclonal immunoglobulin, a decrease in the concentration of a previously elevated class of immunoglobulin, or decrease in rheumatoid factor or beta-2 microglobulin levels. Clinical findings which may indicate malignant change include persistence of parotid swelling, generalized adenopathy, or splenomegaly.

In summary, the management of Sjögren's syndrome is largely symptomatic with careful prophylactic measures to prevent complications in the eyes and mouth, and careful follow-up for the development of systemic complications or malignant degeneration. In addition, treatment of an underlying connective tissue syndrome, if present, may result in improvement in some of the symptoms of Sjögren's syndrome. Patient education and reassurance early on in the disease process may be helpful in avoiding unnecessary diagnostic and therapeutic maneuvers.

References

1. Strand V, Talal N: Advances in the diagnosis and concept of Sjögren's syndrome (autoimmune exocrinopathy). *Bull Rheum Dis* 30:1046-1052, 1980.

2. Kassan SS, Gardy M: Sjögren's syndrome: An update and overview. *Amer Jour Med* 64:1037-1046, 1978.

3. Alspaugh MA, Whaley K: Sjögren's syndrome. In WN KElley, ED Harris, S Ruddy, CB Sledge (eds.), *Textbook of Rheumatology,* 1st Ed. Philadelphia, W.B. Saunders, 1981, pp. 971-999.

4. Chused TM, Kassan SS, Opelz G, Moutsopoulos HM, Terasaki PI: Sjögren's syndrome associated with HLA-DW3. *N Engl J Med* 296:895-897, 1977.

5. Fye KH, Terasaki PI, Michalski JP, Daniels TE, Opelz G, Talal N: Relationship of HLA-DW3 and HLA-B8 to Sjögren's syndrome. *Arthritis Rheum* 21: 337-342, 1978.

6. Fox RI, Carstens SA, Fong S, Robinson CA, Howell F, Vaughn JH: Use of monoclonal antibodies to analyze peripheral blood and salivary gland lymphocyte subsets in Sjögren's syndrome. *Arthritis Rheum* 25:419-426, 1982.

7. Pavlidis NA, Karsh J, Moutsopoulos HM: The clinical picture of primary Sjögren's syndrome: A retrospective study. *J Rheumatol* 9:685-690, 1982.

8. Castro-Poltronieri A, Alarcon-Segovia D: Articular manifestations of primary Sjögren's syndrome. *J Rheumatol* 10:485-488, 1983.

9. Whaley K, Webb J, McAvoy BA, Hughes GRL, Lee P, MacSween RMM, Buchanan WW: Sjögren's syndrome. 2. Clinical associations and immunologic phenomena. *Quart J Med* 42:513-548, 1973.

10. Culp KS, Fleming CR, Duffy J, Baldus WP, Dickson ER: Autoimmune associations in primary biliary cirrhosis. *Mayo Clin Proc* 57:365-370, 1982.

11. Winer RL, Cohen AH, Sawhney AS, Gorman JT: Sjögren's syndrome with immune-complex tubulointerstitial renal disease. *Clin Immunol Immunopath* 8:494-503, 1977.

12. Moutsopoulos HM, Balow JE, Lawley TJ, Stahl NI, Antonovych TT, Chused TM: Immune complex glomerulonephritis in sicca syndrome. *Amer Jour Med* 64:955-960, 1978.

13. Karsh J, Pavlidis N, Weintraub BD, Moutsopoulos HM: Thyroid disease in Sjögren's syndrome. *Arthritis Rheum* 23:1326-1329, 1980.

14. Alexander EL, Provost TT, Stevens MB, Alexander GE: Neurologic complications of primary Sjögren's syndrome. *Medicine* 61:247-257, 1982.

15. Alexander EL, Arnett FC, Provost TT, Stevens MB: Sjögren's syndrome: Association of anti-Ro(SS-A) antibodies with vasculitis, hematologic abnormalities, and serologic hyperreactivity. *Ann Intern Med* 98:115-159, 1983.

16. Moutsopoulos HM, Webber BL, Vlagopoulos TP, Chused TM, Decker JL: Differences in the clinical manifestations of sicca syndrome in the presence and absence of rheumatoid arthritis. *Amer Jour Med* 66:733-736, 1979.

17. Ramos-Niembro F, Alarcon-Segovia D: Development of sicca symptoms in systemic lupus erythematosus patients with existing subclinical abnormalities of lacrimal and/or salivary glands. *Arthritis Rheum* 22:935-936, 1979.

18. Moutsopoulos HM, Klippel JH, Pavlidis N, Wolf RO, Sweet JB, Steinberg AD, Chu FC, Tarpley TM: Correlative histologic and serologic findings of sicca syndrome in patients with systemic lupus erythematosus. *Arthritis Rheum* 23:36-40, 1980.

19. Alarcon-Segovia D, Ibanez G, Hernandez-Ortiz J, Velasquez-Foreso F, Gonzalez-Jiminez Y: Sjögren's syndrome in progressive systemic sclerosis. *Am Jour Med* 57:78-85, 1974.

20. Cipoletti JF, Buckingham RB, Barnes L et al.: Sjögren's syndrome in progressive systemic sclerosis. *Ann Intern Med* 87:535-541, 1977.

21. Gratwohl AA, Moutsopoulos HM, Chused TM et al.: Sjögren's-type syndrome after allogeneic bone-marrow transplanation. *Ann Intern Med* 87:703-706, 1977.

22. Boling EP, Wen J, Reveille JD et al.: Primary Sjögren's syndrome and autoimmune hemolytic anemia in sisters. *Am Jour Med* 74:1066-1071, 1983.

23. Talal N, Schnitzer B: Lymphadenopathy and Sjögren's syndrome. *Clin Rheum Dis* 3:421-432, 1977.

24. Greenspan JS, Daniels TE, Talal N, Sylvester RA: The histopathology of Sjögren's syndrome in labial salivary gland biopsies. *Oral Surg* 37:217-229, 1974.

25. Daniels TE: Labial salivary gland biopsy in Sjögren's syndrome. Assessment as a diagnostic criterion in 362 suspected cases. *Arthritis Rheum* 27:147-156, 1984.

26. Moutsopoulos HM, Karsh J, Wolf RO et al.: Lysozyme determination in parotid saliva from patients with Sjögren's syndrome. *Am Jour Med* 69: 39-41, 1980.

27. Alspaugh M, Talal N, Tan EM: Differentiation and characterization of autoantibodies and their antigens in Sjögren's syndrome. *Arthritis Rheum* 19:216-222, 1976.

28. Alspaugh MA, Buchanan WW, Whaley K: Precipitating antibodies to cellular antigens in Sjögren's syndrome, rheumatoid arthritis, and other organ and nonorgan-specific autoimmune diseases. *Ann Rheum Dis* 37:244-246, 1978.

29. Alexander EL, Hirscht J, Arnett FC, Provost TT, Stevens MB: Ro (SSA) and La (SSB) antibodies in the clinical spectrum of Sjögren's syndrome. *J Rheumatol* 9:239-246, 1982.

30. Dijkstra PF: Classification and differential diagnosis of sialographic characteristics in Sjögren's syndrome. *Semin Arth Rheum* 10:10-17, 1980.

Chapter 16

POLYMYOSITIS AND DERMATOMYOSITIS

Christopher M. Wise, M.D. and
Carlos A. Agudelo, M.D.

Polymyositis and dermatomyositis are terms used to designate inflammatory disease of muscle without known specific cause and frequently associated with autoimmune phenomena. These terms designate a heterogeneous group of conditions which more properly are thought of as syndromes rather than diseases (1). The term polymyositis refers to an inflammatory disease of striated muscle which causes muscle weakness, usually proximally. Dermatomyositis describes the same condition when associated with skin involvement. The distinction between these two entities is somewhat artificial, and much overlap exists. Either condition may occur at any age and may be associated with other connective tissue diseases, such as rheumatoid arthritis, scleroderma, or systemic lupus, and also with various neoplasms.

The earliest descriptions of polymyositis date back to the late nineteenth century, with the first associations with cancer noted in the 1930's. Since the 1950's, several attempts have been made to classify inflammatory muscle disease. Walton and Adams suggested the first such classification in 1958 (2). This particular classification was thought to be overly simplified, and over the next years several more complicated classification schemes were suggested. A recent and more widely accepted classification was proposed by Bohan and Peter (3) (see Table 16.1). This scheme separates polymyositis and dermatomyositis, but leaves a separate category for these conditions when associated with malignancy. Overlap syndromes with connective tissue diseases and childhood disease are considered separately as well.

Inflammatory muscle disease is relatively uncommon, but by no means rare. Large population studies have suggested an annual incidence of 2-5 new cases per million population. This is similar in incidence to muscular dystrophy. When compared to other rheumatic diseases, it is much less common than rheumatoid

TABLE 16.1 Classification of Inflammatory Myopathies [From Bohan and Peter, 1975 (3)]

Group 1 -	Primary idiopathic polymyositis (PM)
Group 2 -	Primary idiopathic dermatomyositis (DM)
Group 3 -	Dermatomyositis or polymyositis associated with malignancy
Group 4 -	Childhood dermatomyositis or polymyositis
Group 5 -	Polymyositis or dermatomyositis associated with connective tissue disease (overlap syndromes)

arthritis and lupus, and is approximately half as common as scleroderma, but twice as common as polyarteritis nodosa. The disease may occur at any age and in both sexes. In the childhood group, males are slightly more frequently affected than females. In adults with polymyositis and dermatomyositis, females are more often affected than men. When myositis is associated with neoplasm, males outnumber females. Overall in adults, the mean age of presentation is about 50 years, although the age tends to be older in those with associated malignancy.

Etiopathogenesis

As with most other rheumatic diseases, the exact cause and pathogenesis of this group of conditions is unknown. Several clinical and laboratory observations have been made which seem to have some bearing on an explanation of etiology and pathogenesis. Any theory of causation of idiopathic inflammatory disease of muscle must take into consideration observed abnormalities in humoral and cellular immunity as well as possible infectious etiologies and association with neoplasm.

A frequent elevation in sedimentation rate and serum immunoglobulins, and the high frequency of autoantibodies in serum suggest that abnormalities in humoral immunity play a role in pathogenesis. Vascular deposits of immunoglobulin and complement have been demonstrated in muscle biopsies in several cases, suggesting that vascular damage from immune complexes is important in the initiation or perpetuation of the condition. Nevertheless, attempts to demonstrate antibodies against skeletal muscle have been inconclusive and nonspecific (1).

Perhaps more convincing is evidence that abnormalities of cell-mediated immunity are important. Peripheral blood lymphocytes from patients with myositis show a higher degree of transformation (as indicated by increased DNA synthesis) than controls when exposed to skeletal muscle. Other studies have shown that activated lymphocytes from patients with myositis are directly toxic to muscle cells in vitro. Mechanisms for this toxicity include release of substances toxic to cells as well as direct attachment and invasion of the muscle fibers themselves (1).

The similarity of polymyositis and dermatomyositis to various types of infectious myositis have led to a search for specific agents that might be responsible for the syndrome. There are several reports of virus-like particles seen in muscle biopsies by electron microscopy, and these have resembled myxovirus and picornavirus. The specificity of these findings has been called into question, since similar structures have been seen in normal muscle. Coxsackie virus has been isolated from muscle in some cases as well. Nevertheless, a lack of consistent isolation of virus or serologic demonstration of prior viral infection have failed to confirm a specific viral etiology for typical polymyositis. The protozoa *toxoplasma gondii* has also been implicated in causation of polymyositis. In addition to isolated case reports of isolation of the organism from muscle tissue, one recent study showed an increased frequency of antibodies to toxoplasma in serum from patients with polymyositis in comparison to controls (4). In this particular study, however, the organism was not isolated, and those with higher titers had more often been treated with high doses of steroids, suggesting that steroid therapy had reactivated latent toxoplasma infection.

Since muscle necrosis can result from a wide variety of forms of vasculopathy, and because of the previously mentioned immune complex deposition in some blood vessels, a primary vascular mechanism has been theorized in the pathogenesis of the condition. Studies showing a loss of capillary area have suggested the importance of this possible mechanism.

In summary then, no specific cause for polymyositis has been found, but it is possible that an immunologic reaction, primarily of cellular origin, may be triggered by a virus or other infectious agent. Activation of lymphocytes which release toxins or cause direct damage to muscle cells then might ensue, resulting in muscle necrosis and weakness (1).

Clinical Features

Clinical Subgroups

Adult Polymyositis

This condition occurs in females more than males with a mean age of presentation of 50 years. Muscle weakness usually has an insidious onset and may or may not be associated with muscle pain. On occasion, there is a preceding history of a viral-like syndrome or fever, and many patients will have experienced joint pain and swelling, stiffness, or Raynaud's phenomenon for several months or years before the onset of muscle weakness. Muscle weakness is usually proximal and occurs in upper and lower limbs. The patient may notice difficulty running, climbing stairs, or arising from a chair. In the upper extremities, difficulty lifting heavy objects or keepting the arms up during activities such as combing the hair may be the first symptoms. Weakness in the muscles of the neck, dysphagia, or weakness in the voice are noted in those with more severe disease. The symptoms of polymyositis generally develop slowly and may be present for several months before a physician is consulted. Systemic symptoms, such as weight loss, are relatively common. The degree of symptoms and muscle weakness at presentation is highly variable. A small number of patients will have such profound muscle weakness that respiratory and pharyngeal functions are severely compromised. On the other hand, some patients have such mild muscle weakness that only a very careful examination will elicit this. Physical examination reveals proximal muscle weakness in the vast majority of patients, and this can be graded as noted

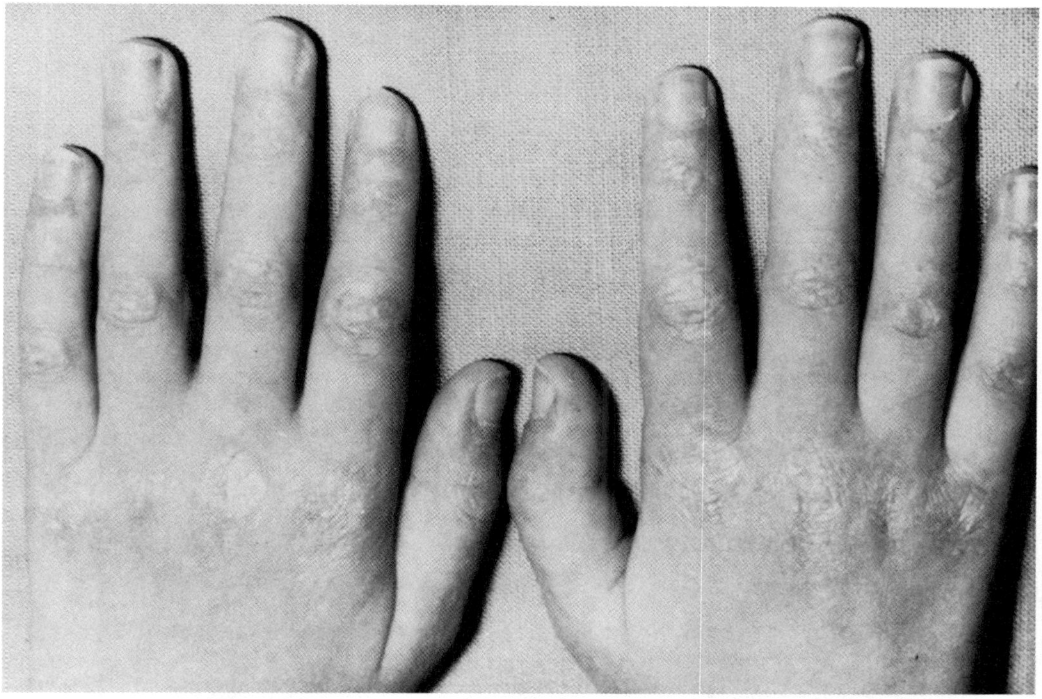

FIGURE 16.1 The erythematous plaques known as Gottron's papules, which typically appear over the knuckles in dermatomyositis. (From the Revised Clinical Slide Collection on the Rheumatic Diseases. Copyright 1981. Used by permission of the Arthritis Foundation.)

in Chapter 1. Muscle tenderness, again more in the proximal muscles, is seen in a minority of patients. Atrophy occurs in about one-third of patients. Muscle contractures may be seen in a small number of patients with long-standing disease.

Adult Dermatomyositis

When dermatologic features coexist with myositis, the condition is known as dermatomyositis. About one-third of all patients in large series are considered to have dermatomyositis. In this group, the muscle disease is identical to that seen in polymyositis. Skin lesions may constitute only a minimal part of the clinical syndrome in a few patients, while in others dermatologic features predominate. Rarely, cutaneous disease may be present without any evidence of muscle disease, but myositis usually becomes evident later (5). A wide variety of skin lesions may be seen in dermatomyositis. The most common areas of involvement are the areas around the eyelids, cheeks, bridge of the nose, and front and back of the chest. The extensor surfaces of the elbows and knees as well as the ankles may be involved. Characteristic erythematous plaques may develop over the knuckles, and these are known as Gottron's papules (Figure 16.1). On occasion the erythema of the skin may take on a red or violaceous hue and is referred to as a heliotrope rash (Figure 16.2). Erythema may be seen without any palpable rash, but when the

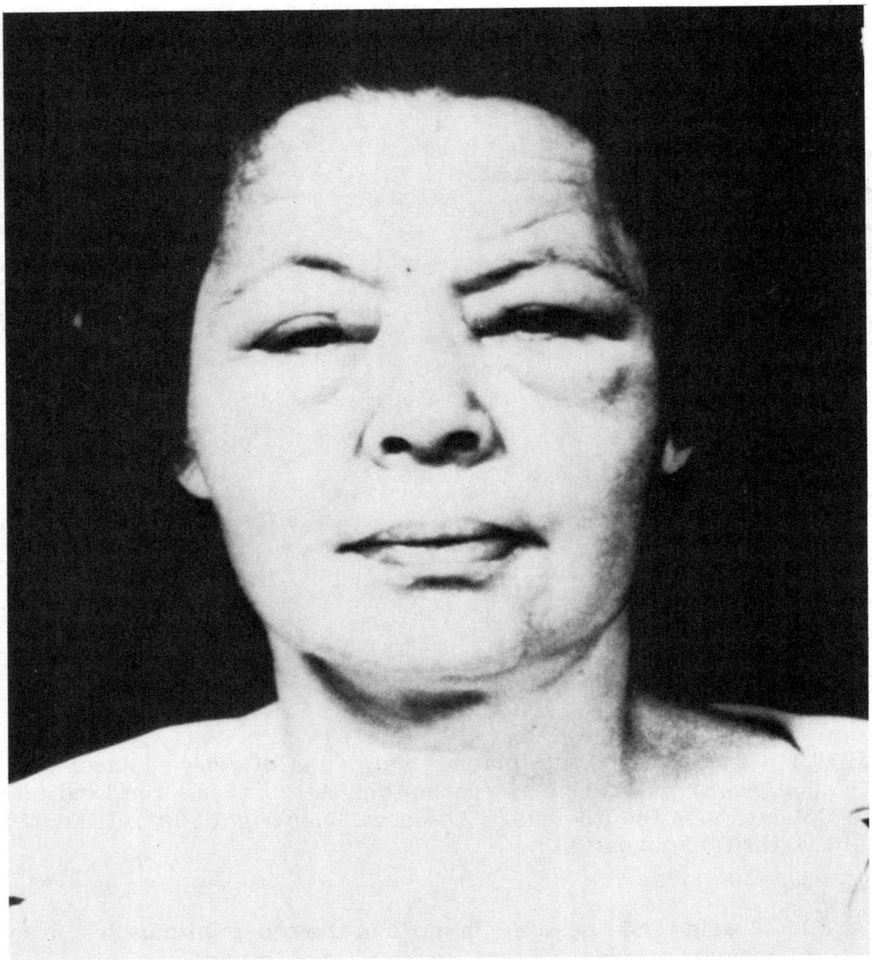

FIGURE 16.2 Periorbital edema and violaceous heliotrope discoloration, typical of dermatomyositis. (From the Arthritis Slide Collection, copyright 1980. Used by permission of the Arthritis Foundation.)

condition is more florid, there may be scaly papules, edema, and tenderness. The rash may be pruritic, but symptoms are often minimal. Erythema around the skin of the nail beds may also be seen in the fingers, and this may be similar to that seen in other connective tissue diseases.

Myositis Associated with Neoplasm

The association of inflammatory myopathy and neoplasm has long been noted, and several studies have suggested that 15–35% of all patients with myositis have an underlying neoplasm. More recent studies have suggested that this number is much too high, and that 5–8% is a more reasonable approximation (1,3). Although any type of neoplasm may be associated with myositis, the most common ones are lung, ovary, breast, and stomach. There is no association between malignancy and myositis in childhood. Malignancy appears to be particularly common in older patients with dermatomyositis, with 15–20% of these patients having an underlying malignancy diagnosed either before or shortly after the diagnosis of dermatomyositis. There is some correlation between response to therapy for the neoplasm and the myopathy, although this is not uniformly the case (6,7). Other than the association with neoplasm, the myositis and/or dermatitis of this group is indistinguishable from that seen in the other subsets.

Myositis of Childhood

Approximately 10–20% of all patients with myositis have the disease during childhood. In this group, males are seen slightly more often than females, and dermatomyositis is about twice as common as polymyositis (1,8). In general, the clinical and laboratory features of myositis in childhood are similar to that in adult disease. The childhood disease seems to be characterized by an increased incidence of vasculitis and calcinosis. Widespread vasculitis has been reported in several children which resulted in gastrointestinal hemorrhage and perforation. Subcutaneous calcification (calcinosis) is seen much more often in childhood disease as well. This may be manifest by palpable subcutaneous areas, and may increase with time, resulting in ulceration through the skin. Most studies suggest that childhood myositis is more mild than adult disease, with death from the condition being extremely uncommon.

Myositis Associated with Other Connective Tissue Disease (Overlap Syndromes)

Inflammatory myositis may occur in the setting of another established connective tissue disease, and this group constitutes about 15–30% of all cases of myositis. The diseases in which it is seen, in decreasing order of frequency, are scleroderma, mixed connective tissue diesease, rheumatoid arthritis, and systemic lupus. Polyarteritis and Sjögren's syndrome may rarely be associated with inflammatory myopathy. The clinical and pathological variation of myositis when associated with other connective tissue syndromes is wide. Muscle weakness and wasting may be minimal, and biopsy findings may show little inflammation. In scleroderma in particular, muscle biopsy may show diffuse fibrosis, and only occasionally extensive inflammatory infiltration. Awareness of the possibility of overlapping of myositis with other connective tissue diseases is extremely important in evaluating patients with other conditions who develop extreme weakness and muscle wasting. This may be particularly true in rheumatoid arthritis or scleroderma, and careful evaluation with enzyme levels, EMG, and muscle biopsy may be necessary to differentiate the causes of weakness in these patients.

Involvement of Other Organ Systems

Arthritis

Synovitis may accompany the muscle disease of polymyositis (9). This often occurs as a presenting symptom, and obviously may be a source of diagnostic confusion early in the course. The arthritis may be inflammatory and mimic rheumatoid arthritis in its symmetry and polyarticular nature. In addition, isolated oligoarticular disease may occur. The arthritis of polymyositis generally causes little or no permanent damage unless there is real coexistent rheumatoid arthritis. Once the diagnosis is established, the articular problems become much less of a problem as the weakness and pain of myopathy predominate.

Vasculopathy

Raynaud's phenomenon occurs with variable frequency in polymyositis and dermatomyositis. It appears to be more common in those patients with overlap syndromes or in those with dermatomyositis. Vasculitis, both cutaneous and widespread involving visceral organs, has been described mostly in children. Periungual erythema, small subcutaneous nodules, and cutaneous ulceration have been described in several patients, although by no means a large proportion. In addition, necrotizing vasculitis presenting with gastrointestinal hemorrhage or perforation has been described in several patients. Although vasculitic lesions have traditionally been thought to be rare in adult patients, one recent study suggested that about 9% of adults may develop vasculitic complications (10). Dermal nodules, periungual infarcts, and digital ulceration were described, and much more frequently seen in those with dermatomyositis or malignancy.

Cardiac Abnormalities

Cardiac abnormalities, both clinically significant and life-threatening, and subclinical, have been increasingly recognized in inflammatory myopathies (11,12, 13,14). Symptomatic cardiac involvement may take several forms, including arrhythmias, congestive heart failure, or even sudden death. The frequency with which symptomatic cardiac disease occurs is probably quite small, with congestive heart failure occurring in less than 5% of patients. Systematic studies have shown a surprising incidence of abnormalities, although many are asymptomatic. Conduction defects resulting from fibrosis have been documented. Histologic evidence of myocarditis and elevation of CPK of cardiac origin (MB) is also surprisingly common even in patients without any clinical evidence of cardiac dysfunction. Although one report attributed the presence of CPK-MB to regenerating skeletal muscle fibers (15), others have suggested that this represents true myocardial damage (13,14).

Pulmonary Disease

Diffuse interstitial lung disease, associated with restrictive pulmonary function changes, is much like that seen in other connective tissue diseases and occurs in about 10% of patients (16,17). Histopathologic evaluation shows a combination of diffuse infiltrates and fibrosis. Although the data are not clear-cut, there is a tendency for this to occur in those with more severe muscle disease. With treatment of the underlying myositis, the pulmonary condition may improve, but this is not uniformly the case.

Diagnostic Criteria

Since polymyositis is a disease of unknown etiology, and probably represents a spectrum of diseases, definitive diagnosis has always been a problem. The diagnosis rests on a combination of clinical, laboratory, electromyographic, and biopsy findings. The most commonly used diagnostic criteria were set forth by Bohan and Peter in 1975 (3), and are summarized in Table 16.2. A definite diagnosis of polymyositis may be made when all of the first four criteria are met, and dermatomyositis when three of these plus the characteristic rash are seen. A probable

TABLE 16.2 Diagnostic Criteria for Polymyositis/Dermatomyositis
[From Bohan and Peter, 1975 (3)]

Symmetric proximal muscle weakness

Muscle biopsy evidence of necrosis, phagocytosis, regeneration, inflammation

Serum muscle enzyme elevation

Electromyographic triad of polyphasic units, fibrillation, and high frequency discharges

Dermatologic features (rash): eyelids, dorsal hands

	Polymyositis	Dermatomyositis
Definite diagnosis:	first four criteria	three to four criteria plus rash
Probable diagnosis:	three criteria	two criteria plus rash
Possible diagnosis:	two criteria	one criterion plus rash

diagnosis can be made with three criteria, and possible by two criteria. Because biopsy findings, electromyographic studies, and serum enzymes may be abnormal in a variety of other conditions, several other conditions must be excluded, and are discussed below under differential diagnoses.

Differential Diagnosis of Polymyositis

Conditions which must be considered in the differential diagnosis of inflammatory myopathies are listed in Table 16.3.

Since the complex of conditions we know as dermatomyositis and polymyositis does not constitute a single homogeneous disease entity and has no specific cause, it is particularly important to consider the various conditions that have similar clinical and pathologic features in any patient that presents with a picture of proximal muscle weakness.

A wide variety of infections may cause inflammation and destruction of muscles that are important to recognize because of potentially definitive treatment (18). The most common viral infections associated with muscle disease are influenza, Coxsackie virus, and hepatitis B. In postinfluenza myositis, pain in the calves and thighs is predominant, muscles are tender, and muscle enzymes are moderately elevated, but his syndrome usually resolves in less than a week. After Coxsackie infection, the term epidemic myalgia or Bornholm's disease has been used. In this syndrome, chest wall pain probably related to muscle involvement is predominant, and this is also self-limited. A typical polymyositis syndrome has been described after hepatitis B infection, but is probably not as common as some of the other better recognized syndromes (essential cryoglobulinemia, polyarteritis nodosa). Bacterial infections of muscle usually occur from a local penetrating wound, gangrene, or spread of infection from a contiguous area. Tropical pyomyositis is an entity usually associated with staphylococcal infections, and may present with crampy muscle pain and fever followed by muscle hardening

TABLE 16.3 The Differential Diagnosis of Polymyositis (see text)

Infectious myositis

Viral:	postinfluenza, Coxsackie, hepatitis B virus
Bacterial:	tropical pyomyositis (staphylococcal), streptococcal, clostridial myonecrosis
Other:	Candida, tuberculosis, leprosy, toxoplasma, trichonosis

Metabolic myopathies

Cushing's syndrome
Hyperthyroidism
Hypothyroidism
Diabetic amyotrophy
Electrolyte disturbance (hypokalemia, hypomagnesemia, etc.)

Drug-induced myopathies (see text)

Exercise-related (enzyme elevations)

Polymyalgia rheumatica

Muscular dystrophies

Neurologic disorders

Myaesthenia gravis
Amyotrophic lateral sclerosis
Other ?

Miscellaneous

Focal nodular myositis
Eosinophilic myositis
Granulomatous myositis

and then localized fluctuance and leukocytosis. This condition is endemic in many tropical areas, and the diagnosis is made by needle aspiration and culture of material obtained. Streptococcal myositis is less common, and may present in a variety of forms, from severe generalized muscle inflammation, septicemia, and a rapid fatal outcome, or a benign localized infection that responds rapidly to incision and drainage. Clostridial myonecrosis (gas gangrene) usually follows major trauma and vascular compromise. Other bacterial infections may be associated with localized muscle disease, including *Hemophilus influenzae, Salmonella typhi,* or syphillis, but these are exceedingly rare. Fungal infections rarely involve muscle, although several cases of myositis associated with Candida have been reported in patients with leukemia. Myopathy has been described associated with chronic mucocutaneous candidiasis, but this appears to be a remote effect of the condition rather than a result of direct infection. Localized muscle infections have also been described in tuberculosis and leprosy, although these two are relatively rare. As noted earlier, patients with typical polymyositis have an increased frequency of serum antibodies to *Toxoplasma gondii*, but it is unclear whether this represents a reactivation of previous infection due to the disease itself or steroid therapy. Actual documentation of myositis caused by toxoplasma by an acute rise in serum antibodies or culture of the organism from muscle tissue is relatively uncommon. Trichinosis is the most common and best known example of muscle involvement by a parasite. This develops when undercooked meat has been contaminated by the larvae of the organism *Trichinella spiralis*. After several days in the gastrointestinal tract, the larvae may reach the circulation and spread to skeletal muscle. Within the muscle, the larvae grow and become encapsulated. Systemic features of fever, weakness, muscle tenderness, edema, and rash occur and eosinophilia is usually prominent. Frequently involved muscles include the diaphragm, extraocular and upper airway muscles, and muscles of the neck, back, abdomen, and limbs. A diagnosis can be made by serologic studies and confirmed by muscle biopsy where encapsulated organisms may be identified.

Myopathy may be a part of several endocrine and metabolic disorders. In Cushing's syndrome, muscle weakness is usually mild, but in severe cases, profound generalized weakness and atrophy may occur. Some of this may be due to the associated hypokalemia, and muscle enzymes are usually minimally elevated or normal. Hyperthyroidism may be associated with a myopathy in which electromyographic studies may show myopathic changes, but biopsy changes are minimal, and serum enzymes are normal. The myopathy of hyperthyroidism is usually relatively mild. In hypothyroidism, muscle weakness may be a prominent part of the presenting symptomatology. In contrast to hyperthyroidism, hypothyroidism is often associated with marked elevation in muscle enzymes, and EMG and pathologic findings may very closely mimic those of idiopathic polymyositis, although inflammatory changes are not usually present on biopsy. On occasion, pseudomyotonia of the muscles may occur. This is a painless swelling that occurs after percussion of a local muscle group (19,20) (see Chapter 23). A syndrome known as diabetic amyotrophy may be seen in poorly controlled diabetics, who present with marked wasting and weakness, primarily affecting the proximal muscles of the legs. This syndrome is usually associated with other evidence of diabetic neuropathy, and electrical studies have shown that muscle wasting and weakness are neurogenic and not due to primary muscle disease. This syndrome may improve with rigid control of the underlying diabetes (21). Electrolyte disturbances, such as severe hypokalemia, hypophosphatemia, or hypomagnesemia, may cause profound muscle weakness, elevation of muscle enzymes, and even acute muscle necrosis (rhabdomyolysis). A long and ever growing list of drugs has been associated with myopathies having a wide range of clinical and laboratory features (22). Alcohol is probably the most common drug associated with myopathies, and may produce either an acute or subacute painful proximal myopathy, acute rhabdomyolysis, or a chronic proximal myopathy. When muscle damage is severe, serum muscle enzymes may be markedly elevated and myoglobulinuria may be present. Drugs which cause hypokalemia, such as diuretics and strong cathartics, may produce weakness and serum enzyme elevations. Corticosteroids and chloroquine can produce a chronic or subacute proximal myopathy with vacuolar changes on biopsy and normal muscle enzymes. Clofibrate, epsilon-amino-caproic acid, heroin, and amphetamines all have been associated with myopathies. A large number of drugs have been associated with myasthenic syndromes, including aminoglycosides, D-penicillamine, propranolol and other beta blockers, procainamide and chlorpromazine. Typical polymyositis has been reported with D-penicillamine, cimetidine, and tamoxifen (23,24).

Prolonged strenuous muscular activity, such as long-distance running, may result in elevations in muscle enzymes (25). Polymyalgia rheumatica is characterized by pain and stiffness in proximal muscles, and on occasion proximal muscles may seem weak on physical examination because of pain in the area. The differentiation of these two syndromes should not be difficult in most cases, since serum muscle enzymes are not elevated in polymyalgia rheumatica.

Slowly progressive unremitting muscle weakness, especially if there is a positive family history or calf enlargement, should suggest the presence of a muscular dystrophy. In these diseases, especially in Duchenne's muscular dystrophy, serum muscle enzymes may be markedly elevated. In other less common types of muscular dystrophy, the findings may not be quite as typical. Muscle biopsy should be helpful in differentiating these disorders, and a poor response to corticosteroid therapy should also suggest a muscular dystrophy. Other neurologic disorders, especially those of motor neurons with resultant muscle denervation and atrophy, may be associated with profound muscle weakness and elevations in muscle enzymes (26,27). A wide variety of motor neuron diseases have been associated with elevated muscle enzymes, including amyotrophic lateral sclerosis, and this has been a source of confusion in many of these patients in whom the eventual diagnosis was delayed and corticosteroid therapy was inappropriately given (28).

Focal nodular myositis is an uncommon condition that may present with local areas of what appears to be typical polymyositis, but without muscle weakness. Granulomatous myositis may occur in sarcoidosis, as an idiopathic condition, or in association with myasthenia gravis and thymoma (1). In general, patients with these syndromes present with mild myalgias and very little muscle weakness or enzyme elevation. Eosinophilic myositis may occur in association with parasitic infection, eosinophilic leukemia, or eosinophilic fasciitis, but a few cases exist of localized idiopathic eosinophilic myositis. This syndrome is associated with peripheral eosinophilia, elevated muscle enzymes and electromyographic changes of myositis, but is a relatively benign disorder without serious sequelae (29).

Laboratory Features

General Laboratory and Antinuclear Antibodies

The general laboratory features of polymyositis and dermatomyositis are relatively nonspecific. Mild anemia may be present. Sedimentation rate is elevated to a mild extent in most patients, and about 20% of patients have an elevation to greater than 50 (1). Nevertheless, about 40% of patients will have a normal sedimentation rate. The urinalysis is generally normal, although in the rare acute case, myoglobulinuria may be present. Antinuclear antibodies are infrequently found, when all categories of polymyositis and dermatomyositis are considered. Although there is some variation from study to study, those patients with overlap syndromes have a high incidence of antinuclear antibodies. Antibodies to native DNA are generally absent, although one study suggests a 25% incidence of this in a selected group of referred patients (30). Antibodies to Sm and RNP are found in a small number of patients, usually in those with syndromes overlapping with other connective tissue diseases. Other antinuclear antibodies have been detected in special preparations that may have more specificity for polymyositis and dermatomyositis, but these are not generally available in most clinical laboratories. Antibodies to the nuclear antigen PM-1 have been detected in roughly half of patients with myositis, and appear to be relatively specific (31). Antibodies to another distinct nuclear antigen, termed Jo-1, have been found in roughly 30-50%

of patients with polymyositis, dermatomyositis, or overlap syndromes, appear to be relatively specific for this group of diseases, and may correlate with the presence of interstitial pulmonary fibrosis (32,33).

Muscle Enzymes

Enzymes are released from injured muscle in polymyositis, and elevated levels of these enzymes in serum are often helpful indicators of the extent of fiber damage. The most frequently elevated enzymes in polymyositis are creatine phosphokinase (CPK), SGOT, and LDH. Serum CPK is elevated at presentation in over 60% of patients, and elevated above the normal range in 99% of patients at some time during the course of their disease (1,6). The CPK level is frequently in the range of 10 times normal, and elevations up to 80 times the normal range may be seen. Although serum CPK levels correlate fairly well with disease activity and response to therapy, it can sometimes be misleading, particularly in patients with widespread atrophy and falsely low serum levels of the enzyme. Nevertheless, the serum CPK level remains a very useful parameter in diagnosis and management of polymyositis, and usually serves as a good laboratory parameter to follow as the condition responds to therapy.

Electrophysiology

Electrophysiologic studies are essential in establishing the diagnosis and ruling out other causes of muscle weakness, such as motor neuron disease. Abnormalities found on electromyogram are summarized in Table 16.4. The classic triad of findings (polyphasic potentials, fibrillation, high frequency discharges) is seen together in about 40% of patients, while 10% have a completely normal EMG, and the rest have at least one of the characteristic abnormalities. Probably the most frequently involved muscles are the paravertebral muscles and, on occasion, abnormalities are found here and nowhere else (3).

Muscle Pathology

Muscle biopsy should be obtained from a painful and weak muscle group, preferably proximal muscles, that have not been previously subjected to electrode insertion, since this can cause a focal inflammatory change by itself. The most common features of the muscle biopsy in polymyositis are muscle fiber degeneration and mononuclear inflammatory infiltrate. Fiber necrosis, regeneration, and fibrosis are seen in a significant but smaller percentage of patients. The inflammatory infiltrate seen in polymyositis is a mononuclear inflammation that is mostly perifascicular. On occasion, vasculitic changes in blood vessels may be seen. The typical pathologic features of polymyositis are illustrated in Figures 16.3, 16.4, and 16.5. About 10-15% of the cases will have a normal muscle biopsy. Changes tend to be more severe in those with more severe disease, but the correlation is not uniform. Biopsy findings tend to improve in most patients as the disease improves with therapy (1,6,34,35).

TABLE 16.4 Electromyographic Findings in Myositis (6)

	Frequency
Polyphasic, short motor unit potentials	90%
Fibrillation, sharp waves, irritability	75%
High frequency discharges	40%
All of above	40%
Normal EMG	10%

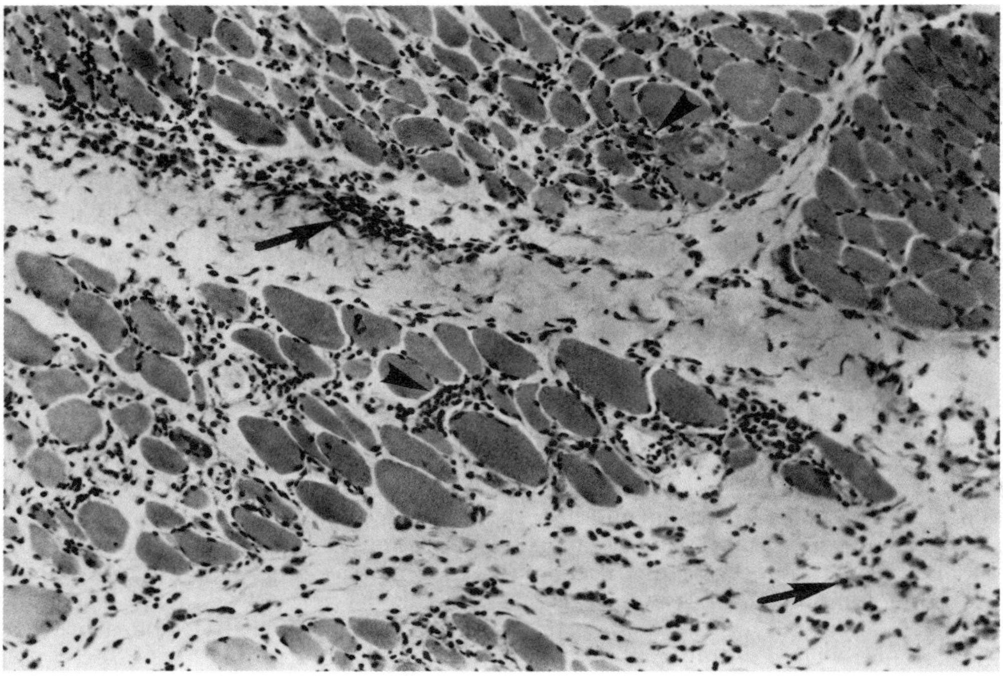

FIGURE 16.3 Low-power photomicrograph of a muscle biopsy in polymyositis, showing interstitial inflammation (arrows) and endomyseal inflammation (arrowhead). There is much rounded atrophy of individual muscle fibers. Mag X 165. (Courtesy of Dr. V.R. Challa, Department of Pathology, Bowman Gray School of Medicine.)

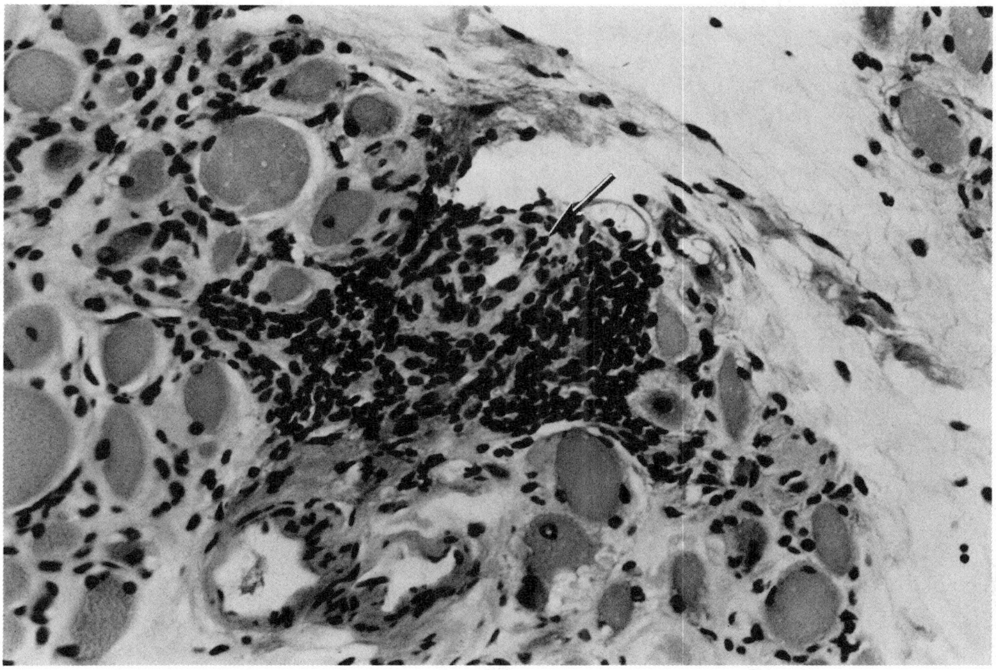

FIGURE 16.4 High-power photomicrograph of a muscle biopsy in polymyositis, showing an endomyseal blood vessel (arrow) surrounded by chronic mononuclear cell infiltrate. Note absence of necrosis in the vessel wall itself. All the muscle fibers in this area appear rounded, atrophic, and surrounded by fibrosis. Mag X 330. (Courtesy of Dr. V.R. Challa, Department of Pathology, Bowman Gray School of Medicine.)

Prognosis and Management

Natural History and Prognostic Features

Polymyositis and dermatomyositis have long been considered devastating and frequently fatal diseases. Studies of mortality prior to the institution of corticosteroid therapy and other supportive measures suggested an overall mortality of 50-60%. In recent years, however, since the introduction of corticosteroids and other forms of therapy, survival has improved, with survival at 5 years of 70-80% (36). There are still wide discrepancies from one study to the next regarding morbidity and mortality, and this probably reflects differences in populations studied, duration of the disease, and forms of therapy. In one recent study of 23 patients in a community hospital, patients were more likely to have mild disease than in other studies, and 41% of patients had discontinued all forms of therapy after approximately 4 years of follow-up.

It is difficult to identify specific prognostic indicators. Those with more severe disease at presentation, and those with associated carcinoma appear to have the highest mortality, and adults do worse than children (36). There is poor correlation of prognosis with degree of enzyme elevation or biopsy findings. Patients with involvement of pharyngeal muscles and aspiration pneumonia have the worst prognosis (37).

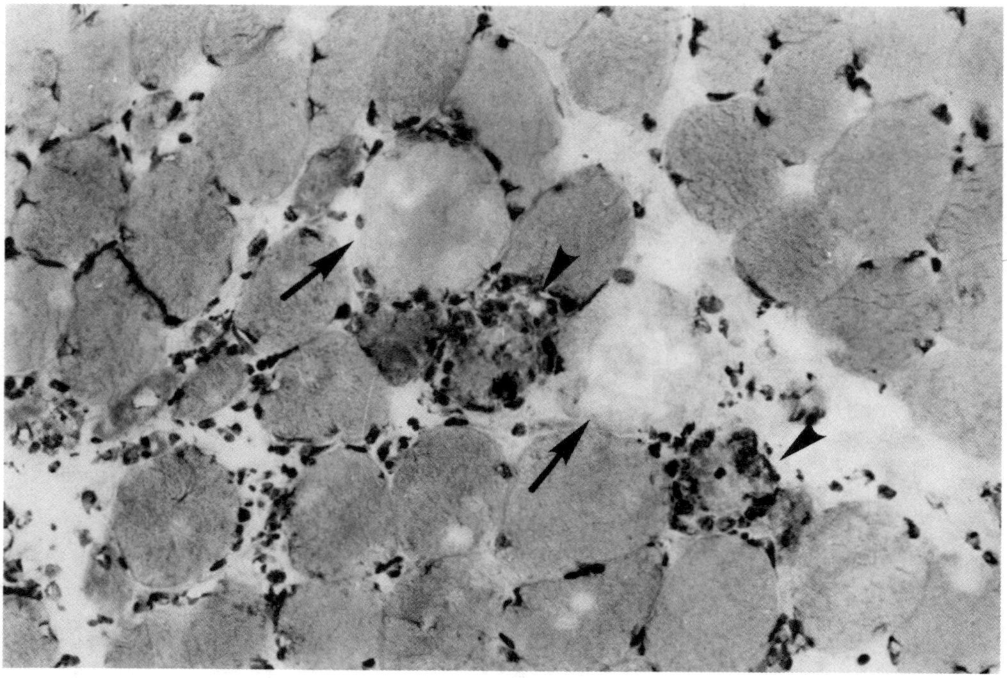

FIGURE 16.5 High-power photomicrograph of a muscle biopsy in polymyositis, showing two necrotic fibers undergoing phagocytosis (arrowheads). Two other fibers in earlier stages of necrosis (arrows). Mag X 330. (Courtesy of Dr. V.R. Challa, Department of Pathology, Bowman Gray School of Medicine.)

Therapy

High-dose corticosteroids are considered the mainstay of therapy for polymyositis and dermatomyositis. Since the institution of this form of therapy for this disease, survival has improved and morbidity has decreased. In spite of this, and general acceptance of this form of therapy, there is no controlled study demonstrating the unequivocal therapeutic benefit of steroids. Prednisone is usually given initially in daily doses of 60–100 mg per day, often in divided doses. After a week of divided dose therapy, a change to a single daily dose is usually made, and eventually therapy may be gradually changed to an alternate day schedule (1). Some authors have suggested the initial use of alternate day therapy in patients with mild disease, and this may be acceptable in those with only mild weakness (38).

Improvement with corticosteroid therapy is relatively slow, with several weeks to months required for a return to near normal muscle strength and serum muscle enzymes. When muscle strength and enzymes have reached a plateau of improvement, careful tapering of steroids may be undertaken as strenth and muscle enzymes are carefully monitored. This condition frequently requires high doses of corticosteroids for several months to years, and the side effects of this therapy are frequent (see Chapter 3).

Immunosuppressive drugs have been used widely in conjunction with corticosteroid therapy. These are usually added to prednisone when the latter has been found to produce an inadequate response after 2-4 months (1). Methotrexate and cyclophosphamide have been reported to be successful in several cases of disease refractory to corticosteroid therapy (1,39). Azathioprine has been studied in a controlled double-blind fashion, comparing azathioprine with prednisone to prednisone alone. After 3 months, no significant difference between the two treatment groups could be demonstrated (40), but after 3 years, the group receiving azathioprine had slightly improved functional disability and less steroid requirement than the group on prednisone alone (41).

Plasmapheresis has also been used with some success in combination with prednisone and/or immunosuppressive drugs after drugs alone had failed to produce a satisfactory response. In a recent report, 35 patients were treated with plasmapheresis, and strength improved in 32 of these (42).

Careful attention to complications of the disease and its therapy is required for a good outcome. Supplemental calcium and vitamin D may retard the development of osteopenia associated with corticosteroids, and early recognition and treatment of infectious complications is important as well. In patients with pharyngeal or upper airway compromise, early recognition and prevention of aspiration are essential, and in those with severe respiratory muscle weakness, supportive ventilation is sometimes necessary. Recognition of cardiac complications is also important. When immunosuppressive drugs are used, monitoring for hematologic side effects and the realization of the low risk of the development of malignancy is important. With methotrexate, the risk of liver fibrosis may be minimized by the use of small doses or by the use of parenteral drug. With careful evaluation, exclusion of other causes of myositis, and aggressive treatment and careful follow-up, the prognosis in polymyositis and dermatomyositis can be quite good, although complications of therapy still remain a significant problem.

References

1. Bradley WG: Inflammatory disease of muscle. In WN Kelley, ED Harris, S Ruddy, CB Sledge (eds.), *Textbook of Rheumatology,* 1st Ed. Philadelphia, W.B. Saunders, 1981, pp. 1255-1276.

2. Walton JN, Adams RD: *Polymyositis.* Baltimore, Williams and Wilkens, 1958.

3. Bohan A, Peter JB: Polymyositis and dermatomyositis. *N Engl J Med* 292: 344-347, 403-407, 1975.

4. Phillips PE, Kassan SS, Kagen LJ: Increased toxoplasma antibodies in idiopathic inflammatory muscle disease. *Arthritis Rheum* 22:209-214, 1979.

5. Krain LS: Dermatomyositis in six patients without initial muscle involvement. *Arch Dermatol*

6. Bohan A, Peter JB, Bowman RL, Pearson CM: A computer-assisted analysis of 153 patients with polymyositis and dermatomyositis. *Medicine* 56:255-286, 1977.

7. Callen JB, Hyla JF, Bole GG, Kay DR: The relationship of dermatomyositis and polymyositis to internal malignancy. *Arch Dermatol* 116:295-298, 1980.

8. Hanissian AS, Masi AT, Pitner SE et al.: Polymyositis and dermatomyositis in children: An epidemiologic and clinical comparative analysis. *J Rheumatol* 9:390-394, 1982.

9. Schumacher HR, Schimmer B, Gordon CV et al.: Articular manifestations of polymyositis and dermatomyositis. *Am Jour Med* 67:287-292, 1982.

10. Feldman D, Hochberg MC, Zizic TM, Stevens MB: Cutaneous vasculitis in adult polymyositis/dermatomyositis. *J Rheumatol* 10:85-89, 1983.

11. Kehoe RF, Bauernfeind R, Tommaso C et al.: Cardiac conduction defects in polymyositis. Electrophysiologic studies in four patients. *Ann Intern Med* 94:41-43, 1981.

12. Denhow CE, Lie JT, Tancredi RG, Bunch TW: Cardiac involvement in polymyositis. A clinicopathologic study of 20 autopsied patients. *Arthritis Rheum* 22:1088-1092, 1979.

13. Strongwater SL, Annesley T, Schnitzer TJ: Myocardial involvement in polymyositis. *J Rheumatol* 10:459-463, 1983.

14. Askari A, Heuttner TL: Cardiac abnormalities in polymyositis/dermatomyositis. *Semin Arth Rheum* 12:208-219, 1982.

15. Larca LJ, Coppola JT, Honig SL: Creatine kinase MB isoenzyme in dermatomyositis: A noncardiac source. *Ann Intern Med* 94:341-343, 1981.

16. Songcharoen S, Raju SF, Pennebaker JB: Interstitial lung disease in polymyositis and dermatomyositis. *J Rheumatol* 7:353-360, 1981.

17. Salmeron G, Greenberg D, Lidsky MD: Polymyositis and diffuse interstitial lung disease. A review of pulmonary histopathologic findings. *Arch Intern Med* 141:1005-1010, 1981.

18. Kallen PB, Louie JS, Nies KM, Bayer AS: Infectious myositis and related syndromes. *Semin Arth Rheum* 11:421-439, 1982.

19. Hochberg MC, Koppes GM, Edwards CO et al.: Hypothyroidism presenting as a polymyositis-like syndrome. *Arthritis Rheum* 19:1363-1366, 1976.

20. Ramsay I: *Thyroid Disease and Muscle Dysfunction*. London, Whitefriars Press, 1974.

21. Casey EB, Harrison MJG: Diabetic amyotrophy: A follow-up study. *Br Med Jour* 1:656-659, 1972.

22. Lane RJM, Mastaglia FL: Drug-induced myopathies in man. *Lancet* 2: 562-566, 1978.

23. Harris AL, Smith IE, Snaith M: Tamoxifen-induced tumor regression associated with dermatomyositis. *Br Med Jour* 284:1674-1675, 1982.

24. Watson AJS, Dalbow MH, Stachura I et al.: Immunologic studies in cimetidine-induced nephropathy and polymyositis. *N Engl J Med* 308:142-145, 1983.

25. Siegel AJ, Silverman LM, Lopez RE: Creatine kinase elevations in marathon runners: Relationship to training and competition. *Yale J Biol Med* 53: 275-279, 1980.

26. Welch KMA, Goldberg DM: Serum creatine phosphokinase in motor neuron disease. *Neurology* 22:697-701, 1972.

27. Edmonds PJ, Ziegler DK: Diagnostic value of serum creatine phosphokinase in motor neuron disease. *South Med Jour* 68:1388-1390, 1975.

28. Harrington TH, Cohen MD, Bartleson JD, Ginsberg WW: Elevation of creatine kinase in amyotrophic lateral sclerosis: Potential confusion with polymyositis. *Arthritis Rheum* 26:201-205, 1983.

29. Sladek GD, Vasey FB, Sieger B et al.: Relapsing eosinophilic myositis. *J Rheumatol* 10:467-470, 1983.

30. Venables PJW, Mumford PA, Main RN: Antibodies to nuclear antigens in polymyositis: Relationship to autoimmune 'overlap syndromes' and carcinoma. *Ann Rheum Dis* 40:217-223, 1981.

31. Wolfe JF, Adelstein E, Sharp GC: Antinuclear antibody with distinct specificity for polymyositis. *J Clin Invest* 59:176-178, 1977.

32. Nishikai M, Reichlin M: Heterogeneity of precipitating antibodies in polymyositis and dermatomyositis. *Arthritis Rheum* 23:881-888, 1980.

33. Yoshida S, Akizuki M. Mimori T et al.: The precipitating antibody to an acidic nuclear protein antigen, the Jo-1, in connective tissue diseases. A marker for a subset of polymyositis with interstitial pulmonary fibrosis. *Arthritis Rheum* 26:604-611, 1983.

34. Schwarz HA, Slavin G, Ward P, Ansell BM: Muscle biopsy in polymyositis and dermatomyositis. *Ann Rheum Dis* 39:500-507, 1980.

35. Bennington JL, Dau PC: Patients with polymyositis and dermatomyositis who undergo plasmapheresis therapy. Pathologic findings. *Arch Neurol* 38:553-560, 1981.

36. DeVere R, Bradley WB: Polymyositis: Its presentation, morbidity and mortality. *Brain* 98:637-666, 1975.

37. Carpenter JR, Bunch TW, Engel AG, O'Brien PC: Survival in polymyositis: Corticosteroids and risk factors. *J Rheumatol* 4:207-214, 1977.

38. Hoffman GS, Franck WA, Raddatz DA, Stallores L: Presentation, treatment and prognosis of idiopathic inflammatory muscle disease in a rural hosptial. *Am Jour Med* 75:433-438, 1983.

39. Metzger AL, Bohan A, Goldberg LS et al.: Polymyositis and dermatomyositis: Combined methotrexate and corticosteroid therapy. *Ann Intern Med* 81:182-194, 1974.

40. Bunch TW, Worthington JW, Combs JJ et al.: Azathioprine with prednisone for polymyositis. A controlled clinical trial. *Ann Intern Med* 92:365-369, 1980.

41. Bunch TW: Prednisone and azathioprine for polymyositis. Long-term follow-up. *Arthritis Rheum* 24:45-48, 1981.

42. Dau PC: Plasmapheresis in idiopathic inflammatory myopathy. Experience with 35 patients. *Arch Neurol* 38:544-552, 1981.

Chapter 17

MIXED CONNECTIVE TISSUE DISEASE

Edward J. Pisko, M.D.

It is quite common for rheumatic disease patients to have features of more than one disease. Overlap syndromes are frequently seen by physicians taking care of patients with rheumatic diseases. In particular, patients with features of both polymyositis and scleroderma (1) and systemic lupus erythematosus and scleroderma (2) have been well described. The descriptions of these overlaps was primarily clinical, but by 1972 advances in autoimmune serological testing allowed Sharp et al. to report 25 cases of an apparently distinct clinical syndrome which they called mixed connective tissue disease (MCTD) (3). These patients had features of systemic lupus erythematosus (SLE), polymyositis (PM), and progressive systemic sclerosis (PSS). The finding of high titers of speckled pattern fluorescent antinuclear antibodies (FANA) and high titers of antibodies to nuclear ribonuclear protein (RNP) by hemagglutination provided a link between their clinical findings and their serological tests (4). These initial MCTD patients appeared to have a relatively benign disease that was readily responsive to corticosteroids.

In the years since the initial description of MCTD, other authors have confirmed Sharp's findings (5-9), but the concept of what constitutes mixed connective tissue disease has gradually evolved (7,10,11). Many patients with MCTD have a quite benign course. These patients may not require hospitalization or aggressive treatment. Some MCTD patients with more severe disease will simultaneously have features of SLE, PSS, and PM as in Sharp's original description, but these patients constitute a minority of MCTD patients. It is more typical for patients with MCTD to appear to have SLE-like disease initially. These patients' disease may then gradually evolve into a PSS-like illness. The SLE-like features of MCTD often will respond to corticosteroids. This explains some of the initial enthusiam for their usage in PSS. However, the PSS-like features of this disease are much more difficult to treat. Although MCTD is often a benign disease, the mortality rate in MCTD appears to be relatively higher than was expected from the original reports (7,10). Despite the changing concepts of what constitutes MCTD, this disease has gradually gained recognition as a distinct clinical entity. Some authors continue to believe that MCTD is a subset of SLE or PSS, but it is clinically useful to make the diagnosis of MCTD because the prognosis of MCTD is different than the prognosis for PSS, SLE, or PM.

Etiopathogenesis

MCTD, like many rheumatic diseases, is a disease of unknown origin. Current thinking about MCTD and similar diseases is that they have an autoimmune origin. However, the precise events leading to the onset of the autoimmune phenomena remain unelucidated. Presumably, environmental events interact with a genetically susceptible host, but these factors are even less well understood than they are in SLE. The high titers of antibodies to RNP found in this disease provide the best evidence that this is an autoimmune disease. Immunological studies have been performed demonstrating that T-suppressor lymphocytes from patients with MCTD are less capable of suppressing in vitro immunoglobulin production (12). This finding is similar to what has been found in SLE and PSS. This decreased suppressor T-cell function provides a possible explanation for the polyclonal increase in immunoglobulin production found in this disease. In addition to antibodies to RNP, many other autoantibodies such as rheumatoid factors are found in MCTD. Decreased T-suppressor function can only partially explain the dramatic increase in antibodies to RNP found in MCTD. More precise genetic and immunologic mechanisms are likely to be responsible for this phenomenon. Autoantibodies contribute to the formation of immune complexes which are frequently found in MCTD (13,14). The case for immune complex-mediated damage in MCTD is not as strong as it is in SLE where antinative DNA-DNA complexes are likely causes of kidney damage, but approximately 25% of patients with MCTD have hypocomplementemia presumably secondary to complement fixation by immune complexes. In addition, antibodies to RNP can also fix complement (15). The pleuropericarditis of MCTD is possibly immune complex-mediated. Renal disease, while not common in MCTD, may in some instances be related to immune complex-mediated damage. Immune complexes may also be playing a role by stimulating inflammatory mononuclear cells to produce inflammatory factors contributing to interstitial lung disease and perhaps also PSS like skin and vascular changes. However, this hypothesis has not been tested in MCTD. It is interesting that reticuloendothelial cell function (16) is not abnormal in MCTD and lymphocytotoxic antibodies are not frequently abnormal in MCTD (17). This emphasizes the differences of this illness from SLE which is characterized by both of these abnormalities.

Experimental in vitro and in vivo work has raised the possibility that antibodies to RNP may be pathogenetic. Antibodies to RNP are capable of entering live cells in culture (18) of skin sections and these antibodies are likely to be responsible for the presence of positive immunofluorescence for IgG antibodies in MCTD skin epithelial cells (19,20). This staining occurs in addition to the staining that has been found at the dermal-epidermal junction (21).

Autopsy studies have demonstrated that patients dying of mixed connective tissue disease often have proliferative endarterial vascular lesions of medium and small arteries (22). These changes are similar to those found in PSS and offer an explanation for why MCTD patients often resemble PSS patients late in their disease course. However, the fibrosis that accompanies these vascular changes is not as prominent as that found in PSS. The patients dying with MCTD will often have lymphocytic infiltration of target organs and this provides further presumptive evidence for an autoimmune etiology for MCTD.

Clinical Features

Diagnostic Criteria

Diagnostic criteria for MCTD have not been formulated by the American Rheumatism Association. A committee assembled to discuss such criteria would have widely differing opinions not only about the criteria, but even whether to call MCTD a specific entity. Table 17.1 is an attempt to develop criteria for MCTD. The criteria emphasize the laboratory features of this disease and, as formulated, MCTD patients must also have features of at least two of three diseases that overlap to form MCTD. Series of patients have been found by two methods. Patients have either been thought clinically to have an overlap syndrome and the diagnosis of MCTD is confirmed by the specific serological tests, or a group of patients is screened and those patients with typical serologies are examined to see if they have an overlap. The former method yields an interesting population of patients who appear to have a rheumatic disease with protean manifestations, which most likely is a distinct entity. The latter method of working back from the serological tests without clinical criteria yields results which are much more confusing (23,24). The proposed criteria are therefore useful because they avoid the problem of the patient with serologies consistent with MCTD who has little or no disease and only mild symptoms and it avoids the occasional patient with typical rheumatoid arthritis who serologically has MCTD but who has no features of an overlap disease. The first criterion is mandatory for MCTD. Patients with MCTD have been defined by their extremely high titers of antibody to ribonucleoprotein (RNP). Patients with MCTD should not have serological markers that are highly specific for systemic lupus erythematosus such as antibodies to SM antigen and native (double-stranded) DNA (criterion 2). Finally, MCTD patients should have features of at least two of the three diseases which overlap to form MCTD (criterion 3).

The titer of antibodies to RNP is very important in making a diagnosis of MCTD. In general, the specificity of any test for a diagnosis increases as the titer increases. This is true for rheumatoid factor in RA and antibodies to native or double-stranded DNA in SLE. With higher titers of antibody to RNP there is an increasing specificity of this test for MCTD. Many patients with antibodies to RNP but not SM antigen who do not have MCTD initially may eventually develop MCTD. Although antibodies to RNP are found in a large variety of rheumatic diseases, the anti-RNP titers tend to be low. The combination of high titers of antibodies to RNP and the absence of other antinuclear antibodies in a patient with an overlap syndrome is the best means of diagnosing MCTD.

In addressing the diagnostic criteria for MCTD, it is important to mention the ongoing debate as to whether MCTD is a distinct clinical entity. Reichlin has argued that antibodies to RNP are frequently found in SLE and he asserts that MCTD patients represent a subset of SLE patients (25,26). MCTD patients often fulfill the American Rheumatism Association criteria for SLE. Reichlin has shown that SLE patients with antibodies to RNP have less renal disease, antibodies to double-stranded or native DNA, and hypocomplementemia. The presence of antibodies to RNP is therefore a marker which implies a more favorable prognosis for renal disease in SLE. However, the presence of PSS-like changes in patients with MCTD is a strong argument for this being a separate disease entity and not

TABLE 17.1 Proposed Criteria for MCTD*

1. Positive antibodies to RNP by immunodiffusion or ≧1:5000 by hemagglutination

2. Negative antibodies to Sm antigen and native DNA by immunodiffusion

3. Three disease features from at least two of the following groups:

   A. Disease features commonly associated with SLE
      1) Malar rash
      2) Discoid rash
      3) Photosensitivity
      4) Oral ulcers
      5) Arthritis
      6) Serositis

   B. Disease features commonly associated with PSS
      1) Diffusely swollen (puffy) hands
      2) Raynaud's phenomenon
      3) Esophageal hypomotility
      4) Bibasilar lung fibrosis
      5) Sclerodermatous skin changes

   C. Clinical myositis (proximal muscle weakness and elevated CPK confirmed by muscle biopsy or typical EMG)

*MCTD can be diagnosed when all three criteria are met.

merely a subset of SLE with a more favorable renal prognosis. Reichlin has argued that the changes consistent with PSS have not been severe or life-threatening. However, more recent studies (7,10,27) have described patients with quite severe organ system involvement (lung and kidney) consistent with PSS. Some authors believe that MCTD is a subset of PSS. Probably, the most cogent argument for calling MCTD a separate disease is the claim by some authors that MCTD is a subset of SLE and by others that it is a subset of PSS.

General Features

The clinical features of PSS are summarized in Table 17.2.

MCTD is predominantly a disease of women. The mean age of all patients is approximately 37. However, men do develop this disease as do children and elderly individuals. The incidence and prevalence of this disease has not been determined, but MCTD is probably somewhat less common than SLE and more common than PSS.

TABLE 17.2 Clinical Characteristics of Mixed Connective Tissue Disease Patients

Characteristic	Percent
Arthritis/arthralgia	95
Raynaud's phenomenon	80
Pulmonary disease	67
Esophageal dysmotility	67
Neuropsychiatric disease	50
Lymphadenopathy	50
Diffuse hand swelling	50
Myositis	40
Cardiac disease	35
Sclerodactyly	35
Telangiectasia	30
Splenomegaly	20
Sjögren's syndrome	15
Renal disease	10
Hashimoto's thyroiditis	5

Presentation and Clinical Course

The onset of MCTD is usually insidious with cutaneous and systemic complaints. MCTD patients often present with Raynaud's phenomenon of long duration and polyarthralgias. Malaise and fatigue frequently accompany the illness at the time of diagnosis and also may be of long duration. Diffuse swelling of the hands is a not uncommon initial complaint. Fever may also be the initial complaint and some patients present with high spiking fevers associated with inflammatory muscle disease. Major organ involvement such as pleuropericarditis or severe interstitial lung disease leading to dyspnea on exertion are uncommon initial complaints. Severe erosive arthritis indistinguishable from RA can occur initially in MCTD and the clinical course of these patients may parallel the disease course of RA. Patients with MCTD are often thought to have RA or SLE on initial presentation; however, MCTD can often be presumptively diagnosed prior to laboratory testing with a careful history and physical examination. This examination should pay careful attention to cutaneous signs, particularly in the hands. Laboratory tests are necessary to confirm the diagnosis.

The clinical course of MCTD is variable. Some patients who are followed with systemic symptoms and serologic features of MCTD may never develop symptomatic internal organ system involvement. The typical course of MCTD is for a patient to present without symptomatic internal organ system involvement. Most patients later develop intermittent periods in which they will have major organ system involvement such as pleuropericarditis, myopathy, or aseptic meningitis. These problems usually resolve with steroid treatment and in general patients do fairly well between disease flares except for chronic problems with fatigue, Raynaud's phenomenon, and polyarthralgias. However, eventually many patients develop pulmonary, esophageal, and cutaneous features of MCTD that resemble PSS. Fortunately, patients rarely die from PSS-like disease complications, and the prognosis does appear to be better than that seen in PSS or SLE.

Cutaneous Manifestations

Raynaud's phenomenon occurs in over 85% of patients and is often an initial complaint. Diffuse hand swelling occurs in approximately 75% of patients. The swelling is often most marked over the dorsum of the hands with extension into the digits sometimes giving a sausage-like appearance. The involved skin can be erythematous and warm, particularly early in the disease course. Skin changes in the hand can resemble those in PSS with thinning and tautness of the skin. These changes as well as digital ulcerations occur, but are not common. Telangiectasia is common and is often most prominent over the hands. The dilated and irregular nailfold capillaries which are seen best on nailfold capillaroscopy (28) can often also be seen with the unaided eye. SLE-like skin lesions including malar rash and alopecia may occur in about half of patients. Diffuse erythematous rashes may also be seen. Heliotrope eruptions of the eyelids and erythema over the knuckles resembling the skin changes of dermatomyositis can occur. Erythema nodosum, erythema multiforme, and toxic epidermal necrolysis have been described in MCTD.

Arthritic Manifestations

The arthritic manifestations of MCTD have been well described (29).

Virtually all patients with MCTD have polyarthralgias and most have arthritis. In general, the arthritis of MCTD is not as severe as that of rheumatoid arthritis and patients primarily have polyarthralgias of varying, but usually mild severity. The MCTD and PIP joints are usually involved. The wrists and MTP joints are involved in about half of patients, and knees, ankles, shoulders and elbows may also be involved. The spine and hips are usually spared. About one-third of patients will have marginal erosions and about one-third of patients will have rheumatoid arthritis-like joint deformities. Joint deformities are usually confined to the hands in MCTD. Arthritis mutilans and erosive distal arthritis have been reported.

Muscular Manifestations

As previously mentioned, MCTD is an overlap between SLE, PSS, and PM. Polymyalgia and muscle tenderness may be present in up to three-fourths of patients. However, only one-third to one-half of patients have myositis defined by EMG, biopsy, and enzyme elevations. In general, the myositis of MCTD is less severe, more responsive to treatment, and more self-limited than the myositis of primary PM. However, occasional patients with serologies consistent with MCTD will have a disease indistinguishable from PM. Elevations of serum muscle enzymes (CPK and aldolase), EMG, and muscle biopsies may be undistinguishable from those seen in PM and SLE. Immunofluorescence studies in muscle biopsy specimens (30) often reveal immunoglobulin deposition in normal blood vessels or muscle fibers. Deposits of immunoglobulin also occur adjacent to or around sarcoplasmic membrane and within perimysial connective tissue. The relationship between these immunoglobulin deposits and the pathological muscle findings is not conclusive, but this gives some credence to there being an autoimmune etiology for MCTD. In some patients an inflammatory myopathy may be associated with intermittent high spiking fevers.

Pulmonary Manifestations

Pulmonary involvement in MCTD is common, but this is rarely the source of severe disability, and indeed most patients do not develop pulmonary symptoms. However, rare patients will present with or develop severe dyspnea on exertion (27). Over 80% of MCTD patients will have either restrictive disease by pulmonary function testing or a reticulonodular interstitial pattern on chest roentgenogram. As in PSS, this interstitial pattern is more common at the lung bases. Decreased carbon monoxide diffusion capacity is common on testing and patients may also have a decreased lung volume on testing. Volume loss may also be seen on chest roentgenogram. Pleural effusions occur in approximately one-third of patients. These tend to be mild and often do not require high-dose prednisone therapy. Pulmonary hypertension is a rare but potentially fatal complication of MCTD. Roentgenograms may reveal cardiomegaly and prominent pulmonary arteries. On biopsy these patients may have severe intimal proliferation and medial hypertrophy. Lung biopsies are more likely to reveal interstitial fibrosis with variable infiltration with mononuclear cells. Fatal pulmonary embolism and lung densities responsive to corticosteroids have also been reported. The latter findings are similar to what has been labelled lupus pneumonia in SLE patients.

Gastrointestinal Manifestations

Esophageal involvement in MCTD is well described (31) and is similar to pulmonary involvement in that most patients have abnormalities in testing but a smaller number of patients will have symptoms. Approximately 70-80% of patients will have esophageal abnormalities by cineesophagram or manometric studies. Decreased peristalsis of the distal two-thirds of the esophagus is common as is a decrease in lower esophageal sphincter pressure. A decrease in upper esophageal sphincter pressure may also be seen. Frank dysphagia is uncommon however. Esophageal abnormalities are related to the duration of the disease and as patients are followed, more severe symptomatic esophageal involvement may occur. This would be in keeping with the tendency of MCTD patients to resemble PSS patients with time. PSS-like bowel changes such as decreased small bowel motility with bacterial overgrowth and malabsorption have been reported and large mouth sacular diverticulae occur. Pneumatosis intestinalis has been reported as a concomitant of MCTD bowel disease.

Cardiac Manifestations

Cardiac disease in MCTD has been well studied (32). Pericarditis is the principal cardiac abnormality in adults with MCTD. The pericarditis is usually relatively benign and transient. High-dose corticosteroids are usually not required for treatment although occasional patients may present with or develop severe pericarditis. Childhood MCTD is associated with more severe interstitial inflammation and/or fibrosis. Intimal thickening and narrowing of small coronary vessels have also been seen.

Neurological Manifestations

Early series of patients with MCTD found a low incidence of neurological complications, but more recent work suggests that MCTD patients frequently develop neurological abnormalities with their illness (33); however, serious and life-threatening neurological manifestations such as seizures and psychosis are fortunately rarer than in SLE. In one series of 20 patients with MCTD (7), four patients developed aseptic meningitis and three patients developed psychosis. Febrile headache, trigeminal neuropathy, and cerebellar ataxia were each described in two patients. The incidence of neurological complications may be lower in an outpatient setting in contrast to this series of patients who required hospitalization. Organic mental syndromes and vascular headache also occur. In general, the neurological findings in MCTD resemble those found in SLE except for there being a probable higher incidence of aseptic meningitis and trigeminal neuropathy in MCTD. The latter finding is also not uncommon in PSS. Cerebral hemorrhage and infarction have been reported, but the relationship between these findings and MCTD is unclear. Arteriosclerosis and hypertension, both possibly exacerbated by corticosteroid usage, were probably involved in these cases.

Renal Manifestations

Renal disease is a fortunately rare cause of serious morbidity or mortality in MCTD. Approximately 10–20% of patients may have renal disease by laboratory testing and/or renal biopsy. The spectrum of histological changes is similar to what is seen in SLE with membranoproliferative changes being a common biopsy finding. Immunofluorescent studies have revealed evidence of immune complex deposition in some biopsy specimens. Renal failure has rarely been the cause of death in MCTD patients. One of the original MCTD patients died after developing renal crisis identical to that seen with PSS. As patients are followed for longer periods of time, PSS-like renal disease may become more common. The occurrence of SLE-like and PSS-like renal disease in MCTD gives further credence to MCTD being a true distinct overlap illness. Fortunately, MCTD patients' risk of developing serious renal disease remains less than for either PSS or SLE.

Miscellaneous Features

Fever is present in about a third to a half of patients with MCTD and is often related to disease activity such as serositis, myositis, or aseptic meningitis. Lymphadenopathy occurs in approximately one-third of patients and hepatosplenomegaly is rare. Hepatic dysfunction is unusual in this illness. Sjögren's syndrome is a not uncommon concomitant of MCTD, and Hashimoto's thyroiditis also occurs with increased frequency in MCTD. Pregnancy is apparently a cause of disease flare in MCTD and there may be a higher than expected incidence of fetal wastage.

Differential Diagnosis

When patients present with features of SLE, PSS, PM, or rheumatoid arthritis, MCTD should be part of the differential diagnosis. MCTD should also be a diagnostic consideration with patients presenting with lymphadenopathy, fever of unknown origin, trigeminal neuropathy, Sjögren's syndrome, Hashimoto's thyroiditis, or digital ulceration. The finding of high titer antibody to RNP as the sole or major antinuclear antibody is the major differentiating test between MCTD and other diseases. Clinically, the presence of Raynaud's phenomenon and swollen hands in patients with an overlap syndrome is the major clue that MCTD is present. However, true overlaps between connective tissue disorders exist in the absence of antibodies to RNP. Undifferentiated connective tissue disease will continue to be found and such cases will be recognized until further diagnostic studies enable us to better characterize these patients. The early phases of many inflammatory illnesses can mimic MCTD.

Laboratory Tests

Immunological Tests

The laboratory findings of MCTD are summarized in Table 17.3. Fluorescent antibody tests (FANA) are virtually always positive in MCTD. This is almost by definition, because the high titers of antibodies to RNP that are the major serological feature of MCTD give a speckled pattern on indirect immunofluorescent testing. Rare patients may have a homogeneous ANA or a negative test at some point in their disease course and ANA titers are occasionally undetectable during disease remission, but all patients will have a speckled FANA at some time during their disease. Antibodies to single-stranded or denatured DNA also can occur in MCTD. These antibodies may be responsible for the rare occurrence of a homogenous pattern of nuclear fluorescence. However, all patients will have a speckled FANA at some time during their disease course.

Hemagglutinating antibodies to extractable nuclear antigen (ENA) are found at some time in all patients with MCTD. ENA consists of a variety of saline extractable nuclear antigens. These antigens include RNP, SM antigen, and probably also SSA and SSB antigens as well as several as yet poorly characterized antigens. Hemagglutination tests are performed with tanned sheep erythrocytes passively coated with ENA. Patients with MCTD have very high anti-ENA titers by hemagglutination with titers ranging from 1:1000 to 1:100,000 and sometimes higher. Titers often remain high throughout a patient's disease course, but the titers tend to parallel the disease course more often than originally thought.

Antibodies to RNP and SM antigen by hemagglutination: MCTD patients do not have antibodies detected by hemagglutination of tanned sheep cells coated with ribonuclease-digested (RNase) ENA. This provided the first evidence that MCTD patients are making antibody to RNP. Approximately half of SLE patients also will have anti-RNP antibodies by hemagglutination. The titers are usually lower in SLE than in MCTD. Antibodies to RNP occur in a variety of other inflammatory connective tissue disorders. The major antigen in RNase-insensitive ENA has been labelled SM antigen. Antibodies to SM antigen are extremely rare in MCTD, but 25% of SLE patients will have antibody to SM.

TABLE 17.3 Laboratory Characteristics of Mixed Connective Tissue Disease

	Percent
Positive RNP antibodies	100
Elevated erythrocyte sedimentation rate	100
Speckled pattern FANA	100
Elevated gamma globulins	75
Anemia	60
Leukopenia	55
Elevated CPK	40
Decreased complement	25
False positive VDRL	10

Determination of antibodies to RNP by immunodiffusion: Patients with MCTD will have antibodies to RNP on testing by immunodiffusion. Immunodiffusion is the most precise method of measuring antibodies to RNP because a sample can be characterized by previously identified reference antisera. This is shown pictorially in Figure 17.1. If a line of identity is seen between the reference sera and the test serum, then the test sample contains anti-RNP antibodies. For these tests extractable nuclear antigen is used either whole or after being digested by RNase.

Immunodiffusion testing for RNP antibodies is quite specific, but this method is not a sensitive means of detecting antibodies to RNP. This lack of sensitivity of immunodiffusion testing for RNP antibodies contributes to the specificity of this test for MCTD. As previously mentioned, the specificity of any test for a disease generally rises with the antibody titer. Immunodiffusion testing generally detects only those sera with relatively high antibody titers and therefore patients with antibodies to RNP alone on immunodiffusion generally have MCTD.

Determination of RNP antibodies by counterimmunoelectrophoresis: This method of detecting antibodies is quite sensitive. When counterimmunoelectrophoresis is utilized, RNP antibodies are found in a wide variety of inflammatory connective tissue diseases. However, the mere presence of anti-RNP antibody is not indicative of MCTD. Only high titers of antibody to RNP in the absence of other antinuclear antibodies is indicative of MCTD.

Disease Activity and Anti-RNP Antibodies

In general the titer of anti-RNP antibodies tends to remain high despite changes in disease activity or treatment. Some patients will have a gradual fall in titer of anti-RNP antibodies especially when this test is performed by hemagglutination. Fortunately, antibodies to RNP performed by immunodiffusion usually continue to be present enabling one to diagnose MCTD serologically. RNP-antibody testing

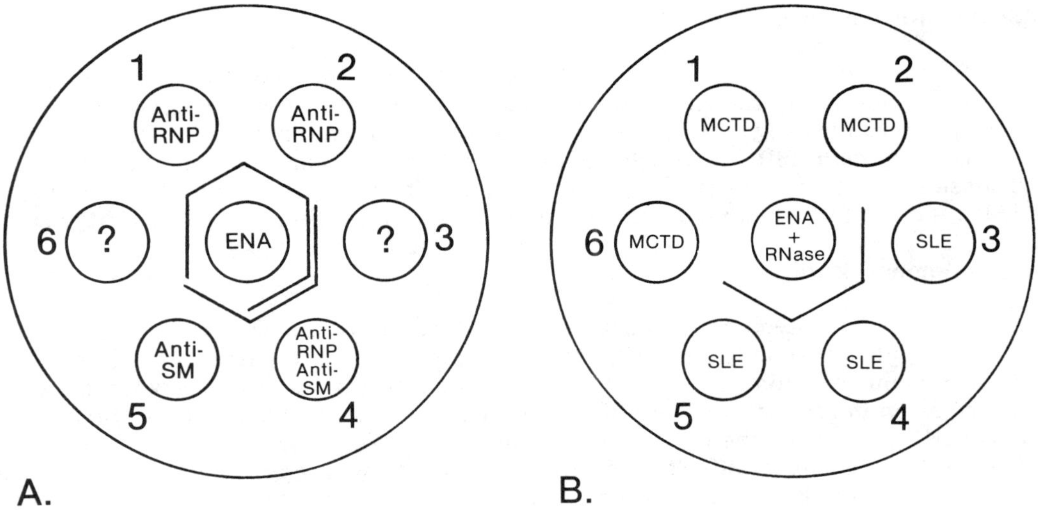

FIGURE 17.1 Immunodiffusion testing for antibodies to RNP and SM antigen. In A, an ouchterlony immunodiffusion plate contains extractable nuclear antigen (ENA) from calf thymus extract. Wells 1 and 2 contain reference sera from patients with anti-RNP antibodies. Well 4 contains reference sera from a patient with antibodies to SM and RNP and well 5 contains anti-SM reference sera. Wells 3 and 6 contain unknown sera. The unknown in well 3 forms two precipitation lines having lines of identity with both anti-SM and anti-RNP reference sera demonstrating the presence of these antibodies in this patient. The unknown sera in well 6 forms a line of identity with the anti-RNP reference sera and therefore has anti-RNP antibody. In B, the center well contains ENA that has been digested with ribonuclease (RNase) to destroy RNP. The sera in B are identical to those in A. The unknown sera in well 3 forms a line of identity with the sera in wells 4 and 5 and therefore contains anti-SM antibody. Patients 3, 4, and 5 have SLE because antibodies to SM are specific for SLE and antibodies to SM are rarely found in other diseases. Sera 1, 2, and 6 are from MCTD patients containing large amounts of anti-RNP antibody and no antibody to SM. ENA or calf thymus extract contains numerous other antigens and reference sera are therefore necessary to identify the antibodies in this system.

therefore continues with time to be diagnostic for MCTD, but is rarely a help in guiding therapy.

Rheumatoid Factors

Rheumatoid factor is present in MCTD patients in about one-fourth to one-half of patients. Both the RA latex and the sheep cell agglutination test (SCAT) may be positive and in general titers are higher and rheumatoid factors are more common than in SLE. An insufficient number of patients have been studied in order to determine if the presence of a high titer of rheumatoid factor by both RA latex and SCAT methods is associated with any particular disease manifestations such as erosive deforming arthritis.

Sedimentation Rate

The erythrocyte sedimentation rate (ESR) is elevated in almost all MCTD patients at some time during their disease course. In general the ESR parallels disease activity but not always. Some patients with only minimal symptoms will have a persistently high ESR. However, many patients have a normal ESR when their disease is inactive and have an increased ESR with disease exacerbation. The ESR tends to fall when vigorous treatment leads to a fall in disease activity.

Complement Studies

Approximately one-quarter to one-third of MCTD patients will have low serum complement determinations. This finding is not associated with any specific disease manifestation such as nephritis although future studies may yield more information in regard to the clinical usefulness of complement testing. Since anti-RNP antibodies themselves are complement fixing, low complement levels may only reflect high anti-RNP antibody levels. Complement fixation by immune complexes may also be playing a role in decreased complement levels.

Immune Complexes

Immune complexes are frequently found in the serum of MCTD patients. Two studies have correlated disease activity with serum immune complex levels (13, 14), but clinical usefulness of immune complex testing is yet to be substantiated.

Other Immunologic Tests

Antibodies to single-stranded (denatured) DNA may occur in up to about one-third of patients. These antibodies are often found nonspecifically in a large variety of autoimmune diseases including MCTD. Hyperglobulinemia occurs in about three-quarters of patients and a false-positive VDRL occurs in about 10%.

Hematological Findings

Mild anemia and leukopenia may be found in up to three-quarters of patients. These findings will sometimes parallel disease activity. Over half of patients may have a positive Coombs test, but Coombs-positive hemolytic anemia and thrombocytopenia rarely occur. Severe thrombocytopenia may be more common in children with MCTD.

Enzyme Determinations

The precise prevalence of an elevated CPK in MCTD is unknown but it may be positive in about half of patients in whom it is tested. The true prevalence of an elevated CPK may be lower because many patients without signs or symptoms of myopathy are not tested. Serum enzymes indicative of hepatic dysfunction are rarely abnormal reflecting the low incidence of liver disease in MCTD.

Roentgenologic Findings

The radiological features of MCTD have been studied in detail by Bennett and O'Connell (7). They found that 60% of their patients had small periarticular as-symetrical, punched-out, cortical erosions in the hands and feet.

Typical rheumatoid-like joint changes with juxtaarticular osteoporosis, erosions, joint-space narrowing, and deformities occur in a small percentage of MCTD patients. Periarticular calcification and ischemic necrosis of bone, particularly the hips, occur in MCTD.

Chest roentgenograms may reveal a bilateral reticulonodular pattern at the bases. Pleural and pericardial effusions may be seen as well as prominent pulmonary arteries in the presence of pulmonary hypertension. Evanescent chest infiltrates such as those seen in SLE may occur.

Wide mouth sacculations (pseudodiverticulae) may be seen on barium enema. Esophageal roentgenograms may reveal decreased peristalsis with dilation, and esophageal stricture may be seen.

Prognosis and Treatment

Prognosis

Several problems exist that preclude precise statements as to the prognosis of MCTD. Clinical criteria have not been established for this disease and few patients have been followed for 10-15 years. However, in general, the prognosis for MCTD appears to be better than for either SLE, PM, or PSS.

In addition, patients are not infrequently seen who have anti-RNP antibodies and nonspecific symptoms such as fatigue, joint and muscle pain, and mild weakness. Many of these patients do not develop major organ involvement consistent with MCTD. The inclusion of such patients in a series looking at mortality in MCTD would lead to the conclusion that MCTD is a much more benign illness than the present literature suggests. Patients rarely die of MCTD although some patients have died with immune-complex-mediated and PSS-like renal disease and pulmonary hypertension and there is excess mortality in MCTD. Cerebral vascular accident, myocardial infarction, and infection have all been responsible for deaths. The role of corticosteroids in causing accelerated atherosclerosis in these patients is undetermined. Corticosteroids and other immunosuppressive drugs are undoubtedly responsible for some deaths secondary to infection. Patients with MCTD have also committed suicide.

Treatment

General

Some patients with MCTD will not require treatment for their illness and other patients will have long periods in which disease manifestations are mild enough to make treatment unnecessary.

Excessive stress, overexertion, poor nutrition, and a lack of proper rest may all play a role in disease exacerbations, but this has not been proven. In general, however, proper diet and rest with avoidance of stress will aid MCTD patients. It is not clear if all factors known to lead to disease exacerbation in SLE will lead to similar disease flares in MCTD. Pregnancy does seem to cause MCTD flares as in SLE (34). MCTD patients with photosensitivity or a typical SLE-like malar rash should probably avoid sun exposure and use sun screens. The role, if any, of sun exposure in other MCTD patients is undetermined.

Drugs that may cause disease exacerbations in SLE should probably also be avoided in MCTD until more data concerning this are available. Birth control pills and sulfa drugs should generally be avoided. Nonsteroidal antiinflammatory agents such as the propionic acid derivative, ibuprofen, should be prescribed with caution in MCTD patients because of the rare occurrence of aseptic meningitis caused by these drugs in MCTD (35), SLE patients, and even normal individuals. The known effects of nonsteroidal antiinflammatory agents causing renal insufficiency through prostaglandin effects and interstitial nephritis are a consideration when giving these drugs to MCTD patients. However, it is not clear that MCTD patients are as sensitive to these drugs as are SLE patients.

Arthritis, Dermatitis and Systemic Complaints

Nonsteroidal antiinflammatory agents are generally sufficient to treat the polymyalgias, polyarthralgias, and mild arthritis that is a common finding in MCTD. These drugs are sometimes insufficient for these disease manifestations and small doses of daily or every-other-day corticosteroids are sometimes added to the treatment regimen. Small doses of corticosteroids may be especially helpful where excessive fatigue is a problem that significantly interferes with activities of daily living. Hydroxychloroquine may be useful for these systemic symptoms, but this drug has not been well studied in MCTD patients. The role of hydroxychloroquine in treating destructive rheumatoid-like arthritis in MCTD has also not been determined. Gold salt therapy is also a therapeutic consideration in the presence of severe destructive arthritis, but the risks and benefits of administrating the drug to MCTD patients have not been determined. Topical corticosteroid creams may benefit some MCTD rashes.

Raynaud's Phenomenon and Digital Ulcerations

Vasodilator therapy may reduce the likelihood of developing Raynaud's phenomenon in MCTD patients. Nifedipine, dibenzyline, and prazosin may all be useful although these drugs are not appreciably more effective than wearing warm gloves. Digital ulcerations may heal more rapidly with vasodilator therapy but this has not been proven. Keeping the ulcerated digit warm will help healing, and immobilization is occasionally helpful in healing refractory ulcers. This is discussed further in the chapter on progressive systemic sclerosis (Chapter 14).

Myositis

The myositis of MCTD is generally more benign than that seen in idiopathic PM. However, high doses of corticosteroids (prednisone 60-80 mg/day) may be necessary in patients with documented myopathy, particularly if they have severe weakness or very high levels of CPK. In general, corticosteroid therapy does not have to be continued for as long as in idiopathic PM. Normalization of muscle strength and the CPK are the keys to tapering corticosteroids.

Pericarditis and Pleuritis

These disease manifestations are often mild and self-limiting; however, pericardial tamponade can occur and caution is warranted especially if pericarditis is present. Only mild temporary increases in corticosteroid therapy may be sufficient to treat these disease manifestations.

Esophageal Dysfunction and Interstitial Lung Disease

The treatment of these disease manifestations which are common in PSS has not been established. It is not clear that corticosteroids will benefit esophageal hypomotility or interstitial lung disease. However, it is possible that the aggressive use of corticosteroids when disease first begins in these regions may prevent progressive changes. Patients with significant esophageal reflux may benefit from the H_2 histamine antagonists (Tagamet and Zantac) and antacids may help prevent esophageal stricture.

Central Nervous System Disease

Aseptic meningitis generally responds to high-dose prednisone therapy. Patients with psychosis and seizures are generally treated with high-dose prednisone although controlled studies have not established the superiority of this treatment compared to more conservative regimens. Azathioprine may be a useful adjunct to the treatment of patients quite ill with disease manifestations such as aseptic meningitis, particularly if these patients also have high fever and myopathy. However, no series of MCTD patients treated with cytotoxic drugs has been published.

References

1. Clark JA, Winkelmann RK, Ward LE: Serologic alterations in scleroderma and sclerodermatomyositis. *Mayo Clin Proc* 46:104-107, 1971.

2. Dubois EL, Chandor S, Friou GJ, Bischel M: Progressive systemic sclerosis (PSS) and localized scleroderma (morphea) with positive LE cell test and unusual systemic manifestations compatible with systemic lupus erythematosus (SLE). *Medicine* 50:199-222, 1971.

3. Sharp GC, Irvin WS, Tan EM, Gould RG, Holman HR: Mixed connective tissue disease: An apparently distinct rheumatic disease syndrome associated with a specific antibody to an extractable nuclear antigen (ENA). *Medicine* 52:148-159, 1972.

4. Sharp GC, Irvin WS, May CM, Holman HR, McDuffie FC, Hess EV, Schmid FR: Association of antibodies to ribonucleoprotein and SM antigens with mixed connective-tissue disease, systemic lupus erythematosus, and other rheumatic diseases. *N Engl J Med* 295:1149-1154, 1976.

5. Leisbarth JH, Persellin RH: Characteristics of patients with serum antibodies to extractable nuclear antigens. *Arthritis and Rheum* 19:851-856, 1976.

6. Bresnihan B, Bunn C, Snaith ML, Hughes GRV: Antiribonucleoprotein antibodies in connective diseases: Estimation by counterimmunoelectrophoresis. *Br Med J* 1:610-611, 1977.

7. Bennett RM, O'Connell DJ: Mixed connective disease: A clinicopathologic study of 20 cases. *Sem Arthritis Rheum* 10:25-51, 1980.

8. Hamburger M, Hodes S, Barland P: The incidence and clinical significance of antibodies to extractable nuclear antigens. *Amer J Med Sci* 273:21-28 1978.

9. Parker MD: Ribonucleoprotein antibodies: Frequencies and clinical significance in systemic lupus erythematosus, scleroderma, and mixed connective tissue disease. *J Lab Clin Med* 82:769-775, 1973.

10. Nimelstein SH, Brody S, McShane D, Holman HR: Mixed connective tissue disease: A subsequent evaluation of the original 25 patients. *Medicine* 59: 239-248, 1980.

11. Sharp GC: Anti-RNP and anti-SM antibodies. *Arthritis Rheum* 25:757-760, 1982.

12. Alarcon-Segovia D, Ruiz-Arguelles A: Suppressor cell loss and dysfunction in mixed connective tissue disease. *Arthritis Rheum* 23:314-318, 1980.

13. Halla JT, Volanakis JE, Schrohenloher RA: Circulating immune complexes in mixed connective tissue disease. *Arthritis Rheum* 22:484-489, 1979.

14. Cunningham PH, Andrews BS, Davis JS: Immunocomplexes in progressive systemic sclerosis and mixed connective tissue disease. *J Rheumatol* 7: 301-308, 1980.

15. Parker MD, Turner RA: Comparison of the complement-fixing activity of antinuclear antibodies in lupus nephritis, mixed connective tissue disease, and scleroderma. *Arthritis Rheum* 19:857-860, 1976.

16. Hamburger MI, Moutsopoulos HM, Lawley TJ, Sharp GC, Frank MM: Reticuloendothelial system Fc receptor function in mixed connective tissue disease. *Arthritis Rheum* 22:618-619, 1979.

17. Schocket AL, Kohler PS: Lymphocytotoxic antibodies in systemic lupus erythematosus and clinically related diseases. *Arthritis Rheum* 22:1060-1063, 1979.

18. Iwatsuki K, Tagami H, Imaizumis Ginoza M, Yamade M: The speckled epidermal nuclear immunofluorescence of mixed connective tissue disease seems to develop as an in vitro phenomenon. *Br J Dermatol* 108:653-657, 1982.

19. Gilliam JN, Prystowksy SD: Mixed connective tissue disease syndrome: Cutaneous manifestations of patients with epidermal nuclear standing in high-titer serum antibody to ribonuclease-sensitive extractable nuclear antigen. *Arch Dermatol* 113:583-587, 1977.

20. Bentley-Phillips CB, Geake TMS: Mixed connective tissue disease characterized by speckled epidermal nuclear IgG deposition of normal skin. *Br J Dermatol* 102:529-533, 1980.

21. Levitin PM, Weary PE, Giuliano VJ: The immunofluorescent "band" test in mixed connective tissue disease. *Ann Int Med* 83:53-55, 1975.

22. Singsen BH, Swanson VL, Bernstein BH, Heuser ET, Hanson V, Landing BH: A histologic evaluation of mixed connective tissue disease in childhood. *Medicine* 68:710-717, 1980.

23. Munves ES, Schur PH: Antibodies to SM and RNP: Prognosticators of disease involvement. *Arthritis Rheum* 26:848-853, 1983.

24. Lemmer JP, Curry NA, Mallory JH, Waller MV: Clinical characteristics and course in patients with high titer anti-RNP antibodies. *J Rheumatol* 9:536-542, 1982.

25. Reichlin M: Problems in differentiating SLE and mixed connective tissue disease. *N Engl J Med* 295:1194-1195, 1976.

26. Reichlin M: Mixed connective tissue disease. In GRV Hughes (ed.), *Modern Topics in Rheumatology.* London, W.H. Heineman, 1976, pp. 157-162.

27. Wiener-Kronish JP, Solinger AM, Warnock ML, Schurg A: Severe pulmonary involvement in mixed connective tissue disease. *Am Rev Respir Dis* 124: 499-503, 1981.

28. Maricq HF, LeRoy EC, D'Angelo WA, Medsger TA Jr, Rodnan GP, Sharp GC, Wolfe JF: Diagnostic potential of in vivo capillary microscopy in scleroderma and related disorders. *Arthritis Rheum* 23:183-189, 1980.

29. Ramos-Ninebro F, Alarcon-Segovia D, Hernandez-Ortiz J: Articular manifestations of mixed connective tissue disease. *Arthritis Rheum* 22:43-51, 1979.

30. Oxenhandler R, Corman HL, Sharp G, Adelstein E: Pathology of skeletal muscle in mixed connective tissue disease. *Arthritis Rheum* 22:43-51, 988, 1977.

31. Gutierrez S, Zalenzuela JE, Ehresmann GR, Quismorio FP: Esophageal dysfunction in patients with mixed connective tissue disease and systemic lupus erythematosus. *Dig Dis Sci* 27:592-597, 1982.

32. Oetgen WH, Mutter ML, Lawless OJ, Davis JE: Cardiac abnormalities in mixed connective tissue disease. *Chest* 83:185-188, 1983.

33. Bennett RM, Spargo BH: Neuropsychiatric problems in mixed connective tissue disease. *Medicine* 65:955-962, 1978.

34. Kausman RL, Kitridou RC: Pregnancy in mixed connective tissue disease: Comparison with systemic lupus erythematosus. *J Rheumatol* 9:549-555, 1982.

35. Burnstein RS: Ibuprofen-related meningitis in mixed connective tissue disease. *Ann Intern Med* 92(2PT.1):206-207, 1980.

Chapter 18

VASCULITIS

Elliott L. Semble, M.D.

Vasculitis is a clinicopathologic process characterized by inflammation and necrosis of blood vessels. Small, medium, and large vessels may be involved at various locations in the body. Vascular damage results in a wide spectrum of clinical manifestations.

Kussmaul and Maier (1) reported the first description of necrotizing vasculitis in 1866 and labelled it periarteritis nodosa. Their patient had inflammation of small and medium-sized arteries with nodular lesions occurring along the course of the arteries. During the next century the diagnostic label periarteritis nodosa or polyarteritis nodosa was used to categorize most patients with findings of vasculitis. In 1952, Zeek (2) formulated a system for the classification of vasculitis. This represented the first attempt to differentiate various types of vasculitis on the basis of clinicopathologic findings.

Several classifications of the vasculitic syndromes have been proposed since the initial system of Zeek. However, since some patients fail to fit into a disease category or have features that overlap several groups, none of these classifications has been totally accepted (3).

Vasculitis may be classified into categories according to clinicopathologic findings (Table 18.1). This chapter will review the major subgroups of the vasculitic disorders.

Polyarteritis Nodosa

Polyarteritis nodosa is a necrotizing vasculitis of small and medium-size muscular arteries. A broad range of organ system involvement may be seen in this clinically and pathologically heterogeneous disorder, resulting in a multiplicity of clinical findings.

TABLE 18.1 Classification of Vasculitis

Polyarteritis nodosa
Allergic granulomatosis and angiitis (Churg-Strauss vasculitis)
Wegener's granulomatosis
Hypersensitivity vasculitis
Vasculitis associated with the rheumatic diseases
Giant cell arteritis
Takayasu's arteritis
Behcet's disease
Thromboangiitis obliterans (Buerger's disease)

Epidemiology

Polyarteritis nodosa occurs infrequently. One study found an annual incidence of 0.3/100,000 persons per year and prevalence of 0.7/100,000 population (4). Polyarteritis nodosa is seen more often in males, with a sex ratio of about 2 to 1. Individuals of all ages are affected, but it is more frequent in the middle-aged population.

Pathogenesis

Polyarteritis nodosa may be an immune complex-mediated disease possibly related to hepatitis B infection. Hepatitis B surface antigen (HB_SAg) may be detected in approximately 30% of patients with polyarteritis nodosa (5,6). Immunoglobulin, complement, and HB_SAg may be found in the walls of involved vessels in patients with polyarteritis nodosa (7). Circulating immune complexes consisting of HB_SAg and antibody directed against this determinant have been demonstrated in patients with polyarteritis nodosa and support the role of immune complexes in the pathogenesis of this disease.

Immune complex mechanisms may also be important in patients with polyarteritis nodosa without hepatitis B antigenemia. Rheumatoid factor, decreased serum complement, cryoglobulins, and immune complexes have been detected in the serum of some of these patients (6).

Pathology

Small and medium-sized arteries are usually involved. The vascular lesions are generally located at the bifurcation points of vessels. There is frequent involvement of the kidneys, heart, and abdominal organs, with sparing of the pulmonary arterial circulation.

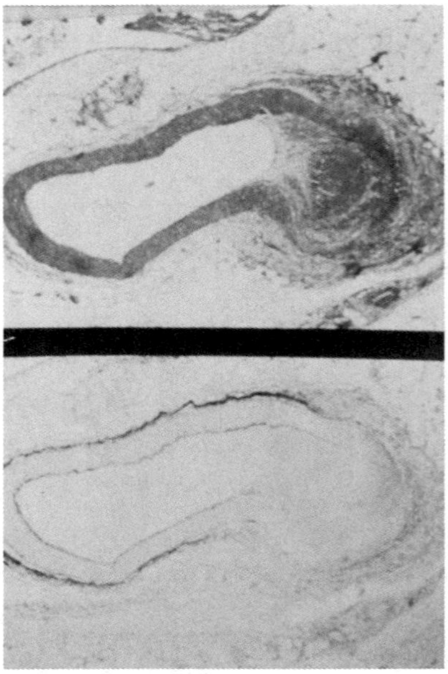

FIGURE 18.1 Polyarteritis nodosa. Most of the arterial wall is normal with well-preserved internal and external elastic laminae. At one pole, however, the lumen is partially obliterated by a thrombus and all portions of the arterial wall are necrotic; elastic laminae have been destroyed in this area. This artery was obtained from a section of infarcted bowel (H&E, left; elastic tissue stain, right; low power). (Reprinted from the Revised Clinical Slide Collection on the Rheumatic Diseases, copyright 1981. Used by permission of the Arthritis Foundation.)

Inflammation in polyarteritis nodosa is characterized by fibrinoid necrosis, and infiltration with polymorphonuclear and mononuclear leukocytes. The elastic laminae are often destroyed, and thrombosis or aneurysmal dilatation may occur at the site of the lesion (Figure 18.1). Lesions at all stages of disease evolution may be found. Healed areas of vasculitis may demonstrate endothelial cell proliferation and fibrosis, occasionally resulting in vascular occlusion.

Clinical Findings

The presenting signs and symptoms of polyarteritis nodosa are variable and almost any organ may be affected. The majority of patients have fever, malaise, and weight loss along with multisystem involvement.

Cutaneous manifestations include maculopapular or purpuric rashes, subcutaneous nodules, or livedo reticularis, a blue-purple net-like mottling of the skin. The majority of patients with polyarteritis nodosa have arthralgias or arthritis. The arthritis is transient and resolves without residual joint damage. Synovial fluid analysis usually reveals evidence of mild inflammation (3).

Peripheral neuropathy occurs in approximately one-half of patients with polyarteritis nodosa. Mononeuritis multiplex, the simultaneous involvement of several peripheral sensory or motor nerves, is the most common pattern of peripheral nerve disease in polyarteritis nodosa. Other patterns include a distal sensory or motor neuropathy.

Central nervous system disease is seen occasionally. Clinical features include cerebrovascular accidents, altered mental status, and seizures.

Kidney involvement occurs in most patients with polyarteritis nodosa. Proteinuria, abnormal urinary sediment, and impaired renal function are frequently seen. Hypertension is a common finding.

Gastrointestinal tract symptoms occur frequently. Nausea, vomiting, abdominal pain, and bloody stools suggest vasculitic involvement of the mesenteric vessels. Liver disease is often seen in autopsy studies, but it rarely presents clinically, except in those cases associated with HB_SAg (3).

The most common cardiac manifestation of polyarteritis nodosa is congestive heart failure (9). It usually results from coronary vasculitis or hypertension. Pericarditis and conduction system disturbances may also be seen.

Pulmonary findings rarely occur in polyarteritis nodosa, but are common in other forms of systemic vasculitis. Other tissues affected by polyarteritis nodosa include the skeletal muscle, eye, and testes.

Laboratory Features

Frequently found laboratory abnormalities in this disease include a polymorphonuclear leukocytosis, normochromic normocytic anemia, and an elevated erythrocyte sedimentation rate. Antinuclear antibodies, low titers of rheumatoid factor, and circulating immune complexes may also be occasionally detected. HB_SAg has been found in 20-30% of patients with polyarteritis nodosa (6). Laboratory tests may be helpful in excluding related diseases, but are not diagnostically specific.

Diagnosis

The diagnosis of polyarteritis nodosa should be suspected in patients with fever, weight loss, malaise, and signs and symptoms of multisystem involvement.

Biopsy evidence of polyarteritis nodosa is necessary to confirm the diagnosis. Clinically involved organs are most likely to reveal vasculitis on pathologic examination. If cutaneous lesions or mononeuritis multiplex is present, a skin or sural nerve biopsy may demonstrate vasculitis. Muscle biopsy may be a useful procedure in detecting vasculitis, but findings are generally present only if clinical involvement is demonstrated (5). Renal biopsies may show vasculitis or, less frequently, a glomerulonephritis.

Abdominal angiography with selective visualization of the celiac, mesenteric, and renal arteries may be a useful procedure for diagnosing polyarteritis nodosa. Saccular or fusiform aneurysms (Figure 18.2) or other vascular irregularities may be demonstrated in approximately 80% of patients (5).

Polyarteritis nodosa may be associated with hepatitis B infection, acute serous otitis media, and intravenous drug abuse. Rheumatoid arthritis and systemic lupus erythematosus may be complicated by a vasculitis, with features identical to that of polyarteritis nodosa. Allergic granulomatosis and angiitis (Churg-Strauss vasculitis) may resemble polyarteritis nodosa, and overlap syndromes consisting of manifestations of both diseases are not uncommon.

Treatment and Prognosis

Corticosteroids have improved the survival rate in patients with polyarteritis nodosa. Initial therapy consists of prednisone in dosages of approximately 60 mg daily. Cytotoxic agents such as cyclophosphamide, azathioprine, or methotrexate may be added in patients whose disease is active and progressive. When the vasculitis is controlled, prednisone is gradually tapered according to the clinical findings and results of the laboratory tests.

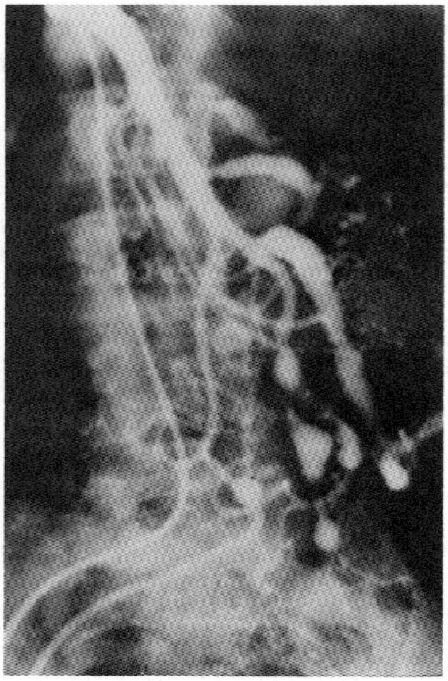

FIGURE 18.2 Polyarteritis nodosa. A selective arteriogram demonstrates multiple small saccular aneurysms in the branches of the superior mesenteric artery. They vary in size and shape. (Reprinted from the Revised Clinical Slide Collection on the Rheumatic Diseases, copyright 1981. Used by permission of the Arthritis Foundation.)

Allergic Granulomatosis and Angiitis (Churg-Strauss Vasculitis)

Allergic granulomatosis and angiitis (Churg-Strauss vasculitis) is a disease characterized by asthma, eosinophilia, vasculitis, and extravascular granulomas.

Epidemiology

Allergic granulomatosis and angiitis is a rare form of vasculitis. Chumbley et al. (10) found only 30 patients with this disease over a 25-year period at the Mayo Clinic. The male-to-female ratio is about 20 to 1 and the age of onset is approximately 50 years.

Pathogenesis

The etiology of allergic granulomatosis and angiitis is unknown. Elevated serum IgE levels have been noted in several patients and may represent a response to an extrinsic antigen.

Pathology

Pathologic findings in allergic granulomatosis and angiitis include necrotizing granulomas as well as necrotizing vasculitis involving small arteries and occasionally veins (11). The granulomas are composed of a core of necrotic cells surrounded radially by macrophages, eosinophils, and multinucleated giant cells.

Arterial lesions in all stages of evolution may be seen. In the acute phase, there is fibrinoid necrosis with infiltration of leukocytes, predominately eosinophils, in the vessel walls and perivascular areas. Healed lesions are characterized by intimal proliferation and fibrosis, resulting in narrowing the lumen.

The lungs, heart, kidneys, skin, and peripheral nerves may also reveal typical lesions consisting of granulomas or vasculitis.

Clinical Findings

The presenting features of allergic granulomatosis and angiitis include fever, weight loss, and pulmonary signs and symptoms. Patients often have a history of asthma, allergic rhinitis, or other atopic diseases. Chest roentgenograms are abnormal in approximately 50% of patients (10) and usually show transient, patchy infiltrates. Noncavitating nodular infiltrates and diffuse interstitial fibrosis are less often seen.

Cutaneous lesions occur in about two-thirds of cases. Purpura and subcutaneous nodules are the two most common manifestations. Peripheral neuropathy, usually mononeuritis multiplex, is seen in a majority of patients. Cardiac, renal, gastrointestinal, and joint involvement also occurs occasionally.

Laboratory Features

Peripheral blood eosinophilia, with absolute counts greater than $1000/mm^3$, is seen in approximately 85% of cases (5,10). An elevated erythrocyte sedimentation rate and anemia are found in the majority of patients. Increased serum IgE levels have also been reported (10).

Diagnosis

Allergic granulomatosis and angiitis should be suspected in middle-aged patients having a recent history of asthma who develop a multisystem disease. The diagnosis is confirmed by a biopsy of involved tissues (e.g., lung) demonstrating eosinophilic, necrotizing, extravascular granulomas and necrotizing vasculitis.

The differential diagnosis of allergic granulomatosis and angiitis includes polyarteritis nodosa, Wegener's granulomatosis, and eosinophilic pneumonia. The findings of pulmonary infiltration, asthma, eosinophilia, and granulomas on biopsy are distinguishing features of allergic granulomatosis and angiitis, but are rarely seen in polyarteritis nodosa. Wegener's granulomatosis may be differentiated from allergic granulomatosis and angiitis by the presence of upper respiratory tract disease and the absence of asthma and eosinophilia. Eosinophilic pneumonia is characterized by pulmonary infiltrates, asthma, and eosinophilia; however, it is usually a more benign and self-limited disorder than allergic granulomatosis and angiitis, and rarely is associated with vasculitis (12).

Treatment and Prognosis

Chumbley et al. (10) have reported a 90% 1-year survival rate and a 62% 5-year survival rate in this disease with corticosteroid therapy. The most common cause of death in their series of patients was from myocardial infarction, followed by congestive heart failure.

Prednisone in dosages between 40 and 60 mg daily is the treatment of choice in allergic granulomatosis and angiitis. Cytotoxic agents may be used if disease suppression is not achieved with corticosteroids, although little information about their beneficial effects is available.

Wegener's Granulomatosis

Wegener's granulomatosis is characterized by necrotizing granulomatous lesions involving the upper and lower respiratory tracts, small vessel vasculitis, and glomerulonephritis. A more limited form of this disorder has been described by Carrington and Liebow who found 16 patients with pulmonary involvement without renal disease (13).

Epidemiology

Wegener's granulomatosis is an uncommon disease. The male-to-female ratio is 2 to 1. The mean age of onset is approximately 40 years.

Pathogenesis

Although the etiology of Wegener's granulomatosis is unknown, immune mechanisms may be important in its pathogenesis. Evidence for hyperreactivity of the immune system consists of increased levels of serum IgA and IgG, and the presence of rheumatoid factor in serum of certain patients with this disorder (14). Circulating immune complexes have been reported in some patients with Wegener's granulomatosis, but their pathogenetic role is uncertain since serum complement levels are generally not diminished.

Pathology

Histopathologic findings of Wegener's granulomatosis include necrotizing granulomas of the upper and lower respiratory tract, necrotizing vasculitis involving both small arteries and veins, and glomerulonephritis (15). The involved vessels show fibrinoid necrosis with mononuclear cell infiltration. Healed vascular lesions with fibrosis may also be seen. Granulomas typically contain a central zone of necrosis, and a peripheral zone of granulation tissue with histiocytes, fibroblasts, and occasional multinucleated giant cells. The granulomas may be within, adjacent to, or separate from the vascular lesions (14).

A variety of renal lesions may be found. The most common is focal and segmental glomerulonephritis. Other patterns include diffuse proliferative glomerulonephritis and interstitial nephritis. Occasionally, a necrotizing vasculitis of small renal arteries may be seen.

The sinuses, ocular tissues, skin, central nervous system, peripheral nerves, and heart may also show histopathologic findings of granulomas or vasculitis.

Clinical Features

The most common presenting complaints in Wegener's granulomatosis involve the upper respiratory tract. Symptoms of sinusitis, rhinitis, and nasal obstruction occur frequently and are often accompanied by fever, weight loss, and anorexia.

Clinical findings related to the lower respiratory tract are seen in a minority of patients and include cough, hemoptysis, dyspnea, and pleuritic chest pain. Although pulmonary symptoms are uncommon, chest roentgenograms are frequently abnormal. Lung involvement may be detected in almost all patients at some time during the course of this disease.

The kidneys are affected in most patients. Renal manifestations include proteinuria, hematuria, red blood cell casts, and renal insufficiency. Hypertension is a rare finding even in patients with extensive renal disease.

Polyarthralgias often occur, but synovitis is less frequent. Cutaneous lesions are found in approximately one-half of patients. The most common dermatologic manifestations include ulcerative and nodular skin lesions (14,16).

Eye involvement occurs frequently and may be a consequence of the direct extension of a purulent sinusitis or result from vasculitis. Ocular findings include proptosis, conjunctivitis, scleritis, episcleritis, retinal artery occlusion, optic neuritis, and dacrocystitis (14).

The central nervous system, peripheral nerves, ears, and heart may also be involved in Wegener's granulomatosis.

Laboratory Tests

The erythrocyte sedimentation rate is usually elevated (often exceeding 100 mm/hr). The majority of patients have a polymorphonuclear leukocytosis without eosinophilia and anemia of chronic disease.

Serum levels of IgA and IgG may be elevated, while IgM is usually normal or slightly diminished. Rheumatoid factor is present in the serum of most patients. Antinuclear antibodies and cryoglobulins are rarely found. Circulating immune complexes have been reported in some patients with Wegener's granulomatosis (17), but serum complement levels are usually normal or elevated.

The findings on chest radiographs in patients with Wegener's granulomatosis include pulmonary infiltrates or nodules. These lesions may be single or multiple, bilateral, and may be found in any lobe of the lung. They may cavitate as seen in Figure 18.3.

Sinus radiographs are abnormal in a majority of patients, and findings include mucosal thickening or pansinusitis with multiple air-fluid levels (14).

Diagnosis

The diagnosis of Wegener's granulomatosis is suggested by the clinical findings of a multisystem disease with upper respiratory tract symptoms, and confirmed by biopsy evidence of necrotizing granulomas with vasculitis (3). If nasopharyngeal or sinus involvement is present, a biopsy from an active lesion may show the typical histopathology. However, chronic inflammation with or without granulomas is often noted, and a lung or renal biopsy may be necessary to establish the definitive diagnosis.

Diseases such as midline granuloma, lymphomatoid granulomatosis, and allergic granulomatosis and angiitis may be confused with Wegener's granulomatosis. Midline granuloma is a locally destructive process involving the upper respiratory tract, but usually spares the lungs and kidneys (18). It is histologically similar to Wegener's granulomatosis, but differs in that vasculitis is usually absent. Midline granuloma generally does not respond to cytotoxic therapy, but is radiosensitive (18).

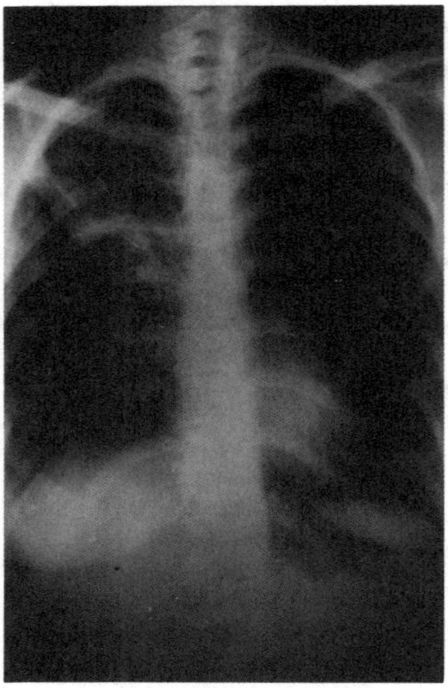

FIGURE 18.3 Wegener's granulomatosis. This posteroanterior projection of the chest from a patient with Wegener's granulomatosis reveals bilateral pulmonary infiltrates, more marked on the right. In the left midlung field there is a solitary cavitating nodule (arrow). (Reprinted from the Revised Clinical Slide Collection on the Rheumatic Diseases, copyright 1981. Used by permission of the Arthritis Foundation.)

Lymphomatoid granulomatosis and Wegener's granulomatosis may be differentiated by histopathologic and clinical findings (19). Upper respiratory tract and sinus involvement suggests the diagnosis of Wegener's granulomatosis. The presence of inflammatory vascular lesions characterized by a pleomorphic mononuclear cell infiltrate containing frequent mitotic figures, supports the diagnosis of lymphomatoid granulomatosis rather than Wegener's granulomatosis (19).

Allergic granulomatosis and angiitis may be differentiated from Wegener's granulomatosis by the findings of an allergic history, peripheral blood eosinophilia, and tissue infiltration with eosinophils.

Treatment and Prognosis

A significant reduction in the mortality rate of Wegener's granulomatosis has been achieved using cytotoxic agents, especially cyclophosphamide (20). Cyclophosphamide is generally given orally in a dose of 1–2 mg/kg/day. The dose is adjusted depending on the clinical response, renal function, and white cell count. Treatment is generally continued until the patient is free of symptoms for one year. Patients treated with cyclophosphamide should be under constant surveillance, inasmuch as severe side-effects may result from the use of this medication. The most serious complications include hemorrhagic cystitis, bladder carcinoma, bone marrow depression, infection, and malignancy.

Hypersensitivity Angiitis

Hypersensitivity angiitis consists of a heterogenous group of clinical syndromes in which the small blood vessels of the skin are predominately involved. Subgroups with distinctive clinicopathologic findings have been recognized in hypersensitivity angiitis, and include Henoch-Schönlein purpura, hypocomplementemic vasculitis, and mixed cryoglobulinemia. They will be discussed in a separate section.

Epidemiology

The incidence and prevalence of hypersensitivity angiitis are unknown. However, it appears to be more common than polyarteritis nodosa (21).

Pathogenesis

Hypersensitivity angiitis may occur after an infection or the administration of drugs, but usually the specific antigen responsible for initiating the process cannot be identified.

Immune complexes may play a role in the pathogenesis of this disorder. Immunoglobulins and complement have been demonstrated in the vasculitic skin lesions in many of these patients, as well as in the vessel walls in biopsies or normal skin in patients with active cutaneous vasculitis (22).

Pathology

Hypersensitivity angiitis affects the small blood vessels of the skin and viscera. The vasculitic process is most pronounced in the postcapillary venules, the smallest and most superficial vessels of the skin (23).

The characteristic lesion has been labeled leukocytoclastic vasculitis and consists of infiltration of the vessel wall with polymorphonuclear leukocytes, leukocytoclasis (presence of nuclear debris), fibrinoid necrosis, and extravasation of erythrocytes (21). The damaged vessels in hypersensitivity vasculitis are generally at the same stage of evolution at any given time. This contrasts with polyarteritis nodosa in which the vasculitic lesions are usually in all stages of evolution at any given time.

Clinical Features

The typical skin lesions of hypersensitivity angiitis are erythematous papules or palpable purpura. This rash usually involves dependent areas, especially the distal lower extremities. The lesions occur in crops lasting approximately 1-4 weeks. Palpable purpura is often associated with pruritus, pain, or a burning sensation, although about one-third of patients may be asymptomatic.

Other dermatologic manifestations of hypersensitivity angiitis include chronic or recurrent urticaria, nonspecific erythematous macular or papular rashes, annular lesions, bullae, plaques, or vesicles. Dependent edema may also be associated with the presence of skin lesions in this disorder.

Arthritis and arthralgias are seen in approximately 40% of patients (21). The most frequently involved joints are the knees, ankles, wrists, and elbows.

Visceral organ involvement may occur in hypersensitivity angiitis. Vasculitis of the kidney is seen frequently and is characterized by hematuria and proteinuria. The gastrointestinal tract is involved occasionally. Clinical findings suggesting bowel disease include abdominal pain and gastrointestinal bleeding. Pulmonary infiltrates on chest radiographs and peripheral neuropathy may also be seen in this disease.

Laboratory Features

A normochromic normocytic anemia, mild peripheral leukocytosis, and an elevated erythrocyte sedimentation rate are the most common laboratory abnormalities. Cryoglobulins and rheumatoid factor may occasionally be present.

Diagnosis

The diagnosis of hypersensitivity angiitis may be suspected clinically by the presence of typical palpable purpuric skin lesions and confirmed by finding small vessel involvement on skin biopsy. Biopsies of involved organs such as the kidneys may also demonstrate small vessel vasculitis.

Hypersensitivity angiitis may be associated with underlying systemic diseases including polyarteritis nodosa, allergic granulomatosis and angiitis, systemic lupus erythematosus, Sjögren's syndrome, and rheumatoid arthritis. It is often difficult to differentiate systemic vasculitis with cutaneous involvement from hypersensitivity angiitis with associated visceral involvement. The term hypersensitivity angiitis should be restricted to small vessel vasculitis predominately affecting the skin.

Treatment and Prognosis

The treatment of an underlying infection or the discontinuation of a drug may result in the resolution of the small vessel vasculitis. Mild cases may not require therapy, but if skin disease is extensive, or if visceral involvement is present, corticosteroid therapy may be necessary. If disease activity is uncontrolled despite corticosteroid therapy, cytotoxic agents or penicillamine may be tried. However the efficacy of these agents has not been clearly demonstrated.

The prognosis in hypersensitivity angiitis is generally good. However, in certain subgroups of this disease significant morbidity and even mortality may occur.

Subgroups of Hypersensitivity Angiitis

Henoch-Schönlein purpura, hypocomplementemic vasculitis, and mixed cryoglobulinemia are distinctive clinical syndromes within the hypersensitivity angiitis group. In this section, clinicopathologic features of these subgroups will be discussed.

Henoch-Schönlein Purpura

Henoch-Schönlein purpura occurs primarily in children, ages 4 to 7, but persons of any age may be affected. Skin biopsies demonstrate histopathologic findings of leukocytoclastic vasculitis. Immunofluorescence studies have shown immunoglobulins, predominately IgA, and complement deposits in skin and kidney lesions (24).

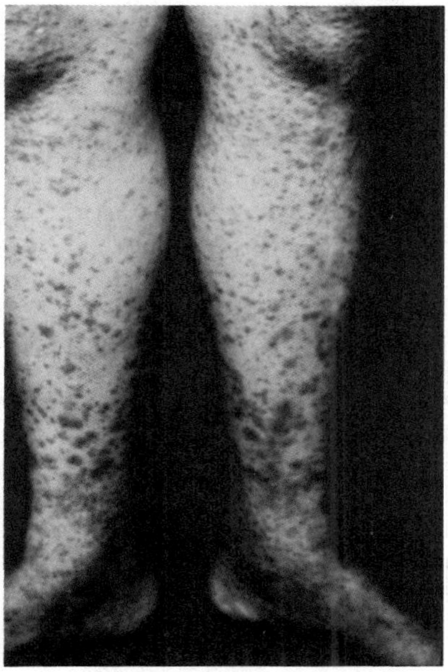

FIGURE 18.4 Henoch-Schönlein purpura. The legs are covered by slightly raised, palpable, purpuric lesions in this patient with Henoch-Schönlein purpura. (Reprinted from the Revised Clinical Slide Collection on the Rheumatic Diseases, copyright 1981. Used by permission of the Arthritis Foundation.)

The disease is frequently preceded by an upper respiratory tract infection. Clinical findings include palpable purpura (Figure 18.4), a transient monoarticular or polyarticular arthritis usually affecting the knees or ankles, abdominal symptoms, and renal involvement.

Henoch-Schönlein purpura is generally self-limited, requiring only supportive care. A small minority of patients with persistent and recurrent disease may develop progressive renal failure. Corticosteroids may be effective in controlling gastrointestinal and joint manifestations, but may not be beneficial in renal disease.

Hypocomplementemic Vasculitis

Clinical manifestations of hypocomplementemic vasculitis include recurrent episodes of urticaria, arthritis, abdominal pain, and renal involvement. Skin biopsies of urticarial lesions usually demonstrate leukocytoclastic vasculitis. Kidney biopsies in patients with renal involvement may show mild glomerulonephritis, with immunoglobulin and complement deposition on glomerular basement membranes.

Diminished levels of serum complement are characteristic of this syndrome. The absence of antinuclear antibodies help differentiate hypocomplementemic vasculitis from systemic lupus erythematosus.

Hypocomplementemic vasculitis appears to be a chronic disease, but severe impairment of renal function has not been described. Patients usually benefit from corticosteroid therapy.

Mixed Cryoglobulinemia

The syndrome of mixed cryoglobulinemia is uncommon. It is characterized by the clinical findings of palpable purpura, arthralgias, and weakness, and by laboratory evidence of a serum cryoglobulin with a mixed pattern. Diffuse glomerulonephritis occurs frequently and may result in renal failure.

Biopsy specimens from skin lesions demonstrate leukocytoclastic vasculitis. Immunofluorescence studies have shown immunoglobulins and complement in the renal and skin biopsies of vasculitic lesions. Serum complement levels may also be decreased. The mixed cryoglobulins contain IgG and IgM, with the IgM component having anti-IgG (rheumatoid factor) activity.

Mixed cryoglobulinemia may have an infectious etiology. Hepatitis B antigen (25), or coccidioidin antigen (26), has been demonstrated in the cryoprecipitates of some patients with this disease.

The clinicopathologic findings may be similar to Henoch-Schönlein purpura, however, the presence of cryoglobulins, positive rheumatoid factor, and decreased levels of complement in the serum of patients with mixed cryoglobulinemia help differentiate these two diseases. The manifestations of mixed cryoglobulinemia may resemble those of systemic lupus erythematosus, but the absence of antibodies to double-stranded DNA and the lack of immunoglobulin deposition at the dermoepidermal junction may help in establishing the diagnosis.

The long-term prognosis of mixed cryoglobulinemia is generally good (21). However, corticosteroids or even cytotoxic therapy may be required in patients with progressive renal failure.

Vasculitis Associated with the Rheumatic Diseases

Vasculitis may occur in rheumatoid arthritis and systemic lupus erythematosus. Vessels of any size may be involved from venules to medium-sized muscular arteries.

The clinicopathologic features of rheumatoid vasculitis reflect involvement of vessels of different sizes (27). Patients having high titers of rheumatoid factor, subcutaneous nodules, and joint erosions are more likely to develop vasculitis.

The clinical features of small artery (e.g., digital artery, vaso nervorum) involvement include peripheral neuropathy, digital gangrene, nailfold infarction, cutaneous ulceration, and bowel infarction (27). Medium-sized artery involvement resembling polyarteritis nodosa may also occur with clinical findings similar to those associated with vasculitis of the small arteries. Rheumatoid vasculitis may affect venules, especially those of the skin. Clinically, venulitis is recognized as palpable purpura involving the lower extremities.

Severe rheumatoid vasculitis should be treated with corticosteroids initially and, if necessary, cytotoxic agents. Penicillamine has also been beneficial in some patients.

Vasculitis is occasionally seen in systemic lupus erythematosus. It may involve the venules or small arteries. Clinical findings include palpable purpura, livedo reticularis, or peripheral gangrene. Lupus vasculitis is more likely to develop in patients with antibodies to double-stranded DNA (28) or the Sm antigen (29).

Corticosteroids are usually required for the treatment of vasculitis associated with systemic lupus erythematosus. Cytotoxic agents may be used in patients unresponsive to corticosteroids.

Giant Cell Arteritis

Giant cell arteritis is an inflammatory necrotizing vasculitis involving medium or large-sized arteries. It usually affects branches of the carotid artery, although involvement may be more widespread.

Epidemiology

Giant cell arteritis is a relatively common disease. The overall incidence of this disease is 2.9/100,000 population/year (30). The incidence rate increases with age, rising from 1.7 in 50-59-year-old patients, to 55.5 for patients over 80 years of age (30). The overall prevalence is 24 cases/100,000 population, but it is 133/100,000 population aged 50 years and older. The prevalence also increases with age and is 843/100,000 population aged 80 years and over (30).

Giant cell arteritis is seen almost exclusively in patients over 50 years of age, although the disease has been reported in young adults. Women are affected more often than men.

Pathogenesis

The etiology of giant cell arteritis is unknown. Familial aggregation of giant cell arteritis (31) and a predilection of this disease for Caucasians (32) suggest a genetic or hereditary predisposition.

The prevalence of HLA-DR3 and DR4 antigens appears to be increased in giant cell arteritis (33). These antigens are also found more frequently in certain autoimmune disorders (HLA-DR3 with systemic lupus erythematosus, HLA-DR4 with rheumatoid arthritis) implicating a role for the immune system in the pathogenesis of giant cell arteritis.

The histopathologic findings in giant cell arteritis suggest that altered cellular immunity may be responsible for the vascular lesions seen in this disease. Although enhancement of cellular immunity has been described in giant cell arteritis, extensive testing has not demonstrated any consistent abnormality (34).

Immune complexes may be important in the pathogenesis of giant cell arteritis. Immunoglobulin and complement deposition have been demonstrated in temporal artery biopsies of patients with active disease (35), and increased levels of immune complexes have been detected in the serum of patients with active giant cell arteritis (36). These observations support a role for immune complexes in this disease; however, additional studies are necessary to further define these complexes.

Pathology

Giant cell arteritis usually involves vessels that originate from the arch of the aorta, but may affect any medium or large-size artery. The superficial temporal, vertebral, ophthalmic, and posterior ciliary arteries are often involved, while the internal carotid, external carotid, and central retinal arteries are less frequently affected. The intracerebral arteries are usually spared.

The histopathologic findings in giant cell arteritis reflect the stage of the inflammatory reaction. The early phase of the disease is characterized by the presence of inflammatory cells at the junction of the media and intima. Intimal thickening often occurs resulting in narrowing of the lumen. Necrosis of portions of the arterial wall (including the elastic laminae) and granulomas containing multinucleated giant cells, epithelioid cells, histocytes, lymphocytes, plasma cells,

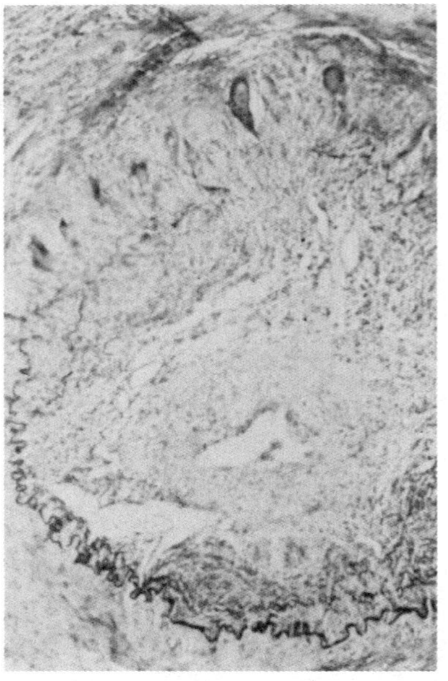

FIGURE 18.5 Giant cell arteritis. In one-half of the field the internal elastic lamina and media of the temporal artery are intact. In the other half both have been destroyed and replaced by a granulomatous reaction including giant cells and epithelioid cells. The exudate extends into the intima where there is extensive necrosis (H&E, elastic tissue stain, low power). (Reprinted from the Revised Clinical Slide Collection on the Rheumatic Diseases, copyright 1981. Used by permission of the Arthritis Foundation.)

and fibroblasts may be found (37) (Figure 18.5). Fibrosis and recanalization of the lumen represent late changes of the disease.

Inflammatory changes in giant cell arteritis affect the vascular walls in a segmental or patchy fashion. Multiple sections along the length of a biopsied vessel may need to be examined before typical pathologic changes are demonstrated (38).

Clinical Findings

The onset of disease may be sudden or insidious over weeks or months. Constitutional symptoms are often present and include fever, weight loss, anorexia, malaise, and depression.

Headache is a common initial symptom in giant cell arteritis. The pain is often severe and frequently involves the areas along the arteries of the scalp. However, the location and type of pain may be more diffuse. Scalp tenderness is a frequent finding and is usually localized to the temporal or occipital arteries (Figure 18.6).

Visual manifestations are common and include ptosis, diplopia, and loss of vision. Visual impairment generally results from ischemia of the optic nerves or tracts secondary to vasculitis of the ophthalmic or posterior ciliary arteries and less often from involvement of the central retinal artery (39). Once established, blindness is usually permanent.

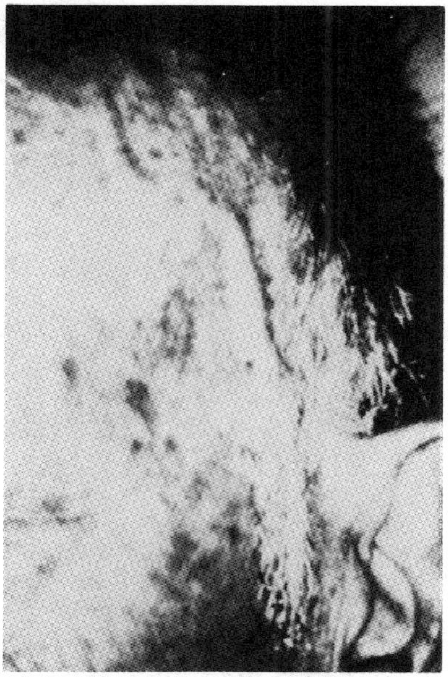

FIGURE 18.6 Giant cell arteritis. A dilated artery can be seen in this patient with giant cell arteritis. It is tender and indurated. (Reprinted from the Revised Clinical Slide Collection on the Rheumatic Diseases. Copyright 1981. Used by permission of the Arthritis Foundation.)

Claudication is occasionally seen and generally affects the jaw, extremities, or tongue. Clinical evidence of large artery involvement occurs in 10-15% of patients (40). Vascular manifestations include upper extremity claudication, bruits over the carotid, subclavian, axillary, and brachial arteries, and/or absent or decreased pulses in the neck or arms (36).

Polymyalgia Rheumatica

Polymyalgia rheumatica is a clinical syndrome occurring in approximately one-half of patients with giant cell arteritis. It is characterized by pain and stiffness involving the neck, shoulder, hip girdles, and the proximal limbs. Morning stiffness and "gelling" after inactivity are common findings. Transient synovitis may occur (42). Constitutional symptoms such as fever, weight loss, and malaise are often seen.

There are no generally accepted diagnostic criteria for polymyalgia rheumatica. However, many studies use the Mason Clinic criteria (32) as a guide in diagnosis (Table 18.2).

Laboratory Features

Giant cell arteritis is characterized by an elevated erythrocyte sedimentation rate with values often over 100 mm/hr. However, cases with normal levels have been reported (43).

TABLE 18.2 Diagnostic Criteria for Polymyalgia Rheumatica

Pain in shoulders and pelvic girdle persisting for at least 1 month, associated with marked morning stiffness and gelling, without muscle atrophy or weakness.
Patients usually older than 55 years.
Erythrocyte sedimentation rate (Westegren) over 50 mm/hr, often 100 mm/hr or more.
Relief of symptoms with 4-5 days of 10 mg prednisone daily.

A mild normochromic normocytic anemia is common during periods of disease activity. Plasma protein alterations may occur including a decrease in albumin concentration and elevations of alpha-2-globulins and fibrinogen. Antinuclear antibody and rheumatoid factor tests are usually negative. Abnormal liver function studies are occasionally seen, but liver biopsies are generally normal.

Diagnosis

The diagnosis of giant cell arteritis should be suspected in patients over 50 years old who have transient or sudden loss of vision, or in elderly patients with fever, polymyalgia rheumatica, and an elevated erythrocyte sedimentation rate (43). Patients should be questioned about present and past symptoms, and a thorough examination of the arteries of the head, neck, upper torso, and arms should be performed.

The diagnosis may be confirmed by an arterial biopsy. The temporal artery is often biopsied, but the occipital or facial artery may also be studied. A symptomatic or clinically abnormal portion of the artery should be chosen for biopsy, since giant cell arteritis is often a segmental disease. The diagnostic yield may be increased if a several centimeter segment of a temporal artery is obtained and serial sections of the specimen are made. Contralateral artery biopsy may be considered if the first side is normal (41).

Giant cell arteritis may be differentiated from other forms of vasculitis by its propensity for affecting large arteries and because of differences in histopathology and organ involvement. Takayasu's arteritis, a chronic vasculitis of the aorta and its primary branches, may be distinguished from giant cell arteritis by its predominance in children and young adults, and different distribution of lesions. However, the histopathologic and angiography findings of Takayasu's arteritis and giant cell arteritis may be identical.

Treatment and Prognosis

Corticosteroid therapy should be started as soon as the diagnosis of giant cell arteritis is established. Since blindness may occur without warning, patients suspected of having giant cell arteritis should be treated immediately without waiting for the results of the temporal artery biopsy.

The initial treatment of giant cell arteritis is 60 mg of prednisone daily. The response to corticosteroid therapy is usually rapid, with systemic and vascular symptoms often resolving within several days. The erythrocyte sedimentation rate may be a useful guide in tapering the dosage of prednisone.

Giant cell arteritis is a self-limited disease lasting from several months to several years. Most patients are able to completely discontinue corticosteroids; however, a small number of patients may require low doses of prednisone for several years. Cytotoxic drugs have not been studied in this disease in a controlled manner.

The treatment of polymyalgia rheumatica consists of prednisone in dosages of 10-15 mg/day. A rapid response to therapy is the rule, and improvement in musculoskeletal pain and stiffness usually occurs within a week.

Polymyalgia rheumatica is a self-limited disease, but prolonged therapy with low doses of prednisone may be necessary. Nonsteroidal antiinflammatory drugs may control symptoms in some patients with polymyalgia rheumatica, but are only indicated if vascular findings are absent or in those patients with normal temporal artery biopsies (36).

Takayasu's Arteritis

Takayasu's arteritis is characterized by inflammation of medium and large-sized arteries with frequent involvement of the aorta and its primary branches.

Epidemiology

Takayasu's arteritis is a rare disease, usually affecting females between the ages of 10 and 30 years. Although most of the reports come from Japan, it has been described in countries all over the world.

Pathogenesis

The etiology of Takayasu's arteritis is unknown. An immunologic cause for this disease has been postulated. A majority of patients have elevated serum immunoglobulins and some patients have antiaorta antibodies in their serum (44). However, the importance of these findings is unclear.

Pathology

Takayasu's arteritis may be restricted to the aortic arch or its branches, involve the ascending thoracic aorta or the abdominal aorta, or diffusely involve the aorta and its branches throughout the chest and abdomen (45). Pulmonary artery disease is occasionally seen.

Takayasu's arteritis is characterized by inflammation of all layers of the arterial wall. Granulomas consisting of lymphocytes, plasma cells, and multinucleated giant cells infiltrate the media and adventitia in the early stages of the disease. With progression of arteritis, intimal proliferation, fragmentation of elastic fibers, and necrosis of smooth muscle occur. Late findings include narrowing or occlusion of the arterial lumen due to intimal thickening and fibrosis, thrombosis, and aneurysm formation.

Clinical Findings

Takayasu's arteritis presents with constitutional symptoms such as fatigue, malaise, weakness, weight loss, and fever. Myalgias, arthralgias, and arthritis may also occur.

Nearly all patients may develop findings of vascular disease in Takayasu's arteritis. Vascular involvement is suggested by complaints of claudication of the upper and lower extremities, pain over an artery, or Raynaud's phenomenon. Physical examination may reveal diminished pulses, vascular bruits, tenderness over vessels, and cool upper extremities.

Hypertension is seen in a majority of patients. Blood pressure readings may be difficult to obtain in the upper extremities due to narrowed or occluded vessels. Lower extremity blood pressure may be measured by use of a wide cuff or other noninvasive methods (1).

Other manifestations of Takayasu's arteritis include dyspnea and hemoptysis resulting from pulmonary artery involvement, and angina pectoris reflecting coronary artery narrowing.

Laboratory Features

A mild anemia or peripheral leukocytosis may be present. The erythrocyte sedimentation rate is usually increased. Immunoglobulin levels are often elevated, while tests for rheumatoid factor and antinuclear antibodies are generally negative (46).

Diagnosis

The diagnosis is suggested by clinical manifestations of vascular insufficiency in young women, and confirmed by typical findings on arteriography. Arteriographic features of Takayasu's arteritis include smooth-walled, tapered, vessel narrowing in association with areas of dilatation (47). The subclavian artery, descending aorta, renal artery, and carotid artery are most often involved (Figure 18.7).

Treatment and Prognosis

Corticosteroids are usually effective in suppressing the systemic symptoms of Takayasu's arteritis, and may be helpful in improving the vascular findings. Prednisone in a dosage of 45-60 mg daily may be given initially, and gradually tapered to a maintenance dose of 5-10 mg daily. The use of a maintenance dosage of corticosteroids may prevent progression of the disease and ameliorate survival (48).

The prognosis of Takayasu's arteritis is guarded since death may occur from congestive heart failure or a cerebrovascular accident (49). However, one study showed an 83% 5-year survival rate (50). The course of the disease is usually protracted with intermittent exacerbations and continued activity for many years.

Behcet's Disease

Behcet's disease is a chronic relapsing syndrome characterized by oral ulceration, genital ulceration, and uveitis. Additional features of this disease include arthritis, cutaneous lesions, and meningoencephalitis.

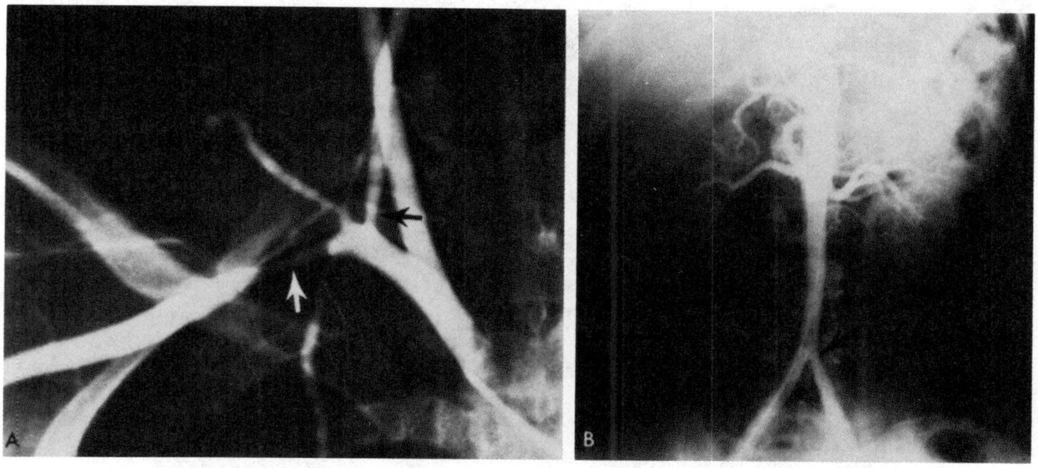

FIGURE 18.7 Takayasu's arteritis. A. Angiogram shows smooth-walled, tapered narrowing of the right subclavian artery (light arrow). Vertebral artery is also narrowed at its origin (dark arrow). B. Abdominal aorta shows smooth-walled tubular narrowing of mid and lower portions and constriction of left common iliac artery at its origin (arrow). (From *Textbook of Rheumatology,* with permission of the authors Gene Hunder and Doyt Conn and W.B. Saunders Co., Philadelphia.)

Epidemiology

Most cases of Behcet's disease have been reported from the eastern Mediterranean countries and Japan. In Japan, the prevalence appears to be 1/10,000 (51) as compared with a point-prevalence in the United States (Olmstead County, Minnesota) of 1/300,000/year (52). There is a male predominance noted in most reported series; however, in North America females are affected more frequently.

Pathogenesis

The etiology of Behcet's disease is unknown, but viral, immune-mediated, and genetic causes have been implicated in its pathogenesis.

A viral etiology is unlikely since the isolation of virus from active lesions in patients with Behcet's disease has been uniformly unsuccessful. Immune complexes may be important in the pathogenesis of this disease. The presence of circulating immune complexes in serum and the deposition of immunoglobulin and complement components in affected tissues (53) support this hypothesis. A genetic predisposition to Behcet's disease may exist as evidenced by the three- to fourfold increase in the histocompatibility marker HLA-B5 in patients with this disease as compared to normal controls (54).

Pathology

The underlying lesion in Behcet's disease appears to be a small vessel vasculitis with a mononuclear cell infiltrate (51). Oral lesions may or may not demonstrate vasculitis, but mononuclear cells are usually present.

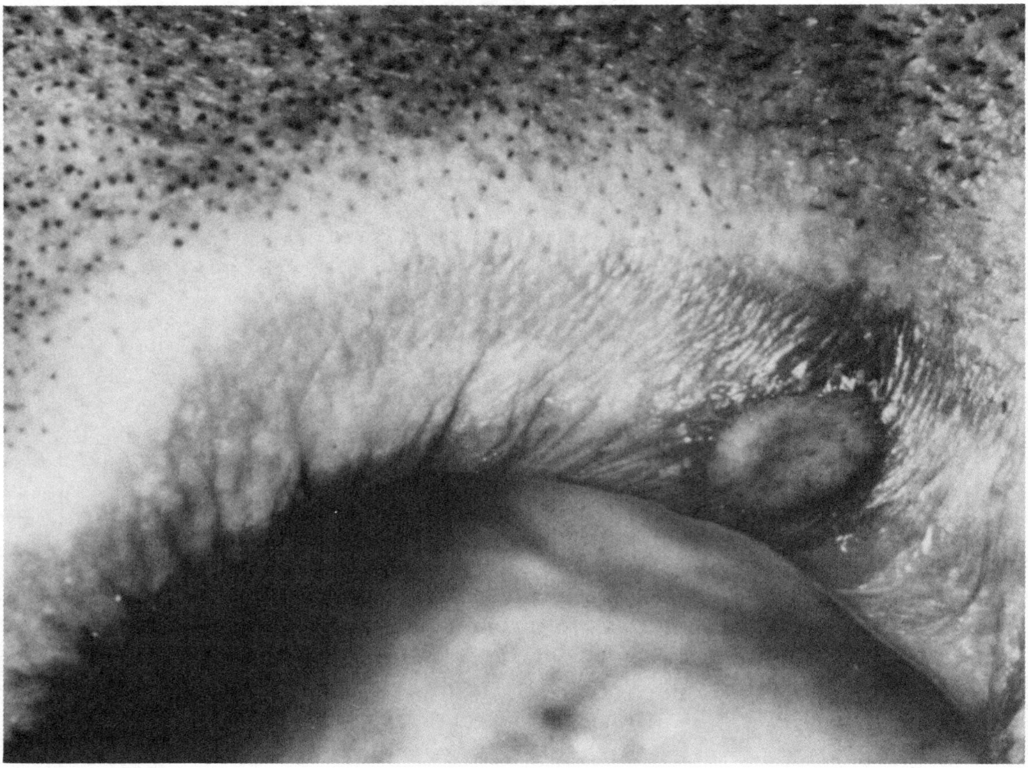

FIGURE 18.8 Behcet's disease. Painful oral aphtha of the upper lip; an erythematous border surrounds a necrotic yellow ulcer. (From *Textbook of Rheumatology,* with permission of the original contributor, Roy Rogers III, the author J Desmond O'Duffy and W.B. Saunders Co., Philadelphia.)

Clinical Findings

Aphthous ulcerations of the oral mucosa are the earliest clinical manifestation of Behcet's disease. The oral lesion, which appears singly or in crops, begins as a slightly raised, reddened area which evolves into a shallow round or oval ulcer with a yellowish necrotic base and erythematous borders (Figure 18.8). The ulcerations usually heal within 10 days. They generally occur on the lips, gingivae, buccal mucosa, and tongue, and usually spare the palate, tonsils, and pharynx.

Genital ulcerations resemble the oral aphthous lesions. They are usually located on the scrotum in males and the vulva in females, but may occur on the penis and in perianal and vaginal mucosa. Genital lesions are generally deeper than oral ulcerations and may heal with scarring.

Uveitis in Behcet's disease involves both the anterior and posterior ocular structures. Anterior uveitis and hypopyon (pus in the anterior chamber) are generally self-limited and resolve without sequelae. Recurrent posterior uveitis with choroiditis and retinal involvement may result in blindness approximately 5-6 years after the onset of ocular symptoms.

Skin lesions occurring in Behcet's disease include pustules, nodules, and papules. Nodular cutaneous lesions resembling erythema nodosum may be seen on the lower extremities.

Arthritis occurs in a majority of patients. Large and small joints may be involved, but the knees and ankles are affected most often. Joint destruction rarely occurs. Sacroiliitis is seen infrequently and only in HLA-B27-positive patients.

Neurologic involvement occurs in a minority of patients and is associated with a poor prognosis (55). Clinical findings include hemiplegia, cranial nerve palsies, cerebellar dysfunction, altered mood, and changes in mental status.

Other manifestations of Behcet's disease include thrombophlebitis, gastrointestinal tract ulcerations, renal abnormalities, and vascular lesions.

Laboratory Features

A peripheral leukocytosis and an elevated erythrocyte sedimentation rate are usually detected during active disease. Synovial fluid white counts average 5000-10,000 cells/mm^3 with a predominance of polymorphonuclear neutrophils. Cerebrospinal fluid findings during episodes of central nervous system involvement include a mild to moderate pleocytosis composed either of mononuclear or polymorphonuclear cells and elevated protein.

Diagnosis

The diagnosis of Behcet's disease is based on clinicopathologic findings. A diagnosis requires that three of the four major clinical criteria be present. These criteria include (51): 1) recurrent oral ulcers; 2) skin lesions; 3) ocular lesions; and 4) genital ulcerations.

Treatment and Prognosis

Prednisone in dosages up to 60 mg daily suppresses skin and joint inflammation, but does not appear to alter the course of the underlying disease. Uveitis has been treated with chlorambucil with some success (56), and chlorambucil may be useful in the therapy of central nervous system disease.

Behcet's disease may result in severe visual impairment or death from central nervous system involvement. Cytotoxic agents may be indicated in life-threatening disease or to prevent blindness. In patients without severe disease manifestations, signs and symptoms of persistent activity, especially oral ulcerations, may continue for many years unaffected by treatment.

Thromboangiitis Obliterans (Buerger's Disease)

Thromboangiitis obliterans (Buerger's disease) is an occlusive vascular disease with an inflammatory component usually affecting small and medium-sized arteries and veins of the extremities.

Epidemiology

Thromboangiitis obliterans is a rare disease generally affecting males in the 20-40-year age group.

Pathogenesis

The etiology of thromboangiitis obliterans is unknown. Since cessation of smoking generally results in disease remission, the use of tobacco has been implicated in its pathogenesis.

Genetic factors may also be important in the etiopathogenesis of thromboangiitis obliterans. An increased incidence of the disease is seen in Oriental populations (57), and Ashkenazi Jews in Israel (58). Moreover, HLA antigens A9 and B5 have an increased incidence in thromboangiitis obliterans as compared to normal controls (59).

Pathology

The vascular lesions of thromboangiitis obliterans involve small and medium-sized arteries and veins of the lower and/or upper extremity. The histopathology has been divided into three stages: acute, subacute, and chronic (60). The acute stage is characterized by polymorphonuclear cell infiltration of the vessel wall with thrombus formation. The vessels rarely show any evidence of necrosis as in polyarteritis nodosa. Mononuclear cells and a few giant cells are found in the subacute stage. The chronic stage is characterized by fibrosis and recanalization of the thrombus.

Clinical Findings

A migratory thrombophlebitis usually involving the lower extremities occurs early in the disease. Clinical manifestations including claudication, numbness, pain, ulceration, or infection may affect the lower legs or feet, but occasionally involve the hands and fingers.

Raynaud's phenomenon is a common complaint in thromboangiitis obliterans. Hyperhydrosis occurs in about one-third of patients (60). Systemic features such as fever, malaise, or arthralgias are usually absent.

Laboratory Findings

Routine laboratory studies are generally normal. Rheumatoid factor and antinuclear antibody tests are usually negative.

Diagnosis

Thromboangiitis obliterans should be suspected in male smokers between the ages of 20 and 40 with symptoms of a migratory thrombophlebitis, claudication, and Raynaud's phenomenon. Physical examination findings of 1) rubor of the feet; 2) absent foot pulses in the presence of a normal femoral or popliteal pulse; and 3) reduction or absence of the radial and/or ulnar pulses may also suggest thromboangiitis obliterans.

The diagnosis is established by biopsy of an involved artery or by angiography. Angiographic findings include segmental symmetric narrowing or occlusion of arteries involving either the lower or upper extremities, or both (58,61). This contrasts with atherosclerosis in which an asymmetric diffuse pattern is seen. Thromboangiitis obliterans may be differentiated from atherosclerosis by pathologic, angiographic, and epidemiologic criteria.

Treatment and Prognosis

The only effective therapy for thromboangiitis obliterans is cessation of smoking (62). Although there is significant morbidity associated with this disorder, including tissue loss or amputation of an extremity, the life span of patients is usually normal.

References

1. Kussmaul A, Maier R: Ueber eine bishir nicht beschriebene eigenthumliche Arterienerkrankung (periarteritis nodosa) die mit morbus Brightii und rapid fortschreitender allgemeiner muskellahmung einhergeht. *Dtsch Arch Klin Med* 1:484-517, 1866.

2. Zeek PM: Periarteritis nodosa: A critical review. *Am J Clin Pathol* 22: 777-790, 1952.

3. Hunder GG, Conn DD: Necrotizing vasculitis. In WN Kelley, ED Harris, S Ruddy, CB Sledge (eds.), *Textbook of Rheumatology,* Philadelphia, W.B. Saunders, 1981, pp. 1165-1202.

4. Kurland LT, Hauser WA, Ferguson RH, Holley KE: Epidemiologic features of diffuse connective tissue disorders in Rochester, Minn., 1951 through 1967, with special reference to systemic lupus erythematosus. *Mayo Clin Proc* 44:649-663, 1969.

5. Cupps TR, Fauci AS: Systemic necrotizing vasculitis of the polyarteritis nodosa group. In LH Smith Jr (ed.), *The Vasculitides.* Philadelphia, W.B. Saunders, 1981, pp. 26-49.

6. Sergent JS, Lockshin MD, Christian CL, Gocke DJ: Vasculitis with hepatitis B antigenemia: Long-term observations in nine patients. *Medicine* (Baltimore) 55:1-18, 1976.

7. Gocke DJ, Hsu K, Morgan C, Bombardieri S, Lockshin M, Christian CL: Association between polyarteritis and Australia antigen. *Lancet* 2:1149-1153, 1970.

8. Conn DL, McDuffie FC, Holley KE, Schroeter AL: Immunologic mechanisms in systemic vasculitis. *Mayo Clin Proc* 51:511-518, 1976.

9. Holsinger DR, Osmundson PJ, Edwards JE: The heart in periarteritis nodosa. *Circulation* 25:610-618, 1962.

10. Chumbley LC, Harrison EG, DeRemee RA: Allergic granulomatosis and angiitis (Churg-Strauss syndrome). *Mayo Clin Proc* 52:477-484, 1977.

11. Churg J, Strauss L: Allergic granulomatosis, allergic angiitis, and periarteritis nodosa. *Am J Pathol* 27:277-294, 1951.

12. Fan PT, Davis JA, Somer T, Kaplan L, Bluestone R: A clinical approach to systemic vasculitis. *Semin Arthritis Rheum* 9:248-304, 1980.

13. Carrington CB, Liebow AA: Limited forms of angiitis and granulomatosis of Wegener's type. *Am J Med* 41:497-527, 1966.

14. Cupps TR, Fauci AS: Wegener's granulomatosis. In LH Smith Jr (ed.), *The Vasculitides*. Philadelphia, W.B. Saunders, 1981, pp. 72-87.

15. Goodman GC, Churg J: Wegener's granulomatosis. Pathology and review of the literature. *Arch Pathol* 58:533-553, 1954.

16. Fauci AS, Wolff SM: Wegener's granulomatosis: Studies in 18 patients and a review of the literature. *Medicine* 52:535-561, 1973.

17. Howell SB, Epstein WV: Circulating immunoglobulin complexes in Wegener's granulomatosis. *Am J Med* 60:259-268, 1976.

18. Fauci AS, Johnson RE, Wolff SM: Radiation therapy of midline granuloma. *Ann Intern Med* 84:140-147, 1976.

19. Cupps TR, Fauci AS: Lymphomatoid granulomatosis. In LH Smith Jr (ed.), *The Vasculitides*. Philadelphia, W.B. Saunders, 1981, pp. 88-98.

20. Wolff SM, Fauci AS, Horn RG, Dale DC: Wegener's granulomatosis. *Ann Intern Med* 81:513-524, 1974.

21. Cupps TR, Fauci AS: Hypersensitivity vasculitis. In LH Smith Jr (ed.), *The Vasculitides*. Philadelphia, W.B. Saunders, 1981, pp. 50-71.

22. Sam WM Jr, Claman HN, Kohler PF, McIntosh RM, Small P, Mass MF: Human necrotizing vasculitis: Immunoglobulins and complement in vessel walls of cutaneous lesions and normal skin. *J Inves Dermatol* 64:441-445, 1975.

23. Gilliam JN, Smiley JD: Cutaneous necrotizing vasculitis and related disorders. *Ann Allergy* 37:328-339, 1976.

24. Levy M, Broyer M, Arsan A, Levy-Bentolila D, Habib R: Anaphylactoid purpura nephritis in childhood: Natural history and immunopathology. *Adv Nephrol* 6:183-228, 1976.

25. Levo Y, Gorevic PD, Kassab HJ, Tobias H, Franklin E: Liver involvement in the syndrome of mixed cryoglobulinemia. *N Engl J Med* 87:287-292, 1977.

26. Gamble CN, Ruggles SW: The immunopathogenesis of glomerulonephritis associated with mixed cryoglobulinemia. *N Engl J Med* 299:81-84, 1978.

27. Glass D, Soter NA, Schur PH: Rheumatoid vasculitis. *Arthritis Rheum* 19:950-952, 1976.

28. Johnson GD, Edmonds JP, Holborow EJ: Precipitating antibody to DNA detected by two-stage electroimmunodiffusion. Study in SLE and in rheumatoid arthritis. *Lancet* 2:883-885, 1973.

29. Dorsch CA, Feinglass EJ, Stevens MB: Clinical significance of antibodies to extractable nuclear antigen (ENA) in systemic lupus erythematosus. *Arthritis Rheum* (abst) 20:114, 1977.

30. Hauser WA, Ferguson RH, Holley KE, Kurland LT: Temporal arteritis in Rochester, Minnesota, 1951 to 1967. *Mayo Clin Proc* 46:597-602, 1971.

31. Liang GC, Simkin PA, Hunder GG, Wilske KR, Healy LA: Familial aggregation of polymyalgia rheumatica and giant cell arteritis. *Arthritis Rheum* 17:19-24, 1974.

32. Healey LA, Parker F, Wilske KR: Polymyalgia rheumatica and giant cell arteritis. *Arthritis Rheum* 14:138-141, 1971.

33. Lowenstein MB, Bridgeford PH, Vasey FB, Germain BF, Espinoza LR: Increased frequency of HLA-DR3 and DR4 in polymyalgia rheumatica and giant cell arteritis. *Arthritis Rheum* 26:925-927, 1983.

34. Papaioannou CC, Hunder GG, McDuffie FC: Cellular immunity in polymyalgia rheumatica and giant cell arteritis. Lack of response to muscle or artery homogenates. *Arthritis Rheum* 22:740-745, 1979.

35. Liang GC, Simkin PA, Mannik M: Immunoglobulins in temporal arteries: An immunofluorescent study. *Ann Intern Med* 81:19-24, 1974.

36. Hunder GG, Hazelman BL: Giant-cell arteritis and polymyalgia rheumatica. In WN Kelley, ED Harris, S Ruddy, CB Sledge (eds.), *Textbook of Rheumatology.* Philadelphia, W.B. Saunders, 1981, pp. 1189-1197.

37. Parker F, Healey LA, Wilske KR, Odland GF: Light and electron microscopic studies on human temporal arteries with special reference to alterations related to senescence, atherosclerosis, and giant cell arteritis. *Am J Pathol* 79:57-72, 1975.

38. Klein RG, Campbell RJ, Hunder GG, Carney JA: Skip lesions in temporal arteritis. *Mayo Clin Proc* 51:504-510, 1976.

39. Wilkinson IMS, Russell RWR: Arteries of the head and neck in giant cell arteritis: A pathological study to show the pattern of arterial involvement. *Arch Neurol* 27:378-391, 1972.

40. Klein RG, Hunder GG, Stanson AW, Sheps SG: Large artery involvement in giant cell (temporal) arteritis. *Ann Intern Med* 83:806-812, 1975.

41. Hunder GG, Allen GL: Giant cell arteritis. A review. *Bull Rheum Dis* 29: 980-987, 1978-9.

42. Hunder GG, Disney TF, Ward LE: Polymyalgia rheumatica. *Mayo Clin Proc* 44:849-875, 1969.

43. Kansu T, Corbett JJ, Savino P, Schatz NJ: Giant cell arteritis with normal sedimentation rate. *Arch Neurol* 34:624-625, 1977.

44. Ueda H, Saito Y, Ito I, Yamaguchi H, Sugiura M, Morooka S: Immunological studies of aortitis syndrome. *Jpn Heart J* 8:4-18, 1967.

45. Nakao K, Ikeda M, Kimata S, Niitani H, Miyahara M, Ishimi Z, Hashiba K, Takeda Y, Ozawa T, Matsushita S, Kuramochi M: Takayasu's arteritis: Clinical report of 84 cases and immunological studies of seven cases. *Circulation* 35:1141-1155, 1967.

46. Asherson RA, Asherson GL, Schrire V: Immunological studies in arteritis of the aorta and great vessels. *Br Med J* 3:589-590, 1968.

47. Lande A, Bard R, Rossi P, Passariello R, Castrucci A: Takayasu's arteritis: A worldwide entity. *NY State J Med* 76:1477-1482, 1976.

48. Fraga A, Mintz G, Valle L, Flores-Izquierdo G: Takayasu's arteritis: Frequency of systemic manifestations (study of 22 patients) and favorable response to maintenance steroid therapy with adrenocorticosteroids (12 patients). *Arthritis Rheum* 15:617-624, 1972.

49. Committee on study of arteritis: Clinical and pathological studies of aortitis syndrome. *Jpn Heart J* 9:76-87, 1968.

50. Ishikawa K: Natural history and classification of occlusive thromboaortopathy (Takayasu's disease). *Circulation* 57:27-35, 1978.

51. Shimizu T, Ehrlich GE, Inaba G, Hayashi K: Behcet disease (Behcet syndrome). *Semin Arthritis Rheum* 8:223-260, 1979.

52. O'Duffy JD: Summary of international symposium on Behcet's disease. *J Rheumatol* 5:229-233, 1978.

53. Gamble CN, Wiesner KB, Shapiro RF, Boyer WJ: The immune complex pathogenesis of glomerulonephritis and pulmonary vasculitis in Behcet's disease. *Am J Med* 66:1031-1039, 1979.

54. Lehner T, Batchelor JR, Challacombe SJ, Kennedy L: An immunogenetic basis for the tissue involvement in Behcet's syndrome. *Immunology* 37: 895-900, 1979.

55. Wolf SM, Schotland DL, Phillips LL: Involvement of nervous system in Behcet's syndrome. *Arch Neurol* 12:315-325, 1965.

56. Tricoulis D: Treatment of Behcet's disease with chlorambucil. *Br J Ophthamol* 60:55-57, 1976.

57. McKusick VA, Harris WS: The Buerger's syndrome in the Orient. *Bull Johns Hopkins Hosp* 109:241-291, 1961.

58. Goodman RM, Elian B, Mozes M, Deutsch V: Buerger's disease in Israel. *Am J Med* 39:601-615, 1965.

59. McLoughlin GA, Helsby CR, Evans LL, Chapman DM: Association of HLA-A9 and HLA-B5 with Buerger's disease. *Br Med J* 2:1165-1166, 1976.

60. Cupps TR, Fauci AS: Thromboangiitis obliterans. In LH Smith Jr (ed.), *The Vasculitides.* Philadelphia, W.B. Saunders, 1981, pp. 133-136.

61. McKusick VA, Harris WS, Ottesen OE, Goodman RM, Shelley WM, Bloodwell RD: Buerger's disease: A distinct clinical and pathologic entity. *JAMA* 181:5-12, 1962.

62. Strandness DE Jr: Vascular diseases of the extremities. In RG Petersdorf, RD Adams, E Braunwald, KJ Isselbacher, JB Martin, JD Wilson (eds.), *Harrison's Principles of Internal Medicine,* 10th Ed. New York, McGraw Hill, 1983, pp. 1494-1495.

Chapter 19

RHEUMATIC DISEASES OF CHILDHOOD

Sara H. Sinal, M.D.

The rheumatic diseases of childhood are a collection of illnesses which involve inflammation of the connective tissue and also belong in the broad category of collagen diseases. There are over 100 diseases recognized by the American Rheumatism Association in which arthritis is a significant manifestation (1). Although these disease states share common symptomatology, they can usually be separated into distinct clinical entities. Precise laboratory tests are not available for the majority of these diseases and diagnosis remains a clinical task. With the decline in the incidence of acute rheumatic fever (ARF), juvenile rheumatoid arthritis (JRA) has become the leading children's rheumatic disease.

Juvenile Rheumatoid Arthritis

Introduction and Definition

Juvenile rheumatoid arthritis (JRA) is the most common rheumatic disease of childhood. In 1963, a subcommittee of the American Rheumatism Association made the first attempt to define and establish specific criteria for JRA. These criteria were published in 1973, and were followed by revised criteria in 1977 (2). Persistent arthritis of one or more joints for 6 weeks is sufficient for the diagnosis of JRA if certain other diseases are excluded. Arthritis is defined as swelling and pain in a joint, or heat, pain, and tenderness with limitation of motion of the joint. Use of these criteria has been very helpful in establishing the correct diagnosis in children with arthritis (Table 19.1).

TABLE 19.1 Criteria for JRA (2)

Arthritis of 6 weeks duration provided certain diseases have been excluded.*
Definition of arthritis: Swelling of a joint or limitation of motion with heat, pain or tenderness. Pain or tenderness alone is not arthritis.
Definition of joint: Joints are counted individually except for the following which are considered one joint each: cervical spine, carpal joints of each hand, tarsal joints of each foot.

*See Table 19-4 for summary of exclusions.

The first report of juvenile chronic polyarthritis was the work of George Frederick Still (3), a pediatrician in training at Great Ormand Street. He reported 22 cases, giving excellent clinical descriptions. Already sensing what others were to write about later, he suggested that chronic polyarthritis in children included a number of different conditions. The term Still's disease was once used for JRA and by some authors for the systemic form of JRA, but to avoid confusion the current recommendation is that the name Still's disease be dropped (2).

Epidemiology

The true prevalence of JRA is not known. The best data available were summarized in 1977 by Baum (4). Based on a number of studies, he estimates a maximum of 200,000 children with JRA in the United States. There appears to be a similar distribution in other western countries. There are studies suggesting a higher prevalence in American Indian children and African blacks, but further data are necessary to confirm this. Approximately 5% of all adult rheumatoid arthritis begins in childhood.

Etiopathogenesis

A number of causes and risk factors for JRA have been suggested but not proved. This list includes infectious agents, immunologic abnormalities of the host, preceding physical trauma to the joints or psychological trauma to the child, and allergy to any substance (5). Since viral infections can cause transient arthritis, the possibility of a preceding or ongoing viral infection has been postulated. Various microorganisms have been cultured from synovial tissues, but none consistently (6). Evidence that an immune mechanism may be involved is based primarily on adult arthritis where rheumatoid factors (antibodies that react with IgG) coexist with typical adult rheumatoid arthritis. In addition, selective IgA deficiency has been associated with JRA and Cassidy et al. (7) have suggested that IgA deficiency may be "only a marker of a more profound but as yet undefined immunologic disturbance involving the cellular immune system." JRA does not appear to be a genetic or familial disease except in the JRA subgroup of older onset pauciarticular arthritis. This subgroup occurs in families with ankylosing spondylitis and is associated with histocompatibility antigen B27 (5).

TABLE 19.2 The Spectrum of Juvenile Rheumatoid Arthritis

	Systemic	Polyarticular	Pauciarticular
Type of Onset	Spiking fever Rheumatoid rash Hepatosplenomegaly Lymphadenopathy Polyserositis Myalgia, arthralgia Leukocytosis, anemia	Symmetrical arthritis 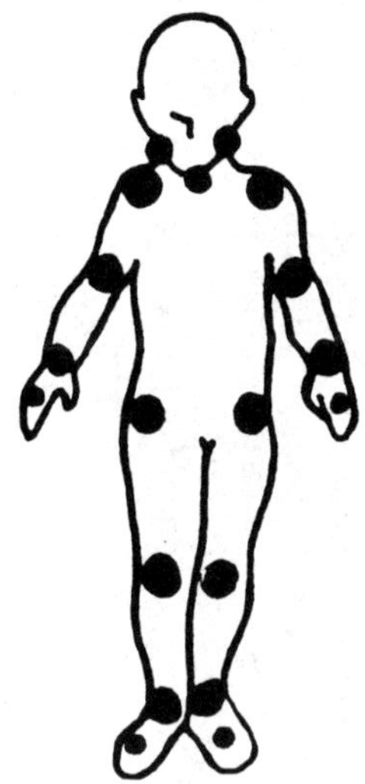	Asymmetrical arthritis 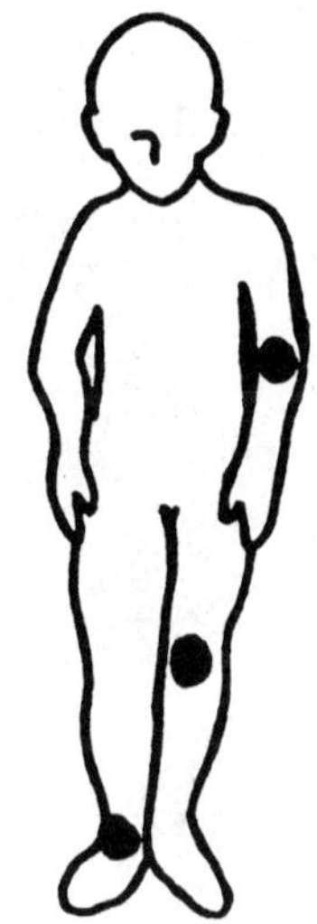
Joint Symptoms	Same as polyarticular JRA	Arthritis involving large and small joints: knees, wrists, hands, ankles, feet, elbows, hips, cervical spine (sparing lumbodorsal spine), jaw, shoulders.	Few joints involved, typically the knee, ankle, elbow, occassionally spotty involvement of other joints as well. In type II, patients frequently have hip girdle involvement.

TABLE 19.2 (Cond't)

	Systemic	Polyarticular Seronegative	Polyarticular Seropositive	Pauciarticular Type I	Pauciarticular Type II
Age of Onset (median)	5 years	3 years	12 years	2 years	10 years
Sex ratio	M-F	F>>M	F>M	F>M	M>>F
Serology: Rheumatoid factor	Absent	Absent	+ in 100%	Absent	Absent
Serology: Antinuclear antibody	Absent	+ in 25%	+ in 75%	+ in 50%	Absent
Course of Joint Disease	Variable (25% severe destructive arthritis)	Remitting RX-responsive May "burn out"	Persistent Rx-negative Chronic Destructive	Joint residua rare	Joint residua those of ankylosing spondylitis
Association with HLA-B27	None	None	None	None	+
Iridocyclitis	Absent or rare	Absent or rare	Absent or rare	Chronic	Acute
Comments	Systemic manifestations self-limited; arthritis may be chronic	Extraarticular manifestations generally mild	Resembles adult RA; subcutaneous rheumatoid nodules	Major cause of morbidity is chronic iridocyclitis	Many patients have early ankylosing spondylitis rather than JRA. Familial pattern

From Wedgewood and Schaller, Hospital Practice, June 1977.

The pathology of joints in JRA is that of inflammation and hypertrophy of the synovium with secretion of increased amounts of joint fluid. Microscopically the synovial tissues show synovial hyperplasia with infiltration of lymphocytes and plasma cells (8). The result is a joint effusion and palpable thickened synovium. With continued synovitis joint destruction may occur. If destruction occurs, there is erosion of subchondral bone, loss of articular cartilage, and deformity. Subluxation or ankylosis of joints may occur (6). Fortunately, children tend to retain the ability to have reversible disease much longer than adults with rheumatoid arthritis, perhaps because the hyaline cartilage is much thicker in children and may protect the joint (8).

Clinical Features

The clinical manifestations of JRA are variable depending on the subgroup involved. It appears that JRA may in fact encompass several disease states. The American Rheumatism Association (3) currently recognizes three distinct subgroups: systemic onset disease, polyarticular onset disease, and pauciarticular onset disease. Rheumatologists are generally divided into two groups: "lumpers" and "splitters." Dr. Jane Schaller (9), who "cheerfully acknowledges" her place among the splitters, has further divided polyarticular disease (rheumatoid factor negative and rheumatoid factor positive) and pauciarticular disease (early childhood onset and late childhood onset). The clinical observations of Dr. Schaller and Dr. Ralph Wedgwood (5,6,9,10) are acknowledged in the description of JRA presented here. The division into subgroups is useful clinically in diagnosis and management of patients. All of the subgroups share chronic synovitis. Table 19.2 summarizes the subgroups.

Systemic Onset JRA

Systemic JRA manifests as JRA with high spiking fevers (daily or twice daily spikes to 39°C or 103°F or higher) (see Table 19.3). There may be an associated rash which is small, macular, and pink or salmon colored; it tends to be evanescent, appearing during the fever spike and rapidly disappearing when the patient becomes afebrile. The rash tends to occur on face, trunk and upper arms, and legs. Most children with systemic JRA will have associated hepatosplenomegaly and lymphadenopathy. The degree of enlargement of organs and nodes may be alarming and lymph node biopsy can resemble lymphoma. One-third to one-half the patients will have pericarditis and pleuritis, but the majority of these patients will have no clinical symptomatology. If symptoms of chest pain, dyspnea or discomfort with breathing should develop, vigorous therapy may be indicated. Children may appear quite ill during fever spikes and by contrast quite playful between them.

Typical fever and rash will be considered probable systemic JRA prior to the onset of joint complaints but arthritis must be present before a definite diagnosis can be established. The majority of patients will develop joint manifestation within a few months of onset of fever. As noted before, pain and tenderness alone do not constitute arthritis and some of the patients will take years to develop frank arthritis. The systemic syndrome may recur but tends to "burn out" after a few months and rarely persists to adulthood.

Systemic JRA occurs in 20% of JRA patients. Male to female ratio is equal. Iridocyclitis is rare in the systemic form. Growth failure is more common in the systemic form of JRA than in the poly- or pauciarticular groups (11).

Table 19.3 Fever Curve in JRA

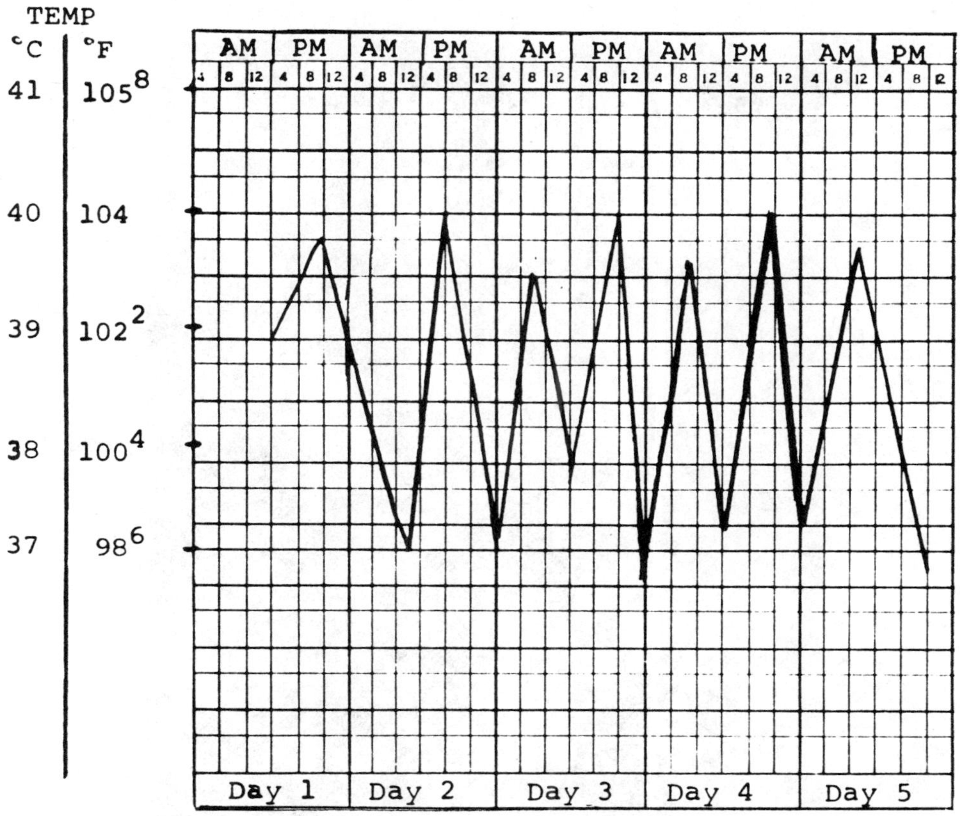

Fever curve during 4 days of hospitalization for a 7-year-old black male with the systemic form of JRA. This demonstrates typical fever spikes once or twice daily with return to normal levels.

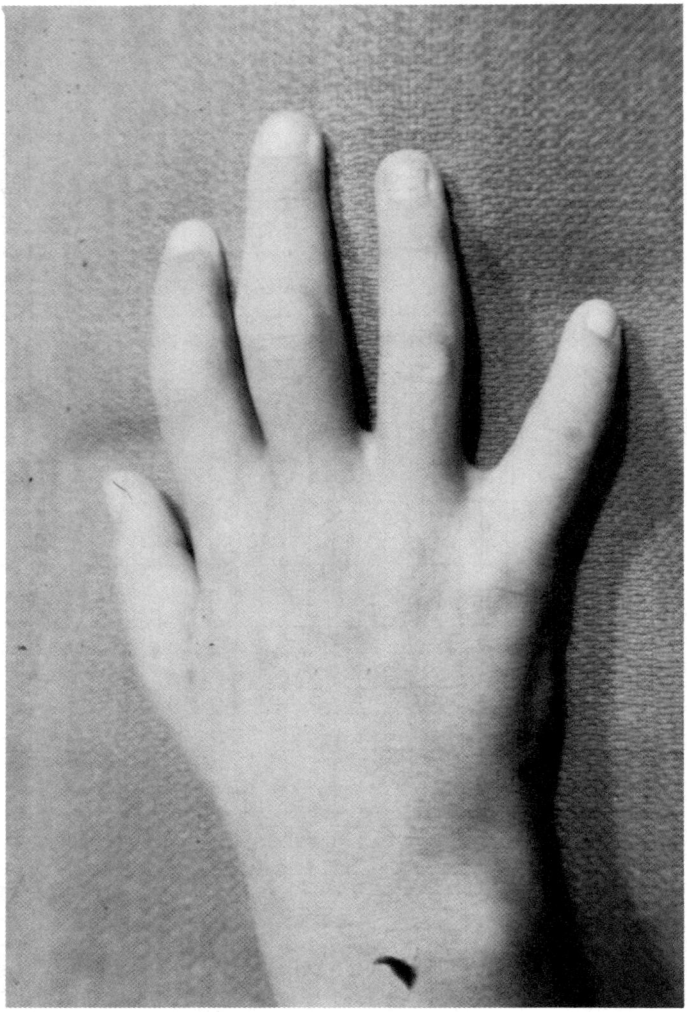

FIGURE 19.1 Characteristic appearance of the hands of an 11-year-old girl with polyarticular JRA. There is swelling of the proximal interphalangeal joints.

Polyarticular JRA

This subgroup manifests as arthritis in five or more joints. Patients with systemic onset are not included in this group although their joint manifestations are similar. Polyarthritis of the small joints of the hands and feet is typical (see Figure 19.1). Wrists, knees, ankles, and elbows are affected in most patients. The shoulders, hips, temporomandibular joints, and neck are affected in half the patients and the lumbodorsal spine is usually spared.

Polyarticular Rheumatoid Factor Negative

This form of JRA may present at any time during childhood, often during early years, and accounts for 25% of JRA patients. Girls are primarily affected by this form. Affected children have an onset of swollen and stiff joints with variable degrees of pain and warmth. Erythema of the joints is rare. Tests for rheumatoid factors are negative and remain so.

Polyarticular Rheumatoid Factor Positive

Children in this subgroup are older, usually over age 8 years at onset, and girls again predominate. This subgroup accounts for 10% of patients and is very similar to typical adult onset rheumatoid arthritis. Subcutaneous nodules are commonly seen on the extensor surfaces (elbows, heels, fingers). Ulcerative skin lesions of the lower extremities may be seen. The arthritis tends to be chronic, progressive, and severely destructive. Permanent joint disability is not uncommon. Iridocyclitis is rare. Two associated syndromes, Felty's syndrome (splenomegaly with leukopenia) and Sjögren's syndrome (parotitis, dry eyes and mouth) may occur as they do in classic adult rheumatoid arthritis.

Pauciarticular Arthritis

This subgroup manifests as arthritis in four or fewer joints, again with systemic onset JRA patients excluded from the subgroups. The large joints are usually the most likely affected and this frequently occurs in asymmetrical distribution. Schaller (5) cautions that small joints can also occasionally be affected and that patients may also fit the subgroup well and yet have more than four joints involved.

Pauciarticular Disease of Early Childhood Onset (Type I)

The majority of patients in this group are young girls who present before the fifth birthday. The subgroup makes up 25% of JRA patients. Approximately 50% of the patients will have antinuclear antibodies.

The joints affected are usually knees, ankles, and elbows. The joints tend to cause less disability than in the polyarticular form of the disease. The majority of patients do not go on to polyarticular disease. Systemic symptoms are rare.

The major morbidity in this subgroup is chronic iridocyclitis with approximately 50% of the patients developing this at some time during the course of their disease. It is especially common if the patient has antinuclear antibodies. The eye disease usually is silent but may cause photophobia, pain in the eye, or an inflamed appearance of the eye. The early changes, detectable only by slitlamp examination, are cells and protein in the anterior chamber. Late changes are posterior synechiae, which cause an irregular pupil; a dense sclera or cornea; cataract formation and even glaucoma; and partial or complete visual loss. Frequent slitlamp exams (4 times per year for the first 10 years) are recommended to detect early eye disease. The eye disease does not correlate with activity of joint disease or elevated sedimentation rate.

Pauciarticular Disease of Later Childhood Onset (Type II)

The patients in this subgroup are boys 8 years of age or older. The subgroup accounts for 15% of JRA patients. They have a pauciarticular arthritis associated with sacroiliitis and HLA-B27 (75%). Many of the patient's family histories will be positive for ankylosing spondylitis or the other spondyloarthropathies (Reiter's disease, pauciarticular arthritis, acute iridocyclitis, spondylitis associated with bowel disease or psoriasis).

The affected joints are those of the lower limbs (hips, knees, ankles, or feet). Onset may be sudden and severe or insidious. The peripheral joints usually do not develop destructive arthritis. Some patients will develop lumbar and thoracic spine involvement during the course of the disease and may go ahead to develop severe progressive disease of the spine. Many of these patients eventually meet the criteria for ankylosing spondylitis (see Chapter 10), but because some patients do not, this subgroup continues to be considered a form of JRA. This subgroup may be associated with acute iridocyclitis (resembling ankylosing spondylitis and Reiter's disease), but because the attacks are usually symptomatic they are treated early and usually do not go ahead to cause permanent eye damage.

Diagnosis and Differential Diagnosis

As discussed before, the diagnosis of JRA is primarily a clinical one. Laboratory tests may be of some value. The 6 weeks time requirement to confirm the diagnosis is valuable since many of the diseases causing transient arthritis will not last this long. If the arthritis meets the established criteria (2) in other ways then the next step is to make the necessary exclusions. A summary of the diseases which should be considered in the differential diagnosis of JRA is in Table 19.4.

In the systemic form of JRA, prior to the onset of arthritis, the differential is similar to that in a fever of unknown origin (FUO) workup. It is extremely important to rule out infectious diseases in these patients and cultures of the blood are necessary. Neoplasia can also present as fever, and routine examination of hemoglobin, white blood cell count and differential, and platelet count may be helpful in ruling out leukemia. A bone marrow aspirate may be helpful for the diagnosis of leukemia, histiocytosis, neuroblastoma, or unusual infectious diseases. Radiographs may help exclude malignancies involving the bone. Although systemic JRA may present with lymphadenopathy, lymph node biopsy may be necessary to rule out malignancy.

In the child with monoarticular arthritis, several conditions must be excluded. Although children with septic arthritis may have more than one joint involved, most frequently the child will have one hot, erythematous, painful joint. Usually the pain is more severe than that of JRA. The swelling is usually of acute onset and the child generally, although not always, has fever and appears toxic. If septic arthritis is suspected a joint aspirate for cell count, gram stain and culture of the synovial fluid is essential. A reactive arthritis secondary to adjacent osteomyelitis is also a concern and may require a technesium bone scan or bone aspirate. Trauma with or without foreign body can classically give a monoarticular arthritis. The traumatic hemarthrosis seen in hemophilia is frequently monoarticular. The absence of fever in monoarticular arthritis is more suggestive of trauma (12).

Polyarticular arthritis is perhaps the most difficult group in establishing a correct diagnosis. As stated earlier septic arthritis may involve more than one joint. Arthritis following viral infections such as rubella, hepatitis, and chicken pox usually involves multiple joints. This is also true of mycoplasma infections

TABLE 19.4 Differential Diagnosis of Juvenile Rheumatoid Arthritis

Infection	Genetic and Metabolic Conditions
Bacterial arthritis	Hemophilia
H. influenza	Osteogenesis imperfecta
S. aureus	Gout (Lesch-Nyan, glycogen storage, disorders of purine metabolism)
N. gonorrheae	Rickets
N. meningococcus	Sickle cell hemoglobinopathies
Salmonella	
Shigella	
Yersinia	**Miscellaneous**
Tuberculous arthritis	Growing pains
	Psychogenic
Viral arthritis	Avascular necrosis
Rubella (including vaccine-related)	Osgood-Schlatter
Varicella	Slipped capital femoral epiphysis
Mumps	Other orthopedic conditions
Adenovirus	
Hepatitis	**Other Rheumatic Diseases of Childhood**
Lyme arthritis	Systemic lupus erythematosus
	Ankylosing spondylitis and other spondyloarthropathies
Neoplasia	Mixed connective tissue disease
Neuroblastoma	Dermatomyositis
Leukemia	Scleroderma
Histiocytosis	Vasculitis syndromes
Lymphoma	Rheumatic fever
Trauma	
Fractures	
Nonaccidental injury (battered child)	

and arthritis following rubella vaccine. A reactive but sterile arthritis has been reported following gastrointestinal infections with Yersinia, Salmonella and Shigella (5). Lyme arthritis which is caused by a tick-borne spirochete, *Treponema borrelia*, can present with polyarthritis. The skin lesion in Lyme arthritis, erythema chronicum migrans, is distinctive and precedes the development of arthritis (13). Malignancy must be excluded in polyarticular arthritis. Other metabolic and genetic conditions, psychogenic arthritis, growing pains, and miscellaneous orthopedic conditions must be considered.

The other childhood rheumatic diseases can be confused with systemic disease, monoarticular or polyarticular JRA. They will be discussed in more detail later in the chapter. Ankylosing spondylitis can usually be diagnosed because of a family history positive for spondylitis and the presence of HLA B27. Reiter syndrome presents with urethritis, conjunctivitis, as well as arthritis. The arthritis of inflammatory bowel disease can generally be identified because of concomitant gastrointestinal complaints, but the arthritis may precede other symptoms. Systemic lupus erythematosus (SLE) may have a distinctive butterfly rash as well as evidence of multisystem disease. Antinuclear antibody is present (usually in high titer) in SLE in almost 100% of patients. These children frequently have anti-DNA antibodies. Dermatomyositis has characteristic skin lesions. Scleroderma causes a distinctive hardening of the skin. The vasculitis syndromes are usually of shorter duration than JRA and have distinctive features. Rheumatic fever is a disease with specific criteria (14). The disease follows streptococcal infection and the evidence of a streptococcal infection plus presence of other major or minor manifestations of rheumatic fever with arthritis can establish the diagnosis.

Laboratory Studies

There is no one laboratory test at the present time to establish the diagnosis of JRA. Several laboratory tests may be helpful. There is frequently a mild anemia, felt to be secondary to chronic disease. The anemia does not respond to iron, though the red blood cells are frequently microcytic and hypochromic. The anemia improves with remission (12). Mild leukocytosis exists in many JRA patients and severe leukemoid reactions have been reported particularly in the systemic form of JRA. Leukopenia is much less likely to occur in JRA and should alert the clinician to the possibility of leukemia or other collagen disease such as SLE. Mild eosinophilia and mild thrombocytosis may occur. Routine urinalysis is usually normal although mild proteinuria can occur. Hematuria has also been reported.

Acute phase reactants such as erythrocyte sedimentation rate and C-reactive protein are not particularly helpful. The sedimentation rate is usually moderately elevated during the active phase of JRA but may be normal. In addition, a number of other conditions such as infection can elevate the sedimentation rate. The C-reactive protein also indicates inflammation but is not specific for JRA.

The special tests for rheumatic disease may be helpful. Rheumatoid factors are antibodies which react with IgG immunoglobulins. The antibodies may react with host or foreign immunoglobulin and are measured by agglutination tests, such as the latex agglutination. Rheumatoid factors measuring IgM antibodies to IgG are classically found in typical adult onset rheumatoid arthritis. As previously discussed, they are found in only a small group (10%) of patients with JRA, the subgroup with rheumatoid factor positive polyarticular disease. Why rheumatoid factors are not positive in the remainder of JRA patients is not known. Rheumatoid factors are nonspecific and may occur in patients with infectious diseases, malignancies, and other conditions.

Antinuclear antibodies (ANA) are antibodies which react with one of several nuclear constituents. Tests to detect their presence are not well standardized and that makes interpretation difficult (6). Brewer et al. (12) found ANA in 68% of cases of pauciarticular disease, 27% of cases of polyarticular disease, and 27% of cases of systemic disease. Schaller reports different values based in part on further breakdowns of JRA into subgroups (5). The ANA is most valuable in recognizing children at risk for chronic iridocyclitis. ANA is not associated with severity of disease.

Measurement of serum immunoglobulins is not helpful in JRA except for identifying children with selective IgA deficiency (12). Circulating complement is usually normal in JRA although complement may be reduced in joint fluid. Histocompatibility antigen B27 can be found in children with late onset pauciarticular JRA but HLA typing is generally not helpful in the diagnosis of JRA.

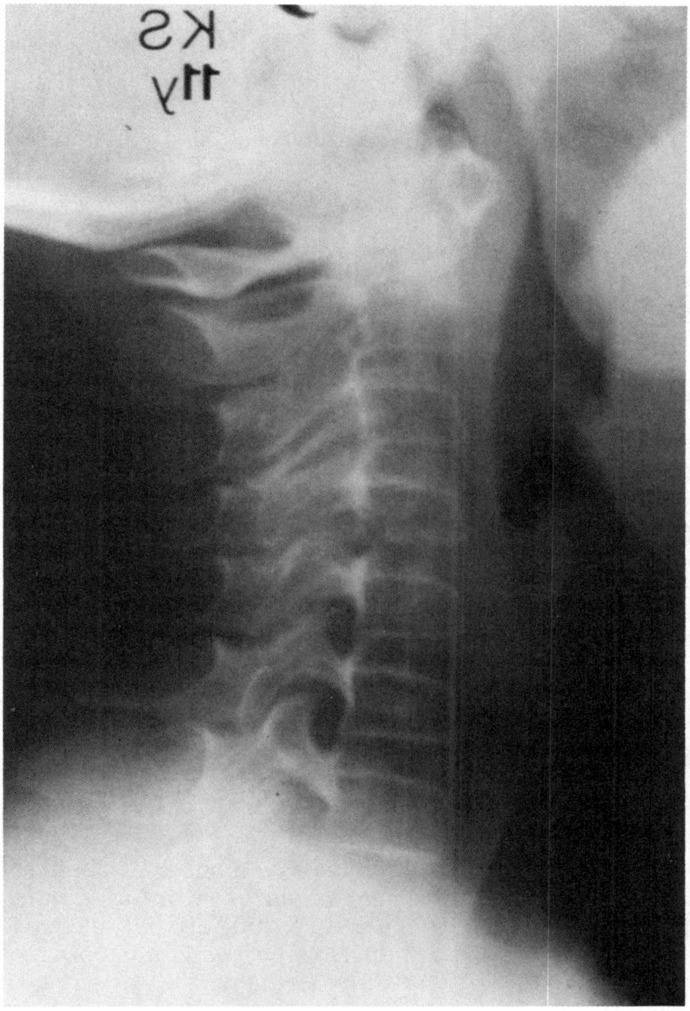

FIGURE 19.2 A radiograph of the cervical spine of an 11-year-old girl with polyarticular JRA. There is early fusion of the posterior elements of the cervical spine with loss of normal mineralization.

Roentgenographic studies of the joints in JRA are important in distinguishing between JRA and other conditions such as trauma, infection, foreign body, and malignancy. Early changes seen in JRA are soft tissue swelling, osteoporosis, and new bone formation. Later changes are those of joint destruction with narrowing of the joint space and erosion of the bone, ankylosis, and subluxation. With severe disease and use of corticosteroid fractures can occur. Isolated abnormalities of bone growth such as micrognathia or under- or overgrowth of long bones can also be detected. Changes can also be seen in the spine with cervical spine involvement seen in all groups (see Figure 19.2), and classical sacroiliac changes seen in late onset pauciarticular disease (12). Chest roentgenograms can be helpful in the diagnosis of pleuritis or pericarditis. However, frequently the echocardiogram can detect a small pericardial effusion in a patient with a normal chest roentgenogram.

Pathologic features are limited primarily to synovial fluid analysis and synovial biopsy. Synovial fluid cell counts in JRA show increased numbers of white cells, primarily polymorphonuclear forms, and total counts may be as high as 80,000-100,000 cells/mm^3. The sugar concentration in joint fluid may be low. The primary value of joint fluid analysis is to rule out a septic joint. In JRA gram stains and cultures are negative. Gout and pseudogout can also be differentiated since the joint fluid in gout contains urate crystals and in pseudogout calcium pyrophosphate crystals. Synovial biopsies are not generally necessary. They show a mononuclear infiltrate and can rule out rare conditions such as pigmented villonodular synovitis (5).

Prognosis

Juvenile rheumatoid arthritis is rarely a fatal condition. Baum and Gutowska (15) report the most common causes of death as renal disease (one-half the total cases), amyloidosis, infection, and heart disease. Most of the renal deaths and many of the infectious and cardiac deaths were also related to amyloidosis. Amyloidosis appears to be a much more common complication of JRA in Europe than in the United States.

Seventy-five to 84% of children who develop JRA will not have serious permanent joint disability. Patients with systemic onset disease and rheumatoid factor positive polyarthritis are at greatest risk for permanent joint deformity. Children with early onset pauciarticular disease are at risk for chronic iridocyclitis which may cause blindness. Children with late onset pauciarticular disease may develop ankylosing spondylitis (5,9).

Management

The management of children with JRA includes a number of phases. Initial careful assessment to make the correct diagnosis and careful follow-up alert to the possibility of changes in the condition are essential. Parent and patient education about JRA, its manifestations, treatment, and generally good prognosis are essential. As in any chronic disease state the stress on the patient and family must be kept in mind and support in this area is crucial for successful management and patient compliance.

The primary goal in the treatment of arthritis is to prevent permanent joint deformity. Physical and occupational therapy are an essential part of the patient management. Parents and children should be given home exercise programs and normal activity should be encouraged whenever possible. Swimming is an excellent form of therapy for children and teenagers. Riding a tricycle is helpful for young children. With joint limitation, physical therapy by a trained therapist may be necessary. Local application of heat can be helpful, and a warm bath prior to the joint exercises can decrease pain and increase joint motion. Night splints for wrists and knees can help prevent deformities (16).

With severe joint disease, orthopedic procedures such as synovectomy and soft tissue releases may be helpful. Total joint replacement is not possible in young children but is sometimes helpful in older age groups (12).

Attention to the possibility of iridocyclitis is important. Children with pauciarticular JRA should have slitlamp exams by an ophthalmologist 4 times per year and those with polyarticular and systemic JRA should be examined at least twice yearly. Iridocyclitis should be treated by an ophthalmologist and initially the therapy is topical steroids and mydriatics. If this therapy is unsuccessful steroid injections in the subconjunctiva or systemic steroids are indicated (5,17).

The mainstay of drug therapy in JRA is salicylates. Two reviews of salicylate therapy summarize their beneficial and undesirable effects (12,18). Aspirin should be given to children in an initial daily dose of 80-100 mg/kg in four divided doses with a total daily starting maximum dose of 3.6 g. Blood levels of salicylate should be documented to achieve maximum therapeutic benefit without toxicity. Usually a serum level of 20-30 mg/100 ml is therapeutic but not toxic. The signs of toxicity in children are drowsiness, irritability, hyperactivity, and hyperventilation. Unlike adults, tinnitus is rarely seen as a sign of toxicity. Some children may complain of stomachaches when taking salicylates. This can be managed by giving the salicylates with food or trying an enteric-coated preparation. Liver enzymes should be measured prior to instituting therapy with salicylates. Salicylates will often cause a definite but mild rise in liver enzyme (transaminase) levels. With evidence of severe liver toxicity (nausea, vomiting, enlarged liver, and dramatic increases in liver enzymes), symptoms resolve if salicylates are withdrawn. Salicylates interfere with platelet aggregation, and increased blood loss during surgery has been reported. Salicylates should be stopped several weeks prior to surgery. Allergic reactions to salicylates are rare but can occur.

If salicylates are not tolerated, tolmetin sodium (Tolectin) is an acceptable antiinflammatory drug which is as effective as salicylates. The recommended daily dosage for children is 15-30 mg/kg in four divided doses with a maximum of 2000 mg/day. Adverse affects are rare (12). Naproxen (Naprosyn) has also been approved for use in JRA at daily dosages of 10 mg/kg in two divided doses with a maximum of 1000 mg/day.

A number of other nonsteroidal antiinflammatory drugs used for adults with arthritis are not approved for use in children. These include phenylbutazone (Butazolidin), indomethacin (Indocin), ibuprofen (Motrin), tenoprofen calcium (Nalfon), and sulindac (Clinoril).

When patients do not respond to the nonsteroidal antiinflammatory agents, therapy with gold salts has been recommended for polyarticular or pauciarticular forms of JRA. The experience with gold in children is not nearly as large as that with salicylates but gold appears to be effective in children. Gold salts are given by weekly intramuscular injections. The starting dose is 2.5-5.0 mg of gold sodium thiomolate (Myochrysine) once weekly for 2 weeks and then a maintenance dose of 1 mg/kg/week (maximum of 25 mg for small children, 50 mg for children over 60 kg) thereafter for several months. The patient must be monitored weekly for any signs of toxicity, including leukopenia, anemia, thrombocytopenia, proteinuria, rash, or mouth ulcers. Response usually requires several months. If the patient responds within 6 months, he is placed on maintenance therapy (6,12).

Antimalarial drugs (chloroquin and hydroxychloroquin) can be used as an alternative to gold but must be monitored very carefully due to possible ocular toxicity. D-penicillamine is still considered an experimental drug in JRA (6,12).

Corticosteroids are indicated for: 1) the severe systemic form of JRA which is unresponsive to salicylates, 2) iridocyclitis unresponsive tc topical therapy, 3) and life-threatening disease such as severe pericarditis. Joint disease alone is rarely an indication for corticosteroids. The significant toxicity of the corticosteroids make them a double-edged sword and the benefit-risk ratio should be weighed carefully before they are prescribed (12) (see Table 19.5 for a summary of drug therapy).

TABLE 19.5 Drug Therapy for Juvenile Rheumatoid Arthritis

Drug Type	Drug	Dosage	Monitors
Nonsteroidal Antiinflammatory Agents	Aspirin	80-100 mg/kg/day 4 divided doses	Serum salicylate levels Acute toxicity (irritability, drowsiness, hyperactivity, GI upset) Chronic toxicity (hepatic)
	Tolmetin Sodium (Tolectin)	15 mg/kg/day starting dose 4 divided doses. Can increase to 30 mg/kg/day (maximum total daily dose 2 g)	
	Naproxen (Naprosyn)	10 mg/kg/day 2 divided doses (maximum total daily dose 1 g)	
Gold Salts	Gold Sodium Thiomolate Myochrysine	Starting dose 2.5-5 mg per week for 2 weeks then maintenance dose 1 mg/kg/week (maximum dose 25 mg for small children, 50 mg for children greater than 60 kg)	Bone marrow and kidney toxicity Rash Mouth ulcers
Antimalarials	Hydroxychloroquine Sulfate (Plaquenil)	6 mg/kg/day (maximum total daily doses not to exceed 200 mg/m^2 of body surface area)	Ocular toxicity
Corticosteroids	Prednisone	Start at maximum of 2 mg/kg/day not exceed 60 mg, rapidly return to as low a dose as possible to control disease—usually 1-6 mg/day	Growth failure Cataracts Osteoporosis

Ankylosing Spondylitis

Ankylosing spondylitis classically involves the sacroiliac joints and lumbodorsal spine resulting in stiffness and pain in the back. It is primarily a disease of young and middle-aged males; however, reports by Ladd (19), Bywaters (20), and Schaller (21) demonstrate that the disease can have its onset in childhood. The male predominance exists in childhood with Ladd reporting that 87% of his patients were male, Bywaters 82%, and Schaller 90%. In all three reports the age of onset was over 8 years in most cases. There is a high association between ankylosing spondylitis and histocompatibility antigen B27 (21).

The etiology of ankylosing spondylitis is not known. Pathologically, inflammatory granulomas are seen in the junction between cartilage and vascular tissue in both peripheral joints and spinal intervertebral disc lesions (20). Synovial pathology is similar to that of JRA. Ankylosing spondylitis is a familial disease.

Clinical Features

Ankylosing spondylitis may present in one of two ways in childhood. The onset may be fairly typical with severe pain and limitation of motion in the back and hip joints. Pain in the spine typically begins in the sacroiliac regions and ascends to the cervical spine. The more common presentation in children is that of peripheral joint involvement with the larger joints of the lower extremities being most typically affected. Heel pain is common. Other joints that can be involved are hands, feet, wrists, and shoulders. Progression of this presentation to the more typical back and hip girdle involvement may take from months to years. Acute iridocyclitis may occur in 25% of patients. Systemic symptoms of growth failure, anemia, and malaise may occur. Rheumatoid nodules are rare.

Although HLA B27 is present in 95% of patients, ANA and rheumatoid factors are classically negative. HLA B27 is not specific for this illness (see Chapters 1 and 10). Mild anemia and elevation of sedimentation rate may be found. Roentgenographic findings of calcification of spinal ligament give a "bamboo spine" appearance which is typical of ankylosing spondylitis but may appear late in the disease (21). Sacroiliac arthritis or fusion on x-ray is also a classical finding of ankylosing spondylitis and may be delayed but tends to appear before spinal changes (19).

The diagnosis of ankylosing spondylitis should be considered in any child with low back and hip girdle pain and stiffness, with or without peripheral arthritis. Loss of lumbar spine flexion and decreased chest expansion are suggestive findings. In addition, in patients with pauciarticular JRA who are HLA B27-positive or have acute uveitis or a positive family history for ankylosing spondylitis the diagnosis must be considered. At times prolonged follow-up may be the only way to establish a definitive diagnosis. Other conditions which should be considered and differentiated in patients with back and hip pain are spinal cord tumors, discitis, Scheuermann's disease, osteomyelitis, slipped capital femoral epiphysis, Legg-Perthes, and the spondyloarthropathies (6,20).

Prognosis and Management

Long-term follow-up is not available on most juvenile ankylosing spondylitis patients. Schaller (21) reported 75% of her patients to have good function 3-20 years after diagnosis. Attention to good posture with posture exercises, breathing exercises, and a firm mattress or bed board are all important in keeping the patient functional. The tendency of the disease is that the spine will develop flexion and cause disability. A brace may become necessary to help maintain good posture (20). Salicylates may be adequate for pain relief. Gold is not effective and corticosteroids are rarely indicated. Indomethacin and phenylbutazone are effective in adults but are not approved for use in children. Radiation of the spine is not suggested for children (6,20).

Other Spondyloarthropathies

Reiter's Disease

The classic triad of Reiter's disease is sterile urethritis, arthritis, and ocular inflammation (conjunctivitis, keratitis, or iritis). Incomplete Reiter's may be any part of the triad but is difficult to diagnose. Other symptoms of Reiter's are skin rash and gastroenteritis. Preceding dysentery seems to be a common feature of childhood Reiter's. Urethritis may be difficult to detect in children and has to be looked for carefully. Mucocutaneous ulcers around the urethral opening may be seen. Symptoms of the triad may occur sporadically making diagnosis of Reiter's less obvious (22). Russell (23), Singsen and Bernstein et al. (22) have reported Reiter's in children following *Yersinia enterocolitica,* Salmonella and Shigella infections. Sexual contact has been reported as a preceding event in adults and probably is in some children also. Gonococcal arthritis should be differentiated. The arthritis usually involves a few larger joints. Achilles tendonitis supports the diagnosis of Reiter's. The affected children are predominantly males. Laboratory tests may show a mild leukocytosis and elevated sedimentation rate. Rheumatoid factor and antinuclear antibodies are negative. HLA B27 is strongly associated. Roentgenographic examinations at the time of presentation are normal.

In general, both eye lesions and skin lesions appear to be milder in children (22). The majority of children will have self-limiting disease that will clear in a few months. A few may progress to ankylosing spondylitis or recurrent arthritis (6). Conjunctivitis and urethritis can also be recurrent. Salicylates are the treatment of choice in young children and other nonsteroidal antiinflammatory agents may be appropriate for older teenagers.

Arthritis of Inflammatory Bowel Disease

Arthritis is a common extraintestinal manifestation of inflammatory bowel disease. The incidence is reported to be 5-25% of patients with inflammatory bowel diseases. The etiology is not known. In a review, Lindsley (24) describes two types of arthritis: 1) the peripheral arthritis of a few larger joints which tends to occur when the intestinal disease is active, and 2) spondylitis which is a much more serious type of arthritis, may be progressive, and is associated with HLA B27 about 75% of the time.

Differential diagnosis is not difficult except when the arthritis precedes the intestinal manifestation. Mucocutaneous lesions may also coexist in inflammatory bowel disease. Laboratory studies reveal an elevated sedimentation rate and the presence of C-reactive protein. There are no antinuclear antibodies or rheumatoid factors present. Anemia frequently occurs and can be a clue to the diagnosis. Roentgenographs show soft tissue swelling and synovial fluid analysis reveals a mild leukocytosis.

The treatment of the peripheral arthritis is to diagnose and treat the inflammatory bowel disease, usually with corticosteroids. If arthritis occurs alone, salicylates may be used. With spondylitis, the treatment is the same as with ankylosing spondylitis.

Reactive Arthritis

Aho (25) reported a sterile arthritis following infection with *Yersinia enterocolitica,* a similar syndrome has been seen with Salmonella and Shigella. The larger peripheral joints are affected and HLA B27 is frequently associated. Whether this is an incomplete Reiter's disease is not known. The arthritis tends to be self-limited, but a few patients go on to develop a spondylitis picture.

Psoriatic Arthritis

Psoriatic arthritis occurs in children uncommonly considering that 35% of psoriasis starts during childhood. A report by Lambert, Ansell et al. (26) summarizes the findings in children. Arthritis usually develops at the same time or later than skin lesions but can precede the skin lesions by months or years. The mean age of onset is 12 years. The arthritis occurs in one or several joints. The most characteristically affected joints are the distal interphalangeal (DIP) joints producing a "sausage digit." The majority of the children with arthritis will have nail pitting. Rheumatoid factors and antinuclear antibodies are absent. In differentiating psoriatic arthritis from JRA, the children with psoriatic arthritis tend to have a later age of onset, DIP involvement, and few systemic manifestations. The majority of patients have a good prognosis although a few will develop ankylosing spondylitis associated with HLA B27. The therapy in children is salicylates and physical therapy.

Systemic Lupus Erythematosus

Systemic lupus erythematosus (SLE) is a progressive systemic collagen disease. The clinical manifestations are highly variable. In 1971, the Diagnostic and Therapeutic Criteria Committee of the American Rheumatism Association (27) published preliminary criteria for the classification of SLE. The proposed revisions of the criteria were published in 1982 (28) and are summarized in Chapter 13.

Epidemiology

SLE is not uncommon in childhood. Meislen and Rothfield (29,30) report that 32% of SLE patients develop symptoms before age 21 and 18% before age 16. SLE is rare in the very young child with perhaps only 5% of childhood SLE cases occurring before age 5 years. It is estimated that 35% of childhood SLE cases develop in the 5-10-year-old age groups, and 60% between the ages of 11 and 15 (31). The female predominance which occurs in adulthood is true for teenagers with a 9 to 1 female to male ratio. In the prepubertal child the ratio is 3 to 1 (30). All races are affected and there may be a slightly increased incidence among blacks (32). SLE has been thought to be a more severe and aggressive disease in children than in adults but recent studies have reported a more favorable outcome in many children (31).

Etiopathogenesis

The etiology of SLE is not known. Evidence suggests a multifactorial etiology with genetic and environmental factors playing important roles. The hallmark of SLE is a generalized excessive autoantibody reaction to a variety of nuclear, cytoplasmic, and serum protein antigens.

There appears to be a familial incidence in SLE with frequent reports of multicase families and identical twins with SLE (33,31). The genetic predisposition may be related to immunological abnormalities of T- and B-cell lymphocyte function. The immunopathology has been reviewed by Kunkel (34).

Environmental factors which have been proposed are ultraviolet light, infectious agents, and drugs (31). Drugs which are known to cause a lupus-like syndrome in children are hydralazine, sulfonamides, procainamide, and a number of anticonvulsants. The lupus-like syndrome is usually reversible when the drug is withdrawn.

The pathology of SLE shows multisystem disease with deposits of hematoxylin-stained material in affected tissues. Fibrinoid, a nonspecific, eosinophilic material, is found in loose connective tissues and blood vessel walls along with a mononuclear cell infiltrate. Granulomas can also be found (6). Renal biopsy material may reveal a variety of findings including minimal glomerulonephritis, mild (focal) segmental glomerulonephritis, severe (diffuse) proliferative glomerulonephritis and membranous nephritis (32).

Clinical Features

The most common presenting features of a child with SLE are fever, malaise, arthritis or arthralgia, and skin rash (30,32). Less specific complaints of weight loss, fatigue, headaches, and alopecia frequently are accompanying symptoms.

The arthritis of SLE is most frequently a polyarthritis involving most of the joints of the body and resembling JRA. However, the arthritis can be monoarticular, migrating (resembling rheumatic fever), or not uncommonly the patient may have pain without objective joint findings. Arthritis is frequently also accompanied by weakness and muscle fatigue (31). Permanent deformity as a result of the arthritis of SLE is rare (6).

The classic skin rash of SLE occurs in the malar areas in a butterfly distribution. The rash itself varies from a blush to bullous type lesions. The skin rash may involve any other part of the body but typically chest and extremities are next most likely to be involved. Nearly one-third of patients first report skin rash following sun exposures. Mucocutaneous lesions occur in nearly one-fourth of children with SLE and the combination of mucosal ulcers and skin rash suggests SLE (30). Alopecia is very frequently associated with the rash. Peripheral vascular changes resulting in macular lesions on the fingertips, palms, and soles occur and can ulcerate (6). Discoid lupus (cutaneous manifestations only) has been reported in children but is rare.

Involvement of the reticuloendothelial system was twice as common in Meislen and Rothfield's (29) series of children versus adults. Enlarged lymph nodes and hepatosplenomegaly are found in nearly 70% of children with SLE at the time of diagnosis (32).

Nervous system involvement is reported in 15-25% of children with SLE (31, 32). Symptoms of central nervous system involvement include chorea, psychosis, extreme muscle weakness, bowel and bladder incontinence, vertigo, tremors, headaches, ataxia, blindness, seizures, paraplegia, personality changes, and cerebral vascular accident. Peripheral neuropathy can also occur.

Other findings are polyserositis (pleurisy, pericarditis, and peritonitis) and cardiac findings including congestive heart failure and myocardial infarction. Pneumonia can occur but should be differentiated from pulmonary hemorrhage or fibrosis. Gastrointestinal findings include abdominal pain, vomiting, diarrhea, and bowel infarction.

Renal disease is probably present in nearly 100% of children with SLE if they are examined by renal biopsy (32). Approximately 70% have renal disease based on abnormal urinalysis (29). Interestingly, it appears that patients can change from one type of renal biopsy lesion to another making it difficult to give a prognosis based on type of lesion found on initial renal biopsy. (Further discussion of renal disease in Chapter 13).

Diagnosis and Differential Diagnosis

Because SLE is a multisystem disease it can be confused with many other disorders. The diagnosis is primarily a clinical one but laboratory tests can be exremely helpful. Antinuclear antibody is present in virtually 100% of SLE patients. The majority of the time it is present in high titer and this is extremely suggestive of the diagnosis of SLE. Renal disease is uncommon in JRA. In the presence of renal disease a renal biopsy may be necessary to differentiate SLE from JRA. Leukopenia and thrombocytopenia are common in SLE and rare in JRA. Other laboratory studies: LE cells, positive Coombs test, hypergammaglobulinemia, anemia, and a false positive test for syphilis may suggest SLE.

Laboratory Features

Anemia, leukopenia, and thrombocytopenia are all seen frequently in SLE. In a routine urinalysis the presence of red cells, white cells, red cell casts, and protein is compatible with SLE. If the urinalysis is normal early in the disease, it should be repeated frequently. Erythrocyte sedimentation rate is elevated in almost all children with active SLE.

The best test to rule out the diagnosis of SLE is the antinuclear antibody since a negative ANA using the child's undiluted serum should alert the clinician to seek another diagnosis (30). A peripheral pattern on the ANA is more specific for SLE, with diffuse and speckled patterns being less specific for SLE. Antibodies to double-stranded DNA and SM antigen are more specific, but less sensitive for SLE. LE preps, VDRL, and complement levels may also be useful in the diagnosis of SLE. The findings are similar to that seen in adults (see Chapter 13). If the diagnosis of SLE is considered clinically the above tests can be very useful in confirming the diagnosis and as a baseline in following the patient (30).

Prognosis and Mangement

Prognosis

The prognosis for children with SLE used to be very poor. Gradually with increased awareness of the spectrum of the disease and drug therapy, survival is improving. A recent study by Abeles (35) reports a 5-year survival of 85% in children with diffuse proliferative lupus nephritis and 100% in children with focal or membranous lupus nephritis. Major causes of death are renal disease, infections, central nervous system LE, and pulmonary LE (31). The risk of infection in SLE patients must be kept in mind by the physician since fatal complications are potentially preventable.

Management

Children with mild SLE and no evidence of renal disease can be managed symptomatically if they are monitored carefully for progressive disease. Arthritis alone may respond to aspirin. The mainstay of therapy for systemic disease is corticosteroids, usually prednisone given initially in a dose of 1.0-2.0 mg/kg/day in four divided doses. The prednisone is then gradually tapered until small daily doses or alternate day doses are achieved. Monitoring serum complement (C_3) levels, the antinuclear antibodies, and the erythrocyte sedimentation rate can be helpful in tapering the drug or anticipating relapse (6,30,33). Immunosuppressive agents have been recommended as therapeutic adjuncts but their use is experimental and should be recommended only in severe disease uncontrolled by corticosteroids.

Mixed Connective Tissue Disease

Mixed connective tissue disease (MCTD) was first described by Sharp (36) in 1970. It is a connective tissue disease which combines features of SLE, scleroderma, dermatomyositis, and rheumatoid arthritis. In addition, antibodies to extractable nuclear antigen (ENA) and high titers of a speckled pattern to antinuclear antibody are detected. A number of children with MCTD have now been reported (33,37). The most common symptoms in children appear to be polyarthritis, skin changes suggesting scleroderma, fever, Raynaud's phenomenon, cardiac involvement (most often pericarditis), rash suggestive of SLE or dermatomyositis, myositis, abnormal esophageal motility, lymphadenopathy, hepatosplenomegaly, pulmonary disease, renal disease, thrombocytopenia, neurological abnormalities, and salivary gland involvement.

There is evidence that MCTD is not a mild disease in many children. Therapy is similar to that for SLE, JRA, or scleroderma. Some children with mild disease can be managed with salicylates alone. Children with severe disease will require corticosteroids (33,37).

Dermatomyositis

Definition and Epidemiology

Dermatomyositis is a disease characterized by nonsuppurative inflammation of the skin and skeletal muscle. The etiology is unknown. Dermatomyositis is classified with the collagen diseases because features such as joint involvement are similar and the pathologic features resemble those of the collagen diseases. Unlike adults, there is no association with malignancy and dermatomyositis in children. Dermatomyositis was first described in adults in 1887 and a number of recent reports have included children (38,39,40). There appears to be a slight female predominance 3:2. The mean age of onset is 6-8 years with the disease being rare in children less than 1 year. There are a few reports of dermatomyositis in siblings.

Polymyositis is rare in children but when it occurs, the clinical course is identical to that of dermatomyositis except for absence of the skin rash. The majority of children have a skin rash and it is not clear whether polymyositis and dermatomyositis are distant entities in children but may, in fact, represent a common disease spectrum (40).

Etiopathogenesis

The etiology of dermatomyositis is uncertain. There is some evidence that a defective cellular immune system is involved (39). Histocompatibility antigen B8 has been found in 72% of children with dermatomyositis (41).

Banker (42) has reported a diffuse vasculitis involving primarily the small arteries, venules, and capillaries of skin, muscle, fat, nerves, and gastrointestinal tract. There may be foci of necrosis resulting from ischemia in the muscle. Areas of muscle regeneration may also be present. In the skin, there is perivascular lymphocytic infiltration and thinning of the epidermis. There is also dermal edema. In the subcutaneous tissues the areas of inflammatory infiltrate also show deposition of calcium, suggesting that the calcific nodules are related to the vasculitis (38). Deposits of IgG, IgM and C_3 have been demonstrated in the walls and blood vessels in dermatomyositis (43).

Clinical Features

The cardinal symptom of dermatomyositis is symmetrical muscle weakness involving the proximal muscles of the limbs. Muscles may also be painful and tender. The onset is most frequently insidious and parents are alarmed when the child suddenly cannot perform normal tasks and begins to fall a lot (33,38). The following are characteristic skin lesions in dermatomyositis: 1) heliotrope hue of upper eyelids, 2) symmetrical, erythematous, or violaceous eruption of extensor surfaces of joints and, 3) a butterfly rash on the face and rash on the chest resembling SLE (see Chapter 16).

Calcinosis occurs usually after a number of months of disease activity in dermatomyositis. Calcium is deposited in the skin, fat, fascia, and subcutaneous tissue in approximately half the patients. The calcinosis can occur in sheets limiting the motion of joints or occur in lumps which can become painful, inflamed and may open and drain calcium.

Fever is another common sign of dermatomyositis in children. Other symptoms which can be seen are dysphagia which can lead to aspiration and death. Arthritis occurs in 25% of children. Gastrointestinal involvement is not uncommon and a serious complication of gut perforation can occur (38). Interstitial pneumonia can be another serious complication. Carditis, retinitis, and renal manifestations can occur but are less common in children.

Diagnosis and Differential Diagnosis

The diagnosis of dermatomyositis is a clinical one. The triad of symmetrical proximal muscle weakness, muscle tenderness, and typical skin rash should make the diagnosis fairly obvious. Elevation of muscle enzymes (CPK and SGOT) are useful supporting laboratory data. Electromyography can also be helpful in diagnosis.

The differential diagnosis includes other inflammatory myopathies such as trichinosis and transient viral myositis which has been reported following influenza A and B, Coxsackie, Epstein Barr, adenovirus, and hepatitis B infections (33). These illnesses do not have skin rashes compatible with the diagnosis of dermatomyositis.

Other collagen diseases can be confused with dermatomyositis. The most likely to be confused are SLE, JRA, and scleroderma but usually careful clinical observation and laboratory studies will distinguish these. Other disorders to be considered are myasthenia gravis, poliomyelitis, Guillain-Barré and muscular dystrophy.

Laboratory Features

Routine laboratory studies are nondiagnostic in dermatomyositis. A mild non-hemolytic, microcytic, hypochromic anemia and leukocytosis may occur. An elevated erythrocyte sedimentation rate occurs in 60% of patients (39). Antinuclear antibodies and rheumatoid factors are present infrequently, and if they occur, are in low titer. Serum enzyme levels of SGOT, CPK, and aldolase are usually elevated. Routine urinalysis is normal but a 24-hour urine collection shows elevated levels of creatinine.

Electromyography findings include fibrillations and positive spike potentials compatible with inflammatory myopathy (39). Electromyography is positive in nearly all patients. Muscle biopsy can be diagnostic but is usually not necessary for diagnosis in typical cases.

Radiographic examinations reveal the presence of calcium in the soft tissues either in sheets or lumps (see Figure 19.3). Technetium bone scan can also identify the presence of calcium in soft tissues.

Prognosis and Management

Prognosis

The prognosis for the majority of children with dermatomyositis is good and appears to be better than the prognosis in adults. Most will survive and very few will not recover normal or near normal function. The improving prognosis is attributable to vigorous and early use of corticosteroids.

Management

Corticosteroids are the mainstay of therapy. Dubowitz (44) has summarized the successful use of steroids: "1) high-dosage corticosteroid is essential to produce remission, 2) initial high-dosage therapy needs to be continued until full remission is produced, 3) subsequent long-term, low-dosage maintenance therapy is essential to prevent relapse, and 4) response to therapy can be monitored by the fall in serum enzyme levels." Prednisone is used in dosages of 1-2 mg/kg/day or 60 mg/M^2/day. With this therapy, muscle enzymes will usually return to normal in 2 weeks and patients will seem well at the end of several months. The prednisone is then tapered slowly. If muscle weakness or elevation of enzymes recur the corticosteroids should be increased. Therapy with steroids will usually be needed for 1-2 years. Other immunosuppressive agents are rarely necessary.

During the acute phase of the disease, the muscles of respiration and swallowing may be weak. Supportive care and monitoring are extremely important during this time. Physical therapy to increase muscle strength and prevent joint deformity is important.

Scleroderma

Scleroderma is the name for a group of disorders that have as their primary feature a hardening of the skin and subcutaneous tissue. It is believed to be a chronic inflammation of the connective tissue. At least two-thirds of children with scleroderma are female. The etiology of scleroderma is unknown. Scleroderma, in general, is rare in children. There are two types of scleroderma: localized scleroderma and progressive systemic sclerosis. The latter form is the classic adult form and occasionally does occur in children (33).

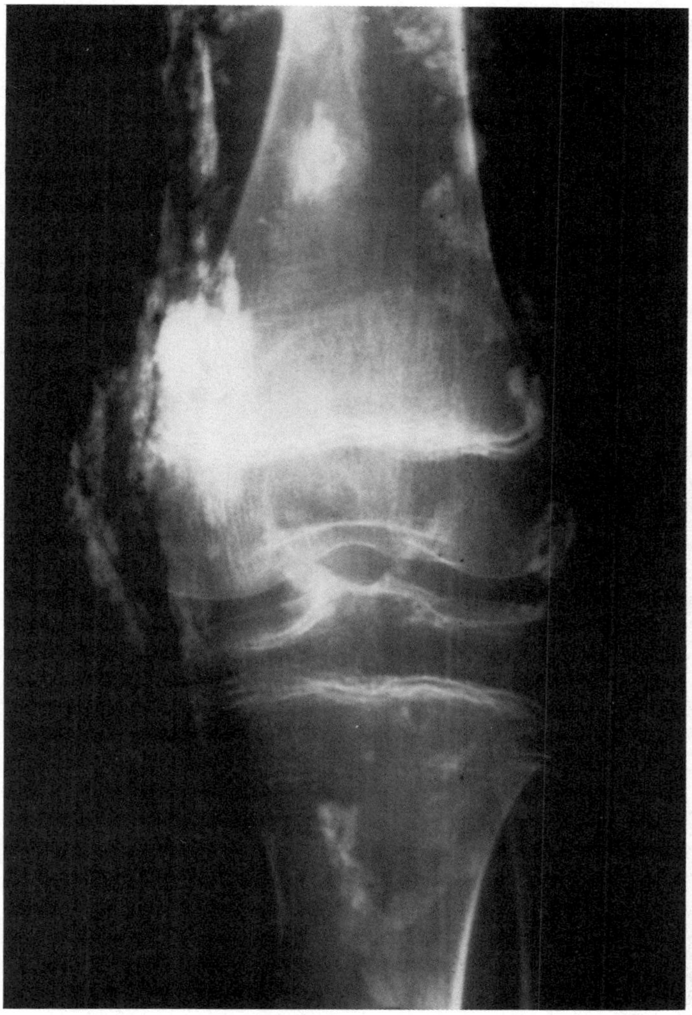

FIGURE 19.3 A radiograph demonstrating soft tissue calcification around the knee in an 8-year-old boy with dermatomyositis.

Clinical Manifestations

Localized Scleroderma, Linear Scleroderma, Morphea

The skin lesion of localized scleroderma starts as an indurated, erythematous or bluish area or lump. Pruritis may be associated with the lesion. The lesion gradually progresses to a hardened and thickened area with increased or decreased pigmentation. The lesion may become linear and progress to involve an entire extremity. Ulcerations may occur in the distal part of the extremity and with severe involvement the limb may wither and amputation may be necessary. In the final stages, the skin lesion atrophies and softens leaving the skin thin, and superificial veins are prominently seen (38) (see Figure 19.4).

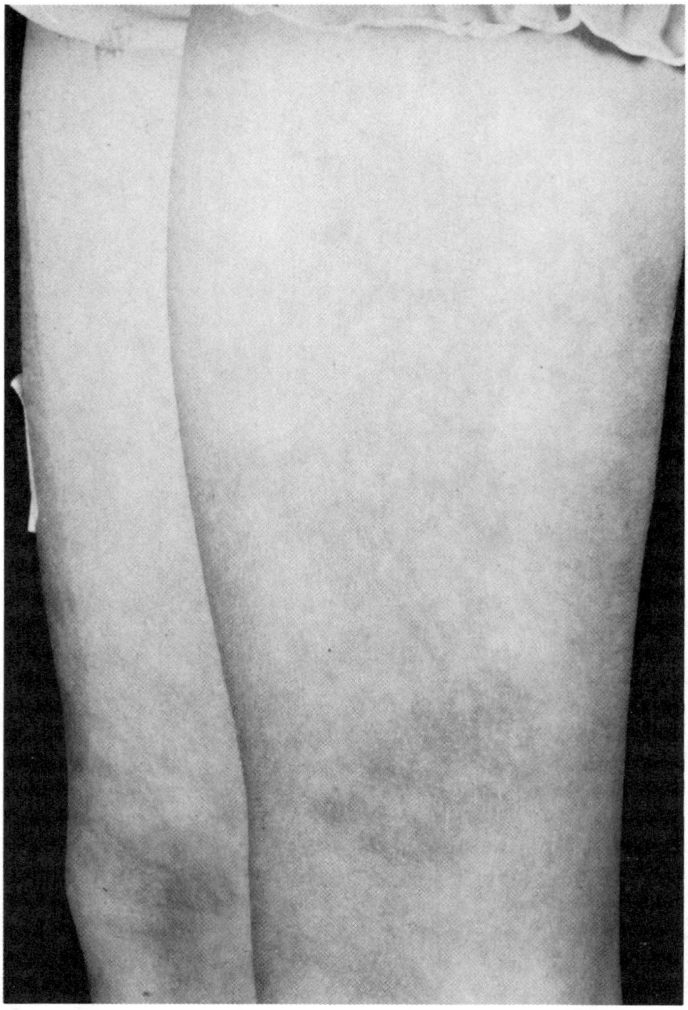

FIGURE 19.4 The final stages of localized scleroderm in a 13-year-old girl. There is atrophy of the skin with prominence of the superficial veins.

Localized scleroderma may occur on the trunk, face and scalp as well as on an extremity. The lesions on the extremities tend to be the most severe, although the *coup de sabre* lesion of the scalp and face can be quite disfiguring. Children with localized scleroderma can present with polyarthritis, usually less symptomatic than the arthritis seen in JRA.

The underlying tissue including subcutaneous tissue, muscle, bone, synovium, and blood vessels may become involved. Very rarely the disease may progress to the systemic sclerosis form. In general, the prognosis for localized scleroderma is good for normal life expectancy but significant disability and disfigurement may occur. There is a tendency toward improvement after 2-3 years but the disease may smolder for years and new lesions may occur later in the course of the disease (38,45,46).

Progressive Systemic Sclerosis (PSS)

This condition is rare in children but does occur and when it occurs the course is indistinguishable from that of the adult with PSS. Preliminary criteria for the diagnosis of PSS were published in 1980 (47). To summarize, the criteria include the major criterion of proximal scleroderma or two or more of the minor criteria: sclerodactyly, pitting scars of the fingertips or loss of distal finger pads, or bilateral basilar pulmonary fibrosis.

Presenting symptoms frequently include diffuse hardening of the skin, most commonly of the fingers and face, Raynaud's phenomenon, contractures of the joints, and arthralgias. Dysphagia, subcutaneous calcification, dyspnea, and muscle weakness are found less commonly (48). As the disease progresses any organ system can become involved. Extensive diagnostic testing such as barium studies of the gastrointestinal tract, esophageal motility studies, pulmonary function tests, and plethysmography can help reveal the extent of the disease. The true prognosis for PSS in children is probably not known due to the rarity of the condition. Mortality figures from 20 to 40% are quoted. Involvement of lung, heart, or kidneys is the usual cause of death in fatal cases. Sudden spontaneous improvements later in the course of the disease have been noted (38,45,48).

Laboratory Manifestations

No specific laboratory tests exist for either localized or systemic forms of scleroderma. Routine laboratory values are normal. Rheumatoid factors and antinuclear antibodies are common. The skin biopsy in both localized and systemic scleroderma reveals large amounts of collagen in and beneath the dermis and a mononuclear cell infiltrate (38).

Diagnosis and Differential Diagnosis

The diagnosis of both forms of scleroderma is a clinical one. Usually the appearance of the skin, clinical course, and skin biopsy can distinguish between scleroderma and other similar-appearing diseases such as subcutaneous fat necrosis or Weber-Christian nonsuppuratic panniculitis. The arthritis of scleroderma is not as severe as that of JRA, and the skin lesions of dermatomyositis are quite different from those of scleroderma. Scleroderma adultorum is seen following infections, usually streptococcal infections, and produces a self-limiting induration of the skin of the neck, upper trunk, and arms (6). Eosinophilic fasciitis has been reported as a type of scleroderma that is very responsive to corticosteroids. It can usually be distinguished from scleroderma by the rapidly progressive fasciitis and the eosinophilia seen in peripheral blood and bone marrow (33,49).

Treatment

There is no known effective treatment for scleroderma. Localized scleroderma has been treated with topical corticosteroids. Severe systemic sclerosis can be treated with corticosteroids, penicillamine, or immunosuppressive agents (azathioprine or cyclophosphamide). There is no conclusive evidence that these drugs are effective. Supportive treatment as well as vigorous occupational and physical therapy are definitely recommended (45). Surgical treatment of localized scleroderma is controversial.

Vasculitis Syndromes

Inflammation of the blood vessels is the cause of the vasculitis syndromes. The rheumatic diseases discussed in this chapter all have vasculitis as a part of a complex disease process. In the vasculitis syndromes, the predominant pathologic process is vasculitis and the clinical manifestations are a result of the damage resulting from the vasculitis. The cause of these disorders is not fully known although exposure to foreign substances, drugs, or allergens can play a part in serum sickness, Schönlein-Henoch purpura, and polyarteritis. The vasculitis syndromes include allergic vasculitis (Schönlein-Henoch purpura, serum-sickness-like reactions), Wegener's granulomatosis, giant cell arthritis (Takayashu's disease), Behcet's syndrome, polyarteritis nodosa, Kawasaki's disease, and others. The vasculitis syndromes are reviewed in detail by Schaller and Wedgewood (6), and Jacobs (33). There is some overlap of the syndromes. Four of the more common vasculitis syndromes will be discussed here.

Schönlein-Henoch Vasculitis

Schönlein-Henoch vasculitis, also called anaphylactoid purpura or allergic purpura, is by far the most common vasculitis syndrome in children. Allergy or drug sensitivity can be implicated in some cases but in the majority of patients the cause is not known. Pathologically, there is inflammation of the small blood vessels of the skin, joints, gastrointestinal tract, and kidneys. The disease can occur at any age but tends to occur in young children with a peak age of 5 years. Males are affected 2:1 over females. Symptoms may last from a few days to several months.

Clinical Features

The rash of Schönlein-Henoch purpura is the most typical feature and best clue to diagnosis. The location of the rash is primarily on the buttocks and legs. Occasionally the rash may extend to include the face, arms, and trunk. The rash may take many forms with a mixture of petechiae, urticaria, purpura, and fading brown spots being typical (see Figure 19.5). Occasionally, bullous lesions can occur. Localized patches of edema also occur with involvement of the dorsum of hands and feet, ankles, face, and scalp being fairly typical locations. Edema of the genitalia can occur.

Arthritis occurs in over 50% of children with Schönlein-Henoch purpura. Joints typically involved are knees and ankles, and the arthritis may be migratory. The arthritis usually spontaneously resolves in a few days but may recur if the disease remains active.

Abdominal pain occurs due to the vasculitis of the gastrointestinal tract. Cramping can be severe and blood in the stools is common although significant blood loss is rare. An area of vasculitis can serve as a lead point for an intussusception. If abdominal pain occurs before the onset of other symptoms the diagnosis can be very difficult and may lead to surgical exploration.

Microscopic hematuria occurs in nearly half of the patients with Schönlein-Henoch purpura. Occasionally, nephritis with hematuria, proteinuria, and hypertension can occur but usually has a good prognosis. Nephrotic syndrome can be associated infrequently and has a poor prognosis. Serious renal disease tends to occur more commonly in older patients and in those whose other clinical symptoms are more severe (50).

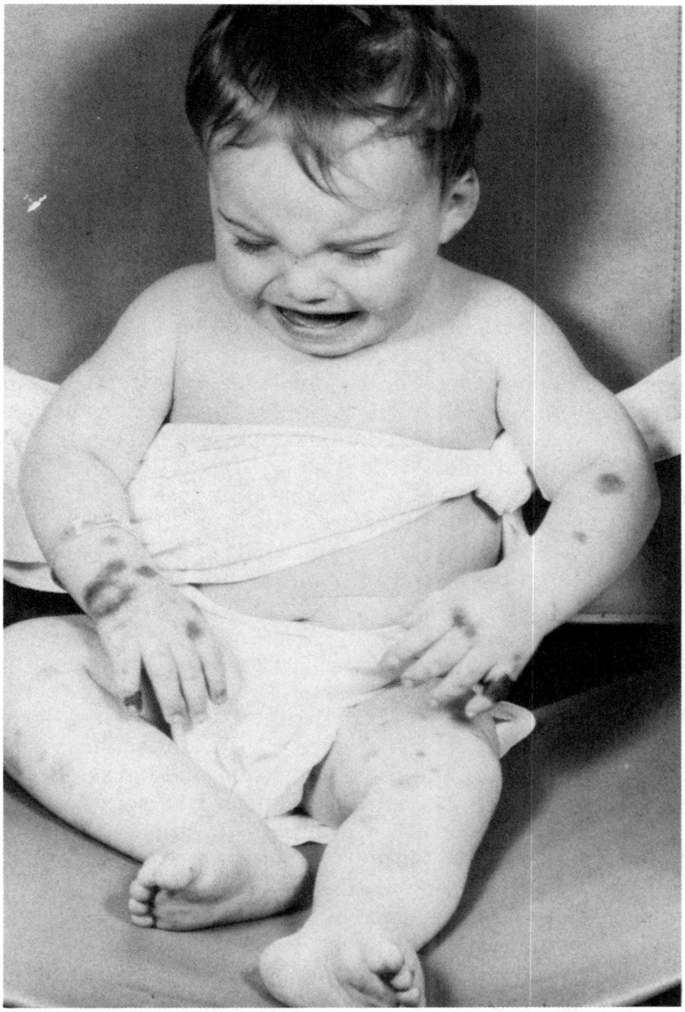

FIGURE 19.5 A 12-month-old boy with the skin rash of Schönlein-Henoch vasculitis. The photograph demonstrates the typical location of the rash on the extremities and the many forms of the rash including petechiae, purpura, and fading brown macules.

Diagnosis and Differential Diagnosis

The diagnosis of Schönlein-Henoch purpura is a clinical one and, if the typical rash is present, is not difficult. Laboratory studies can differentiate idiopathic thrombocytopenic purpura. The arthritis does not usually last long enough to be confused with JRA. The absence of antinuclear antibody distinguishes Schönlein-Henoch purpura from SLE.

Laboratory Findings

Laboratory studies in Schönlein-Henoch purpura are most helpful in eliminating other disease states. Normal platelet counts and coagulation studies are reassuring. A routine urinalysis may reveal blood and/or protein. Immunofluorescent studies of the skin may reveal deposits of immunoglobulin (51). If severe kidney disease occurs, renal biopsy material may also reveal deposits of immunoglobulin, complement, and fibrin around the glomerular basement membrane (50).

Prognosis and Management

The prognosis for Schönlein-Henoch purpura is excellent. Except for occasional patients who develop chronic nephritis, the symptoms are self-limiting. Treatment of this disease is supportive therapy only in the majority of cases. Corticosteroids are not helpful in treatment of the nephritis. In chronic progressive nephritis a renal biopsy is necessary. Immunosuppressive agents may be tried although there are no good studies to document efficacy of this treatment. With severe abdominal pain and bleeding, prednisone in a dose of 1-2 mg/kg/day is helpful. Symptoms generally subside rapidly and steroids should be tapered within a few weeks (51). In our experience, tapering of the steroids may lead to recurrence of the abdominal pain and we prefer not to use steroids unless pain is very severe.

Serum Sickness

An allergy induced by exposure to foreign protein such as horse serum can cause an immediate or delayed reaction. The classic form of serum sickness occurs 8-12 days following injection of the foreign protein and causes fever, rash, and pain and swelling of the joints. The serum sickness-like reactions seen today are more likely to be due to a drug or other allergen which may or may not be identified. These patients present with urticaria or erythema multiforme lesions. They frequently have angioneurotic type swelling of hands and feet and may have swelling, pain, and stiffness of the large joints. The joints are usually without heat or erythema. The erythrocyte sedimentation rate is usually normal.

Most of the serum sickness-like reactions are self-limiting after a few days. Antihistamines will help control the rash and aspirin can be used for painful joints. Corticosteroids are rarely indicated (33,50).

Polyarteritis Nodosa

Polyarteritis nodosa is a vasculitis involving the small and medium-sized arteries. It is rare in children but can affect any age group. The cause of polyarteritis nodosa is unknown but allergy to drugs or response to viral or streptococcal infections has been suggested in some cases (6).

The involved arteries, such as coronary, which have been studied show four stages of the vasculitis: 1) necrosis, edema, and fibrin deposition in the media, 2) intense infiltrate with neutrophils, macrophages, and plasma cells of the entire arterial wall and adventitia with rapid formation of aneurysms, 3) proliferation and regenerative change, and 4) scarring and healing. Deposition of gamma globulin and complement has been seen and suggests a possible immunopathogenic mechanism (38).

In children common clinical findings are fever, leukocytosis, abdominal pain, skin rash, hypertension, and arthralgia. However, a wide variety of symptoms can be produced depending on the organ system involved (6,38).

The diagnosis of polyarteritis is best made by biopsy, EKG or renal arteriographic studies. Prognosis is generally poor. Treatment with corticosteroids is indicated in proven cases and antihypertensive medication should be used if hypertension occurs.

Kawasaki Syndrome

Kawasaki syndrome was first described in Japan in 1967 and was called mucocutaneous lymph node syndrome. The first report from the United States was by Melish et al. (52). Although the disease has occurred worldwide, it has a marked prevalence for Japanese children. The disease occurs primarily in young children with half of the patients being less than 2 years of age and 80% less than 4 years of age. Males predominate in a ratio of 1.5:1. A number of possible etiologies have been proposed but to date the cause of Kawasaki syndrome is unknown. Outbreaks do occur primarily in late winter and spring (53,54). The pathology is identical to the infantile form of polyarteritis nodosa.

A set of diagnostic criteria have been established by the Center for Disease Control. A patient must have five of the six clinical criteria: "1) fever for more than 5 days; 2) bulbar conjunctival injection; 3) changes in the mouth (erythema, fissuring, and crusting of the lips; strawberry tongue, diffuse oropharyngeal erythema); 4) changes in the peripheral extremities (induration of hands and feet, erythema of palms and soles, desquamation of tips of fingers and toes approximately 2 weeks from onset of illness, transverse grooves across fingernails 2-3 months after onset of illness); 5) erythematous rash on trunk and/or extremities; 6) enlarged lymph node mass > 1.5 cm in diameter" (54). Ninety percent of patients will have the first five criteria and 50% will have lymph node enlargement. Other associated clinical findings include pyuria, arthralgia or arthritis, diarrhea, abdominal pain, aseptic meningitis, carditis, hepatitis, obstructive jaundice, and hydrops of the gallbladder. The clinical symptoms occur in three phases. The first phase consists of fever, conjunctival injection, mouth lesions, edema of hands and feet, rash, and lymph node enlargement. In the second phase, approximately 10 days after onset of illness, the rash and fever tend to subside and arthritis and carditis can develop. During the second phase death may occur from coronary artery aneurysm. The third phase starts approximately 25 days after onset and is a convalescent phase with gradual return of the erythrocyte sedimentation rate to normal.

The diagnosis of Kawasaki syndrome is a clinical one and is not difficult if criteria are strictly followed. A number of infectious diseases including leptospirosis, streptococcal disease, Rocky Mountain spotted fever, and measles can be included in the differential diagnosis. Appropriate cultures and serologic tests should be performed to help in the differential.

Laboratory studies in Kawasaki syndrome are too variable to be diagnostic. During the early phase, total white blood cell counts are usually elevated, frequently to the 20,000-30,000 mm^3 range with an increase in polymorphonuclear forms. Sedimentation rate and C-reactive protein are elevated during the febrile phase and gradually return to normal in about 6-10 weeks. During the second phase of the illness, thrombocytosis occurs with platelet counts from 600,000 to 1.8 million. Quantitative immunoglobulins may show an acute rise (54).

Prognosis is good for full recovery except in the case of cardiac involvement. Nearly 20% of children will show some evidence of cardiac disease. Two-dimensional echocardiography or cornonary angiography can help diagnose coronary artery aneurysms. Two percent of patients will die from massive myocardial infarction due to coronary artery involvement. Another 5% have been reported to have persistent coronary artery disease. The treatment of Kawasaki syndrome is salicylates. Salicylates are recommended at 80-100 mg/kg/day and can produce defervescence usually in 2-3 days. After the fever has disappeared or the platelet count has risen, salicylate dosage should be reduced to 20 mg/kg/day. Corticosteroids are believed to be contraindicated by some because of a possible increase in coronary artery aneurysms following the use of steroids (33). Careful monitoring of the patient during the acute illness for development of carditis is indicated and prolonged follow-up of children with coronary aneurysms is recommended (54).

Rheumatic Fever

Introduction and Definition

Rheumatic fever (RF) is an inflammatory disease which is a nonsuppurative complication of a group A streptococcal pharyngitis. It tends to involve primarily the joints and heart. There has been a marked decrease in the incidence of rheumatic fever in the developed nations of the world in the past 10 years. In addition, when the disease occurs now it is a milder form of the disease than was once seen. Reasons for the decline are not totally understood but include a combination of factors: improving socioeconomic conditions, use of antibiotics to treat streptococcal infections and prevent recurrences of RF, and decreasing rheumatogenic potential of a group A beta hemolytic streptococcus. However, it should be noted that RF continues to be a major source of morbidity and mortality in the third world nations and among the disadvantaged in the United States (55,56,57).

Historical Aspects

Rheumatic fever was described in the seventeenth century as acute articular rheumatism but it was 1836 before the description of RF and heart disease was published. Cheadle described the major manifestations of RF 50 years later and in 1931 the streptococcal etiology was established. The relationship between treating streptococcal infection and preventing rheumatic fever was reported within the next 20 years (56). Jones formulated criteria for the diagnosis of RF in 1944. These were modified in 1955 and 1965 by the American Heart Association's Council on Rheumatic Fever and Congenital Heart Disease (14) (Table 19.6).

Epidemiology

The current incidence of RF in the United States is 10/100,000 or less (58). As was alluded to in the introduction, the annual incidence in Denmark fell from 200/100,000 in 1862 to 70/100,000 in 1940 and 10/100,000 in 1962 (55).

The incidence of acute RF and rheumatic heart disease continues to be quite high in less developed nations. In Egypt where crowding is common, rheumatic fever is frequent and reported mortality for acute RF is 1.0/100,000 and for rheumatic heart disease it is 27.5/100,000 (57).

TABLE 19.6 Jones Criteria for the Diagnosis of Rheumatic Fever (Revised) (20)

Major Manifestations:	Minor Manifestations:
Carditis	Clinical
Polyarthritis	Fever
Chorea	Arthralgia
Erythema margination	Previous rheumatic fever or rheumatic heart disease
Subcutaneous nodules	Laboratory
	Elevated ESR or positive CRP or leukocytosis
	Prolonged PR interval

Plus

Supporting evidence of preceding streptococcal infection: recent scarlet fever; positive throat culture for group A streptococcus; increased titers of antistreptococcal antibodies.

Rheumatic fever is rare in children under age 2 years. The peak incidence is in the 5-15-year age group, or school-aged child. The incidence is highest in late winter and early spring, parelleling the incidence of streptococcal pharyngitis. RF does have a familial tendency. Although the reasons for this are not known, it would appear that genetic and environmental factors are involved (56). Incidence in males and females is equal. There does not appear to be a higher incidence of RF in blacks if environmental factors are controlled. Living in poverty is a high risk factor for RF (59).

Etiopathogenesis

Both initial and recurrent attacks of rheumatic fever result from group A streptococcal infections of the upper respiratory tract. Streptococcal skin infections, particularly impetigo, can result in acute glomerulonephritis but not rheumatic fever. There is a 2-5 week latent period between the streptococcal infection and the onset of RF; therefore, it may be difficult to culture the organism. The preceding streptococcal infection can be documented by comfirming the presence of an elevated streptococcal antibody titer (56).

There are a number of theories regarding how streptococci cause rheumatic fever. These have been reviewed by McCarty (60). One of the theories is that there is actual bacterial invasion of the affected tissues by streptococci, but this theory has never been proved and is less popular than it once was.

Another theory is that one of the streptococcal substances such as streptolysin S causes a direct toxic effect on involved tissues. No evidence has been found to support this hypothesis. Another thought is that streptolysin O combines with antibody to form antigen-antibody complex and that the streptolysin O is released after the latent period to damage tissues. Supporting evidence for this theory is the knowledge that RF does not follow streptococcal skin infections and that the antistreptolysin O (ASO) titer in skin infections is only mildly elevated. In addition, streptolysin O is cardiotoxic in tissue cultures and in animals (55).

The most favored theory is that RF is an autoimmune disease. There are now a number of examples of antibodies produced in response to streptococcal antigens that cross-react with natural antigens in human tissues. Whether in fact these shared antigens cause tissue damage is not clear (55).

Clinical Features

The major and minor clinical manifestations of RF are outlined in Table 19.6. The variability in the clinical findings is determined by the sites involved, the time of appearance during the course of illness, and when the patient presents for examination (59).

Seventy-five percent of RF patients will present acutely with joint complaints. These vary from arthralgia to frank arthritis. The knees, ankles, elbows, and wrists are most commonly involved. The joint findings are frequently disproportionate to the pain. Joints are often exquisitely tender with the slightest applied pressure causing the child to cry with pain. Classically, the joint involvement is a migratory polyarthritis with each joint being involved for 1-5 days but several joints may be involved at one time. If antiinflammatory agents are used the migratory picture can be obscured. The joint findings usually subside in 2-4 weeks without treatment and RF never causes permanent joint deformity with the rare exception of Jaccoud's deformity. Jaccoud's deformity occurs so rarely that its relationship to rheumatic fever is not clearly understood. Children with severe arthritis are less likely to develop carditis (59).

Carditis is by far the most serious manifestation because of the potential for acute mortality as well as long-term morbidity or mortality. Carditis occurs in 40-50% of cases of acute RF. The appearance of carditis is variable. It may be obvious on first examination or may appear within the first 2 weeks. Rarely, carditis may be diagnosed late in the course of acute RF or as a heart murmur after the acute disease has passed, apparently undetected. The incidence and severity of carditis are greater in the patient with insidious onset than in the patient with frank arthritis and high fever. Occasionally, active carditis may be detected in a patient who presents with chorea.

The classical signs of carditis are: 1) significant new murmurs, 2) cardiac enlargement, 3) cardiac failure, and 4) pericardial friction rub or effusion (59). A tachycardia out of proportion to that seen with fever is also suggestive of RF. The classical murmurs found in acute RF are the apical high pitched, blowing, holosystolic murmur of mitral valvulitis which may be accompanied by a low-pitched middiastolic (Carey-Coombs) murmur. A decrescendo diastolic murmur along the left sternal border indicates aortic regurgitation and is less frequent. Carditis generally lasts from 6 weeks to 6 months.

Chorea may occur in conjunction with other manifestations of RF or as the sole manifestation. The incidence of chorea in RF has declined from 52 to 10% over the past 40-50 years. Because chorea is frequently a late manifestation, patients are usually afebrile and acute phase reactants are normal. The latent period for chorea can be from 1 to 6 months after the streptococcal infection and streptococcal antibodies are also frequently absent. Emotional instability, deteriorating school performance, and personality changes are frequently noted prior to the onset of frank chorea. Difficulty in writing is frequently an early finding. Gradually, incoordination develops followed by spasmodic, jerky, and rapid movements. The upper extremities and face are most commonly involved. Weakness may also occur. Speech is indistinct. Mild cases of chorea can last only a week with severe cases lasting 6 months to 1 year. Chorea does not occur in children under age 3 and is rare after puberty. It most often occurs in females (57,59).

Subcutaneous nodules are also relatively rare, occurring in only 5-10% of RF cases. They usually occur in association with severe carditis. The nodules are hard, painless, freely moveable and range in size from a B-B to that of a marble. The common locations are over the extensor surfaces of the joints (elbows, knuckles, knees, ankles) and over the scalp and shoulder blades (57,59).

Erythema marginatum occurs in fewer than 5% of children with RF. It is a characteristic skin rash which starts as a small, pink, slightly raised macule and takes the form of an enlarging ring or coalescing wavy lines. The rash occurs primarily on the trunk, buttocks, and extremities. Like subcutaneous nodules, it tends to occur in the presence of carditis (56,57).

Fever in an acute attack varies from 38.3 to 40°C (101-104°F) in no particular pattern. It may be low grade in the insidious form of RF. Abdominal pain and epistaxis are two less common manifestations (56).

Diagnosis and Differential Diagnosis

The modified Jones criteria (Table 19.6) are an excellent guide to the correct diagnosis of RF. The criteria required are two of the major criteria (carditis, polyarthritis, chorea, erythema marginatum, and subcutaneous nodules) or one major and two minor (fever, arthralgia, previous RF or rheumatic heart disease, elevated ESR or positive CRP or leukocytosis, prolonged PR interval) plus evidence of a preceding streptococcal infection. It is true that any set of criteria is not perfect and there are probably patients with RF who do not meet the Jones criteria and those who meet the Jones criteria but do not have RF. However, if careful clinical observation is combined with the criteria, they will be accurate in most cases (57).

With the decline in carditis, subcutaneous nodules, chorea, and erythema marginatum, there are increasing numbers of RF patients who will have arthritis alone as a major criterion. In these cases, care must be taken to rule out other causes. In children less than 3 years of age, arthritis is much more likely to be JRA. Teenagers are at high risk for gonococcal arthritis. Many common infections, viral and bacterial, as discussed in the differential of JRA, must be eliminated. The polyarthritis of RF tends to respond much more quickly to salicylates than JRA and that can be useful in the differential. In addition, JRA patients will frequently have a less migratory pattern of arthritis, associated symptoms of typical fever curves, lymphadenopathy, and splenomegaly. Nonspecific joint and muscle pains and common orthopedic problems can frequently be differentiated because of lack of fever and normal sedimentation rate (56).

In diagnosing carditis, innocent murmurs must be distinguished. Viral myocarditis occurs in young children but does not produce valvular disease seen in RF. Isolated pericarditis is rare in RF. Isolated mitral and aortic valve diseases are less likely to be diagnosed as rheumatic in origin than in the past (55,56,57).

The differential diagnosis of chorea in the absence of other evidence of RF includes nervous tics, tic of Gilles de la Tourette, and Huntington's chorea. These usually are not difficult to differentiate.

Clinical Laboratory Features

The most important laboratory studies in RF are those that confirm the presence of a preceding streptococcal infection. Throat cultures should be obtained but are frequently negative due to the latent period. Streptococcal antibody tests are more useful and reach their peak about the same time as the onset of RF. An antistreptolysin O (ASO) titer of 400 units is positive. If the ASO titer is borderline (250 or 333), serial measurements may detect a two-dilution fall in titer which is suggestive of recent streptococcal infection. If the ASO is negative, other streptococcal antibodies (antihyaluronidase, anti-DNase B, antistreptokinase and anti-NADase) should be measured. The Streptozyme test is a multiple antibody test that is commercially available and is used in lieu of other antibody tests in many laboratories. The ASO remains as the most reliable test (56,57). Because insidious isolated carditis and chorea may not be diagnosed until months after the streptococcal infection, the streptococcal antibody tests may have returned to normal.

The erythrocyte sedimentation rate (ESR) and the C-reactive protein (CRP) are nonsepcific tests for inflammation. They are usually elevated in RF and may be useful in following disease activity and monitoring medications. Leukocytosis suggests inflammation but leukocyte counts are so variable that they are not very helpful.

Electrocardiographic changes may be found in RF. A prolonged PR interval is seen in one-third of patients with RF and is a minor criterion. It is not equivalent to a diagnosis of carditis. With myocarditis, T waves can be flattened or inverted and with pericarditis there may be elevation of the S-T segment (56).

Radiographic Features

Chest roentgenograms may show cardiac enlargement. If pericardial effusion is suspected, echocardiography is the diagnostic tool that is most useful.

Pathologic Features

The basic pathologic changes seen in RF are exudative and proliferative inflammatory reactions in mesenchymal supporting tissues of the heart, joints, blood vessels, and subcutaneous tissues. These changes are nonspecific. The pathologic feature that is specific for RF is the Aschoff body. It is oval and is a perivascular gathering of large cells with polymorphous nuclei and basophilic cytoplasm. These cells are arranged in a rosette formation around an avascular core of fibrinoid material. The Aschoff body is found in the myocardium. Rheumatic endocarditis results in several pathologic findings. The left atrium develops a thickened rough area above the base of the posterior mitral valve leaflet. This is known as MacCallum's patch. Rheumatic vegetations develop on the edge of the valve causing scarred fibrotic cusps. The pathology of the subcutaneous nodule resembles the Aschoff body (59).

Prognosis and Management

Prognosis

Rheumatic fever without carditis is self-limiting and therefore has an excellent prognosis. With carditis, the prognosis varies depending on the severity of the carditis. Death during acute rheumatic fever is now quite rare. If congestive heart failure is present during the acute attack, 75% of these patients will have chronic valvular disease 10 years later. In cases of mild carditis, if recurrences are prevented, the majority of patients will have complete healing. The 10-year mortality for RF has dropped from 30 to 4% since 1950 (56).

Management

Treatment for acute RF consists of bedrest and antiinflammatory agents. During the first 2 weeks of acute rheumatic fever without carditis, activity should be restricted. Whether strict bed rest is essential is controversial. Many clinicians believe that if the acute symptoms of polyarthritis and fever are brought under control that strict bedrest can be liberalized to include bathroom privileges, sitting up for meals, and sitting in a chair several hours per day. Bedrest should be continued if joint symptoms, new murmurs, enlarged heart, elevated sleeping pulse (>100), or subcutaneous nodules are present. If the above signs and carditis are not present, then ambulation is gradually achieved. If carditis is present, bedrest should continue for 4 weeks to 3 months (56).

Antiinflammatory agents are very effective in acute RF. If the diagnosis is in question, they should be withheld during a period of observation. Patients with arthritis or carditis without cardiomegaly should be treated with salicylates 100 mg/kg/day in divided doses for 2 weeks, and 75 mg/kg/day for the next 4-6 weeks.

If carditis is moderate to severe, prednisone should be used because patients respond more rapidly to steroids: a daily dose of 2 mg/kg/day in divided doses for 2 weeks and then gradually tapered by 5 mg every 2-3 days. Aspirin should be instituted during the tapering of prednisone and continued for 1 month after prednisone is stopped to prevent rebound. There is no evidence that steroids decrease the incidence of residual heart disease. Congestive heart failure should be additionally treated with oxygen, fluid restriction, digitalis, and diuretics. Chorea can be treated with barbiturates, chlorpromazine, or haloperidol (56).

Prevention of recurrent attacks of RF is one of the most important aspects of therapy as far as controlling morbidity and mortality. Patients who have had one attack are more susceptible to recurrent attacks. Following the diagnosis of RF, continuous antibiotic prophylaxis is recommended to prevent streptococcal infection. The most effective prophylactic regime is intramuscular benzathine penicillin 1.2 million units once a month. Oral penicillin is also effective in a dose of 200,000 U twice a day. Compliance is a problem with oral therapy. Sulfadiazine 0.5 g once daily in children <30 kg and 1.0 g in larger children is recommended for patients allergic to penicillin (56,59). Prophylaxis is recommended throughout childhood and, in most cases, in adult life also.

Prevention of the first attack of RF is possible with proper recognition and treatment of streptococcal pharyngitis. Improved medical care for the poor is an important part of this task. Ten days of antibiotic therapy is necessary to eradicate streptococcus from the pharynx. Benzathine penicillin intramuscularly is again the treatment of choice. Oral penicillin is effective if compliance is good. Erythromycin is the drug of choice for patients allergic to penicillin.

References

1. Rodnan GP, McEwen C, Wallace SL (eds.): *Primer on Rheumatic Diseases,* 7th Ed. *JAMA* 224:661-812, 1973.

2. Brewer EJ, Bass J, Baum J et al.: Current proposed revision of JRA criteria. *Arthritis Rheum* 20:195-199, 1977.

3. Still GF: On a form of chronic joint disease in children. *Med Chir Trans* 80:47, 1897.

4. Baum J: Epidemiology of juvenile rheumatoid arthritis (JRA). *Arthritis Rheum* 20:158-160, 1977.

5. Schaller JG: Juvenile rheumatoid arthritis. *Pediatr Rev* 2:163-174, 1980.

6. Schaller JG, Wedgewood RJ: Rheumatic diseases (inflammatory diseases of connective tissues, collagen diseases). In RE Behrman, VC Vaughan (eds.), *Nelson Textbook of Pediatrics,* 12th Ed. Philadelphia, W.B. Saunders, 1983, pp. 561-588.

7. Cassidy JT, Petty RE, Sullivan DB: Occurrence of selective IgA deficiency in children with juvenile rheumatoid arthritis. *Arthritis Rheum* 20:181-183, 1977.

8. Bywaters EGL: Pathologic aspects of juvenile chronic polyarthritis. *Arthritis Rheum* 20:271-276, 1977.

9. Schaller JG: Juvenile rheumatoid arthritis. *Arthritis Rheum* 20:165-170, 1977.

10. Wedgewood RJ, Schaller JG: The pediatric arthritides. *Hospital Practice* 12:83-97, 1977.

11. Bernstein BH, Stobie D, Singsen BH et al.: Growth retardation in juvenile rheumatoid arthritis (JRA). *Arthritis Rheum* 20:212-216, 1977.

12. Brewer EJ, Giannini EH, Person DA: *Juvenile Rheumatoid Arthritis.* Philadelphia, W.B. Saunders, 1982.

13. Steere AC, Malawista SE, Hardin JA et al.: Erythema chronicum migrans and lyme arthritis. The enlarging clinical spectrum. *Ann Int Med* 86:685, 1977.

14. Stollerman GH, Markowitz M, Toranta A et al.: Report of the ad hoc committee of the American Heart Association Council on Rheumatic Fever and Congenital Heart Disease. *Circulation* 32:664-668, 1965.

15. Baum J, Gutowski G: Death in juvenile rheumatoid arthritis. *Arthritis Rheum* 20:253, 1977.

16. Donovan WH: Physical measure in treatment of juvenile rheumatic arthritis. *Arthritis Rheum* 20:553-557, 1977.

17. Cassidy JT, Sullivan DB, Petty RE: Clinical patterns of chronic iridocyclitis in children with juvenile rheumatoid arthritis. *Arthritis Rheum* 20:224-227, 1977.

18. Baum J: Aspirin in the treatment of juvenile arthritis. In L Lasagna, M Gilbert (eds.), New Perspectives in Aspirin Therapy, Proceedings of a Symposium. *Amer J Med* 74:10-15, 1983.

19. Ladd JR, Cassidy JT, Martel W: Juvenile ankylosing spondylitis. *Arthritis Rheum* 14:579-590, 1971.

20. Bywaters EGL: Ankylosing spondylitis in childhood. In BM Ansell (ed.), *Clinics in Rheumatic Diseases.* London, W.B. Saunders, 1976, Vol. 2, No. 2, pp. 387-396.

21. Schaller JG: Ankylosing spondylitis of childhood onset. *Arthritis Rheum* 20:398-401, 1977.

22. Singsen BH, Bernstein BH, Koster-King KG et al.: Reiter's syndrome in childhood. *Arthritis Rheum* 20:402-407, 1977.

23. Russell AS: Reiter's syndrome in children following infection with Yersinia enterocolitica and shigella. *Arthritis Rheum* 20:471-472, 1977.

24. Lindsley CB: Arthritis in inflammatory bowel disease in children. *Arthritis Rheum* 20:411-413, 1977.

25. Aho K, Ahvonen P, Lassus A et al.: HL-A27 in reactive arthritis. *Arthritis Rheum* 17:521-526, 1974.

26. Lambert JR, Ansell BM, Stephenson E et al.: Psoriatic arthritis in childhood. In BM Ansell (ed.), *Clinics in Rheumatic Diseases.* London, W.B. Saunders, 1976, Vol 2, No. 2, pp. 339-352.

27. Cohen AS, Reynolds WE, Franklin EC et al.: Preliminary criteria for classification of systemic lupus erythematosus. *Bull Rheum Dis* 21:643-648, 1971.

28. Page H: New criteria for diagnosing SLE. *JAMA* 248:622, 1982.

29. Meislin AG, Rothfield N: Systemic lupus erythematosus in childhood: Analysis of 42 cases with comparative data on adult cases followed concurrently. *Pediatrics* 42:37-49, 1968.

30. Rothfield N: Systemic lupus erythematosus. *Pediatr Ann* 11:397-402, 1982.

31. Kornreich H: Systemic lupus erythematosus in childhood. In BM Ansell (ed.), *Clinics in Rheumatic Diseases.* London, W.B. Saunders, 1976, Vol 2, No. 2, pp. 429-443.

32. King KK, Kornreich HK, Bernstein BH et al.: The clinical spectrum of systemic lupus erythematosus in childhood. *Arthritis Rheum* 20:287-294, 1977.

33. Jacobs JC: *Pediatric Rheumatology for the Practitioner.* New York, Springer-Verlog, 1982.

34. Kunkel HG: The immunopathology of SLE. *Hosp Pract* 15:47-56, 1980.

35. Abeles M: Systemic lupus erythematosus in the younger patient: Survival studies. *J Rheumatol* 7:515-522, 1980.

36. Sharp GC: Mixed connective tissue disease. *Bull Rheum Dis* 25:828-831, 1974-1975.

37. Singsen BH, Kornreich HK, Koster-King KG et al.: Mixed connective tissue disease in children. *Arthritis Rheum* 20:355-360, 1977.

38. Hanson V: Dermatomyositis, scleroderma, and polyarteritis nodosa. In BM Ansell (ed.), *Clinics in Rheumatic Diseases.* London, W.B. Saunders, 1976, Vol 2, No. 2, pp. 445-467.

39. Sullivan DP, Cassidy JT, Petty R: Dermatomyositis in the pediatric patient. *Arthritis Rheum* 20:327-331, 1977.

40. Hanissian AS, Masi AT: Comparison of 12 childhood polymyositis and 30 childhood dermatomyositis patients. *Arthritis Rheum* 20:341-342, 1977.

41. Packman LM, Cooks N: Juvenile dermatomyositis: A clinical and immunologic study. *J Pediatr* 96:226-234, 1980.

42. Banker BQ, Victor M: Dermatomyositis (systemic angiopathy of childhood). *Medicine* 45:261-289, 1966.

43. Whitaker JN, Engel WK: Vascular deposits of immunoglobulin and complement in idiopathic inflammatory myopathy. *N Engl J Med* 286:333-338, 1972.

44. Dubowitz V: *Muscle Disorders in Childhood.* London, W.B. Saunders, 1978.

45. Kornreich HK, King KK, Bernstein BH et al.: Scleroderma in childhood. *Arthritis Rheum* 20:343-350, 1977.

46. Kesler RW, McDonald TD, Balasubramaniam M: Linear scleroderma in children. *Am J Dis Child* 135:738-740, 1981.

47. Masi AT et al.: Preliminary criteria for the classification of systemic sclerosis (scleroderma). *Arthritis Rheum* 23:581-590, 1980.

48. Cassidy JT, Sullivan DB, Dabich L et al.: Scleroderma in children. *Arthritis Rheum* 20:351-354, 1977.

49. Britt WJ, Duray PH, Dahl MV et al.: Diffuse fasciitis with eosinophilia: A steroid responsive scleroderma. *J Pediatr* 97:432-434, 1980.

50. West RJ: Acute polyarthritis: Diagnosis and management. In BM Ansell (ed.), *Clinics in Rheumatic Diseases.* London, W.B. Saunders, 1976, Vol 2, No. 2, pp. 305-337.

51. Emery H, Larter W, Schaller J: Henoch-Schönlein vasculitis. *Arthritis Rheum* 20:385-388, 1977.

52. Melish ME, Hicks RM, Larson EJ: Mucocutaneous lymph node syndrome in the United States. *Am J Dis Child* 130:599-607, 1976.

53. Bell DM, Morens DM, Holman RC et al.: Kawasaki syndrome in the United States. *Am J Dis Child* 137:211-214, 1983.

54. Melish ME, Hicks RV, Reddy V: Kawasaki syndrome: An update. *Hosp Prac*:99-106, 1982.

55. Markowitz M: The changing picture of rheumatic fever. *Arthritis Rheum* 20:369-374, 1977.

56. Markowitz M: Rheumatic fever. In RE Behrman, VC Vaughan (eds.), *Nelson Textbook of Pediatrics,* 12th Ed. Philadelphia, W.B. Saunders, 1983, pp. 588-594.

57. DiSciascio G, Taranta A: Rheumatic fever in children. *Am Heart J* 99: 635-658, 1980.

58. Land MA, Bismo AL: Acute rheumatic fever—A vanishing disease in suburbia. *JAMA* 249:895-898, 1983.

59. Markowitz M, Gordis L: *Rheumatic fever.* 2nd Ed. Philadelphia, W.B. Saunders, 1972.

60. McCarty M: Theories of pathogenesis of streptococcal complications. In LW Wannamaker, JM Matsen (eds.), *Streptococci and Streptococcal Disease—Recognition, Understanding and Management.* New York, Academic Press, 1972, pp. 517-526.

Chapter 20

HERITABLE AND METABOLIC DISEASES OF CONNECTIVE TISSUE AND BONE

K. Patrick Ober, M.D. and John Hennessy, M.D.

Form and structure within the human body depend on specific cell lines which produce and maintain the lattice work that connects and protects other cells. Depending upon the desired goal, this lattice work, composed of a variety of proteinaceous complexes, may be flexible (to provide mobility) or rigid (to provide a stable structure offering form and protection). This lattice work of material is collectively referred to as connective tissue, a term which literally describes its primary function, the connecting together of the body's various cellular components. This chapter will deal with problems that can arise when disorders in maintaining and producing this "body glue" occur. Particular attention will be placed on bone diseases. Nearly all metabolic bone diseases can be understood best if there is some appreciation of normal mechanisms by which specialized cells in bone produce and maintain a rigid (calcified) form of connective tissue. In this regard, bone should be viewed as a specialized form of connective tissue in which the cellular components have developed a unique capacity to induce a state of rigidity to what would otherwise be a very pliable collagen matrix.

Extracellular Matrix (1,2,3,4,5)

The major component of most connective tissues is a fibrous protein, usually collagen or elastin. Collagen is the major fibrillar protein in most connective tissues, and in bone it accounts for about 95% of the total organic material. Although the use of terms such as collagen vascular disease may lead to the concept that collagen is predominantly a component of cartilage, tendon, fascia, and joint capsules, it is important to note that all organs have some connective tissue component that is responsible not only for form but for mechanical function. Collagen is the most abundant protein in the human body.

Collagen represents a class of protein that is characterized by its amino acid composition (every third amino acid is glycine) and its structural organization (three chains intertwined in a triple helix, with each of the three chains composed of about 1000 amino acid residues). Outside of bone, the synthesis of collagen is principally the responsibility of fibroblasts; in bone, the osteoblast or osteocyte is responsible. The synthesis of collagen is illustrated in Figure 20.1. The alpha chain precursor, preprocollagen, is synthesized on the ribosomes in the rough endoplasmic reticulum. The amino acid sequence is controlled by chromosomal DNA (as in the case with protein synthesis in general). Procollagen is formed by removal of the amino terminal leader sequence of the newly synthesized protein. After production of the alpha chain, further modifications take place. These changes in the structure are not determined by DNA or RNA (and are therefore referred to as posttranslational modifications). Specific enzymes cause the hydroxylation of proline and lysine residues, leading to formation of hydroxyproline and hydroxylysine. The hydroxylysine can be further modified by the addition of sugar groups. The addition of galactose to hydroxylysine is also under enzymatic control; in some cases, a second glycosylation enzyme will add glucose to the galactosylhydroxylysine. The basic amino acid sequence of the alpha chain confers special stereochemical properties which result in helix formation. The posttranslational changes lead to stabilization of the helical structure, and eventually contribute to cross-links from one collagen molecule to another. After the release of the alpha chain precursor from the ribosomes, interchain disulfide bonds form at the carboxyterminal end of the molecules. This initiates triple helix formation, with three alpha chains combining and intertwining into a single unit. The procollagen product is then secreted by the cell after packaging into membranous vesicles. Outside of the cell, enzymes cleave the amino and carboxypropeptide extensions of the collagen molecule. This results in formation of insoluble collagen molecules, which subsequently organize themselves into fibrils. The fibrils of collagen aggregate along the long axis with a staggered pattern. This leaves occasional voids or holes, which become sites for mineral deposition in skeletal tissue. In order to develop appropriate tensile strength, however, the immature fibrils need to be cross-linked by a series of covalent bonds. This involves several enzymatic steps, including the conversion of specific lysine and hydroxylysine residues to reactive aldehydes by lysyl oxidase. These reactive aldehydes then generate the formation of more stable cross-links between the chains, resulting in formation of what is often referred to as mature collagen molecule.

The breakdown of collagen begins soon after its synthesis. In bone, where the collagen is mineralized, the breakdown of matrix collagen begins with resorption of the mineralized bone by osteoclasts. The degradation of collagen is performed by proteolytic enzymes which are referred to as collagenases. The collagen polypeptide eventually is broken down into shorter peptides and finally to the constituent amino acids. Since the posttranslationally modified amino acids (hydroxyproline and hydroxylysine) cannot be reutilized, they are either catabolized or excreted in the urine. About 85 or 90% of the hydroxyproline is oxidized. The remainder is excreted in the urine; this urinary hydroxyproline is easily measured, and is used clinically to assess the dynamics of collagen turnover.

Depending on the genetic message in a particular cell, the production of several distinct alpha chains is possible. Each of these chains varies in is amino acid composition, which then gives each type of alpha chain some unique properties. The structural variation causes differing degrees of pliability, resistance to breakdown, and other mechanical attributes. This is obviously of great importance, since different properties of connective tissue are needed in different tissues (strength in tendons, rigidity in bone, flexibility in skin, etc.). There are five major alpha chains (in addition to some less common forms): α_1(I), α_1(II), α_1(III),

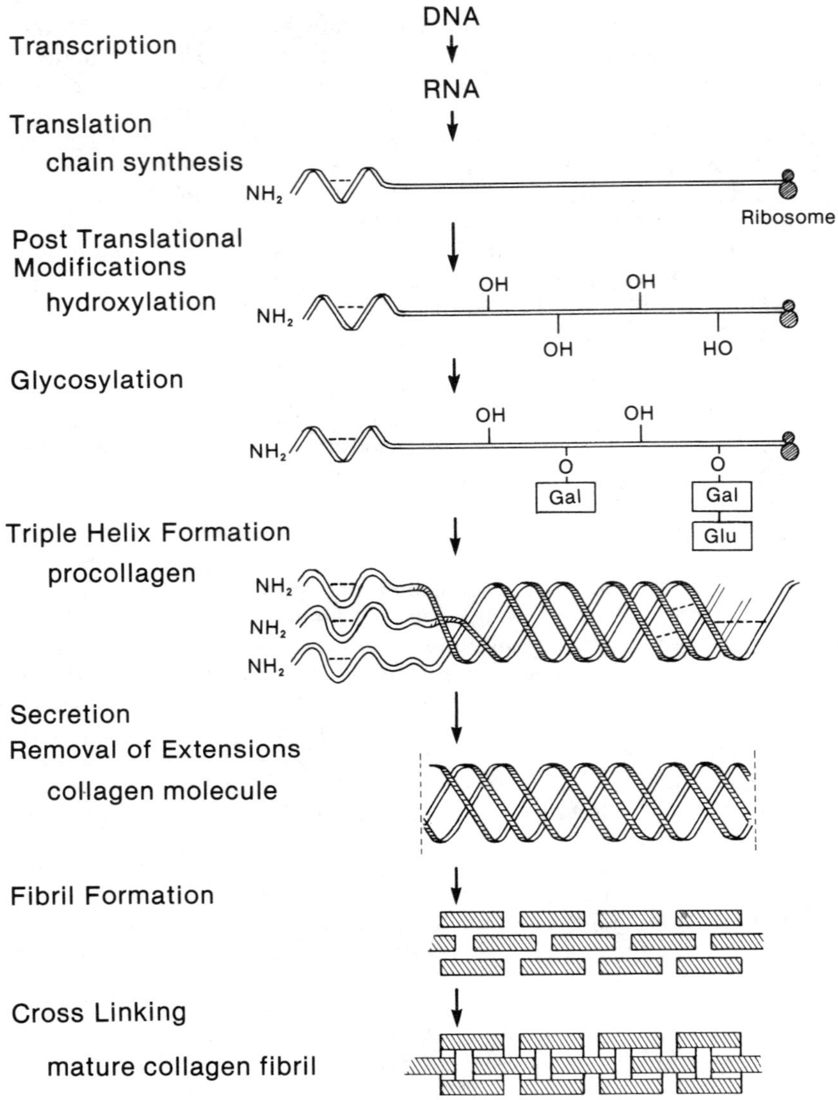

FIGURE 20.1 Collagen synthesis. As described in the text, collagen synthesis begins with production of the alpha chain. The amino acid sequence is dictated by the genetic message of the nucleic acids (DNA and RNA). Posttranslational modifications include the hydroxylation of proline and lysine residues, and the addition of sugar groups (Gal = galactose, Glu = glucose). Three alpha chains intertwine to form a triple helix; this process is initiated by the formation of interchain disulfide bonds at the carboxyterminal end of the molecule, denoted by the dashed lines on the right side of the triple helix. The procollagen product is then secreted by the cell. After cleavage of the amino and carboxyterminal extensions by enzymes, the insoluble collagen molecules aggregate along the long axis in a staggered pattern to form fibrils. Later, cross-linking by covalent bonds provides the stability and tensile strength of the mature collagen molecule.

α_1(IV), and α_2. Since each collagen molecule is comprised of three alpha chains, a number of combinations is possible. At this time, at least nine unique collagen chains have been identified. Because of some similarities, these nine collagen chains are classified into five different types of collagen. The most common type of collagen, found in skin, bone dentin, ligament, fascia, and sclera, is type I collagen. This is predominantly composed of two α_1(I) chains and one α_2 chain. Type II collagen consists of three identical chains of α_1(II), and this represents the type of collagen found in hyaline cartilage. Type III collagen is made of three α_1(III) chains, and is found in skin, blood vessel walls, and uterus. Type IV collagen is made of three chains of α_1(IV), and is found predominantly in basement membranes. Type V collagen is the most recently described. It is widely distributed as a component of pericellular membrane and basement membranes, but makes up only a small fraction of the total collagen content. (See Table 20.1.)

A number of human genetic diseases are characterized by defects in connective tissue synthesis. The prototype for this sort of disorder is osteogenesis imperfecta. At least six different subtypes have been described, and they vary on the basis of inheritance, clinical manifestations, and severity of the defect, as well as in terms of the underlying biochemical abnormality (which has not been completely defined in all cases). The classic dominant form of osteogenesis imperfecta is associated with a decrease in the synthesis of type I collagen. As might be expected, considering the distribution of type I collagen, the main tissues involved are bone, skin, sclerae, and dentin. The bone abnormality leads to an increased risk of fractures, and the term brittle bone syndrome has been applied to this disease. These patients may also have thin and atrophic skin, hypoplastic teeth, and a striking feature of blue sclerae (caused by visualization of the underlying pigmented retina through the thinned-out sclerae). Patients may also have otosclerosis and cardiovascular abnormalities. (See Table 20.2.)

The Ehlers-Danlos syndrome represents another group of disorders related to defects in collagen biosynthesis. This disease has been classified into nine types. Similar to the situation with osteogenesis imperfecta, these various types differ in terms of their inheritance, major clinical features, and biochemical defect (which has not been fully elucidated in all cases). In general, Ehlers-Danlos syndrome is associated with hyperextensible skin and joints, easily bruised skin,

TABLE 20.1 Types of Collagen

Type	Molecular Form	Tissue
I	$[\alpha_1(I)]_2\alpha_2$	Skin, bone, tendon, sclera
II	$[\alpha_1(II)]_3$	Hyaline cartilage
III	$[\alpha_1(III)]_3$	Skin, arterial walls, uterus
IV	$[\alpha_1(IV)]_3$	Basement membrane
V	$[\alpha_1(V)]_3$, others	Pericellular membranes

TABLE 20.2 Osteogenesis Imperfecta

Type	Inheritance	Clinical Features	Biochemical Defect
IA	Autosomal dominant	Blue sclerae; deafness; hypermobile joints; easy bruising; moderate severity	↓ Ratio of type I/ type III collagen in skin
IB	Autosomal dominant	Same as IA, plus dental abnormalities	?
II	Autosomal recessive	Severe lethal form with multiple fractures, intra-uterine or early childhood death; blue sclerae	↓ Type I collagen synthesis; ↑ hydroxy-lysine content of bone collagen
III	Autosomal recessive	Congenital and early childhood fractures with progressive deformities; dental involvement; blue sclerae at birth lighten with age	Heterogeneous, including ↓ type I collagen synthesis, absence of α_2(I) chain
IVA	Autosomal dominant	Variable bone fragility, white sclerae	?
IVB	Autosomal dominant	Same as IVA, plus dental abnormalities	?

poor tissue strength, and poor wound healing. Unlike osteogenesis imperfecta, bone abnormalities are uncommon. Patients with Ehlers-Danlos syndrome are susceptible to arterial rupture and gastrointestinal perforation which can lead to a catastrophic demise of afflicted patients. Mitral valve prolapse and other cardiac abnormalities have been described. Some patients suffer from emphysema, and problems with hernias (inguinal and umbilical) are common. Among the defects that have been described in the various types of Ehlers-Danlos syndrome are diminished production of type III collagen, lysyl hydroxylase deficiency (with subsequent impairment in hydroxylysine formation), lysyl oxidase deficiency (with impairment of collagen cross-linking), and deficient procollagen aminoprotease (with a resultant incomplete conversion of procollagen to collagen). (See Table 20.3.)

Cutis laxa is a rare collection of disorders in which the skin is loose and redundant, but without the hyperextensibility or other features of the Ehlers-Danlos syndrome. Emphysema, hernias, tortuous blood vessels, and other abnormalities indicative of a connective tissue problem may be seen. In some of these patients, lysyl oxidase activity in the skin is diminished with subsequent impairment in the cross-linking of collagen.

TABLE 20.3 Ehlers-Danlos Syndrome

Type	Inheritance	Clinical Features	Biochemical Defect
I	Autosomal dominant	Marked skin hyperextensibility and fragility, easy bruising, joint hypermobility, poor healing	?
II	Autosomal dominant	Mild, with hypermobility limited to digits	?
III	Autosomal dominant	Marked hypermobility of large joints with minimal skin involvement	?
IV	Autosomal dominant and autosomal recessive types	Fragile skin with marked bruisability, arterial rupture, intestinal perforation, sudden death	Heterogenous including ↓ type III collagen synthesis (? ↓ secretion in some)
V	X-linked	Hyperextensible and fragile skin, hernias, mitral and tricuspid prolapse	Lysyl oxidase deficiency
VI	Autosomal recessive	Joint hypermobility, recurrent joint dislocations, ocular fragility(ruptured globes)	Lysyl hydroxylase deficiency
VII	Autosomal recessive	Marked joint hypermobility and dislocations, short stature, peculiar facies	Heterogeneous, including procollagen aminoprotease deficiency, structural defects in $\alpha 2$ chain
VIII	Autosomal dominant	Premature and severe periodontal disease, marked skin extensibility and bruising	?
IX	Autosomal recessive	Mental retardation, hernias, hypermobile joints, fragile skin	?

Other metabolic disorders can lead to abnormalities in the production of mature collagen. In Menkes' syndrome, decreased intestinal absorption of copper leads to deficiencies of copper-dependent enzymes. These patients have various neurologic, pigmentary, and hair abnormalities related to copper deficiency, but also suffer from a bone disease that is described as osteoporosis, and resembles the bone disease found in scurvy. Lysyl oxidase is a copper-dependent enzyme, responsible for the production of aldehydes which initiate the cross-linking process, and deficiency of this enzymatic activity results in the subsequent bone disorder.

Abnormalities in cross-linking of collagen fibers may also be seen in other metabolic disorders. In homocystinuria, caused by a deficiency in cystathionine synthase, the accumulation of homocysteine may chelate the aldehydes involved in cross-linking. The resultant abnormal collagen contributes to the clinical picture of ectopia lentis, long thin extremities, osteoporosis, deformed chest, and high arched palate. Drugs such as penicillamine may have a homocysteine-like effect on collagen, causing fragile skin and delayed wound healing.

Alkaptonuria is a genetic disorder in which decreased activity of the enzyme homogentisic acid oxidase leads to accumulation of homogentisic acid with deposition of pigment in connective tissue (ochronosis) and degenerative joint changes. Polymers of a homogentisic acid metabolite have high affinity for collagen-containing tissue, and homogentisic acid has been shown to inhibit hydroxylysine formation and subsequent formation of collagen cross-links. This abnormality may be responsible for the early arthritis in the larger joints seen with this disease.

Marfan's syndrome is a connective tissue disorder in which skeletal, eye, and cardiovascular problems are common. Patients with this syndrome are usually tall and thin, have long and thin fingers (arachnodactyly), hypotonic muscles, ectopia lentis (with the lens displaced upward), and degeneration of the media of the aorta (leading to aortic insufficiency, aortic aneurysm, and frequently aortic rupture). Mitral valve prolapse is also frequently seen. Although the specific connective tissue defect of Marfan's syndrome has not been fully described, various abnormalities in collagen synthesis have been suggested. It is of interest that Marfanoid features are seen in other connective tissue disorders, including the hydroxylysine-deficient subtype of Ehlers-Danlos syndrome and homocystinuria.

In addition to these genetic diseases, vitamin deficiencies can also influence posttranslational steps of collagen metabolism. In vitamin C deficiency (scurvy), there is decreased hydroxylation of proline. With low hydroxyproline content, the alpha chains cannot form a stable triple helix, and secretion of a nonfunctional collagen is delayed. Clinically, this is reflected in poor wound healing, thin connective tissue providing poor vascular support, and abnormal bone. Vitamin D deficiency, which has its most striking effect on bone mineralization (as will be discussed later), leads to increased lysyl hydroxylation, producing an abnormal type of collagen which may be resistant to calcification, resulting in buildup of unmineralized osteoid.

Elastic fibers, like collagen, represent another major fibrillar component of connective tissue. The major component of elastic fibers is an amorphous elastin, which has a characteristic amino acid composition that is similar in some ways to collagen, with approximately one-third of amino acids consisting of lysine. However, there are differences in terms of amino acid makeup which give the elastin different physical properties. Elastic fibers do not show any of the ordered structure of periodicity found in collagen. Elastin is predominantly a product of the smooth muscle cell. There are several disease states in which abnormalities in elastin structure or synthesis are likely . In pseudoxanthoma elasticum, skin lesions (skin folds and yellowish plaques), angioid streaks in the fundus, and vascular abnormalities (arterial calcification, occlusion, and hypertension) are the major components. As noted previously, there is evidence that Marfan's syndrome may be related to an abnormality in collagen; however, since a major component of the pathology consists of the disruption of elastic fibers in the aortic media, it is possible that this disease process may be related to abnormalities in elastic fiber. Similarly, in type V Ehlers-Danlos syndrome, characterized by extreme extensibility of the skin and prolapsing cardiac valves, there is evidence of an increased turnover in the elastin. This type of Ehlers-Danlos syndrome has been associated with low lysyl oxidase activity, leading to decreased collagen cross-links; it is likely that lysyl oxidase is also required for synthesis of cross-links in elastin.

In addition to the fibrillar components of connective tissue (collagen and elastic fiber), other major components of connective tissue are complex carbohydrates which make up the so-called ground substance. Although these complex polysaccharides were formerly referred to as mucopolysaccharides, they are known as glycosaminoglycan and proteoglycan by current terminology. Abnormalities in the metabolism of these substances are caused by a variety of enzyme defects, which cause the so-called mucopolysaccharide storage diseases. These metabolic diseases are not usually considered connective tissue disorders in the strictest sense, and will not be discussed further in this chapter.

The Skeletal System

Outside of bone tissue, the cellular components responsible for collagen formation are collectively referred to as fibroblasts. However, compared to other connective tissues, bone has some unique requirements because of its function in providing a rigid framework for body form, point of attachment for ligaments, tendons, and muscles, and as a protective covering. Because these special requirements demand mineralization of the underlying protein matrix, a series of specialized cells are required to accomplish the calcification of bone. Although at first glance the skeleton might be considered to be very stable and static tissue, it is actually undergoing continuous remodeling, which to some extent is affected by mechanical stress, hormonal influences, and other factors. Specialized cells are also required for this ongoing remodeling activity. In consideration of the overall process of bone remodeling, it is important to realize that the mineral component, deposited within the collagen matrix, provides bone its unique mechanical and tensile properties, giving it most of its strength and rigidity. The mineral phase of the skeleton consists of several different types of calcium phosphate salts. The predominant salt is hydroxyapatite, which has relatively small crystals, but other salts of calcium and phosphate are also found in normal skeleton. Approximately 500 mg of calcium enter and leave the skeleton daily as a result of bone formation and resorption. Thus, while bone itself is a static collection of protein fibrils and salts, the skeletal system is an extremely dynamic system which must remain responsive to changing physical and chemical demands. The constant physical demands call for remodeling or reshaping of the bone, while chemical demands may be independently placed on the skeleton's vast reservoir of calcium salts.

Bone Remodeling (6,7,8)

The process of bone remodeling follows an orderly sequence which starts with resorption of old bone, which is then followed by formation of new bone within the resorption cavity (Figure 20.2). In the process of bone resorption, both mineral and protein matrix are removed. With new bone formation, the protein matrix is deposited first, and then later calcified. Thus, the finding of an increased amount of unmineralized bone (osteoid) always indicates a failure of normal mineralization, rather than a selective removal of mineral from previously calcified bone.

The bone remodeling process begins with the osteoprogenitor cell, which represents the fundamental cell line from which more specialized cells are derived. These cells are found within the cellular lining material of all bones, and their subsequent differentiation into more specialized cells results from various hormonal and metabolic stimuli.

The osteoprogenitor cells collect together and become large multinucleated cells known as osteoclasts. These cells elaborate the degradative lysosomal enzymes which are necessary to mobilize the minerals surrounding the collagen fibrils, and also secrete the enzymes and organic acids which are responsible for the local dissolution of bone. This resorptive process is usually very intense, and involves relatively few cells.

The next cell to appear in this sequence is the osteoblast. This is the single-nucleated cell which generates the bone collagen or osteoid, which subsequently becomes calcified. The deposition of bone involves more cells than the resorption process, and formation of new bone usually is a lengthier process than the resorptive phase. Appropriate mineralization of the osteoid requires synthesis of a specific type of bone matrix, consisting of type I collagen with specific posttranslational modifications. The precipitation of the mineral phase requires optimal concentrations of calcium and phosphate at the mineralization site; as will be seen later, inadequate levels of calcium and/or phosphate will lead to mineralization defects. It is likely that the extracellular fluid is normally supersaturated in respect to the bone mineral phase. It is only the presence of specific inhibitors of calcification (such as inorganic pyrophosphates) which prevent mineralization of other collagenous matrices. It is possible that enzymes such as pyrophosphatases may be required locally to overcome this inhibition and promote mineralization.

After the formation of new osteoid is generated by the osteoblasts, and the first areas of calcification are started, the osteoid osteocyte becomes the predominant cell. As these cells mineralize the osteoid, they virtually encase themselves with the now fully calcified osteoid matrix. At that point, the primary function of the osteocyte appears to be maintenance of the structural integrity of the calcified unit; at the same time, the osteocyte retains its responsiveness to the body's demands for calcium through mobilization of mineral stores.

The process of bone remodeling should not be considered as a series of isolated, independent, or unrelated steps. More appropriately, it should be looked upon as a continuum, with an orderly sequence of closely linked events, each of which is dependent on the preceding step. Thus, within each bone remodeling unit, activation of the cell line leading to osteoclasts is followed by bone resorption. Bone resorption in turn is followed by a reversal phase in which the osteoblast becomes the most important cell. The osteoblast then is responsible for new matrix formation, at which point the osteoid osteocyte becomes the predominant cell and causes mineralization. In general, because of this close coupling, any factor that alters the rate of bone resorption will alter the rate of new bone formation to a similar degree. Thus, in patients with mild hyperparathyroidism, there is a significant

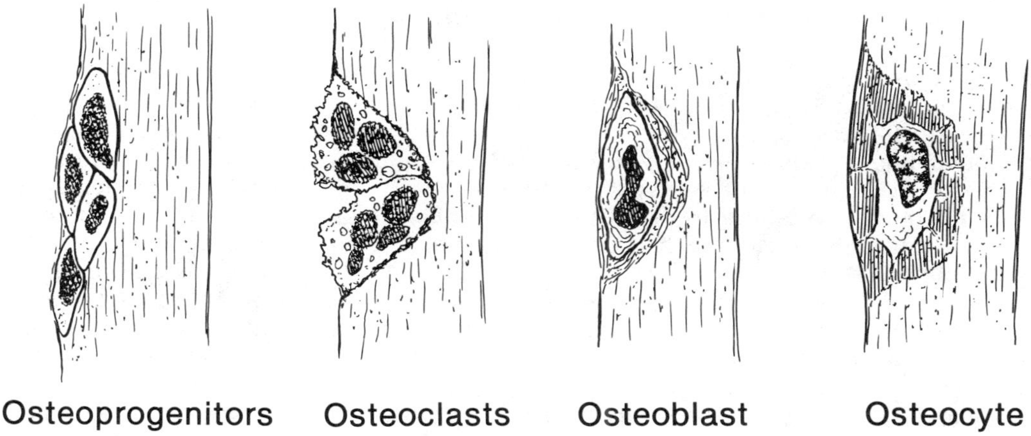

FIGURE 20.2 Bone remodeling. The process of bone remodeling begins with osteoprogenitor cells; these cells join together to form multinucleated osteoclasts. The osteoclasts resorb previously formed bone, setting the stage for new bone formation. Following the resorptive stage, the osteoblast is the next cell to appear on the scene. The single-nucleated osteoblasts (only one is shown here for illustrative purposes) produce new bone collagen, or osteoid, at the site of previous resorption. The process of new bone formation is complete by the calcification of the newly deposited osteoid, a process which is controlled by osteocytes, the final cells to appear in the remodeling sequence. After mineralization of the osteoid, the osteocytes are responsible for the maintenance of the calcified tissue.

increase in the overall rate of bone remodeling and bone turnover without a change in bone mass. Although this in general is a very balanced state of affairs, it can lead to problems in providing medical therapy for the patient with diminished bone mass (any maneuver to increase new bone formation will also tend to increase bone resorption, and any approach that slows down bone resorption will also eventually decrease bone formation). The close linkage between resorption and formation does not necessarily imply that all the cells involved come from the same source. It is possible that osteoclasts and osteoblasts arise from separate precursor pools. It has been suggested that osteoclasts may arise from blood-borne cells, perhaps a subclass of monocytes, while osteoblasts may arise independently from bone tissue cells. Regardless of their origin, the most important factor in the bone remodeling process is the functional interrelationship of these cell types. However, over the years, there tends to develop some slight dissociation between the resorptive phase and the formation phase. With each remodeling cycle, the resorbed bone is not quite entirely replaced during the subsequent formation phase. Thus, there is a slow but progressive loss in skeletal mass at a rate of about 0.5% annually from the time of maximum skeletal maturity; this loss of skeletal mass is accelerated in women at the time of menopause. This process will be discussed in more detail later.

Mineral Metabolism (9,10,11,12,13)

As noted previously, bone represents a specialized type of connective tissue in which mineralization of the underlying matrix results in formation of a fairly rigid material. Because of this mineral deposition, the skeleton has a great potential for becoming a major source of calcium for the whole organism. Over 90% of total body calcium is in the skeleton and, as a result, the skeleton is frequently called upon to contribute to overall calcium homeostasis. At times, the demand on the skeleton as a calcium source is excessive, and the structural integrity of the skeleton may eventually be sacrificed, leading to the development of metabolic bone disease. The clinical aspects of metabolic bone disease will be considered in a later section in this chapter. However, prior to consideration of these problems, it is necessary to review the overall control of calcium and phosphate metabolism.

Among the body's various homeostatic functions, maintenance of the serum calcium concentration within the limits of a fairly narrow physiologic range is critical to life. The calcium ion plays an extremely important role in neuromuscular excitability, membrane function, enzyme action, hormone effects, and a multitude of other life-sustaining actions. Ideally, the body's calcium needs should be met through dietary intake of calcium. However, dietary intake represents an erratic and inconsistent source for repletion of circulating calcium levels; there is a great deal of variability in calcium content of various foods, timing of meals, etc., which may not correspond at all to the body's calcium demand at any given time. Therefore, it becomes necessary to have a potential endogenous source of calcium to meet calcium needs when other sources (dietary) are not readily available. The skeleton serves as this reservoir of calcium with the calcium-regulating hormones (parathyroid hormone, vitamin D, calcitonin) determining the net flow of calcium into and out of bone. Although mineral may be borrowed from the bone from time to time as needed, under optimal conditions it is eventually replaced when calcium becomes available in excess of the organism's needs. However, in some situations, a portion of the calcium withdrawn from bone is never completely replaced. This persistently negative calcium balance may lead to the development of metabolic bone disease. The flux of calcium in and out of bone is largely controlled by hormonal signals, as discussed below.

Parathyroid Hormone (PTH)

Parathyroid hormone is one of the more important regulators of calcium homeostasis. Because of the very important role of calcium in cell function, an elaborate system exists to maintain the serum calcium within a physiologic range, and parathyroid hormone is one of the central determinants of the calcium level. Parathyroid hormone is a polypeptide of 84 amino acids (although the precursor molecule made by the parathyroid gland is somewhat larger). Promptly after secretion, the parathyroid hormone molecule is cleaved into multiple fragments. The most important fragment is the N-terminal end, composed of amino acids 1-34. The biologic activity of the molecule seems to be localized in this fragment, which typically has low plasma levels and a very short half-life. Other fragments are produced, including a C-terminal fragment of amino acids 35-84, which are present in higher quantity and have a longer half-life, but are biologically inactive. The multiple fragments of PTH in the circulation have led to some difficulties in correlating PTH as measured by radioimmunoassay with the biologic activity of the hormone.

As might be expected, hypocalcemia is the major stimulus for secretion of PTH. In turn, PTH has effects (directly or indirectly) on the three major organs involved in calcium regulation: bone, kidney, and intestine (Figure 20.3). In bone, PTH stimulates all cell types (osteoclasts, osteocytes, and osteoblasts). This leads to an increase in the rate of bone remodeling, but not necessarily to a loss of bone mineral, as long as dietary calcium intake is adequate. However, if calcium intake is inadequate and a calcium deficiency state exists (which frequently is the case when PTH levels are increased), the resultant imbalance between bone resorption and the formation of new bone can eventually lead to a decrease in skeletal mass. In the kidney, PTH has three primary functions which serve to maintain calcium homeostasis. In the distal tubule, PTH enhances reabsorption of calcium, supporting calcium retention and decreased calcium excretion by the kidney. PTH also inhibits reabsorption of phosphate by the tubule, leading to a lowering of the serum phosphate level. Since calcium can complex with phosphate to cause relatively insoluble crystals (which is essential to skeletal calcification, but potentially deleterious if these crystals are deposited in soft tissue), the lowering of serum phosphate by PTH promotes calcium solubility and the maintenance of calcium levels. The third action of PTH on the kidney is the stimulation of the 1-hydroxylase enzyme which converts 25-hydroxyvitamin D to the active product, 1,25-hydroxyvitamin D, which in turn regulates intestinal absorption of calcium.

Vitamin D

Vitamin D and its metabolites also play a pivotal role in calcium homeostasis. The vitamin D molecule can occur in at least two forms, each of which undergoes the same metabolism and has equivalent biologic effects. The naturally occurring animal vitamin D is D_3 (cholecalciferol). Vitamin D_3 is produced in the skin from its sterol precursor, 7-dehydrocholesterol; this conversion occurs under the influence of ultraviolet light exposure. The other form of vitamin D is vitamin D_2 (ergocalciferol), which is derived from a plant sterol, and is used for fortification of foods. In temperate areas such as the United States, 90% of all vitamin D comes from endogenous production, so that in the strictest sense vitamin D is not truly a vitamin (except in situations where there is inadequate sunlight exposure). It is more appropriately looked upon as a prohormone, since its metabolites (produced by the liver and kidney) are metabolically active factors.

After production of vitamin D by the skin, the compound is either carried in the plasma by a sterol-binding protein or stored in fat tissue. The first important step in its metabolism is the conversion to 25-hydroxyvitamin D by the liver. This compound has some physiologuc activity, including a direct action on bone of increasing bone resorption. However, more important than any intrinsic function it may have, 25-hydroxyvitamin D serves as a precursor for other vitamin D forms, including 1,25-dihydroxyvitamin D, 24,25-dihydroxyvitamin D, and a series of other metabolites. With the exception of 1,25-dihydroxyvitamin D (and to a lesser extent 24,25-dihydroxyvitamin D) very little is known of these metabolites and their function in calcium homeostasis.

1,25-dihydroxyvitamin D is produced in the kidney. Parathyroid hormone stimulates the 1-hydroxylase enzyme which leads to formation of this vitamin D metabolite. The other major controlling factor is plasma phosphate; a fall in plasma phosphate will stimulate production of 1,25-dihydroxyvitamin D, while increased phosphate levels suppress its formation. The intestine and bone represent the two major end organs for the action of 1,25-dihydroxyvitamin D. At the gut level, the hormone stimulates active absorption of both calcium and phos-

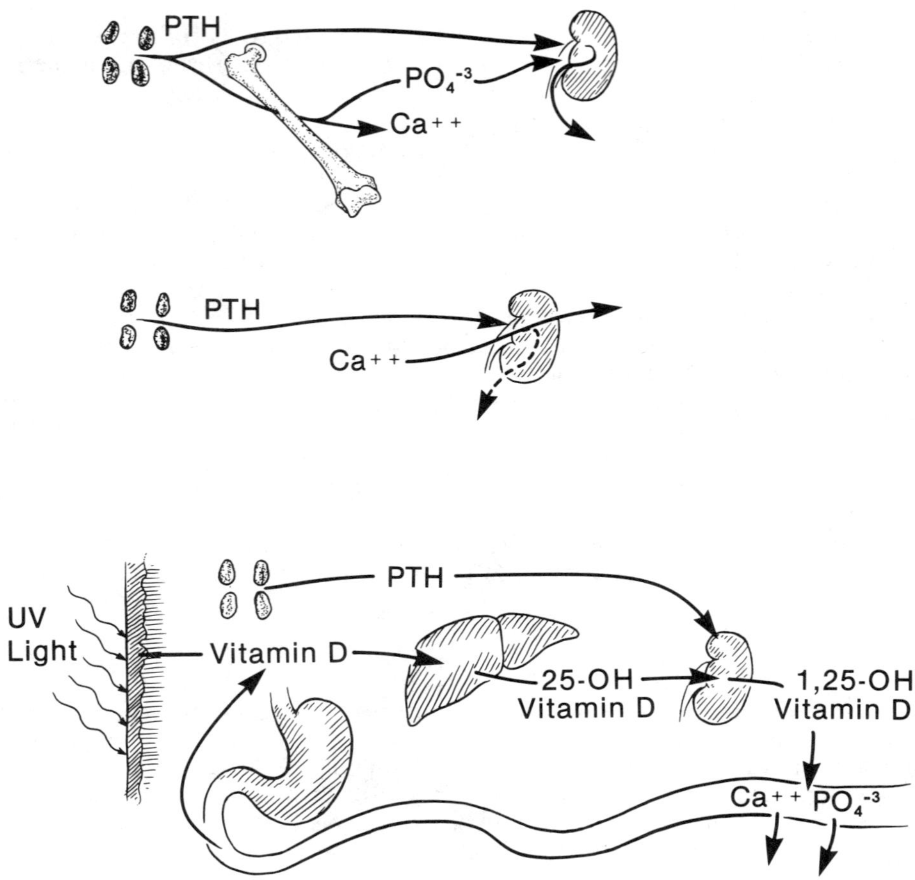

FIGURE 20.3 Hormonal control of mineral homeostasis. Maintenance of calcium and phosphorus homeostasis is a complicated undertaking, requiring the interaction of several hormonal messengers with a number of organ systems, as shown here. The top illustration portrays the effect of PTH on bone, where enhanced resorption leads to increased availability of calcium and phosphorus. The major goal of PTH is to provide calcium to the system, and the simultaneous release of phosphorus is a largely undesirable side effect of PTH's action on bone; the newly available but unwanted phosphorus is cleared by the kidneys, an action that is promoted by a separate effect of PTH on the renal tubule. The middle illustration shows a second renal effect of PTH, enhanced calcium reabsorption, which also contributes to overall calcium balance. The lower illustration demonstrates the complexities of vitamin D metabolism. The parent vitamin D molecule can be produced by skin (under the stimulus of ultraviolet irradiation), or can be obtained from dietary sources and absorbed by the intestinal tract. This precursor vitamin D is 25-hydroxylated by the liver, and then converted to the active hormone (1,25-dihydroxyvitamin D) by a 1-hydroxylase enzyme in the kidney; this enzyme is stimulated by PTH. The final goal of this sequence of vitamin D activation is enhanced intestinal absorption of calcium (and phosphorus), an action promoted by the end product 1,25-dihydroxyvitamin D.

phate. In addition, 1,25-dihydroxyvitamin D stimulates the resorption of bone with liberation of both calcium and phosphate. On a mole for mole basis, 1,25-dihydroxyvitamin D is at least as potent as parathyroid hormone in causing bone resorption.

Although 1,25-dihydroxyvitamin D is considered to be the active and most important metabolite of vitamin D, there has been some evidence to suggest that 24,25-dihydroxyvitamin D also plays an important physiologic role. This substance is also a metabolite of 25-hydroxyvitamin D, formed by the kidney in situations where calcium is readily available and PTH levels are not elevated (opposite from the circumstances which lead to 1,25-dihydroxyvitamin D production). Although some would suggest that 24,25-dihydroxyvitamin D is an inactive metabolite, there is evidence that the molecule has physiologic functions which include suppression of PTH secretion and stimulation of bone mineralization.

Calcitonin

Calcitonin is a 32 amino acid peptide which is produced by the parafollicular cells (C-cells) in the thyroid gland. Calcitonin serves as a hypocalcemic hormone, and its levels are increased in the setting of hypercalcemia. Its principal effect on the skeleton is an inhibition of osteoclastic bone resorption. Calcitonin may also have effects on the kidney and gastrointestinal tract, although these are not as clearly defined as its skeletal action. The importance of calcitonin in calcium regulation in the human being is open to question, since hypercalcemia does not occur in the thyroidectomized patient, and no clinical syndrome attributable to calcitonin deficiency has ever been described. Some studies have shown lower basal calcitonin levels in women than in men, and other studies have shown a decreased calcitonin reserve in some women, suggesting that a relative calcitonin deficiency might be a predisposing factor for development of postmenopausal osteoporosis. However, this is currently more a matter of speculation than of proven fact.

Coordination of Mineral-Regulating System

Obviously, with two, and perhaps three, major hormonal regulators of calcium metabolism (PTH, vitamin D, and calcitonin), and three major end organs for the action of these hormones (bone, kidney, and intestinal tract), the overall coordination and interaction of this system are of major importance. The major interactions are shown in Figure 20.3. To illustrate the interactions among the various components in this system, it might be worthwhile to consider a situation in which the supply of dietary calcium is inadequate. Because of decreased availability of calcium, the serum ionized calcium level will fall. This hypocalcemic stimulus leads to an increased secretion of PTH. Parathyroid hormone's action on the bone will increase the availability of both calcium and phosphate. The liberation of calcium from bone is the major goal, and the simultaneous release of phosphate from the bone is not of any particular advantage. In fact, the increased phosphate levels will decrease calcium availability, as noted previously. However, this PTH-mediated release of phosphate from the bone is counteracted by the effect of PTH on the kidney: parathyroid hormone leads to increased urinary loss of phosphate, thus serving to get rid of the extra phosphate that was released from the bone. In general, all states of increased parathyroid hormone secretion will ultimately lead to phosphate wasting (assuming renal function is normal). PTH also acts on the kidney to increase reabsorption of calcium, which is of obvious benefit in a situation of decreased calcium availability. Finally, the effect of PTH on the 1-hydroxylase enzyme in the kidney leads to increased production of 1,25-dihydroxyvitamin D. This in turn has an effect at the intestinal level to increase absorption of calcium, serving to counteract the effect of the initial insult (deficient calcium intake). On the basis of these interactions, it should be possible to predict the expected changes that occur in response to defects anywhere in the calcium homeostatic system (vitamin D deficiency, parathyroid hormone deficiency, etc.). Familiarity with these various interactions becomes important in the understanding of clinical states of metabolic bone disease, in which the skeleton frequently bears the brunt of the system's attempt to regulate calcium metabolism.

Disorders of Bone Metabolism (14,15,16,17,18,19,20)

Osteopenia, defined as a decrease in the absolute volume of mineralized bone, is a very common clinical finding. Many times, this is an incidental finding on a chest x-ray or abdominal film obtained for unrelated reasons. On other occassions, the patient may be symptomatic with the sudden onset of pain following physical activity associated with the radiographic finding of a fracture in the setting of generalized bone loss.

In the patient with a decreased volume of mineralized bone (osteopenia), it is important to make a differentiation between the terms osteoporosis and osteomalacia, since this distinction will have a major impact on the evaluation and treatment of the patient. The term osteopenia makes no assumptions as to the nature or cause of the state of decreased bone mass, but simply acknowledges that such a state exists. Since the development of osteopenia parallels the aging process, most human beings will show evidence of osteopenia if they live long enough, and it is frequently difficult to distinguish between normal age-related bone loss and the more severe bone loss which manifests itself with fractures and deformity. Osteoporosis is the most common type of osteopenia; in this situation, the total bone mass is decreased, but there is a normal ratio of bone mineral to bone protein matrix, and the composition of the bone is normal. Osteoporosis is to be distinguished from osteomalacia, which represents a disorder of mineralization of the bone matrix, so that the ratio of mineral to matrix is decreased. In some patients with osteomalacia, x-rays may demonstrate linear areas of localized mineral loss known as Looser's zones or pseudofractures, but in the vast majority of patients it is impossible to distinguish osteoporosis from osteomalacia on the basis of x-ray examinations. In most cases, there are specific clinical and biochemical clues that suggest the possibility of osteomalacia. In general, it is advisable to use the term osteopenia in the patient with decreased bone mass, at least until the possibility of osteomalacia has been considered and excluded. This is of great importance to the patient, since osteomalacia can easily be overlooked, and yet it represents one of the types of metabolic bone disease that is most responsive to appropriate therapy.

Osteoporosis

Osteoporosis is by far the most common metabolic bone disease. It is estimated that approximately 1 million fractures occur each year in the United States among women with osteoporosis. Osteoporosis can result in significant morbidity and its complications are a significant cause of death in the elderly. The costs of osteoporosis are measured not only in terms of the need for medical, nursing, and rehabilitative care, but also in terms of the chronic suffering, physical restriction, and general deterioration of quality of life that frequently is associated with the disorder.

As previously described, in the normal process of bone remodeling, there is a close link between the resorption of previously formed bone and the subsequent formation of new organic matrix and deposition of mineral. Because of this strict association between loss of old bone and formation of new bone, it would seem that skeletal mass should remain constant, and that osteoporosis should not be nearly as common as it actually is. However, the tightly coupled formation and resorption of bone are not an absolute and, through the years, new bone formation does not quite keep up with the amount of bone removed, resulting in a slow but progressive loss of skeletal mass with aging. Therefore, to some extent osteoporosis can be looked upon as a natural consequence of the aging process, with most individuals showing some loss of bone mass after the age of 40. Whether or not this disorder progresses to the point of symptomatic osteoporosis, with its painful bone fractures, skeletal deformity, and related abnormalities, is dependent upon a variety of factors. The absolute amount of bone that is formed at maturity seems to be a critical feature; people with the greatest bone mass are better able to withstand age-related bone loss because of their larger skeletal reserve. Skeletal mass is usually greater in blacks than in whites, and in men than in women, so that symptomatic osteoporosis is extremely rare in black men, but very common in white women. In addition, there are a number of factors that determine the rate of decline in bone mass through the years, including dietary factors, hormonal effects, exercise, and numerous other variables. It seems certain that osteoporosis is not a single disease process, and various disorders may affect the process of normal skeletal remodeling in a number of ways. However, in the final analysis, whenever the net rate of bone reabsorption exceeds the net rate of bone formation, there will predictably be a loss of bone mass, and osteoporosis will follow. The absolute rates of bone formation and bone resorption may be increased, decreased or normal; it is the imbalance between these two processes that causes osteoporosis.

The most common causes of osteoporosis are listed in Table 20.4 and will be discussed here in further detail.

Postmenopausal osteoporosis is the most common cause of decreased skeletal mass. In the early 1940's, Dr. Fuller Albright noted that the vast majority of osteoporotic patients were postmenopausal women. Although there has been some controversy as to which menopause-related factors lead to the development of osteoporosis, the bulk of the available information indicates a primary role for estrogen deficiency. With the loss of ovarian function (either by natural menopause or by oophorectomy), bone mass is seen to decrease, accompanied by an increase in urinary calcium and hydroxyproline secretion, presumably reflecting accelerated bone resorption. Hypercalciuria can also be seen at this time. These changes are reversed by administration of exogenous estrogen. In addition, administration of estrogen at the time of menopause or oophorectomy will dramatically retard bone loss. (This effect may not be seen if the initial administration of estrogen is delayed for several years.) In the premenopausal woman, estrogen seems to inhibit the bone resorption that is caused by parathyroid hormone. With loss of estrogen, the bone becomes more sensitive to the action of PTH and calcium homeostasis is probably maintained with lower levels of PTH. With lowered PTH levels, the reabsorption of calcium by the kidney which is normally promoted by PTH declines. Hypercalciuria follows, and the increased calcium wasting contributes to the negative calcium balance. In addition, since the renal hydroxylase which converts 25-hydroxyvitamin D to the active 1,25-dihydroxyvitamin D is PTH-dependent, the estrogen-deficient patient has lower levels of

TABLE 20.4 Causes of Osteoporosis

Endocrine

- Postmenopausal
- Hyperparathyroidism
- Hyperthyroidism
- Hypogonadism
- Hypopituitarism
- Cushing's syndrome
- (Pregnancy/lactation)
- (Diabetes mellitus)

Nutritional

- Calcium deficiency
- Protein deficiency
- Vitamin C deficiency

Bone marrow replacement

- Multiple myeloma
- Waldenström's macroglobulinemia
- Leukemia
- Lymphoma
- Mast cell disease
- Gaucher's disease

Drugs

- Heparin
- Methotrexate
- Ethanol

Genetic connective tissue disorders

- Osteogenesis imperfecta
- Homocystinuria
- Menkes' syndrome

Immobilization

Idiopathic (primary)

- Involutional (senile)
- Adult
- Juvenile

Miscellaneous

- Chronic obstructive lung disease
- Postgastrectomy
- Chronic liver disease
- Rheumatoid arthritis

Localized

- Posttraumatic (Sudek's osteodystrophy)
- Disuse
- Regional (migratory) osteolysis

1,25-dihydroxyvitamin D. This ultimately results in decreased gastrointestinal absorption of calcium, adding further insult to the imbalances of calcium homeostasis. Thus, with estrogen deficiency, the renal and intestinal contributions to calcium balance are diminished, and the bones (with their increased sensitivity to PTH) become increasingly important in the maintenance of normal circulating calcium levels. Chronically, this continued dependence on the skeleton as a calcium source leads to osteoporosis.

In addition to the consequences of lowered estrogen production, other factors almost certainly contribute to the osteoporosis of many postmenopausal patients. Deficient dietary calcium intake may be a major factor. It has been estimated that most postmenopausal women require about 1500 mg of elemental calcium daily; however, very few women actually meet this requirement. Dairy products constitute the major dietary source of calcium, and these foods are frequently avoided by many adults. In addition, there is a high dietary consumption of phosphorus in developed countries (from meat and soft drinks) which could have an adverse effect on calcium metabolism, and potentially also lead to an increased acid load which might contribute to osteopenia. Calcium supplementation of the diet has been shown to reduce bone loss in postmenopausal women. Dietary deficiency of vitamin D may also be a contributing factor in some patients, although problems with conversion of vitamin D to its active forms is a more likely problem. A relative calcitonin deficiency in women has also been postulated as playing a role in the development of osteoporosis. In addition, decreased physical activity is another risk factor; physical activity to some extent determines the bone mass that develops before maturation, and physical inactivity may contribute to bone loss. Immobilization will lead to bone loss, and an exercise program for postmenopausal women will result in a positive calcium balance (contrasted to the negative balance shown in nonexercising controls). Other factors may also contribute to osteoporosis. There seems to be a strong relationship between osteoporosis and thinness, for uncertain reasons. Obese postmenopausal women have higher estrogen levels than their thin counterparts, so it is possible that this is an estrogen-related phenomenon; alternatively, increased forces on the skeleton caused by the need for weight-bearing may serve to strengthen bone in these patients. Cigarette smoking also seems to be an important risk factor.

There is no specific test for postmenopausal osteoporosis and the diagnosis is a diagnosis of exclusion. It cannot be assumed a priori that any bone disease seen in an elderly woman results from this disorder, and it is always necessary to exclude other causes of osteopenia in the postmenopausal woman before making the diagnosis. Since there are no historical, clinical, or radiographic findings which are specific for postmenopausal osteoporosis, premature assumptions regarding the diagnosis can lead to erroneous and inappropriate patient management.

Hyperparathyroidism leads to accelerated bone remodeling. This is associated with an increased bone resorption, and frequently a negative skeletal calcium balance. Primary hyperparathyroidism is associated with elevated levels of serum calcium, and frequently with hypophosphatemia and a hyperchloremic acidosis. It is obviously important to differentiate hyperparathyroidism from other disorders which may cause an elevated calcium and bone disease (such as multiple myeloma). Measurement of parathyroid hormone by radioimmunoassay and determination of the nephrogenous component of urinary cyclic AMP are commonly used, but neither method is foolproof. In the final analysis, the definitive diagnosis of hyperparathyroidism rests on surgical resection of abnormal parathyroid tissue with return of the serum calcium to normal.

Hyperthyroidism is a hypermetabolic state that is associated with increased bone resorption. Thyrotoxicosis can decrease the bone density in any patient, but the more severe changes, including increased incidence of fractures, are seen in women over the age of 50. Typical clinical features of hyperthyroidism may be obscured in the elderly patient (so-called apathetic thyrotoxicosis). The diagnosis is confirmed by documenting elevated levels of thyroid hormone.

Hypogonadism is another cause of decreased bone mass. The role of sex hormone deficiency in promotion of osteoporosis has been mentioned under the discussion of postmenopausal osteoporosis. In addition, sex steroids are probably important in the development of full skeletal mass at the time of maturity. Patients with Turner's syndrome or Klinefelter's syndrome are at risk for osteoporosis, perhaps because they never develop optimal skeletal mass. Theoretically, sex hormone replacement should deter the development of advanced osteoporosis in these patients.

Hypopituitarism can also be associated with severe osteopenia. This seems to be related to the gonadal insufficiency that accompanies the pituitary dysfunction.

Cushing's syndrome, whether caused by exogenous steroid therapy or by endogenous overproduction of glucocorticoids, can lead to osteopenia. Corticosteroids can directly inhibit bone formation, but also inhibit intestinal calcium absorption, leading to increased PTH levels and increased bone resorption. In addition, exogenous steroids suppress adrenal function, which ultimately leads to a decreased level of estrone. Since adrenal-derived estrone is the predominant estrogen in the postmenopausal woman, steroid therapy may contribute to the estrogen deficiency state in these patients.

Pregnancy and lactation have been associated with severe osteoporosis in some young women. Although there is a significant drain on maternal calcium balance because of the need for fetal skeletal formation and because of the demands of lactation, this loss is usually compensated for by increased intestinal calcium absorption, which in turn is mediated by increased synthesis of 1,25-dihydroxyvitamin D. The finding of osteoporosis is uncommon during pregnancy and lactation, and there is no documentation that multiparity or repeated periods of lactation are related to fracture incidence in later life. It has been proposed that women who present with osteoporosis during pregnancy actually have another underlying skeletal disorder that is made clinically apparent during the time of increased calcium needs.

Diabetes mellitus is also associated with a high incidence of osteopenia, although the etiology is obscure. Some studies have indicated that this may not be clinically important, as reflected by the incidence of fractures. A number of these patients have hypercalciuria, and it has been suggested that there is excessive calcium loss through the urinary tract in conjunction with poor glucose control and glycosuria. Other studies have suggested that there may be some imbalance between calcium absorption, PTH, and vitamin D metabolism, resulting in defective bone remodeling.

Nutritional factors might also be responsible for osteoporosis in some subjects. Dietary calcium deficiency can lead to osteoporosis in some animals. It is not clear whether or not this also happens in humans. In general, with reduced dietary calcium intake, the ability of the human being to absorb calcium is increased through compensatory changes in PTH and 1,25-dihydroxyvitamin D formation. However, decreased intestinal calcium absorption has been documented in patients with osteoporosis, as well as with aging and with postmenopausal status. Patients with lactose intolerance (who therefore avoid dairy products) have an increased incidence of osteoporosis. Increased calcium intake has been shown to slow the loss of skeletal mass in postmenopausal patients. Protein deficiency has also been suggested as a cause of osteoporosis, but this has not been well documented. Obviously, in most patients with malnutrition or malabsorption, a number of deficiencies (in addition to protein deficiency) are present. In fact, it has also been suggested that high protein intake can lead to osteoporosis by introduction of large amounts of acid-ash which is buffered at the expense of bone mineral, leading to hypercalciuria and negative calcium balance. Similarly, increased dietary phosphate (caused by consumption of meat and soft drinks) has been suggested to decrease serum calcium and promote secondary hyperparathyroidism and increased skeletal resorption. The overall significance of this has also been questioned. Vitamin C deficiency (scurvy) can lead to abnormalities of collagen synthesis, as discussed previously, which can then contribute to osteoporosis.

Bone marrow replacement should always be considered in the osteopenic patient. Although many malignancies are metastatic to bone, most of them cause a localized loss of bone. However, there are some malignancies (especially those which involve the marrow space) which can cause a generalized loss of bone mass and which may be indistinguishable from so-called primary osteoporosis. Multiple myeloma, Waldenström's macroglobulinemia, monocytic leukemia, and some lymphomas are the disorders most likely to be associated with this problem. These cells have been shown to secrete a peptide, osteoclast-activating factor (OAF), which stimulates osteoclastic resorption of bone. With multiple myeloma, bone pain is commonly seen; the most frequently involved sites include the vertebral column, ribs, and pelvis, in addition to fairly frequent skull involvement. Although demonstration of abnormal protein production on electrophoresis is helpful in making the diagnosis, at times a direct examination of the bone marrow is necessary. Mast cell disease and Gaucher's disease have also been associated with osteoporosis.

Several drugs have been associated with the development of osteopenia. Long-term heparin therapy can lead to osteoporosis with associated fractures, with some improvement after withdrawal of the drug. Heparin potentiates the effect of PTH on bone, and may also inhibit crystal aggregation and activation of collagenase. A heparin-related effect may explain the association of osteoporosis with systemic mast cell disease. In addition, it has been noted that bone marrow mast cells are increased in elderly individuals, suggesting that the effects of heparin may be another contributing factor to the osteoporosis of advancing age. Osteoporosis has also been reported with methotrexate therapy, which causes intestinal calcium malabsorption and increased urinary calcium loss. Ethanol has also been linked to the development of metabolic bone disease, although the mechanisms of its effect are not all clear. Anticonvulsant drugs such as phenytoin and phenobarbital are also associated with osteopenia, but the skeletal abnormality in these cases is usually osteomalacia (as will be discussed later).

As discussed in an earlier section, osteoporosis can be a manifestation of several genetic connective tissue disorders, including osteogenesis imperfecta, homocystinuria, and Menkes' syndrome. These have all been discussed earlier in this chapter.

Immobilization can lead to severe osteoporosis; it has been estimated that bone loss during immobilization occurs at 5-20 times the rate that is seen in other demineralizing conditions. Gravitational forces are important in the maintenance of skeletal mass. Muscle mass, muscle tone, and related physical forces are important in the regulation of bone remodeling and bone formation. Patients at prolonged bedrest demonstrate an increase in osteoclastic bone resorption and a decrease in osteoblastic bone formation. Immobilization is accompanied by calcium malabsorption, hypercalciuria, and increased urinary hydroxyproline excretion. Similar changes have been documented in astronauts who are exposed to decreased gravitational forces, as well as in patients with neurologic disorders in which paralysis of an extremity is associated with localized bone loss. After mobilization, most of the skeletal changes seem to be reversible, although this is not always true in elderly patients with preexisting osteopenia.

Involutional (or senile) osteoporosis is a relatively nonspecific term that is applied to osteoporosis seen in elderly patients. In all likelihood, there are probably multifactorial causes of this disorder. As discussed previously, there is a progressive loss in bone mass after the maximal skeletal mass has been achieved in early adult life. Many factors may influence this loss of bone mass, including the maximal amount of bone mass that has been achieved at the time of maturity, calcium intake, physical activity, estrogen status, genetic factors, 1,25-dihydroxyvitamin D levels, etc. As with postmenopausal osteoporosis, other contributing factors need to be sought out and identified where possible. Obviously, any type of osteoporosis that is defined by the age of the patient is somewhat arbitrary and artificial. Thus, similar to "senile osteoporosis," the terms "juvenile osteoporosis" and "idiopathic osteoporosis in young adults" have been used, although with little insight into the mechanisms of the bone disorder. Some of these younger patients may have osteogenesis imperfecta or some other genetic disorder, but in general the exact cause of osteoporosis in many younger individuals remains obscure.

In addition, a number of miscellaneous causes of osteoporosis have been noted. Associated disorders include chronic metabolic acidosis, chronic obstructive pulmonary disease, postgastrectomy status, chronic liver disease, and rheumatoid arthritis. In many of these disorders, the link between the underlying disease process and osteoporosis is unclear, and in some cases has not been definitely established.

In some unusual cases, the osteoporosis seems to be a localized process. Osteoporosis on a regional basis can be seen with disuse of an extremity, similar to what is seen in a more generalized form with immobilization. In addition, there is a posttraumatic type of osteodystrophy (Sudek's) in which there is evidence of increased bone turnover as well as autonomic dysfunction with increased sweating. In another disorder, regional migratory osteoporosis, there is increased bone turnover on a localized basis, with successive regions of the legs becoming involved with redness, heat, and swelling of the soft tissue, in addition to progressive bone loss. The cause of this disorder is unknown.

Treatment of osteoporosis is centered around the identification and treatment of the causative disorder, where such a disorder can be identified (i.e., parathyroidectomy for hyperparathyroidism, normalization of thyroid hormone levels in hyperthyroidism, etc.). In some situations, the underlying problem may not be reversible. For instance, some patients require pharmacologic doses of steroids for severe systemic disorders, and it is not always appropriate to decrease the steroid dosage. In this situation, however, supplementation with additional calcium and vitamin D will overcome some of the negative effects of glucocorticoids on calcium absorption, and serve to protect the skeleton against excessive calcium loss. There remains a great deal of controversy in regard to the most appropriate treatment for the most common type of osteoporosis, that which is seen in the postmenopausal woman. As discussed, estrogen deficiency seems to be a major component of this disorder, and estrogen therapy has in fact been shown to decrease the accelerated rate of bone resorption seen in these patients. However, some studies suggest that the estrogen therapy may not be effective if it is delayed beyond 3 years after menopause. There has also been some concern about potential side effects, including hyperplastic and even neoplastic changes in the endometrium (which can probably be avoided if the estrogen is given cyclically, or if progestational agents are used episodically to cause endometrial shedding). Alternatively, calcium therapy can also help maintain skeletal mass. In postmenopausal women, about 1500 mg of elemental calcium is required daily to maintain normal calcium balance. A routine program of graded physical activity can also help maintain skeletal mass in the postmenopausal patient. Calcium supplementation of the diet and exercise are reasonable recommendations in any woman who is approaching menopause in an effort to prevent accelerated bone loss. However, in the patient who presents with fractures and significant loss of bone mass, none of these treatment regimens will restore the bone mass already lost. In recent years, it has been shown that fluoride therapy may have the ability to restore skeletal mass; used alone, fluoride produces poorly mineralized bone, but with calcium supplementation it seems to promote increased bone mass and decreased risk of fractures. Unfortunately, at the relatively high doses required to achieve this action, fluoride therapy is associated with frequent gastrointestinal and rheumatological side effects. Additionally, it should be noted that fluoride remains an investigational drug at this time and has not been approved for use in the treatment of osteoporosis.

Osteomalacia

Although osteomalacia is less common than osteoporosis, there is a greater understanding of its pathophysiology, and therapy tends to be more specific. If the diagnosis of osteomalacia is not considered, it is readily overlooked; this is unfortunate because osteomalacia generally responds well to therapy, which is certainly not the case in many forms of metabolic bone disease.

Osteomalacia represents a failure of normal mineralization of bone collagen. In children, prior to fusion of the epiphyseal growth plates, there is defective cartilage mineralization as well as impaired bone mineralization, and the resultant growth retardation and skeletal deformities constitute the disorder known as rickets. In adults, osteomalacia may be asymptomatic. As noted previously, osteomalacia may be indistinguishable from osteoporosis on the basis of clinical presentation and radiographic findings, and the two disorders may often coexist in the same patient. Clinically, however, patients with osteomalacia may have diffuse skeletal pain, while bone pain is not usually seen with osteoporosis except at the site of a fracture. In addition, patients with osteomalacia may demonstrate severe proximal muscle weakness, at times associated with a waddling gait. This is most commonly seen in patients with profound hypophosphatemia.

Several different disorders can lead to defective bone collagen mineralization and osteomalacia. Most commonly, there is an abnormality in vitamin D metabolism or a deficiency of phosphate. Although hypocalcemia is frequently associated with osteomalacia, it is not an essential component in all cases of osteomalacia. In order to definitely establish the diagnosis of osteomalacia, it is necessary to examine undermineralized sections of bone biopsy specimens; this examination should document the presence of increased osteoid in the absence of a mineralization (calcification) front. Prior ingestion of tetracycline by the patient at timed intervals aids in the demonstration of impaired mineralization. However, in many clinical situations the diagnosis of osteomalacia may be very obvious, and biopsy is not essential in all cases.

A classification of the disorders that can lead to osteomalacia is seen in Table 20.5.

Vitamin D deficiency is rarely seen in developed countries. Dairy products are fortified with vitamin D, and multivitamin preparations are commonly used. Only in populations of extremely malnourished individuals or in food faddists is vitamin D deficiency likely to be encountered. In fact, even with very poor dietary vitamin D intake, vitamin D deficiency is still unlikely to develop unless the patient is also deprived of ultraviolet irradiation (in the United States, 90% of circulating 25-hydroxyvitamin D is derived from skin production rather than dietary intake, and typical vitamin D deficiency has been cured with sunlight exposure alone). Thus, vitamin D deficiency is usually associated with poor dietary intake combined with inadequate sunlight exposure. This has been described in Asian immigrants to Britain, where climatic factors combined with cultural use of extensive clothing and avoidance of sunshine are associated with dietary deficiency of vitamin D, aggravated by a diet which is high in phytate (which further interferes with calcium absorption). Dietary vitamin D deficiency might also be seen in home-ridden elderly patients with poor dietary habits.

TABLE 20.5 Causes of Osteomalacia

Vitamin D deficiency (diet, sunlight)

Vitamin D malabsorption

Impaired 25-hydroxylation (liver)

Accelerated 25-hydroxyvitamin D catabolism/excretion (anticonvulsants, nephrotic syndrome)

Impaired 1-hydroxylation
- Genetic enzyme defect (vitamin D-dependent rickets)
- Acquired (chronic renal failure, PTH deficiency)

Phosphate depletion states
- ↑PTH/↓ vitamin D
- Malabsorption, phosphate binders
- X-linked hypophosphatemic rickets (vitamin D-resistant rickets)
- Sporadic hypophosphatemic rickets (oncogenic osteomalacia)
- Renal tubular disorders (Fanconi syndrome)
- Metabolic acidosis (renal tubular acidosis, ureterosigmoidostomy)

Inhibitors of mineralization (diphosphonates, fluoride, aluminum)

Hypophosphatasia

Miscellaneous
- Fibrogenesis imperfecta ossium
- Axial osteomalacia

Since vitamin D is a fat-soluble vitamin which is absorbed in the upper part of the small intestine, virtually any malabsorptive disorder can be associated with vitamin D malabsorption. Osteomalacia has been described as a complication of gastrectomy, although the mechanisms for this disorder are not completely clear. Vitamin D malabsorption can also be seen with sprue or other small bowel diseases, small bowel resection or bypass, or pancreatic insufficiency. In addition, since 25-hydroxyvitamin D is excreted in the biliary tract and reabsorbed in the small intestine, biliary tract disease can interrupt the normal enterohepatic circulation of this vitamin D metabolite and lead to deficient vitamin D levels.

Considering that 25-hydroxylation of vitamin D represents the initial step in activation of vitamin D, it is not surprising that impaired 25-hydroxylation by the liver has been described in alcoholic hepatitis, cirrhosis, and primary biliary cirrhosis, and contributes to the development of osteomalacia in these disorders. As is the case in malabsorptive disorders, other factors such as malnutrition, hypoproteinemia, and deficiencies of other nutrients may also play a role in causing the decreased bone mass.

Osteomalacia may also result from accelerated breakdown or excretion of 25-hydroxyvitamin D. This is most frequently seen in patients who are on long-term anticonvulsant therapy (phenytoin, phenobarbital, etc.). These drugs induce liver microsomal enzymes, leading to increased catabolism of vitamin D metabolites. Levels of 25-hydroxyvitamin D are typically low, although there does not seen to be any impairment of 1,25-dihydroxyvitamin D production. Vitamin D loss can also be seen with the nephrotic syndrome, in which the loss of vitamin D binding protein into the urine is associated with increased excretion of 25-hydroxyvitamin D.

Osteomalacia can also be seen as a result of impaired 1-hydroxylation of 25-hydroxyvitamin D. This disorder can be on the basis of congenital enzyme deficiency; in vitamin D-dependent rickets (or pseudovitamin D deficiency), plasma levels of 1,25-dihydroxyvitamin D are low and do not increase even after pharmacologic doses of vitamin D or 25-hydroxyvitamin D. However, replacement with physiologic doses of 1,25-dihydroxyvitamin D improve the hypocalcemia and mineralization disorder. (It should be noted that there is a clinically similar disorder in which levels of 1,25-dihydroxyvitamin D are actually elevated, but there is an apparent end-organ defect in responsiveness to the vitamin D.) More commonly, however, impaired 1-hydroxylation is seen with renal disease. With renal insufficiency, impaired phosphate clearance leads to hyperphosphatemia which then suppresses the 1-hydroxylase enzyme. In addition, since 1-hydroxylation is an activity of the renal cortex, in advanced renal insufficiency there may simply be an inadequate amount of enzyme to hydroxylate 25-hydroxyvitamin D to the active form. Although patients with hypoparathyroidism also have impaired 1-hydroxylation capability, metabolic bone disease in this state is extremely rare.

Hypophosphatemic states are frequently associated with osteomalacia. Apatites, which are the constituents of bone mineral, are essentially phosphate crystals. The organization of the phosphate groups is the most important determinant of the structural characteristics of the crystals. Therefore, phosphorus plays a crucial role in the mineralization of bone, and any state of phosphate depletion can potentially lead to a mineralization defect (osteomalacia). Since 1,25-dihydroxyvitamin D is involved in the intestinal absorption of phosphate, any state of vitamin D deficiency or impaired vitamin D function will lead to decreased phosphate availability. In addition, states of vitamin D deficiency, vitamin D resistance, and other hypocalcemia states lead to secondary hyperparathyroidism, which then promotes increased renal phosphate loss. Phosphate depletion may be seen as a consequence of decreased dietary intake or use of phosphate-binding antacids. Renal phosphate wasting can also be seen on a congenital basis, as is the cases with x-linked hypophosphatemic rickets (vitamin D-resistant rickets). This is a familial disorder which is characterized by renal phosphate wasting and subsequent hypophosphatemia, short stature, and abnormal mineralization of bone. In contrast to other forms of rickets, calcium levels are usually normal. There is some controversy as to whether vitamin D abnormalities are involved in this disorder; 1,25-dihydroxyvitamin D levels are normal, but in the setting of hypophosphatemia and phosphate loss, increased levels would be anticipated. A similar disorder, in which renal phosphate wasting leads to osteomalacia, can occur on an acquired basis. This phosphate-wasting disorder is associated with various malignancies (usually mesenchymal tumors), and the osteomalacia may heal after resection of the tumor. In addition to the phosphate wasting, these patients have been shown to have low levels of 1,25-hydroxyvitamin D. It has been suggested that these tumors make some humoral substance which causes renal phosphate wasting as well as impaired 1-hydroxylation of 25-hydroxyvitamin D, but this proposed substance has not yet been identified. Finally, a number of renal tubular disorders can lead to hypophosphatemia and eventually to osteomalacia. These disorders may include hereditary disorders or acquired lesions (caused by heavy metal poisoning, paraproteinemias, or related to toxicity from drugs). A number of these tubular disorders are also associated with a metabolic acidosis, which seems to be an additional risk factor for osteomalacia. The effect of acidosis is not well understood. It is probably much more complex than the simplistic concept of a leaching of mineral from bone. The low pH seems to have local effects on mineralization of newly formed matrix, and affects phosphate metabolism by altering renal tubular transport. In addition, acidosis may interfere with vitamin D metabolism. In many cases, it is difficult to dissociate the effects of acidosis from those of phosphate depletion.

Several drugs are inhibitors of mineralization. Diphosphonates (such as etidronate) are analogs of pyrophosphate and inhibit mineral deposition and bone resorption. These drugs are used in treatment of skeletal disorders such as Paget's disease and in high doses can impair mineralization and lead to osteomalacia. In addition, long-term administration of fluoride can cause an accumulation of unmineralized matrix. In most regimens in which fluoride is used to treate osteoporosis, calcium supplementation is usually employed to avoid this problem. Aluminum toxicity can also lead to osteomalacia; it has been suggested that this is a major factor in the osteomalacia that is seen in dialysis patients.

Osteomalacia can also be seen with hypophosphatasia, a deficiency of the enzyme alkaline phosphatase. This enzyme may be necessary to break down the organic phosphate compounds which inhibit mineralization.

In some rare circumstances, osteomalacia may not develop from a disorder of mineral metabolism, but instead may be caused by a tissue abnormality which prevents effective mineralization of the matrix. Fibrogenesis imperfecta ossium is a rare disorder in which the polarization of collagen fibers is abnormal, leading to defective mineralization. Similarly, in axial osteomalacia, there does not seem to be any generalized disturbance of mineral metabolism. Instead, a bone cell defect may be responsible for this disease in which the appendicular skeleton is normal, but osteoid accumulation occurs in the axial skeleton.

Therapy of osteomalacia varies, depending on the underlying abnormality. With simple vitamin D deficiency, administration of physiologic doses of vitamin D or ultraviolet irradiation can normalize circulating vitamin D levels. In the case of vitamin D malabsorption, the most appropriate approach is to identify and treat the underlying condition. Pharmacologic doses of vitamin D may be necessary in refractory conditions. Similarly, it is probably possible to compensate for the accelerated vitamin D catabolism in patients on anticonvulsants by administering supplemental vitamin D and calcium. In patients with impaired 1-hydroxylation of vitamin D, it is possible to give either physiologic doses of 1,25-dihydroxyvitamin D, or pharmacologic doses of parent vitamin D. Although it might be argued that the former is more physiologic, the latter approach is less expensive. In addition, the possibility that metabolites of vitamin D other than 1,25-dihydroxyvitamin D are also important suggests that the precursor parent vitamin D may represent more appropriate treatment. In patients with x-linked hypophosphatemic rickets, therapy consists of oral phosphorus supplementation in addition to vitamin D; optimal therapy of this condition has not yet been clearly established. In a patient with apparent acquired hypophosphatemic rickets, the possibility of oncogenic osteomalacia arises, and it is appropriate to search for an underlying malignancy. Resection of a tumor frequently leads to improvement of the bone disease. In patients with unresectable tumor, phosphorus supplementation and 1,25-dihydroxyvitamin D therapy may prove useful. In patients where acidosis is a major component of the problem (as in renal tubular acidosis), alkalization is effective and useful therapy. For some conditions, such as hypophosphatasia, no known effective therapy exists.

Other Disorders of Bone/Mineral Metabolism

There are several other specific disorders of connective tissue and mineral metabolism which do not fit cleanly into any of the previously described categories. However, some of these disorders are relatively common (Paget's disease), and they all have the potential of giving further insight into specific aspects of connective tissue and mineral metabolism, so they will be discussed here.

Paget's Disease (21)

Paget's disease is a relatively common bone disorder, afflicting 3-4% of the population over the age of 45, and perhaps as much as 10% of the population by the ninth decade. Strictly speaking, Paget's disease is not a metabolic bone disease; bone involvement is focal, and some portions of the skeleton are always spared. Paget's disease is a process in which there is basically an increased remodeling of the bone, leading to pain, skeletal deformities, and structurally abnormal and weakened bone. The etiology of the disease is unknown. The possibility of a viral cause has been suggested, but this has never been well documented, and a number of other possibilities have also been suggested. Paget's disease starts with increased osteoclastic resorption of normal bone by giant multinucleated cells. This is a haphazard process, leading to irregularly shaped resorption cavities. This increased resorption is followed by an accelerated osteoblastic response with formation of primitive or woven bone in association with increased connective tissue reaction. This accelerated and disorganized process of bone remodeling leads to formation of distorted and abnormal bone. The pelvic bones are most commonly involved, but Paget's disease also frequently involves the femur, skull, tibia, and lumbosacral spine. Disease may also be seen in the dorsal spine, clavicles, and ribs, but smaller bones are less frequently involved.

Most patients with radiographic evidence of Paget's disease are asymptomatic. Pain is one of the more common symptoms of Paget's disease, but in many cases it is difficult to tell whether the pain is coming from the Paget's disease per se or from osteoarthritis which frequently occurs in major joints near areas of skeletal involvement with Paget's disease. Because of the increased remodeling and formation of abnormal bone, bony deformities (enlarged skull, kyphosis, and bowing of the lower extremities) and pathologic fractures can be seen. New bone growth can lead to nerve compression; this commonly involves cranial nerves, and can lead to optic atrophy and decreased hearing. With vertebral involvement, pressure on the spinal cord and nerve roots can lead to neurologic impairment. Hypercalcemia secondary to increased bone turnover represents another complication of Paget's disease. In addition, some patients will develop a high-output cardiac failure. Patients with Paget's disease are also at an increased risk of developing osteogenic sarcoma.

Laboratory investigation will demonstrate findings that are compatible with increased bone turnover. Biochemically, an elevated alkaline phosphatase correlates with the extensiveness of the skeletal involvement, and increased urinary hydroxyproline reflects the increased bone resorption. Bone scans are positive in the area of involved bone, and bone x-rays may show lytic areas as well as sclerotic areas. In some cases, x-rays may suggest the possibility of metastatic cancer.

Several forms of therapy are available for Paget's disease. In an asymptomatic patient with minimal disease, no specific therapy may be required. If pain is present, analgesics may be the only treatment that is needed. However, in the case of more extensive disease (especially when associated with complications), an effort to decrease the rapid bone turnover is worthwhile.

Calcitonin has been shown to be effective treatment for Paget's disease, leading to a reduction in pain and lowering of alkaline phosphatase and hydroxyproline levels. The action of calcitonin on bone formation has been discussed previously. Its major handicap is that it must be given parenterally, and is not uncommonly associated with antibody formation (since the clinically available calcitonin preparation is salmon calcitonin). Synthetic salmon calcitonin is usually administered in a dose of 100 U subcutaneously once a day, but may be reduced to 50 U 3 times a week if there is a good response.

More recently, disphosphonates (such as etidronate) have been shown to be effective. These drugs are analogs of pyrophosphate and have the advantage of being administered orally. At very high doses, however, etidronate can interfere with bone mineralization and cause osteomalacia. Etidronate is usually given in a dosage of approximately 5 mg/kg/day, limited to 6-month courses of therapy, which may be repeated if necessary after a 3-6-month interval of not taking the drug.

Fibrous Dysplasia

Fibrous dysplasia represents another poorly understood process which may simulate a number of other metabolic bone diseases. In this disorder, proliferating fibrous tissue replaces mature bone in one or more areas of the skeleton. Localized cartilage formation may appear within areas of fibrous tissue proliferation, and areas of bone destruction (appearing as bone cysts on x-rays) may also be seen. Bony deformity and pathologic fractures can occur, and sarcomatous changes have even been described. The skull, femur, and tibia are the most commonly involved sites. The disease may involve only a portion of one bone, or may involve several bones. Polyostotic fibrous dysplasia is associated with irregular café au lait spots which end at the midline, and at times is associated with endocrine disturbances such as sexual precocity, hyperthyroidism, or acromegaly.

Osteosclerosis

Osteosclerosis represents an increase in radiodensity, reflecting an increased amount of mineralized bone. This may occur because of a failure in bone resorption or from the presence of excessive amounts of partially mineralized osteoid tissue. Localized forms may be seen due to metastatic cancer (breast, prostate, lymphoma) or infection, but some generalized forms also exist. Osteopetrosis is a childhood disorder in which a bone marrow cavity eventually becomes obliterated, leading to severe anemia; a milder form has also be described in adults. In these patients, there seems to be a defect in the ability of osteoclasts to normally resorb bone. Osteosclerosis can also be seen with myelofibrosis. This usually occurs with blood disorders such as leukemia or polycythemia vera, where fibroblast and osteoblast proliferation may be part of the basic hematologic disease. Osteosclerosis is also seen in osteofluorosis, where fluoride ingestion results in the formation of bone crystals that are larger and more resistant to bone resorption than the normal bone crystal. In addition, fluoride causes an increase in osteoid. If this is coupled with adequate calcium intake, it can lead to increased osteoid mineralization and osteosclerosis. As mentioned previously, sclerotic lesions are also seen in Paget's disease, and occasionally diffuse sclerosis may be the only manifestation of the disease. Rarely, osteosclerosis has been described in hyperparathyroidism, hypoparathyroidism, hypophosphatemic rickets, axial osteomalacia, and fibrogenesis imperfecta ossium.

Tumoral Calcinosis

Tumoral calcinosis is a rare disorder of mineral metabolism. In this disease, large deposits of calcium phosphate occur adjacent to large joints. Serum levels of calcium are normal, but phosphate levels are increased. The hyperphosphatemia seems to be responsible for the precipitation of calcium and phosphate into soft tissue, and efforts to decrease serum phosphorus have led to regression of the calcified deposits. No abnormalities of PTH or vitamin D have been documented, and it appears that there is an abnormality in renal tubular transport of phosphorus independent of PTH status.

References

1. Krane M: Connective tissue. In LH Smith Jr, SO Thier (eds.), *Pathophysiology: The Biological Principles of Disease.* Philadelphia, W.B. Saunders, 1981, pp. 755-798.

2. Miller EJ: The structure of collagen. In BM Watner, R Fleischmager, N Kaufman (eds.), *Connective Tissue Diseases.* Baltimore, Williams and Wilkins, 1983, pp. 4-15.

3. Pinnell SR, Murad S: Disorders of collagen. In JB Stanbury, JB Wyngaarden, DS Fredrickson, JL Goldstein, MS Brown (eds.), *The Metabolic Basis of Inherited Disease,* 5th Ed. New York, McGraw-Hill, 1983, pp. 1425-1449.

4. Prockop DJ, Kivirikko KI, Tuderman L, Guzman NA: The biosynthesis of collagen and its disorders. *N Engl J Med* 301:13-23, 77-85, 1979.

5. Smith R: Collagen and disorders of bone. *Clin Sci* 59:215-223, 1980.

6. Canalis E: The hormonal and local regulation of bone formation. *Endocr Rev* 4:62-77, 1983.

7. Lutwak L, Singer FR, Urist MR: Current concepts of bone metabolism. *Ann Int Med* 80:630-644, 1974.

8. Raisz LG, Kream BE: Regulation of bone formation. *N Engl J Med* 309: 29-35, 83-89, 1983.

9. Agus ZS, Wasserstein A, Goldfarb S: Disorders of calcium and magnesium homeostasis. *Amer J Med* 72:473-488, 1982.

10. Harrison JE, Hitchman AJW, Hitchman A, Hasany SA, McNeill KG, Tam CS: Differences between the effects of phosphate deficiency and vitamin D deficiency on bone metabolism. *Metabolism* 29:1225-1233, 1980.

11. Mawer EB: Clinical implications of measurements of circulating vitamin D metabolites. *Clin Endocr and Metab* 9:63-79, 1980.

12. Norman AW, Roth J, Orci L: The vitamin D endocrine system: Steroid metabolism, hormone receptors, and biological response (calcium binding proteins). *Endocr Rev* 3:331-366, 1982.

13. Stoff JS: Phosphate homeostasis and hypophosphatemia. *Amer J Med* 72: 489-495, 1982.

14. Cordy PE, Mills DM: The early detection and treatment of renal osteodystrophy. *Mineral Electrolyte Metab* 5:311-320, 1981.

15. Frame B, Parfitt AM: Osteomalacia: Current concepts. *Ann Int Med* 89: 966-982, 1978.

16. Goldring SR, Krane SM: Metabolic bone disease, osteoporosis and osteomalacia. *Disease-A-Month* Vol 27 (No. 7):1-103, 1981.

17. Hahn TJ: Drug-induced disorders of vitamin D and mineral metabolism. *Clin Endocr and Metab* 9:107-129, 1980.

18. Meredith SC, Rosenburg IH: Gastrointestinal-hepatic disorders and osteomalacia. *Clin Endocr and Metab* 9:131-150, 1980.

19. Teitelbaum SL: Pathological manifestations of osteomalacia and rickets. *Clin Endocr and Metab* 9:43-62, 1980.

20. Thomson DL, Frame B: Involutional osteopenia: Current concepts. *Ann Int Med* 85:789-803, 1976.

21. Ryan WG: Pathophysiology and modern management of Paget's disease. *Comprehensive Ther* (No. 9):64-69, 1983.

Chapter 21

INFECTIOUS ARTHRITIS

Elliott L. Semble, M.D. and Carlos A. Agudelo, M.D.

Acute Bacterial Arthritis

Acute bacterial arthritis (septic arthritis) is a medical emergency requiring the prompt initiation of appropriate antibiotic therapy. Almost any organism can cause septic arthritis, but a limited number of agents are usually responsible for most infections.

Disease Susceptibility

Diabetes mellitus, cirrhosis of the liver, neoplasms, chronic renal failure, and rheumatoid arthritis may predispose patients to acute bacterial arthritis. Intravenous drug abusers and immunosuppressed patients are also at increased risk for septic arthritis.

Drugs used in the treatment of rheumatic diseases including corticosteroids and cytotoxic agents may compromise host resistance resulting in an increased incidence of acute bacterial arthritis.

Local factors such as underlying joint disease have been implicated in the development of septic arthritis. Rheumatoid arthritis, osteoarthritis, trauma, gout, pseudogout, and neuropathic joint disease cause local anatomic abnormalities which may result in an increased risk of sepsis in affected joints. Joint infection may be a consequence of direct trauma to a joint or may occur after an intra-articular corticosteroid injection.

Pathogenesis

Acute bacterial arthritis occurs most often by hematogenous dissemination from a primary focus of infection. However, joint sepsis may also result from the extension of an adjacent soft tissue infection or adjoining osteomyelitis.

If a joint infection is not eradicated early, it may result in joint destruction. Three stages of cartilage destruction have been identified in septic arthritis (1). The initial events are characterized by a release of lysosomal enzymes from activated polymorphonuclear leukocytes and proliferating synovial lining cells. These enzymes result in a loss of proteoglycan from cartilage. If the infectious process is halted during this early stage, a restoration of proteoglycan matrix may be achieved and chondrocyte injury avoided. During the second stage, increased mechanical stress and inadequate nutrition result in chondrocyte damage. In the last stage, enzymes released from polymorphonuclear leukocytes and proliferating synovium along with altered joint mechanics gradually destroy the collagen network. When the collagen framework has been destroyed, major structural modifications occur resulting in joint deformity.

Clinical Features

Septic arthritis usually affects one joint, but may involve two or more joints. The involved joint is generally warm, painful, swollen, red, and limited in motion. The hips and knees are involved most often, but any joint may become infected.

Systemic features of acute bacterial arthritis include fever, which is often low grade, and chills. Signs and symptoms of a primary infection may also be present. A careful physical examination may reveal an infectious focus involving any site, but the usual sources include the skin, nasopharynx, sinuses, lungs, cervix, and rectum.

Infections involving the sacroiliac or spinal apophyseal joints are difficult to detect since clinical findings may be absent. Elderly patients and immunosuppressed individuals may demonstrate less evidence of inflammation with septic arthritis despite their greater risk for this disease. Patients with underlying joint disease (e.g., rheumatoid arthritis) have an increased incidence of superimposed joint infection. Acute bacterial arthritis may be suspected in these patients when a single joint is more severely involved than other joints.

The differential diagnosis of septic arthritis includes crystal-induced synovitis, viral arthritis, and traumatic arthritis. Monoarticular rheumatoid arthritis and Reiter's syndrome occasionally may be confused with acute bacterial arthritis; however, rheumatoid disease and Reiter's syndrome usually have a more insidious onset. If several joints are affected at the same time, acute rheumatic fever, gout, viral arthritis, and serum sickness may be considered along with septic arthritis (1).

Laboratory Tests

Peripheral leukocytosis occurs in a majority of patients with acute bacterial arthritis. An elevated erythrocyte sedimentation rate is generally found in this disease.

Patients suspected of having acute bacterial arthritis should have blood and urine cultures performed prior to the initiation of antibiotic therapy. Blood cultures are mandatory since they may be positive in approximately 75% of patients (2). Sputum, nasopharyngeal, and wound cultures may be obtained if clinically indicated.

The diagnosis of septic arthritis is established by a positive synovial fluid culture. A typical joint infection demonstrates a purulent effusion with a synovial fluid white count of greater than 50,000 cells/mm^3 and more than 90% polymorphonuclear leukocytes (3). Synovial fluid leukocyte counts are often greater than 100,000 cells/mm^3 in septic arthritis, but occasionally white counts in the 5000 to 10,000 cells/mm^3 range may be associated with acute bacterial arthritis (4).

Synovial fluid glucose levels may be low in acute bacterial arthritis. The normal plasma-synovial fluid glucose differential obtained simultaneously in the fasting state is less than 40 mg/dl. This difference is often greater than 90 mg/dl in septic arthritis. However, synovial fluid glucose levels may also be low in rheumatoid arthritis which limits the utility of the test.

Gram-stain and culture of the synovial fluid are obligatory when infection is suspected. The gram stain may be positive in one-half (4) to two-thirds (3) of patients with septic arthritis. A positive synovial fluid culture confirms the diagnosis and identifies the offending agent, while sensitivity testing provides the basis for appropriate therapy by assaying the antimicrobial activity of the organism. Synovial fluid should either be plated at the bedside or hand-delivered to the laboratory by the physician. Aerobic cultures should be obtained routinely. Cultures of *Neisseria gonorrhoeae, Hemophilus influenzae,* and anaerobes require the use of special media.

Radiographic examination of affected joints may reveal only soft tissue swelling early in the course of septic arthritis. However, roentgenograms should be obtained initially to document the presence and extent of prior joint damage. Juxtaarticular osteopenia appears about 7-10 days after the onset of joint infection. If the joint infection is not eradicated, progressive joint space narrowing may develop. Late radiographic findings in septic arthritis include subluxation and eventual joint destruction.

Additional laboratory procedures may be useful in the diagnosis of acute bacterial arthritis. Gas chromatography has been employed to detect microbial metabolites in synovial fluid and may yield results in approximately 4 hours (5). Synovial fluid lactic acid levels have been utilized to differentiate septic from nonseptic arthritis, and gonococcal from nongonococcal arthritis (6). However, this test has limited utility since synovial fluid lactic acid values in gonococcal arthritis are not significantly different from those in rheumatoid arthritis, systemic lupus erythematosus, or gout (7).

Counterimmunoelectrophoresis is a rapid procedure (1-2 hours) for the detection of bacterial antigens in joint fluid (5). It may be positive even if the synovial fluid is sterile. The technique has been useful in the identification of pneumococcal, meningococcal, and *H. influenzae* joint infections.

Radioisotope scanning techniques may be helpful in localizing unsuspected sites of infection in acute bacterial arthritis, and in differentiating soft tissue infections from septic arthritis or osteomyelitis (1). However, the findings on scintigraphy are not specific and radionuclide imaging of the musculoskeletal systems generally has little role in the initial evaluation of acute bacterial arthritis (7).

Causative Organisms in Septic Arthritis

Neisseria gonorrhoeae is responsible for approximately one-half of septic arthritis in adults (Table 21.1). Gram-positive organisms account for about 90% of nongonococcal acute bacterial arthritis and staphylococci are responsible for three-quarters of these. Gram-negative bacilli account for a small percentage

TABLE 21.1 Incidence of Organisms in Acute Bacterial Arthritis in Adults

Organism	Incidence (%)
Gram-positive cocci	
Staphylococcus aureus	35
Streptococcus pyogenes viridans, pneumoniae	10
Gram-negative cocci	
Neisseria gonorrhoeae	50
Gram-negative bacilli (*Escherichia coli,* Salmonella, Pseudomonas, etc.)	5

From Ihman RD: Infectious arthritis. In JF Beary III, CL Christian, TP Sculco (eds.), *Manual of Rheumatology and Outpatient Orthopedic Disorders. Diagnosis and Therapy.* Boston, Little, Brown and Co., 1981, pp. 151-157.

of the cases of septic arthritis, although their incidence appears to be increasing. Because of differences in clinical presentation and management, infectious arthritis due to *Neisseria* (gonococcal and meningococcal) species are considered separately.

Gram-Positive Organisms

Septic arthritis due to staphylococci involves a single joint or several joints in a patient with a primary infectious focus located elsewhere, most often a cutaneous source (e.g., furuncle).

Streptococci acount for approximately 10% of septic arthritis in adults (Table 21.1). Streptococcal arthritis usually originates from an infection in the upper respiratory tract or skin. Acute bacterial arthritis due to *Streptococcus pneumoniae* generally results from hematogenous dissemination from a primary pulmonary source, or less often, from meningeal, upper respiratory, or endocardial sites (9).

Gram-Negative Organisms

Gram-negative bacilli are responsible for approximately 5% of septic arthritis in adults (Table 21.1). *Escherichia coli, Pseudomonas aeruginosa,* and *Serratia marcescens* are the most frequent offending organisms. *E. coli* most often originates from the urinary tract, while *Pseudomonas* and *Serratia* joint infections usually result from intravenous drug abuse (10). Salmonella, *Hemophilus influenzae,* and anaerobic bacteria have also been reported to cause septic arthritis in adults.

Treatment

The management of bacterial arthritis should begin immediately after the suspicion and/or confirmation of the diagnosis. Successful therapy of septic arthritis requires the use of appropriate antibiotics and the mechanical drainage of purulent fluid.

The antibiotic should be chosen primarily on the basis of the results of the synovial fluid gram-stain. If the gram-stain is negative, the choice of antibiotic depends on the clinical setting. The antibiotic may be changed depending on the results of cultures (Table 21.2). Parenterally administered antibiotics achieve bactericidal concentrations in joint fluid and the direct instillation of antibiotics into the joint space is unnecessary.

The antibacterial activity of synovial fluid during antibiotic therapy may be monitored by a tube-dilution technique. A margin of bactericidal effect 10 or more times that found in undiluted joint fluid provides adquate antimicrobial action.

The duration of antibiotic treatment for septic arthritis depends on the nature of the offending organism and the response to therapy (Table 21.2). Gonococcal arthritis may be treated systemically until improvement occurs (several days usually), followed by oral antibiotics to complete 7 days of treatment (see later in chapter). Streptococcal joint infections should be treated for several weeks, while staphylococcal arthritis requires at least 3 weeks of therapy. Gram-negative articular infections should be treated for a minimum of 4 weeks.

Closed-needle aspiration should be performed at least once daily to drain the affected joint. Open surgical drainage is indicated in hip and sacroiliac joint infections or if there is a lack of response to therapy (i.e., joint fluid cultures persistently positive or patients remaining febrile after 3-4 days of antibiotic therapy).

The infected joint should be kept at rest. A splint provides complete immobilization and helps to reduce pain and trauma to the cartilage. As joint symptoms resolve, passive range of motion exercises should be started to avoid joint contracture. Weight-bearing should be deferred until inflammation has completely resolved.

General measures used to treat septicemia should also be included in the therapy of acute bacterial arthritis. Daily assessment of the patient's fluid and nutritional needs is necessary. Pain control may be accomplished by the use of analgesics that do not affect fever. Antiinflammatory drugs (e.g., aspirin) should not be given until the early response to antibiotic therapy can be evaluated. The early diagnosis and treatment of septic arthritis results in an improved outcome.

Gonococcal Arthritis

Gonococcal arthritis is the most common form of acute bacterial arthritis. Joint involvement usually occurs during dissemination of the gonococcal infection.

Clinical Manifestations

Arthritis is a major feature of disseminated gonococcal infection. Prior to the antibiotic era, gonococcal arthritis was more common in males than females. However, recent studies have noted a higher incidence in young females (11,12), especially if they are pregnant or menstruating. Most patients with gonococcal arthritis are less than 40 years of age, but newborn infants, children, and older adults may be affected.

TABLE 21.2 Antibiotic Therapy of Acute Bacterial Arthritis in Adults Based on Culture Identification of Organism

Organism	Antibiotic of Choice	Alternate Drug(s)	Duration of Treatment
Staphylococci	Nafcillin 8-12 g/day	Cephalothin 6-8 g/day	3-4 weeks
Streptococci	Penicillin G 10 million U/day	Erythromycin 2-4 g/day*	2-3 weeks
Neisseria gonorrhoeae (penicillinase negative)	Penicillin G 6-10 million U/day	Tetracycline 2 g/day*	7 days
Gram-negative bacilli (*E. coli*, *Proteus* species, *Serratia marcescens*, etc.)	Tobramycin 3-5 mg/kg/day or Another aminoglycoside	2nd/3rd generation cephalosporin depending on sensitivities	4-6 weeks
Pseduomonas aeruginosa	Ticarcillin 12 g/day and Tobramycin 5 mg/kg/day	Synergy using an anti-pseudomonal and an aminoglycoside is preferred, but with contraindications regimens should be selected according to the results of the sensitivities	4-6 weeks

*Medication may be administered orally or parenterally.

The usual sites of primary gonococcal infection are the urethra in males, cervix in females, and pharynx and rectum in both sexes. These primary sources for dissemination of gonoccocal infection should be cultured in all patients suspected of having gonococcal arthritis.

Patients with gonococcal arthritis may have systemic findings of infection such as fever and chills. A low-grade fever is seen most often, but occasionally higher temperature elevations may be detected in patients with bacteremia.

A migratory polyarthritis is the most common initial joint manifestation in gonococcal arthritis. Subsequently, findings may localize to one or several joints. The knees, wrists, small joints of the hands, ankles, and elbows are affected most often, but any joint may be involved.

Periarticular pain and swelling are common (13). Tenosynovitis is found in a significant number of patients with disseminated gonococcal infection, and is recognized as a major clinical feature of the disease. The dorsum of the hands and feet, wrist, or Achilles' tendons are most often involved (11).

Typical skin lesions are a frequent manifestation of disseminated gonococcal infection. They generally begin as small, erythematous macules, that either disappear or develop into vesicopustular lesions characterized by a gray, necrotic center and a hemorrhagic base (Figure 21.1).

Laboratory Tests

Peripheral leukocyte counts may be normal or moderately elevated in gonococcal arthritis. Synovial fluid analysis generally reveals an inflammatory fluid with a variable number of white cells ranging from a few thousand to several hundred thousand per cubic millimeter. Joint fluid cultures are positive in less than one-half of all patients even under ideal culture conditions (13).

Pathogenesis

A direct toxic effect of gonococci on tissues is the most likely pathogenetic mechanism in disseminated gonococcal infection (13). However, the host's immune response to the gonococcal organism may be important in the pathogenesis of joint and cutaneous inflammation (14). The role of immune complexes in this disorder has not been resolved and requires further study (1,13).

Keiser et al. (15) have described two clinical forms of gonococcal arthritis. The septic form is characterized by fever, chills, polyarthritis, skin lesions, and little joint effusion. The nonseptic form is manifested by monoarticular joint effusions from which gonococci are frequently recovered, but with few systemic findings such as fever or chills. However, subsequent investigators have been unable to identify different subgroups in gonococcal arthritis (11,16), and little clinical evidence is available to support such a distinction.

Diagnosis

Disseminated gonococcal infection should be suspected in young, sexually active females who develop a migratory polyarthritis, tenosynovitis, and/or characteristic skin lesions. Bacteriologic studies are necessary to confirm the diagnosis. Cultures should be obtained from the cervix, urethra, rectum, pharynx, blood, and affected joints.

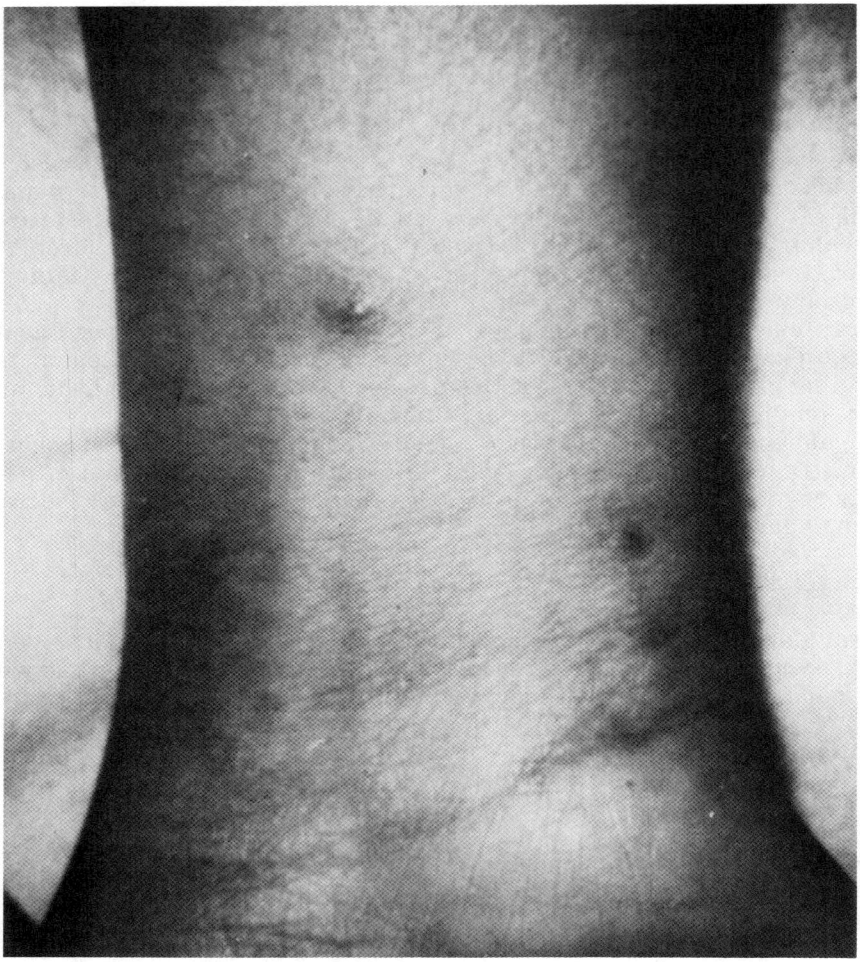

FIGURE 21.1 Skin lesions of disseminated gonococcal infection. The major lesion is vesicopustular, surmounting a hemorrhagic base. The other two, smaller lesions appear more necrotic and probably represent older lesions. (From *Textbook of Rheumatology,* with permission of the author Alan Myers, and W.B. Saunders Co.)

The gonococcus is a fastidious organism. The successful isolating of gonococcus requires proper handling of cultures. Special culture medium (e.g., chocolate agar) should be used for blood or synovial fluid cultures, while Thayer-Martin medium is recommended for contaminated areas such as the cervix, rectum, and pharynx.

Additional diagnostic tests which may be useful in identifying the gonococcus include fluorescent antibody techniques (16), and counterimmunoelectrophoresis of serum and synovial fluid (17).

The differential diagnosis of gonococcal arthritis includes septic arthritis resulting from other organisms, and rheumatologic disorders such as rheumatic fever, Reiter's syndrome, gout, rheumatoid arthritis, and systemic lupus erythematosus. A therapeutic trial of procaine penicillin after appropriate cultures have been obtained may distinguish between gonococcal arthritis and rheumatic fever or Reiter's syndrome (18). Gout is diagnosed by its typical clinical findings and the presence of negatively birefringent crystals in synovial fluid. However, septic and crystal-induced arthritis may simultaneously occur. The finding of crystals in synovial fluid should not dissuade the physician from searching for infection (19). Patients with rheumatoid arthritis or systemic lupus erythematosus may occasionally develop gonococcal or nongonococcal bacterial arthritis. Septic arthritis should be suspected in these patients when fever, chills, or increased local joint inflammation occurs.

Treatment

The management of gonococcal arthritis includes antibiotics, joint aspiration, and splinting. Penicillin is the drug of choice in nonallergic patients. The recommended dosage is 6-10 million units daily of aqueous penicillin G intravenously in divided doses every 4 hours until improvement occurs, followed by oral ampicillin 0.5 g 4 times daily to complete a 7-day course. Alternative treatment programs include oral ampicillin 3.5 g or amoxicillin 3.0 g orally, each with probenecid 1.0 g, followed by ampicillin 0.5 g or amoxicillin 0.5 g orally 4 times daily for 7 days, or spectinomycin 2.0 g intramuscularly twice daily for 3 days (7).

A low-dose regimen of penicillin (procaine penicillin G, 600,000 U intramuscularly every 12 hours for 10 days) has also been found to be as effective as high-dose penicillin therapy (20). In patients allergic to penicillin, tetracycline 0.5 g or erythromycin 0.5 g is given orally 4 times daily for 7 days.

Hospitalization is indicated for patients who are unable to follow or tolerate an outpatient regimen or who have purulent synovial effusions (7). Joint drainage by closed-needle aspiration should be performed daily on all hospitalized patients as long as the joint effusion persists. Immobilization of the affected joint by splinting may also be helpful in providing pain relief. As joint symptoms improve, passive range of motion exercises should begin. When inflammation has subsided, active exercises and weight-bearing may be instituted.

The response to therapy generally occurs within 2-3 days. The prognosis for full recovery of joint function is good if appropriate treatment is instituted early in the course of the disease.

Meningococcal Arthritis

Arthritis is a relatively common complication of meningococcal infection. It generally involves several joints and appears as the meningeal infection is improving (21). The most frequently involved joints include the knees, ankles, and elbows. Skin lesions may be identical to those seen with disseminated gonococcal infection (22), but the absence of tenosynovitis helps to differentiate meningococcal from gonococcal disease.

Joint effusions may be mildly inflammatory or purulent, but often are culture-negative. The principles that guide the diagnosis of meningococcal arthritis are the same as for gonococcal disease. Penicillin G is the antibiotic of choice in meningococcal arthritis and should be given in high doses intravenously.

TABLE 21.3 Incidence of Organisms in Childhood Septic Arthritis

Organism	Incidence (%)
Gram-positive cocci	
Staphylococcus aureus	45
Streptococcus pyogenes, Viridans, pneumoniae	25
Gram-negative cocci	
Neisseria gonorrhoeae	5
Gram-negative bacilli	<15
*Hemophilus influenzae**	10

**H. influenzae* has been separated from the rest of the gram-negative bacillary group since its frequency is so high in the pediatric age group.

Childhood Septic Arthritis

Acute bacterial arthritis occurs in all age groups in children and is frequently seen in those under 2 years old (23). Males are affected 2-3 times more often than females. The hip and knee joints are usually involved.

The incidence of offending organisms in acute bacterial arthritis in children is illustrated in Table 21.3. Staphylococci or gram-negative bacilli are usually responsible for infected joints in children under 6 months of age. *H. influenzae,* streptococci, or staphylococci are generally responsible for acute bacterial arthritis in children younger than 5 years of age (24).

Acute bacterial arthritis in childhood may present after an infection or recent trauma. The disease usually begins suddenly with pain involving the affected extremity. A high fever may accompany the joint symptoms. Examination of the infected joint generally reveals warmth, swelling, and limitation of motion. A peripheral leukocytosis or an elevation of the erythrocyte sedimentation rate may be noted on laboratory testing. Radiographs may show distension of the joint cavity with adjacent soft tissue swelling early in the course of the disease. Destructive changes of the joint may be noted on roentgenograms in advanced infection.

Confirmation of the diagnosis of chilhood septic arthritis is dependent on the identification of the causative agent. If acute bacterial arthritis is suspected, Gram-stained smears and cultures of possible sources of infection and synovial fluid should be performed. The choice of antibiotic depends on the results of the synovial fluid gram-stain. If the gram-stain is negative, cefuroxime should be used. The antibiotic may be switched depending upon the results of the cultures (Table 21.4).

Parenteral antibiotics should be given for at least 2 weeks in *H. Influenzae* and streptococcal joint infections. Staphylococci and gram-negative bacillary arthritis require at least 3 weeks of treatment. Daily joint aspiration of the infected joint should be performed to drain the purulent effusion. Immobilization of the affected limb is helpful in reducing pain and controlling inflammation.

TABLE 21.4 Antibiotic Therapy of Childhood Septic Arthritis Based on Culture Identification of Organism

Organism	Antiobiotic of Choice	Alternate Drug(s)**	Duration of Treatment
Staphylococci	Nafcillin 150 mg/kg/day	Cefuroxime* 75 mg/kg/day	3-4 weeks
Streptococci	Penicillin G 100,000 U/kg/day	Cefuroxime 75 mg/kg/day	2-3 weeks
Neisseria gonorrhoeae	Penicillin G 100,000 U/kg/day	Cefuroxime 75 mg/kg/day	7 days
Gram-negative bacilli	Gentamicin 6-7.5 mg/kg/day	Other aminoglycosides or 2nd/3rd generation cephalosporins	3-4 weeks
Hemophilus influenzae	Ampicillin 150 mg/kg/day or Cefuroxime 75 mg/kg/day	Chloramphenicol 75 mg/kg/day	2-3 weeks

*From Nelson JD: Cefuroxime: A cephalosporin with unique applicability to pediatric practice. *Ped Infect Dis* 2:394-396, 1983.
**Other antibiotics may be used depending on organism sensitivity.

Surgical drainage should be considered early in the course of septic arthritis of the hip in children, since closed-needle aspiration may provide inadequate joint drainage and may result in vascular injury. Open drainage may also be indicated for other affected joints if closed-needle aspiration is not successful in reducing the effusion, or if fever persists for 48 hours despite appropriate antibiotic therapy.

The prognosis of childhood septic arthritis depends on the duration of the disease prior to therapy and the presence of hip involvement. Significant morbidity from hip infections is not uncommon in infants or children, and early diagnosis and treatment may prevent joint damage.

Viral Arthritis

Viral arthritis often begins with nonspecific symptoms such as malaise and fatigue, chills and fever, headache, stiff neck, sore throat, or nausea and vomiting. Signs of a viral illness may include a low-grade temperature and regional lymphadenopathy. Joint involvement in viral arthritis is generally polyarticular, but occasionally a single joint or several joints may be affected. Viral arthritis is usually of short duration and rarely results in joint damage. Tenosynovitis may accompany joint inflammation in viral disorders. Cutaneous, neurologic, and cardiac abnormalities may also occur.

Laboratory tests are nonspecific. Patients may be mildly anemic or have a few atypical lymphocytes. An elevated erythrocyte sedimentation rate is often found. Rheumatoid factor tests are usually negative (except in rubella) and antinuclear antibodies are almost always absent. Serum cryoprecipitates are occasionally found and may be associated with decreased complement levels. Synovial effusions range from noninflammatory to septic with predominately polymorphonuclear leukocytes.

Viral arthritis is difficult to recognize since many of the clinical and laboratory findings are nonspecific. A history of drug abuse suggests the diagnosis of hepatitis B infection, while a history of recent immunization for rubella suggests this organism as the causative agent.

Hepatitis B Viral Arthritis

Joint manifestations are seen in 10–30% of patients with hepatitis B infection. Adolescents and young adults are at greater risk of developing arthritis with males and females affected equally.

Clinical Features

There is often a prodrome of malaise, anorexia, nausea and vomiting, chills and fever, or myalgia, 1 day to 12 weeks prior to the onset of arthritis (25). Patients may develop an acute, symmetrical arthritis affecting multiple joints simultaneously, or less often, a migratory polyarthritis. The small joints of the hands are frequently involved, but the large peripheral joints may also be affected. Joint findings generally resolve in several weeks, but may last up to 6 months. Tenosynovitis or bursitis may be associated with arthritis in some patients.

The arthritis is frequently accompanied by an urticarial skin rash, often pruritic, and usually on the lower extremities. The skin lesions may last from several days to many weeks. Joint manifestations generally disappear before the onset of jaundice, although most patients remain anicteric.

Laboratory Findings

Most patients with hepatitis B infection have normal hematocrits and peripheral white cell counts. Occasionally, a relative lymphocytosis or a few atypical lymphocytes may be seen. Synovial fluid white counts are variable ranging from 465 to 90,000 cells/mm^3 (25).

Patients with acute polyarthritis generally have hepatitis B surface antigen (HB_sAg) in their sera. HB_sAg has also been found in synovial fluid (25). As joint inflammation improves, HB_sAg usually disappears from the serum and its antibody (anti-HB_s) may be detectable.

As the onset of polyarthritis, decreased levels of the complement components C3 and C4 may be found in the serum of some patients with hepatitis B infection. Higher concentrations of HB_sAg may be associated with lower values of C4.

Pathogenesis

The arthritis of hepatitis B infection may involve circulating immune complexes. Serum cryoprecipitates, which may derive from large, circulating immune complexes may be found during active joint and skin disease. These precipitates may contain HB_sAg, antibody to HB_s, immunoglobulins, and complement components. Serum complement levels are often depressed during acute joint inflammation.

Hepatitis B virus may also cause tissue damage by a direct toxic effect. It may invade and replicate in the synovium. Particles resembling virus have been seen in synovial tissues in the electron microscope (26).

Treatment

The polyarthritis of hepatitis B infection is generally self-limited regardless of therapy. Some patients may have resolution of the arthritis with salicylate therapy.

Rubella Arthritis

The arthritis associated with rubella may occur in natural rubella infection or after immunization with live attenuated virus.

Clinical Features

Joint involvement is more common in postpubescent girls and women in both natural rubella and in vaccine-induced rubella. The joint symptoms are similar in both disorders. The onset of arthritis is generally abrupt, affecting the fingers, knees, and wrists symmetrically. Pain on motion and stiffness may be the only signs of joint inflammation.

The arthritis occurs from 6 days before to 6 days after the rash in natural rubella. Joint symptoms may last up to 30 days, but residual articular damage has not been reported. The arthritis associated with vaccine-induced rubella usually occurs 2-4 weeks after immunization. Recurrent joint inflammation involving the knees has been seen in several patients with vaccine-induced rubella up to 5 years after the immunization (27).

Patients with natural rubella infection often have a rash, cough, sore throat, posterior cervical lymphadenopathy, low-grade fever, malaise, and fatigue. Similar manifestations occur in vaccine-induced rubella; however, rash is less common.

Laboratory Findings

Complete blood counts are normal in most patients with either natural or vaccine-induced rubella. Occasionally, patients may have a mild leukocytosis or an elevated erythrocyte sedimentation rate. Tests for serum rheumatoid factor may be positive in natural rubella infection, but are generally negative in vaccine-induced rubella. Synovial fluid white counts ranged from 14,600 to 27,000 cells/mm^3 in three patients with natural rubella infection (28).

Pathogenesis

Rubella vaccines have been associated with arthritis in 5-10% of patients. However, mean serum rubella titers are not significantly different in those patients who develop vaccine-induced arthritis compared to those who do not (29).

The pathogenesis of vaccine-induced rubella arthritis is unknown. Since rubella virus has been cultured from the synovial fluid in several patients (30), it has been hypothesized that the organism may invade and replicate in synovium. Immune complex formation has also been suggested as a pathogenetic mechanism in vaccine-induced rubella; however, evidence of circulating immune complexes, cryoprecipitates, and diminished complement levels have not been reported.

Treatment

Salicylates may provide relief of symptoms in both natural rubella and vaccine-induced rubella arthritis.

Lyme Arthritis

Lyme disease was first recognized as a distinct clinical entity in 1975 because of a close geographic clustering of cases in Lyme, Connecticut (31). This presumably tick-transmitted disorder is characterized by brief, recurrent attacks of arthritis.

Arthritis occurs in approximately one-half of patients with Lyme disease. The initial attack of arthritis may involve a single, several, or many large joints. The attacks usually last about 1 week. Recurrent episodes of joint pain and swelling may be seen in about two-thirds of patients. A chronic arthritis has also been described in Lyme disease usually developing 6-12 months after the initial manifestation of the disorder (32).

The most common clinical finding in Lyme disease is the skin rash, erythema chronicum migrans. This cutaneous lesion occurs about 4-20 days after a tick bite, which the patient may have forgotten. A red macule or papule forms at the site of the bite and expands to form an annular lesion (Figure 21.2). Erythema chronicum migrans is often associated with systemic symptoms including malaise, fatigue, headache, and stiff neck. Neurologic and cardiac abnormalities may also occur in some patients.

The erythrocyte sedimentation rate is often elevated in Lyme disease. Synovial fluid white blood cell counts range from 500 to 98,000 cells/mm^3 during acute attacks of arthritis (31). Synovial fluid white counts in patients with chronic arthritis range from 5000 to 76,000 cells/mm^3. Synovial biopsies from patients with acute arthritis reveal nonspecific findings of an inflammatory arthritis, while synovium from four patients with chronic arthritis demonstrated

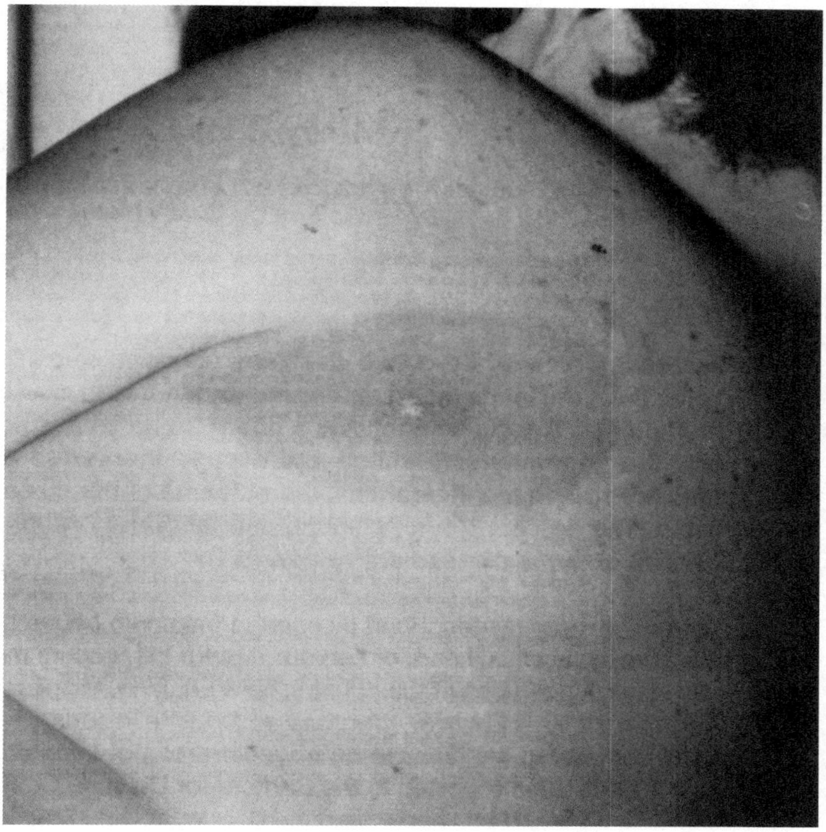

FIGURE 21.2 A patient with erythema chronicum migrans. The lesion on the left scapula was warm to touch and was 6 x 15 cm in size. There was a 4 x 1 cm central area that was desquamating. (Illustration reproduced with permission of Meyerhoff J. *Am J Med* 75:663-670, 1983, and Technical Publishing Co.)

pathological changes identical to that of rheumatoid arthritis (34). Cryoprecipitates and immune complexes may be detected in joint fluid or serum early in the course of Lyme disease, and may recur before or during attacks of arthritis.

Lyme disease appears to be transmitted by the bite of an Ixodes tick (33). A recent study described the presence of spirochetal organisms in Ixodes ticks (35), while another report identified a spirochetal organism in the blood of two patients with Lyme disease (36).

Patients with erythema chronicum migrans should be treated with either penicillin or tetracycline for 7 to 10 days. These drugs may accelerate the healing of the skin lesions and reduce the number and duration of arthritic attacks (37).

The arthritis associated with Lyme disease is generally short-lived. Patients with acute arthritis may be treated with nonsteroidal antiinflammatory drugs. Chronic arthritis with persistent synovial effusions may require injections of intraarticular steroids or synovectomy, if functional disability occurs (37).

Mycobacterial Bone and Joint Infections

Skeletal tuberculosis is an important, serious and common extrapulmonary form of tuberculosis occurring in approximately 1-2.6% of patients with tuberculosis (38,39). Early diagnosis is essential, before joint or bone destruction occurs, since excellent therapy is available. Unfortunately, the diagnosis of skeletal tuberculosis is often delayed as it is not considered in the differential diagnosis of chronic monoarthritis or back pain.

It is generally believed that skeletal tuberculosis is caused by dissemination of bacilli by hematogenous spread or lymphatic drainage from another area of tuberculosis. Since weight-bearing joints are most frequently affected, it is suspected that trauma may play a role in pathogenesis (39). Patients may present with a chronic monoarthritis, spondylitis, or osteomyelitis. There is no sex preference and it is more common in adults. In a study of 99 cases with skeletal tuberculosis (39) mean age at diagnosis was 48 years (1-91 years).

Tuberculosis arthritis most frequently involves large weight-bearing joints and is usually monoarticular. Hips, knees, wrists, elbows, and shoulders are involved in decreasing frequency. Usual presentation is that of an adult with monoarticular pain and swelling for several months. A draining sinus may occasionally occur and a history of trauma is elicited in about 30% of the patients. Some may have had intraarticular corticosteroid injections. Synovial fluid shows decreased mucin clot and viscosity with a white count ranging from 4000 to 50,000 in most patients. Synovial fluid and synovial biopsy culture establish the diagnosis in over 90% of the cases. A positive tuberculin skin test is obtained in most patients and in about 50% a previous personal or family history of tuberculosis is present. Synovial pathology reveals a chronic granulomatous reaction with giant, Langhans cell type, infiltration. Acid-fast stains in the synovial fluid or tissue may reveal organisms.

Roentgenologically, the affected joint may reveal only soft tissue swelling or more advanced changes with destruction of periarticular bone, narrowing of joint space, and osteoporosis. In patients with spondylitis, narrowing of disc spaces, vertebral destruction with earliest changes demonstrable at the anterior vertebral bodies, and evidence of paravertebral abscess may be seen. Chest x-ray abnormalities, suggestive of past or present tuberculosis, may be present in 50% of the patients.

Spine involvement occurs most frequently in the lower thoracic and lumbar areas. Earliest changes may be seen at the anterior vertebral bodies with erosive, destructive changes, disc space narrowing, and anterior collapse which may lead to spinal kyphosis. Unilateral sacroiliac involvement may occur.

A history of chronic monoarticular pain and swelling, usually of lower extremity joints, or back pain, with a high sedimentation rate, in a person with a family or personal history of tuberculosis is highly suggestive of skeletal tuberculosis. A search for the organism including synovial fluid and synovial tissue cultures should be done. Treatment is the same as for other forms of tuberculosis, with two or three different antituberculous medications required for approximately 18 months.

Atypical mycobacteria may affect joints or bursae in a similar manner to skeletal tuberculosis.

Fungal Arthritis

A wide variety of fungi may cause joint infections. These may arise either from a direct extension from a focus of osteomyelitis or by hematogenous dissemination (40). Although fungal arthritis may occasionally present in an acute fashion, the clinical presentation is usually quite similar to that seen in tuberculous arthritis. The condition is usually mono- or pauciarticular, most often in large weight-bearing joints, and generally follows a chronic, indolent course characterized by long delays in correct diagnosis. Synovial fluid analysis is highly variable, ranging from noninflammatory to grossly purulent. Synovial fluid culture may be negative, particularly with organisms that are difficult to culture.

Fungi that may be associated with infectious arthritis may be grouped as superficial or deep organisms (40). Among the superficial fungi associated with joint disease are sporotrichosis, candida, and actinomycosis (actually a fungus-like bacterium). Among the deep fungi are aspergillus, histoplasma, cryptococcus, coccidioides, and blastomycoses.

Although normal hosts may develop disseminated fungal infections with septic arthritis, there is usually some predisposing factor that increases susceptibility to infection. Among these factors are compromised immune function due to underlying malignancy or immunosuppressive therapy, alcoholism, or a chronic indwelling catheter or hyperalimentation line that affords access for hematogenous spread.

Fungal arthritis should be suspected in acute arthritis in immunocompromised hosts or in any chronic unexplained mono- or pauciarticular arthritis. The diagnosis can be made only by culturing the organism from synovial fluid, or from synovial tissue obtained at surgery or by percutaneous biopsy. Treatment usually involves the use of amphotericin-B, 5-flurocytosine or other newly developed antifungal agents, depending on organism susceptibility. Therapy may be unsatisfactory due to the delay in recognition of the process, underlying host factors, or toxicity from antifungal drugs.

References

1. Myers AR: Septic arthritis caused by bacteria. In WN Kelley, ED Harris, S Ruddy, CB Sledge (eds.), *A Textbook of Rheumatology*. Philadelphia, W.B. Saunders, 1981, pp. 1551-1572.

2. Argen RJ, Wilson CH, Wood P: Suppurative arthritis. Clinical features of 42 cases. *Arch Intern Med* 117:661-666, 1966.

3. Goldenberg DL, Cohen AS: Acute infectious arthritis. A review of patients with nongonococcal joint infections (with emphasis on therapy and prognosis). *Am J Med* 60:369-377, 1976.

4. Newman JH: Review of septic arthritis throughout the antibiotic era. *Ann Rheum Dis* 35:198-205, 1976.

5. Rytel MW: Microbial antigen detection in infectious arthritis. *Clin Rheum Dis* 4:83-93, 1978.

6. Reza MJ, Brook I, Finegold SM, Bluestone R: Joint fluid lactic acid: A diagnostic aid in septic arthritis. *Abstracts, XIV International Congress of Rheumatology.* San Francisco, 1977, p. 155.

7. Inman RD: Infectious arthritis. In JF Beary III, CL Christian, TP Sulco (eds.), *Manual of Rheumatology and Outpatient Orthopedic Disorders. Diagnosis and Therapy.* Boston, Little, Brown and Co., 1981, pp. 151-157.

8. Schmid FR: Bacterial arthritis. In DJ McCarty (ed.), *Arthritis and Allied Conditions,* 9th Ed. Philadelphia, Lea and Febiger, 1979, pp. 1363-1379.

9. Kluge R, Schmidt M, Barth WF: Pneumococcal arthritis. *Ann Rheum Dis* 32:21-24, 1973.

10. Goldenberg DL, Cohen AS: Arthritis due to Gram-negative bacilli. *Clin Rheum Dis* 4:197-210, 1978.

11. Brogadir SP, Schimmer BM, Myers AR: Spectrum of the gonococcal arthritis-dermatitis syndrome. *Semin Arthritis Rheum* 8:177-183, 1979.

12. Sharp JT: Gonococcal arthritis. In DJ McCarty (ed.), *Arthritis and Allied Conditions,* 9th Ed. Philadelphia, Lea and Febiger, 1979, pp. 1353-1362.

13. Munoz AF: Gonococcal and meningococcal arthritides. *Clin Rheum Dis* 4:169-180, 1978.

14. Holmes KK, Counts GW, Beaty HN: Disseminated gonococcal infection. *Ann Intern Med* 74:979-993, 1971.

15. Keiser H, Ruben FL, Wolinsky E, Kushner I: Clinical forms of gonococcal arthritis. *N Engl J Med* 279:234-240, 1968.

16. Barr J, Danielsson D: Septic gonococcal dermatitis. *Br Med J* 1:482-485, 1971.

17. Ludivico CL, Myers AR: Survery for immune complexes in disseminated gonococcal arthritis-dermatitis syndrome. *Arthritis Rheum* 22:19-24, 1979.

18. Garcia-Kutzbuch A, Dismulce SE, Masi AT: Gonococcal arthritis: Clinical features and results of penicillin therapy. *J Rheumatol* 1:210-221, 1974.

19. McConville JH, Potosky RS, Calia FM, Pachas WN: Septic and crystalline joint disease. A simultaneous occurrence. *JAMA* 231:841-842, 1975.

20. Trentham DE, McCrarey JW, Masi AT: Low-dose penicillin for gonococcal arthritis: A comparative therapy trial. *JAMA* 236:2410-2412, 1976.

21. Pinals RS, Ropes MW: Meningococcal arthritis. *Arthritis Rheum* 7:241-258, 1964.

22. Pinals RS: Meningococcemia presenting as an acute polyarthritis. *J Rheumatol* 4:420-424, 1977.

23. Nelson JD: The bacterial etiology and antibiotic management of septic arthritis in infants and children. *Pediatrics* 50:437-440, 1972.

24. Nelson JD: Cefuroxime: A cephalosporin with unique applicability to pediatric practice. *Ped Infect Dis* 2:394-396, 1983.

25. Duffy J, Lidsky MD, Sharp JT, Davis JS, Person DA, Hollinger FB, Min KW: Polyarthritis, polyarteritis, and hepatitis B. *Medicine* 55:19-37, 1976.

26. Schumacher HR, Gall EP: Arthritis in acute hepatitis and chronic active hepatitis. Pathology of the synovial membrane with evidence for the presence of Australia antigen in synovial membranes. *Am J Med* 57:655-664, 1974.

27. Spruane SL, Metcalf R, Smith CB, Griffiths MM, Ward JR: Chronic arthropathy associated with rubella vaccination. *Arthritis Rheum* 20:741-747, 1977.

28. Yanez JE, Thompson GR, Milckelsen WM, Bartholonew LE: Rubella arthritis. *Ann Intern Med* 64:772-777, 1966.

29. Thompson GR, Weiss JJ, Eloise MI, Shills JL, Brackett RG: Intermittent arthritis following rubella vaccination. *Am J Dis Child* 125:526-530, 1973.

30. Ogra PL, Herd JK: Arthritis associated with induced rubella infection. *J Immunol* 107:810-813, 1971.

31. Steere AC, Malawista SE, Syndman DR, Shope RE, Andimon WA, Ross MR, Steele FM: Lyme arthritis: An epidemic of oligoarticular arthritis in children and adults in three Connecticut communities. *Arthritis Rheum* 20:7-17, 1977.

32. Steere AC, Broderick TF, Malawista SE: Erythema chronicum migrans and Lyme arthritis: Epidemiologic evidence for a tick vector. *Am J Epidemiol* 108:312-321, 1978.

33. Steere AC, Gibofsky A, Patarrayo ME, Winchester RJ, Hardin JA, Malawista SE: Chronic Lyme arthritis. *Ann Intern Med* 93:1-8, 1979.

34. Steere AC, Malawista SE, Hardin JA, Ruddy S, Askenase PW, Andiman WA: Erythema chronicum migrans and Lyme arthritis. *Ann Intern Med* 86:685-698, 1977.

35. Burgdorfer W, Barbour AG, Hayes SF, Benach JL, Brunwaldt E, Davis JP: Lyme disease - A tick-borne spirochetosis. *Science* 216:1317-1319, 1982.

36. Benach JL, Bosler EM, Hanrahan JP, Coleman JL, Habicht GS, Bast TF, Cameron DJ, Ziegler JL, Barbour AG, Burgdorfer W, Edelman R, Kaslow RA: Spirochetes isolated from the blood of two patients with Lyme disease. *N Engl J Med* 308:740-742, 1983.

37. Steere AC, Malawista SE, Newman JH, Spieler PN, Bartenhagen NH: Antibiotic therapy in Lyme disease. *Ann Intern Med* 90:896-901, 1979.

38. Davidson PT, Horowitz I: Skeletal tuberculosis. A review with patient presentations and discussion. *Am J Med* 48:77-84, 1970.

39. Enarson DA, Fujii EM, Nakielna MB, Grzybowski MD: Bone and joint tuberculosis: A continuing problem. *Can Med Ass J* 20:139-145, 1979.

40. Hoffman GS: Mycobacterial and fungal infections of bones and joints. In WN Kelley, ED Harris, S Ruddy, CB Sledge (eds.), *Textbook of Rheumatology.* Philadelphia, W.B. Saunders, 1981, pp. 1573-1585.

Chapter 22

TUMORS OF BONES AND JOINTS

Ivan L. Holleman, M.D.

Introduction

Primary tumors of bones and joints generally are uncommon. The major exceptions are the leukemias and plasma cell myeloma. Secondary (metastatic) malignant neoplasms are more common than primary tumors in the skeleton. Primary tumors may arise from any of the tissues which make up the bones and joints and there are fairly numerous types of such tumors. This makes classification complex and specific diagnosis is often difficult. The malignant skeletal tumors are neoplasms classified as sarcomas (i.e., malignant neoplasms of mesenchymal deviation). Some of the benign tumors may be neoplasms but most probably are developmental malformations, hamartomas, hyperplastic, dysplastic, or reactive tumors.

Classification

Skeletal tumors are classified in the same way as tumors of other organ systems. Basic pathologic classification (pathologic diagnosis) includes three features of the tumor: natural behavior, histology or histogenesis, and anatomic location.

Natural behavior, whether the tumor is benign or malignant, is the most important classifiable feature of a tumor because prognosis and therapy largely depend on this quality of the tumor. Gross, microscopic, and radiographic study of the anatomy of a tumor and clinical findings all play a variable part in behavioristic classification. Some tumors cannot be reliably classified as benign or malignant by available means. Time may be necessary to determine their behavior.

Histologic classification is based on determination of the type of tissue which forms the parenchyma of the tumor. Histogenetic classification depends on the type of tissue from which the parenchyma of the tumor developed. The histologic and histogenetic classifications of a tumor may or may not be the same. Diagnostic classification is most often histologic. As with the behavioristic classification, the parenchymal cell or tissue type of a tumor cannot always be definitely classified by available techniques. For example, the cells of a malignant neoplasm may be so undifferentiated that they cannot be recognized as being cells of a specific type. This is sometimes true even with the most advanced techniques of light and electron microscopy, tissue culture, and immunologic study.

The anatomic location of a tumor is obviously important practical information for prognostic and therapeutic purposes.

Chondrosarcoma of the femur is an example of tumor classification (pathologic diagnosis). *Chondro* indicates that the parenchyma of the tumor is cartilage (histologic and possibly histogenetic classification); *sarcoma* indicates that it is a malignant neoplasm (behavioristic classification) and *of the femur* indicates the anatomic location.

Other information, in addition to the basic classification, is important for therapy and prognosis of tumors. Grading or the determination that a malignant neoplasm is of low, intermediate, or high degree (or grade) of aggressiveness (malignancy) can be done for some tumors and in such cases is valuable for prognosis and treatment. In a case of femoral chondrosarcoma, for example, grading is helpful in predicting the course of the disease. Low-grade (grade 1 or well differentiated) chondrosarcomas tend to grow slowly and metastasize late whereas high-grade (grade 3 to 4 or poorly differentiated) chondrosarcomas often grow fast and metastasize early. Grading of tumors usually is based primarily on histology and cytology but clinical information, location, rapidity of growth, and the radiographic findings are also important. Grading of malignancy varies in reliability and prognostic value among different neoplasms. Many types of tumors do not show predictable differences in behavior from case to case and cannot, therefore, be subclassified into variable grades of malignancy. Some tumors, such as central osteosarcoma and Ewing's sarcoma, are uniformly high-grade malignant neoplasms.

Additional information needed for staging of a tumor and necessary for diagnosis, prognosis, and therapy includes the size of the tumor, its relationship to important or vital anatomic structures, the rapidity of its growth, its invasiveness, and whether it has metastasized or not and if so to what organ.

Diagnosis

In practice the specific diagnosis (i.e., classification) of some skeletal tumors is easy and of others very difficult. Commonly the diagnosis, or at least a determination that a tumor probably is either benign or malignant, can be made from clinical and radiographic findings. Often, however, biopsy is necessary for specific classification of a tumor. Diagnosis may be very difficult and sometimes is uncertain even when all available diagnostic techniques, including microscopic study, are used.

Microscopic examination of lesional tissue is a mainstay for the diagnosis of bone and joint tumors. Often, however, microscopic examination alone is not adequate for diagnosis of skeletal tumors and it is extremely important that physicians involved in diagnosis and treatment of skeletal lesions know this and act accordingly. The pathologist needs the pertinent clinical data including the radiographic findings in addition to the microscopic findings in order to make a correct diagnosis. The histologic features of many skeletal tumors overlap so that specific diagnosis by microscopy alone may be uncertain or impossible. Most importantly, the histologic features of some benign and malignant skeletal tumors are so similar that they may be easily confused. It is likely to be tragic for a patient if his benign tumor is classified as malignant or vice versa. It is imperative, therefore, that the pathologist, the radiologist, and the clinician fully consider with each other the findings in any case in which there is question as to whether a tumor is benign or malignant. Consultation with other experienced diagnosticians should be obtained if reasonable doubt as to the correct diagnosis cannot be resolved.

It is helpful in differential diagnosis of skeletal tumors to remember that many of the lesions have peculiarities of clinical presentation and/or typical radiographic features that support a particular diagnosis over other possibilities or at least very often place a lesion into a group having similar characteristics. Some tumors typically occur in a certain age range and/or in particular anatomic sites and/or have typical symptoms and/or have typical radiologic findings.

Manifestations

Patients with bone tumors most often complain of the presence of a mass or of pain. Pain often is a primary symptom of malignant tumors. Benign tumors often are asymptomatic but some are painful because of a pathologic fracture involving the lesion. Some benign bone tumors, such as the osteoid osteoma, however, may be painful without a complicating fracture. Bone tumors may also cause pain and effusion in adjacent joints on occasion.

Patients with tumors of joints commonly complain of swelling, pain, and loss of mobility.

Treatment

It is not within the scope of this chapter to consider details of therapy of skeletal tumors. Conservative and radical surgery, radiotherapy, and chemotherapy all have a place.

One principle of therapy, however, should be emphasized. Accurate diagnosis and staging of the tumor are necessary to plan the correct treatment. Radical treatment for cancer requires an assured diagnosis. In most cases biopsy confirmation of the clinical and radiologic diagnosis of malignancy should be obtained before a primary bone tumor is treated as cancer.

Tumors of Bones

Tumors may arise from or be composed of any of the tissues which comprise the bones. Thus, not all tumors of the bones have bone tissue (i.e., osteoblasts and osteoid matrix) as a component. The common histologic components of primary tumors of the bones (excluding leukemias, lymphomas, and plasmacytoma) are bone tissue, cartilage, fibrohistiocytic tissue (including multinucleated giant cells), and blood vessels. Some tumors of bones are benign, some are malignant (see Table 22.1). Sometimes benign tumors undergo malignant transformation. The cause of most bone tumors is not known. Some are genetic (e.g., hereditary multiple exostoses), some complicate other diseases (e.g., sarcoma complicating Paget's disease of bone), and some are induced by ionizing radiation (e.g., some osteosarcomas).

TABLE 22.1 Tumors of Bones

Benign Tumors
Osteochondroma (osteocartilaginous exostosis)
Fibroma (nonossifying fibroma and fibrous cortical defect)
Fibrous dysplasia
Ossifying fibroma (osteogenic fibroma)
Enchondroma (central chondroma)
Osteoid osteoma
Solitary bone cyst (unicameral bone cyst)
Aneurysmal bone cyst
Hemangioma
Chondromyxoid fibroma
Chondroblastoma
Malignant Tumors
Osteosarcoma (osteogenic sarcoma)
Chondrosarcoma
Ewing's sarcoma
Fibrosarcoma
Malignant fibrous histiocytoma
Malignant plasmacytoma (plasma cell myeloma)
Malignant lymphoma
Intermediate Tumors
Giant cell tumor (osteoclastoma)
Chordoma

Benign Tumors

Most benign tumors of bones are developmental malformations, hamartomas, hyperplastic or dysplastic masses rather than true neoplasms.

Osteochondroma (Osteocartilaginous Exostosis)

Osteochondroma is one of the most common of the bone tumors. It may be solitary or multiple. It tends to involve the metaphyses of long bones, most often the distal femoral, the proximal humeral or proximal tibial metaphyses but may involve flat bones (e.g., the pelvis and scapula). The lesion forms a mass on the surface of the parent bone. It is composed of cortical and cancellous bone, continuous with those parts of the parent bone, covered by a cap of cartilage (Figure 22.1). These tumors tend to develop and grow during the period of normal skeletal growth. In size they range from about 1 to 10 cm in diameter. These lesions may be asymptomatic but sometimes they are painful. Rarely, chondrosarcoma develops in the cap of a solitary osteochondroma. Multiple osteochondromas characterize the uncommon dominantly inherited condition named hereditary multiple

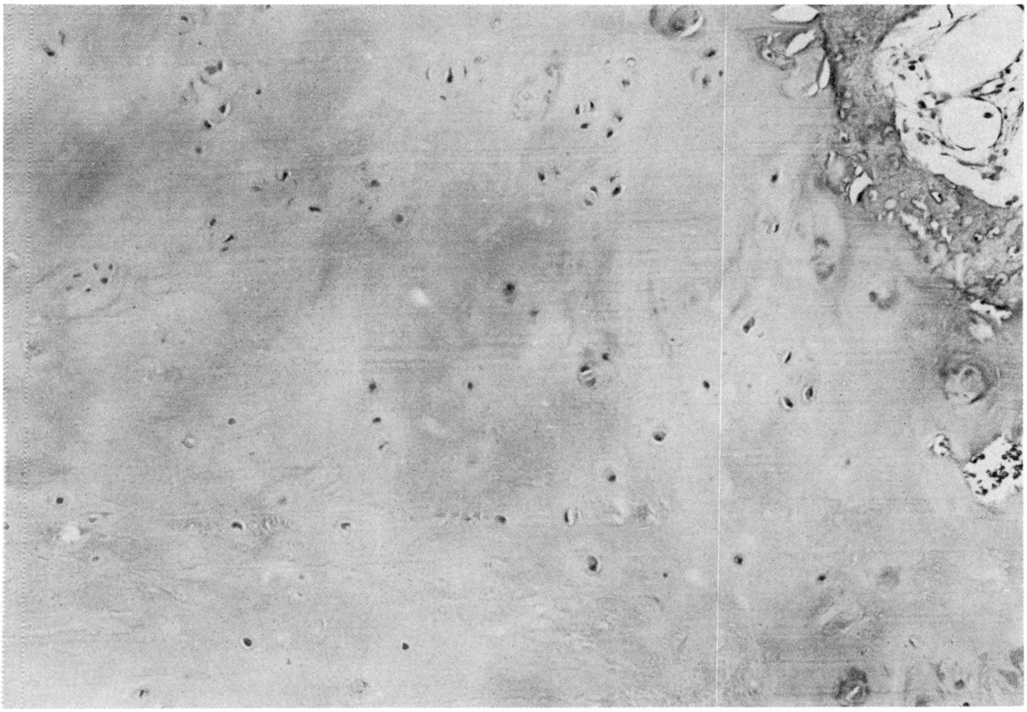

FIGURE 22.1 Osteochondroma. H & E X 170

exostoses. In this condition chondrosarcoma arises in one or more of the lesions in 10-20% of cases. Osteochondroma does not necessarily require treatment. Indications for therapy are pain, the presence of an unsightly mass, abnormal or continual rapid growth, or radiographic findings suggestive of malignancy. When indicated, the usual treatment is total excision of the lesion.

Fibroma (Nonossifying Fibroma and
Fibrous Cortical Defect)

This is another of the relatively common bone tumors which tend to occur during the period of normal skeletal growth. It characteristically involves the metaphysis of a long bone, most often the distal femur or distal tibia. The fibrous cortical defect is a common, asymptomatic, small, intracortical, circumscribed radiolucent lesion which usually is an incidental radiographic finding in children. It tends to resolve spontaneously. The nonossifying fibroma is a larger, eccentric, circumscribed lucent lesion which involves the medulla of the bone as well as the cortex and also may resolve spontaneously. Growth of a fibrous cortical defect may give rise to a nonossifying fibroma. Both are composed basically of fibroblastic tissue containing multinucleated giant cells (Figure 22.2). Frequently in nonossifying fibroma there are hemorrhage, hemosiderin deposition, and histiocytic foam cells. These lesions typically are longer than they are wide and their radiographic features are usually characteristic. These lesions may be asymptomatic or they may cause pain and swelling in the involved area. Sometimes pain is

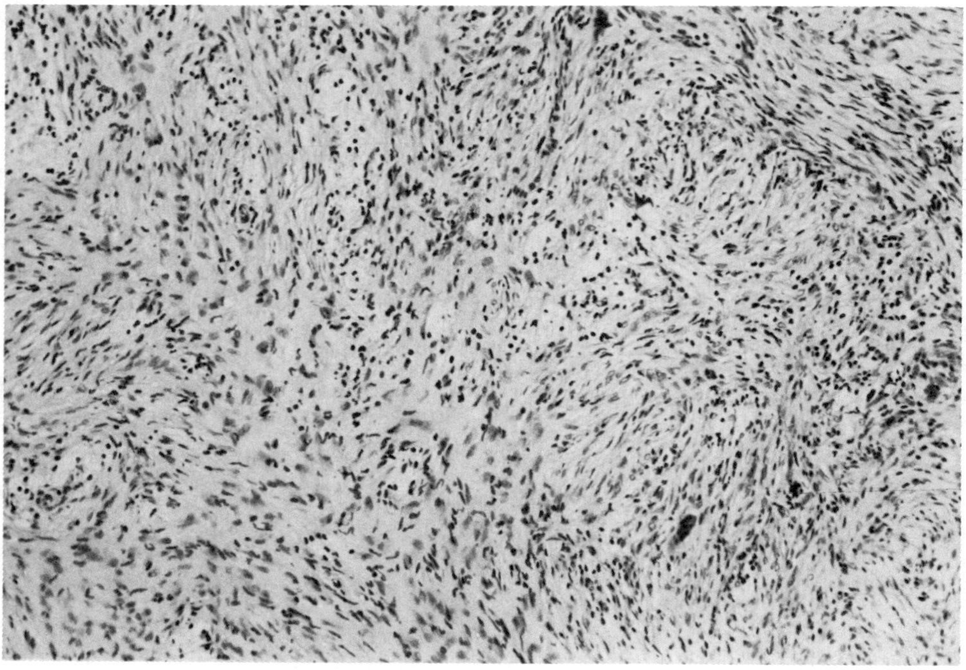

FIGURE 22.2 Fibroma. H&E X 170

secondary to fracture through the lesions. These tumors are benign and rarely if ever undergo malignant transformation. Fibrous cortical defect usually is not treated. Nonossifying fibroma is successfully treated by curettage.

Fibrous Dysplasia

This is a fairly common tumor composed of fibrous tissue in which woven osteoid matrix is formed by metaplasia from the fibrous component (Figure 22.3). Most often it involves one bone (monostotic) but it may involve several bones (polyostotic). It may involve most any bone, but a rib and the jaw are the most common sites. The tumor replaces normal bone tissue and expands the bone in which it is situated. Monostotic cases may be asymptomatic or there may be pain and swelling if the lesion is fractured. Involvement of the bones of the face may lead to asymmetry. Polyostotic tumors tend to be more deforming, more often painful and cause more disturbance of function than monostotic lesions. Polyostotic fibrous dysplasia may be associated with other manifestations, particularly foci of abnormal cutaneous pigmentation and, in females, precocious puberty in which case it is commonly referred to as Albright's syndrome. Fibrous dysplasia probably develops during childhood or adolescence but may be manifest at any age depending on location and severity of involvement. Development of sarcoma is an uncommon complication. Curettage or resection is the usual method of treatment.

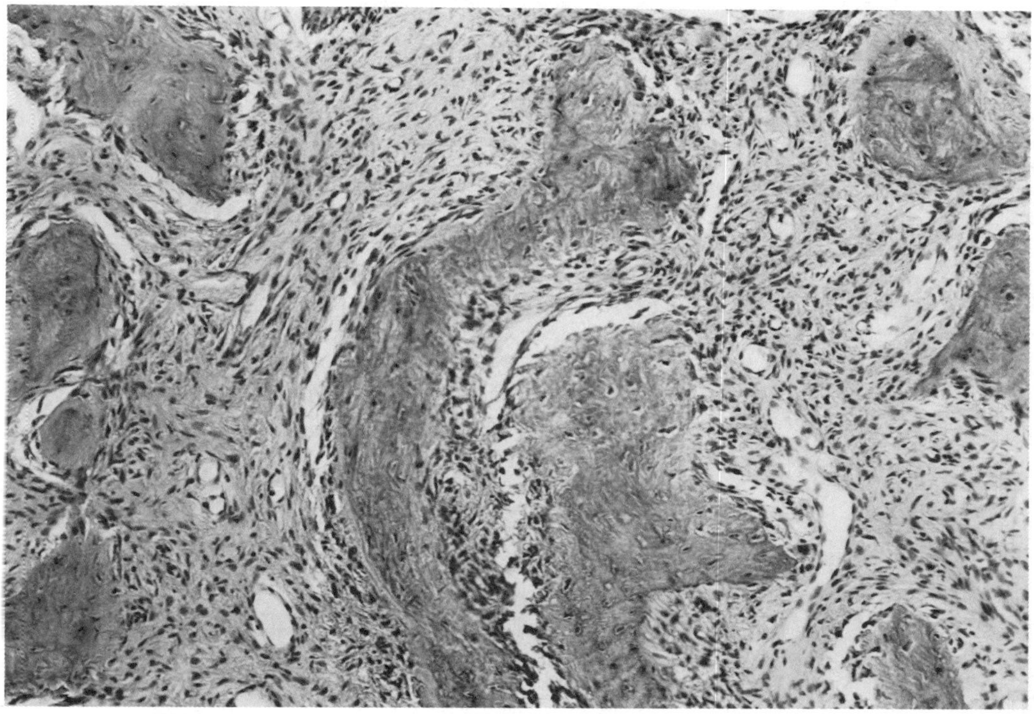

FIGURE 22.3 Fibrous dysplasia. H&E X 170

Ossifying Fibroma (Osteogenic Fibroma)

This is a fibroosseous tumor which some authors believe is a variant of fibrous dysplasia and others believe to be a distinct entity. The latter consider it to be separable from fibrous dysplasia microscopically by the presence of osteoblasts rimming the lesional osteoid and the lamellar appearance of the osteoid trabeculae which they believe are not features of fibrous dysplasia. Ossifying fibroma typically involves the jaw bones but some cases involving long bones have been reported. Ossifying fibroma tends to grow slowly. Curettage or resection is the usual method of treatment.

Enchondroma (Central Chondroma)

This is a benign tumor composed of cartilage located within a bone. Solitary enchondroma most often involves a tubular bone of the hand or foot but it may occur in other bones, most often a humerus or femur. Solitary enchondroma is usually detected between the third and fifth decades of life and is rarely diagnosed in children before 10 years of age. Solitary enchondroma tends to grow slowly, may be asymptomatic but sometimes is painful or forms a palpable mass. Pathologic fracture may be a presenting complication. Solitary central cartilaginous tumors in the small bones of the hands and feet are nearly always benign. Central cartilaginous tumors located elsewhere are more often malignant and differential diagnosis between benign enchondroma and well-differentiated central chondrosarcoma in such locations often is difficult.

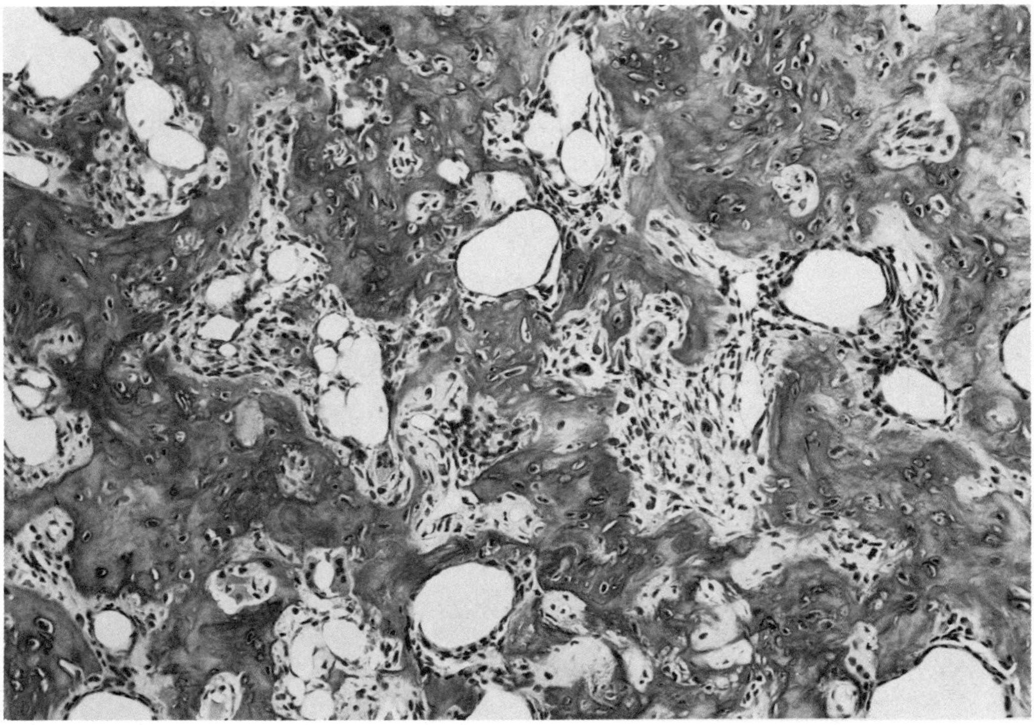

FIGURE 22.4 Osteoid osteoma. H&E X 170

Multiple enchondromatosis (Ollier's disease) is a nonfamilial disorder characterized by the presence of multiple enchondromas in multiple bones. This disease varies in severity but may be very deforming. Chondrosarcoma ultimately complicates about 50% of the cases of Ollier's disease.

Maffucci's syndrome is a nonfamilial disorder characterized by multiple skeletal enchondromas and multiple hemangiomas of the soft tissue.

Enchrondroma is usually treated by curettage.

Osteoid Osteoma

Osteoid osteoma may involve any bone but most often occurs in a tibia or femur. Most cases occur between the ages of 5 and 25 years. Typically, osteoid osteoma is a small lesion less than 2 cm in diameter. It is characterized by abnormal bone formation in a fibrovascular stroma (Figure 22.4). The abnormal bone trabeculae may be variably mineralized. This lesion is characterized by a radiolucent to radiodense nidus surrounded by a radiodense zone. Osteoid osteoma tends to be painful. When located near a joint it may cause effusion in the joint. Excision is the usual treatment. These lesions may involute spontaneously.

Benign Osteoblastoma (Giant Osteoid Osteoma)

This is a rare neoplasm which histologically is very similar to osteoid osteoma but tends to become larger than 2 cm in diameter. This is a benign tumor which may be easily confused diagnostically with osteosarcoma, a malignant tumor, because of the prominent osteoblastic activity and osteoid formation which characterize both types of tumor.

Solitary Bone Cyst (Unicameral Bone Cyst)

This is a fluid-filled cavity lined by a thin layer of fibrous tissue rather than a solid tumor. Most patients with solitary cyst are children or adolescents. These lesions tend to occur in a metaphysis of a long tubular bone, most often the proximal humerus. As the bone grows in length the cyst becomes more diaphyseal in location. The usual symptom is pain secondary to pathologic fracture involving the cyst. These lesions usually heal readily when curetted and filled with bone chips.

Aneurysmal Bone Cyst

Lesions of this type are anatomically complex and of controversial pathogenesis and cause. Some believe this to be an entity, others think it represents one of a number of lesions, tumorous or traumatic, complicated by an unusual vascular proliferative change. Aneurysmal bone cyst may involve most any bone: vertebrae, flat bones, and tubular bones. It is an osteolytic lesion which causes aneurysmal enlargement of the affected area of the involved bone and ultimately may reach large size, involve nerves and joints, and interfere with function. These tumors tend to be characterized by swelling, tenderness, and pain. Histologically, aneurysmal bone cyst is composed of large blood-filled spaces with connective tissue walls in which multinucleated giant cells are often present. These tumors may be confused with giant cell tumor or even telangiectatic osteosarcoma. These lesions may occur at any age but most are found before the age of 30 years. Curettage is the usual treatment for accessible lesions but about 50% recur one or more times. En-bloc resection, amputation, and radiotherapy may be necessary in some cases. Radiotherapy carries the risk of radiation-induced sarcoma after a latent period.

Hemangioma

Hemangioma is a benign hamartoma of blood vessels (Figure 22.5) which may occur in any organ. Hemangiomas are uncommon in bones. In most cases hemangioma of bone is solitary and involves the skull or a vertebra. It may occur at any age but most often is found between the ages of 20 and 60 years. Sometimes hemangiomas may become large, produce a palpable mass, lead to pathologic fracture, and be painful. Vertebral hemangiomas sometimes cause spinal cord or nerve compression. Excision and irradiation are employed in treatment. Hemorrhage may complicate resection.

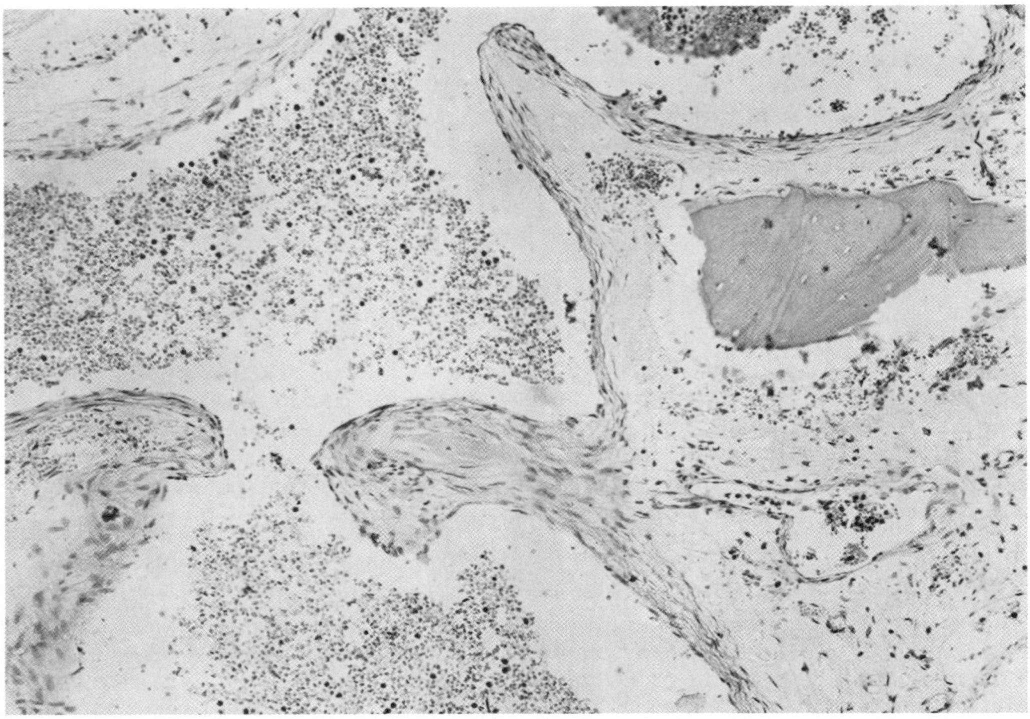

FIGURE 22.5 Hemangioma. H&E X 170

Chondromyxoid Fibroma

This is a rare benign neoplasm which may occur from early childhood to old age but is most common between the ages of 10 and 30 years. Most any bone may be involved, but the proximal tibia and distal femur are the most common sites, together being the location of about one-third of such tumors. Pain, swelling, and restriction of movement are the most common symptoms and signs. These tend to be lytic lesions and are composed of fibrous, myxoid, and chondroid tissues. Histologically, these tumors may be mistaken for some type of sarcoma because of their cellularity. In most cases these tumors are successfully treated by curettage. Occasionally there is local recurrence following curettage.

Chondroblastoma

This rare neoplasm is also known as Codman's tumor, as epiphyseal chondromatous giant cell tumor, and as calcifying giant cell tumor. Chondroblastoma may occur at most any age but in about two-thirds of the cases the patient is in the second decade at the time the lesion is discovered. Chondroblastoma tends to occur in the epiphysis of a long limb bone. The most common sites are the proximal humerus, the distal femur, and the proximal tibia. Somewhat more than half of all cases are in one of these locations. The usual presenting signs and symptoms are pain, swelling, limitation of motion, and joint effusion. Radiographically, these tend to be lytic lesions with punctate calcification and well-circumscribed sclerotic margins. Histologically, these tumors are composed of uniform polygonal cells (chondroblasts), multinucleated osteoclast-like giant cells, chondroid matrix, and foci of calcification. Nearly all of these tumors are benign and can be cured by curettage. However, in an occasional case the tumor may recur, have aggressive local growth and, rarely, metastasize.

Malignant Tumors

As currently defined malignant tumors are neoplasms. There is no single completely satisfactory definition of malignant neoplasia. In general, malignant neoplasms are those tumors which by nature tend to kill their host. Malignant tumors of the skeleton do this by aggressive, invasive local growth or by metastasis thereby causing lethal interference with vital functions. Some neoplasms are by nature highly malignant, others are much less aggressive and are referred to variously as low-grade malignant neoplasms, tumors of borderline malignancy, or intermediate tumors. There is, therefore, a range in aggressiveness or malignancy of neoplasms and the behavior of neoplasms in individual cases cannot always be accurately predicted. Not only are there differences in the degree of malignancy between tumors of different histologic types but tumors of the same histologic type may vary in malignancy. For example, well-differentiated chondrosarcomas of bone tend to grow slowly and metastasize late and are slow to kill the host whereas poorly differentiated chondrosarcomas tend to grow more rapidly, metastasize earlier, and kill much more quickly than the well-differentiated tumors.

Neoplasms are composed of parenchyma and stroma. The stroma is the non-neoplastic fibrovascular supportive tissue of the tumor. The parenchyma is made up of the neoplastic cells which have undergone the malignant mutation. Classification of a malignant neoplasm is based on the nature of its parenchyma. Neoplastic malignant mutation of cells is often associated with abnormalities in the morphology of the cells, commonly referred to as anaplasia, which is one of the useful microscopic features in determining that a particular neoplasm is malignant and in predicting its degree of malignancy. The degree of anaplasia or morphologic abnormality of the cells is a reflection of the degree of differentiation of the neoplasm. As indicated previously, degree of differentiation is a feature often useful in predicting the degree of malignancy or grade of a neoplasm.

The parenchyma of most malignant neoplasms is composed of one type of cell. Identification of the cell type is the basis of the histologic classification of this type of tumor. Some neoplasms, however, have a parenchyma composed of two or more different types of cells or tissues. These are mixed neoplasms and histologic classification of them is variable.

Osteosarcoma (Osteogenic Sarcoma)

This is the most common primary malignant neoplasm of the skeleton (excepting the leukemias, plasma cell myeloma, and lymphomas). Osteosarcoma may arise within the bone or on the surface of a bone. Classic primary intramedullary (central) osteosarcoma is a highly malignant neoplasm which typically is a tumor of young persons. About 75% of cases occur between 10 and 25 years of age. Male to female ratio is about 2:1. Such tumors most often involve the metaphysis of a long tubular bone. The distal femur and the proximal tibia are the sites of about 50% of such tumors and the proximal humerus is the site of about 10%.

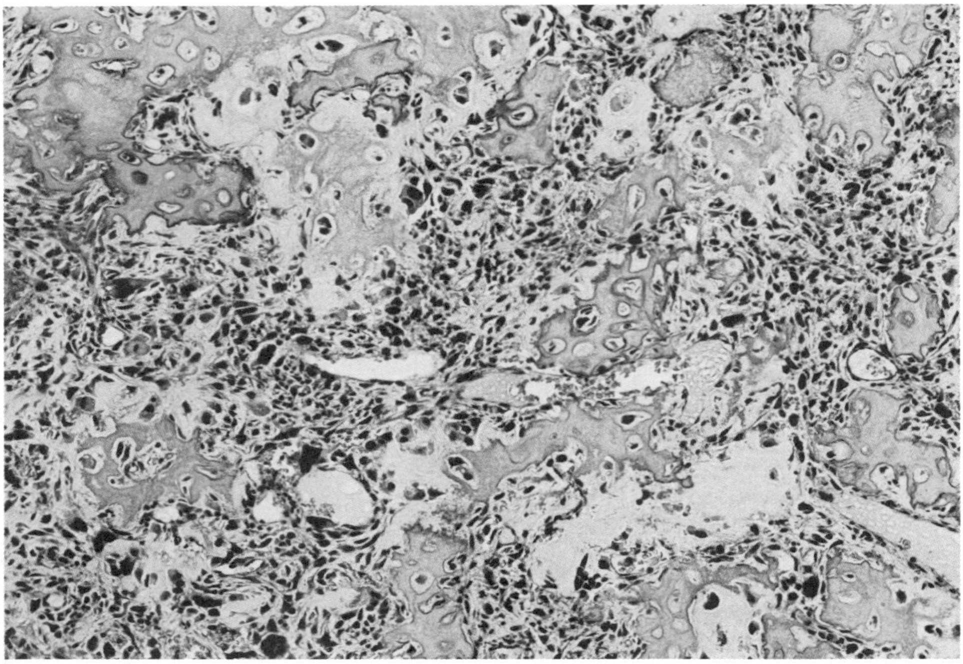

FIGURE 22.6 Osteosarcoma. H&E X 170

Osteosarcomas in general are malignant, mixed mesodermal tumors, neoplastic components of which variably include fibrosarcoma, malignant fibrous histiocytoma, giant cell tumor, angiosarcoma, undifferentiated sarcomatous tissue, very often chondrosarcoma, and always malignant osteoblastic tissue (Figure 22.6). The identification of malignant osteoblastic tissue is necessary to classify a tumor as osteosarcoma no matter what other histologic components are present.

Primary intramedullary osteosarcoma usually presents as a painful, tender mass. Alkaline phosphatase levels in the blood may be elevated. The tumor tends to grow rapidly, destroys normal bone, invades surrounding soft tissue, and tends to metastasize early and widely. The metastatic lesions are usually detected first in the lungs. The radiographic findings at the primary site reflect the anatomic features resulting from the aggressive local growth of the tumor. There is destruction of normal bone by a variably lytic to slcerotic lesion, the latter feature depending on the amount of mineralized neoplastic tissue produced by the tumor. As the tumor growth progresses, cortical destruction, periosteal elevation and destruction, Codman's triangle formation, and a mass in the soft tissue are seen in the radiograph. Such radiographic and clinical features are typical of classic osteosarcoma; however, biopsy confirmation should be obtained before definitive therapy. Treatment modalities include chemotherapy, radiation therapy, and surgery. Recent advances in therapy have considerably improved survival rates from the previous 5-10% rate attained by amputation.

The cause of the classic primary type of central osteosarcoma described above in most cases is unknown. Some cases, however, are known to occur as complications of Paget's disease of bone in persons older than 40 years. Depending on the severity of the Paget's disease, the risk of developing complicating sarcoma is between 1 and 10%. Other cases of osteosarcoma are induced by the effect of ionizing radiation on bone. Such tumors may occur any time from about 3 to 50 years after the radiation exposure. The incidence of radiation-induced bone sarcoma is low and in general is proportional to the dose of radiation (i.e., the higher the dose the higher the incidence of complicating sarcoma). Osteosarcomas complicating Paget's disease or induced by ionizing radiation are sometimes referred to as secondary osteosarcoma.

Osteosarcomas arising on the surface of a bone are variously named juxtacortical, parosteal or periosteal osteosarcoma. They are rare and somewhat more common in females than in males. Most cases occur between the ages of 20 and 50 years. Over half of such tumors involve the distal femur and another fourth involve the proximal tibia or humerus. About three-fourths of juxtacortical osteosarcomas are well differentiated, grow slowly but inexorably, and are late to metastasize. This type of tumor is referred to by some authors as parosteal osteosarcoma. About a fourth of the juxtacortical tumors show greater anaplasia and are more malignant than the well-differentiated parosteal tumors but generally less so than classic intramedullary osteosarcoma. Some of these latter juxtacortical tumors are named periosteal osteosarcoma by the same authors. Well-differentiated parosteal osteosarcomas are usually treated by complete excision of the tumor either en-bloc or by amputation.

Chondrosarcoma

Chondrosarcoma may arise within a bone (central chondrosarcoma) or on the surface of a bone (peripheral chondrosarcoma). Chondrosarcoma is next in frequency to osteosarcoma among the primary malignant bone tumors. The bones of the pelvis are the most common site followed by the metadiaphyseal parts of the proximal and distal femur and proximal tibia, fibula, and humerus. Chondrosarcoma may arise de novo (primary chondrosarcoma) or from a preexisting enchondroma or osteochondroma, or less often as a complication of some other condition such as Paget's disease or fibrous dysplasia (secondary chondrosarcoma). Solitary primary chondrosarcoma tends to occur on average about 2 decades later than classic osteosarcoma.

Radiographically, central chondrosarcomas typically are destructive lesions with mottled calcification. Chondrosarcomas are composed of anaplastic cartilage (Figure 22.7) and may range from very well to poorly differentiated. In general, the degree of differentiation has a correlation with the degree of malignancy of the tumor (i.e., the poorly differentiated tumors are highly malignant and vice versa). Well-differentiated tumors tend to grow slowly and metastasize late but they recur locally if incompletely excised and can be transplanted to other sites by surgery.

One of the difficult problems in histopathology is to determine whether a well-differentiated cartilaginous tumor is a benign chondroma or a well-differentiated chondrosarcoma. Central cartilaginous tumors of the small tubular bones of the hands and feet are likely to be benign enchondroma. Well-differentiated central cartilaginous tumors of the long tubular bones or flat bones are more likely to be well-differentiated chondrosarcoma than benign enchondroma. As previously noted there is a significant danger of central chondrosarcoma developing in cases of multiple enchondromatosis and of peripheral chondrosarcoma com-

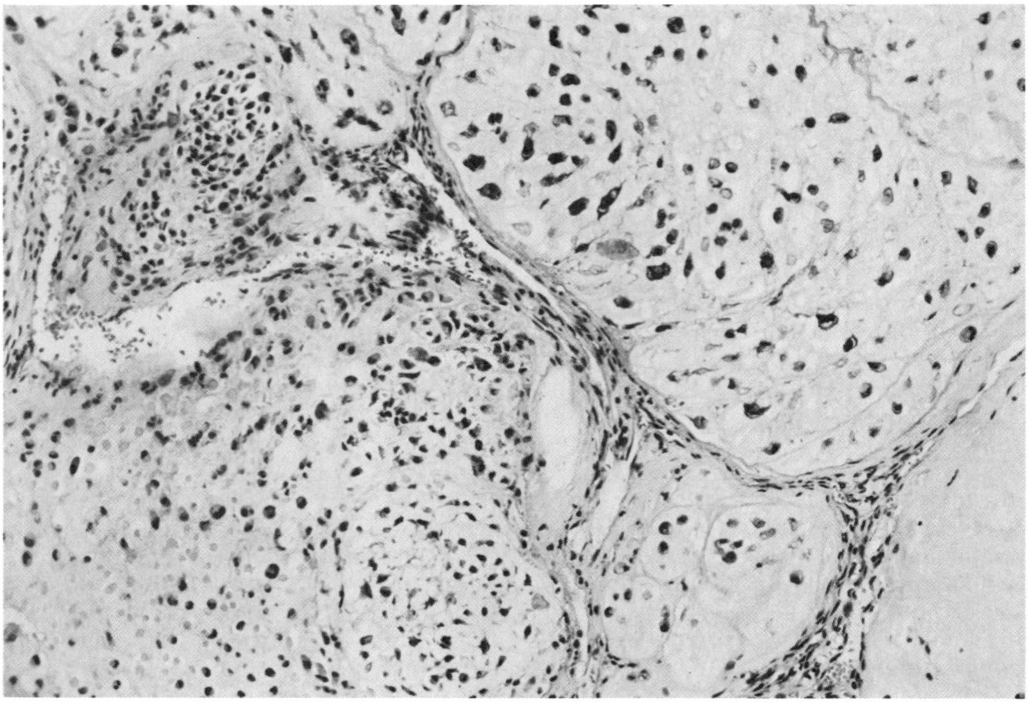

FIGURE 22.7 Chondrosarcoma, moderately differentiated. H&E X 170

plicating multiple hereditary exostoses. Occasionally, well- or moderately differentiated chondrosarcomas may undergo a transformation into a much more highly malignant neoplasm in which osteosarcoma or some other type of sarcoma develops. This is known as dedifferentiated chondrosarcoma. A rare variant of chondrosarcoma is the mesenchymal chondrosarcoma which is composed of a mixture of anaplastic cartilage and undifferentiated mesenchymal cells. In general, complete surgical excision is the primary treatment of choice for chondrosarcoma.

Ewing's Sarcoma

This is an uncommon, highly malignant neoplasm of uncertain histogenesis which, however, probably arises from undifferentiated mesenchymal cells in bones. It occurs most often between the ages of 5 and 15 years, may involve most any bone but is most common in the diaphysis of a femur, tibia, or humerus. Local pain, a tender mass, and an infection-like syndrome with fever, leukocytosis, anemia, and increased erythrocyte sedimentation rate are common presenting features. This neoplasm is composed of relatively small, uniform cells (Figure 22.8) similar to the parenchymal cells of reticulum cell sarcoma, lymphoma, neuroblastoma, and poorly differentiated carcinoma all of which may be histopathologic differential diagnostic considerations. This tumor is highly malignant and tends to metastasize early and widely. Radiographically, the findings are nonspecific and basically are those of an osteolytic lesion consistent with a variety of malignant neoplasms or osteomyelitis. Definitive diagnosis requires biopsy in conjunction with the clinical and radiographic findings. Recent advances in com-

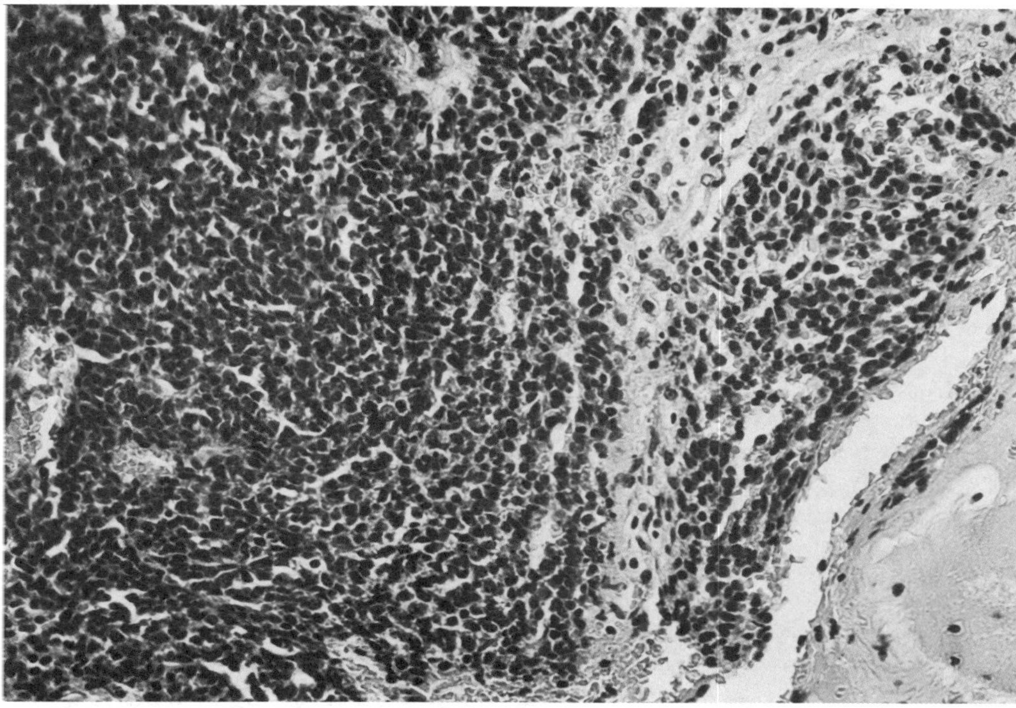

FIGURE 22.8 Ewing's sarcoma. H&E X 338

bined chemotherapy and radiotherapy have increased 5-year survival from about 10 to about 50%.

Fibrosarcoma

This is an uncommon intramedullary malignant neoplasm composed of anaplastic fibroblasts. Fibrosarcomas may occur at any age but most do so between the ages of 10 and 60 years. Any bone may be involved but the distal femoral metaphysis and the proximal tibial metaphysis are the most common sites. These tumors histologically range from well to poorly differentiated with a corresponding variation in degree of malignancy. The more poorly differentiated tumors may be mistaken for osteosarcoma, malignant fibrous histiocytoma, and other sarcomas. Resection is the usual treatment.

Malignant Fibrous Histiocytoma

Tumors of this type have been recognized as a distinct variety of soft tissue neoplasm relatively recently and were first described as a primary bone neoplasm in 1972. Previously, these tumors apparently had usually been classified as fibrosarcoma or osteosarcoma. The parenchyma is composed of both fibroblastic and mononuclear and multinuclear histiocytic anaplastic cells. These tumors may occur at any age. Males are afflicted somewhat more commonly than females. A significant number of cases complicate other skeletal abnormalities such as infarcts and Paget's disease or arise in irradiated bone. In about half of the cases

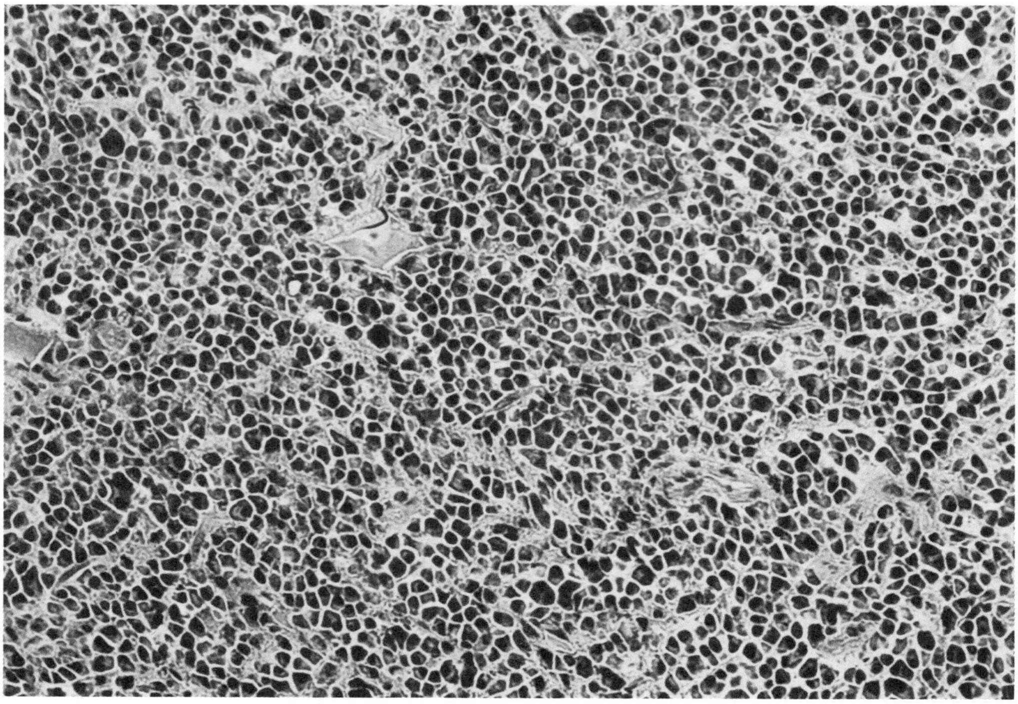

FIGURE 22.9 Malignant plasmacytoma. H&E X 338

the tumor involves either the distal femoral or proximal tibial metaphysis. Any other bone may be involved. Sometimes the tumor invades a joint. These are lytic, generally radiolucent, tumors. Resection is the usual primary treatment.

Malignant Plasmacytoma (Plasma Cell Myeloma)

This is a malignant neoplasm of plasma cells and is histogenetically a type of B-cell lymphoma. Multiple myeloma is the most common primary bone neoplasm in adults. About 85% of the cases occur between the ages of 40 and 70 years with a peak incidence between 50 and 60 years of age. Male to female ratio of occurrence is about 2:1. The parenchyma of this type of tumor is composed of malignant plasma cells (Figure 22.9) which may vary from well to poorly differentiated in different cases. This tumor may involve any bone and commonly is multifocal (multiple myeloma) although occasionally there may be only one lesion (solitary myeloma). Ultimately, solitary myeloma usually becomes disseminated with multiple lesions developing. The skull, spine, ribs, and sternum are involved most frequently. The tumors destroy bone and typically produce radiolucent lesions often with a circumscribed or punched-out appearance. The most common presenting symptoms are bone pain and malaise. Common important laboratory findings are anemia, malignant monoclonal gammopathy, and Bence Jones proteinuria. Secondary amyloidosis and renal failure are important complications. Chemotherapy and radiation therapy are the usual modes of treatment.

Malignant Lymphoma

The bone marrow is commonly involved by non-Hodgkin's malignant lymphomas of various cell types and by Hodgkin's disease, usually as a component of disseminated disease. Occasionally, however, non-Hodgkin's malignant lymphoma of large cell (histiocytic) or mixed large and small cell type (mixed histiocytic and lymphocytic type) is primary in a bone where it forms a lytic tumor. Such lesions are commonly called reticulum cell sarcoma of bone. This type of tumor may occur from childhood to old age and may involve any bone. The long tubular bones, particularly the femur, and the bones of the pelvis are most often involved. Pain, tenderness, and swelling secondary to the tumor are the usual presenting complaints. This neoplasm tends to be locally destructive, may invade surrounding soft tissue and an adjacent joint. Histologically, this tumor may be confused with Ewing's sarcoma or metastatic carcinoma or neuroblastoma. Primary reticulum cell sarcoma of bone may remain localized to the region of the primary site for a variable period of time but ultimately it tends to disseminate to regional and distant lymph nodes, other bones, and other organs. Radiation therapy, chemotherapy, and sometimes surgery are the methods of treatment. With appropriate therapy 5-year survival is 50% or better.

Intermediate Tumors

The tumors included in this group are those whose behavior is often difficult to predict, or are sometimes classified as borderline or low-grade malignant neoplasms. In general, they are tumors which are variably aggressive locally, tend to recur locally, and sometimes metastasize although not distinctly anaplastic.

Giant Cell Tumor (Osteoclastoma)

There has been a great deal of controversy about this tumor as to its histogenesis, the nature of its parenchymal cells, criteria which differentiate it from other tumors which contain numerous multinucleated giant cells with which it may be confused, and the value of histologic grading in predicting its behavior. There has even been controversy as to whether or not there is such an entity. Most authors now accept giant cell tumor as an entity although controversy continues over some other aspects of the lesion. Giant cell tumor typically arises in the epiphyseal area of a bone formed by enchondral ossification. The distal femur and proximal tibia are the most common sites followed by the distal radius and ulna. Multiple tumors are rare. Most cases occur between the ages of 20 and 40 years. Occasionally, it occurs in teenagers but in such cases the patient usually has relatively advanced bone age. The tumor rarely occurs before closure of the involved epiphysis. Histologically, giant cell tumor is composed of numerous osteoclast-like giant cells in a parenchymal matrix of fibrohistiocyte-like tissue (Figure 22.10). Histologic grading of the tumor based on the degree of atypia of this parenchymal matrix (commonly but incorrectly referred to as the stroma) has been proposed as a guide for prognosis and therapy. In general, the less atypical this tissue is the lower the grade and the less aggressive the tumor is. Even low-grade (nonatypical) giant cell tumors, however, often recur locally after curettage and sometimes metastasize. Anaplastic (high-grade) giant cell tumors are fully malignant neoplasms. Giant cell tumors tend to grow progressively, destroy and expand the involved part of the bone, and produce a trabeculated radiolucent mass radiographically. Local pain and swelling and limitation of motion of the adjacent joint are the usual presenting complaints. Surgery

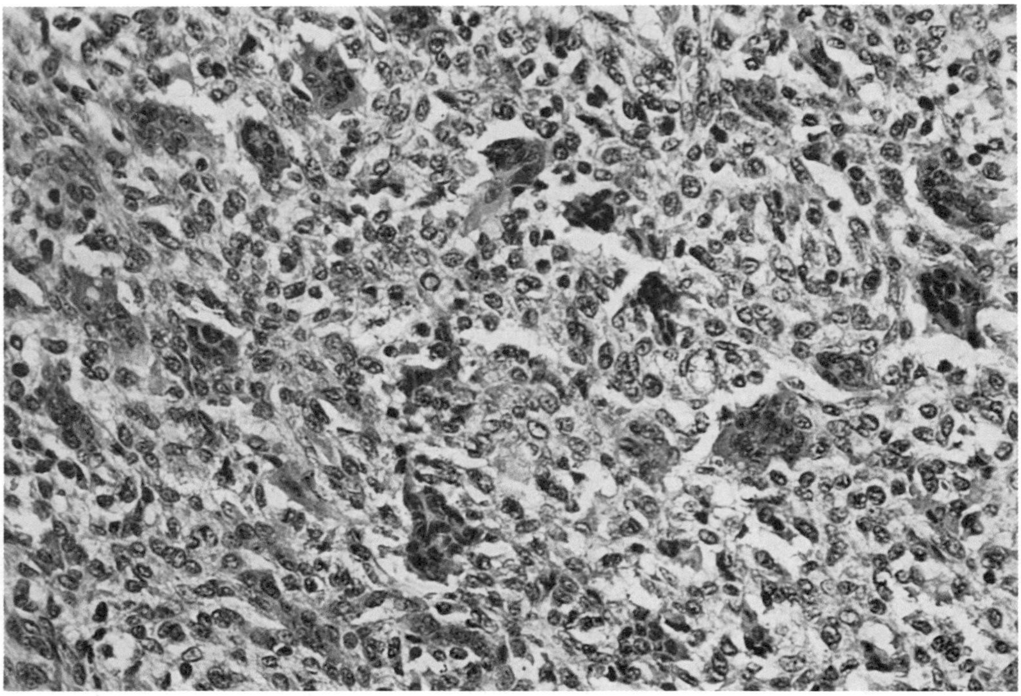

FIGURE 22.10 Giant cell tumor. H&E X 338

(curettage, en-bloc resection, or amputation) and radiation therapy are the usual means of treatment depending on the circumstances in each case.

Chordoma

Chordoma is a rare neoplasm which arises from the notocord and involves the spine, most often the sacrum-coccyx and the base of the skull. About 90% of cases occur in these two areas. This tumor may occur at any age but most cases occur between the ages of 30 and 70 years. There is approximately equal sex incidence of tumors at the base of the skull but sacrococcygeal tumors are more frequent in males. In general, chordoma is a slow-growing but locally invasive and destructive lesion which may metastasize. Metastasis, however, usually occurs only late in the course of the disease if at all. Histologically, the tumor is composed of vacuolated cells in a myxoid or chondroid matrix. The main histologic differential diagnostic considerations are metastatic adenocarcinoma, chondrosarcoma, and liposarcoma. Primary treatment is surgical excision or high-dose radiation therapy. In most cases the tumors have reached such an advanced stage by the time diagnosis is made that they cannot be completely excised. In general, therefore, the long-term prognosis is poor. Radiation therapy is also used for palliation as is chemotherapy.

TABLE 22.2 Tumors of Joints

Benign Tumors
Pigmented villonodular synovitis
Synovial chondrometaplasia
Chrondroma
Hemangioma
Lipoma
Synovial cyst
Ganglion
Cyst of meniscus
Malignant Tumors
Synovial sarcoma

Tumors of Joints

There are not as many types of primary tumors of joints as there are of bones but like tumors in other parts of the skeleton those that involve the joints include neoplastic and nonneoplastic, benign and malignant lesions (see Table 22.2). Most primary tumors of the joints arise in the synovium. A joint may be secondarily involved by a tumor arising in an adjacent bone or by a metastatic tumor.

Common presenting signs and symptoms of joint tumors are pain, tenderness, swelling, effusion, palpable mass, and dysfunction.

Benign Tumors

Most benign tumors and tumor-like lesions of joints are not neoplasms although the nature of some is debated. Pathogenetically, most or all probably are hyperplastic, hamartomatous, inflammatory, retrogressive (degenerative), or metaplastic masses.

Pigmented Villonodular Synovitis

This lesion of undetermined cause and uncertain pathogenesis involves the synovium of joints, tendon sheaths, and bursae. It may vary from a diffuse villous (papillary) or villonodular growth involving the synovium to a single nodule or tumor. The villonodular type of growth is most common in joints, most often the knee, whereas the localized distinct nodule (tumor) tends to involve tendon sheaths, most often in the fingers. The localized nodular or tumorous variety of the lesion is commonly called giant cell tumor of synovium or localized nodular synovitis. These lesions have also been called benign synovioma, myeloplaxoma, xanthoma, xanthogranuloma, and fibrous histiocytoma of synovium. This localized nodular type of lesion occasionally occurs in a joint, usually the knee.

As the various names imply, it is uncertain whether this disease is inflammatory, hyperplastic, or neoplastic.

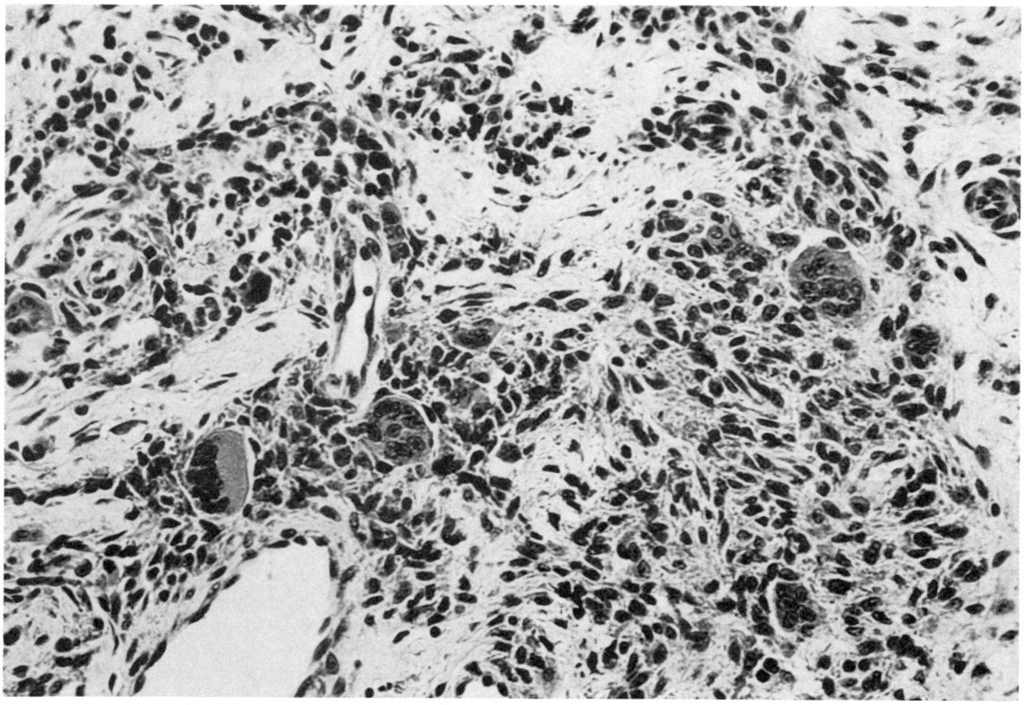

FIGURE 22.11 Synovial giant cell tumor (pigmented villonodular synovitis). H&E X 338

The histologic features are essentially the same whatever the gross appearance of the lesion - villous, villonodular, or nodular. These lesions are characterized by proliferation of mononuclear cells which probably are synovial cells, the presence of multinucleated giant cells, histiocytes, fibrosis, hyalinization, vascular proliferation, and hemosiderin deposition (Figure 22.11).

Villonodular synovitis of the joints tends to occur in adults most often between the ages of 30 and 50 years and is somewhat more common in men than in women. Any synovial joint may be affected but either the knee or hip is involved in more than 80% of cases. The presenting complaint usually is pain. There may or may not be swelling of the joint. Locking of the knee sometimes occurs. The usual treatment is excision of the involved synovium. The disease has a tendency to recur. Sometimes the lesion may invade a bone or bones adjacent to the joint in which case it is referred to as invasive or intraosseous villonodular synovitis. This is still a benign lesion but invasion of the bone may lead to diagnostic confusion.

Synovial Chondrometaplasia

This disease is also known as synovial chondromatosis and osteochondromatosis. It is characterized by multiple cartilaginous or osteocartilaginous nodules in the synovium formed through metaplasia from the stroma. These commonly give rise to numerous cartilaginous and osteocartilaginous loose bodies in the involved joint (sometimes called joint mice or rice bodies). The knee is the most commonly affected joint but the hip, elbow, shoulder, and occasionally some other joint may be involved. Usually only one joint is involved. This condition is somewhat more common in males than in females and tends to occur in young or middle-aged adults. Pain, swelling, and joint dysfunction are the usual complaints. The calcified cartilaginous and osteocartilaginous bodies may be seen radiographically.

Treatment usually is removal of the loose bodies and excision of the involved synovium. The lesion may recur but it also may undergo spontaneous regression. Rarely chondrosarcoma has been reported to complicate synovial chondrometaplasia.

Chondroma

Rarely, a mass of cartilage may develop in the fibrous capsule of a joint, possibly through metaplasia. This type of tumor is called intracapsular or paraarticular chondroma. Such lesions vary from 1 to 2 cm in diameter in small joints to as much as 5 cm in diameter in a large joint such as the knee. The patient is usually a young adult.

Hemangioma

Vascular hamartomas are uncommon in joints. Nearly always the affected joint is a knee. These are capillary, cavernous, or venous hemangiomas which may be circumscribed or diffusely involve the joint and also adjacent soft tissues and bone. They occur most often in adolescents and young adults. The circumscribed type of hemangioma can usually be cured by excision. Diffuse hemangioma is difficult to completely excise and attempted excision may be complicated by hemorrhage.

Lipoma

This tumor rarely occurs in joints. It occurs most often in a knee or ankle joint. Lipoma may arise from the subsynovial fat of the articular capsule. Lipomas are usually no more than 3 or 4 cm in greatest dimension.

Synovial Cyst

Cysts lined by a synovial membrane develop by herniation of synovium through a joint capsule. A common site for such lesions is the popliteal space where the cyst forms following herniation of synovium through the posterior capsule of the knee joint. In the popliteal space the cyst tends to develop a thick fibrous wall. Lesions of this type are commonly called Baker's cyst. If communication with the joint space is closed, as by inflammation of fibrosis, the synovial lining of such cysts tends to atrophy and may disappear and the cyst content tends to become mucoid. Synovial cysts may arise from joints other than the knee, most often in the wrist, the fingers, and the ankle. These lesions may form a palpable mass which may be tender or painful.

Ganglion

This is a peculiar cavitary lesion which tends to develop in or adjacent to joint capsules and tendon sheaths. It consists of a cavity or cavities in the connective tissue filled with mucoid material. The cause and pathogenesis of ganglia are uncertain. Probably in most cases they result from localized mucinous degeneration of the connective tissue. Pathogenetically, however, some probably are synovial cysts. Ganglia tend to be small, usually 1-2 cm in diameter. They form a palpable mass and may be painful and tender. The dorsum of the wrist is a common site. Ganglia may be excised. Sometimes they recur. They may regress spontaneously.

Cyst of Meniscus

This uncommon lesion is similar anatomically to a ganglion in that it consists of a cavity or cavities filled with mucoid material but is located in a semilunar knee cartilage. These lesions also probably arise through mucinous degeneration of the tissue in the involved area. Meniscal cysts vary from a few millimeters to 2 or 3 cm in diameter and usually involve the peripheral part of the anterior two-thirds of a lateral meniscus. These lesions may cause chronic ache, swelling, and dysfunction, such as locking of the knee. They usually are cured by complete excision but may recur after incomplete excision or aspiration.

Malignant Tumors

Primary malignant neoplasms of the joints are uncommon. Synovial sarcoma is the most common and important. Rarely, chondrosarcoma arises in a joint. Other primary malignant neoplasms of joints are very rare.

Synovial Sarcoma

Synovial sarcoma is a malignant neoplasm which usually but not always occurs in paraarticular regions and which has a parenchyma of anaplastic synovial-like tissue. About 10% of these tumors occur within joints where they arise from the synovial lining. Most of the others arise in soft tissues adjacent to joint capcules, tendon sheaths, or bursae. Occasionally, they arise in soft tissues away from joints as in the abdominal wall. In more than 80% of cases the tumor is located in an extremity, most commonly the lower. The sites most commonly affected are the knee (about half of all cases), ankle, foot, wrist, hand, shoulder, and elbow. This tumor may occur at and age but most often develops in young adults and adolescents. About 90% of cases occur between the ages of 10 and 50 years. In individual cases the course of the disease is difficult to predict. In general, synovial sarcoma tends to grow relatively slowly but commonly recurs locally following excision and ultimately metastasizes. Metastasis often occurs late in the course of the disease but sometimes is an early manifestation. Metastases, usually in the lungs, may be detectable at the time of initial diagnosis of the primary tumor or local reucrrence, or metastases may first become manifest as long as 20 years after original diagnosis. Average 5-year survival rate is about 45% and average 10-year survival rate is about 20%.

The usual presenting complaint of the patients is the presence of a deep palpable mass which may be painful or tender. Sometimes there is limitation of motion of the involved joint.

Histologically, synovial sarcoma characteristically has two parenchymal components: a spindle-cell fibrosarcoma-like tumor and cuboidal or columnar epithelial cells which line slits or gland-like spaces in the spindle cell component (Figure 22.12). There is variation in the amount and distribution of these two types of parenchymal tissue in different tumors or in different areas of one tumor so that the histologic findings are quite variable. In some tumors there is very little epithelial parenchyma. Less frequently, most of the tumor is epithelial with little

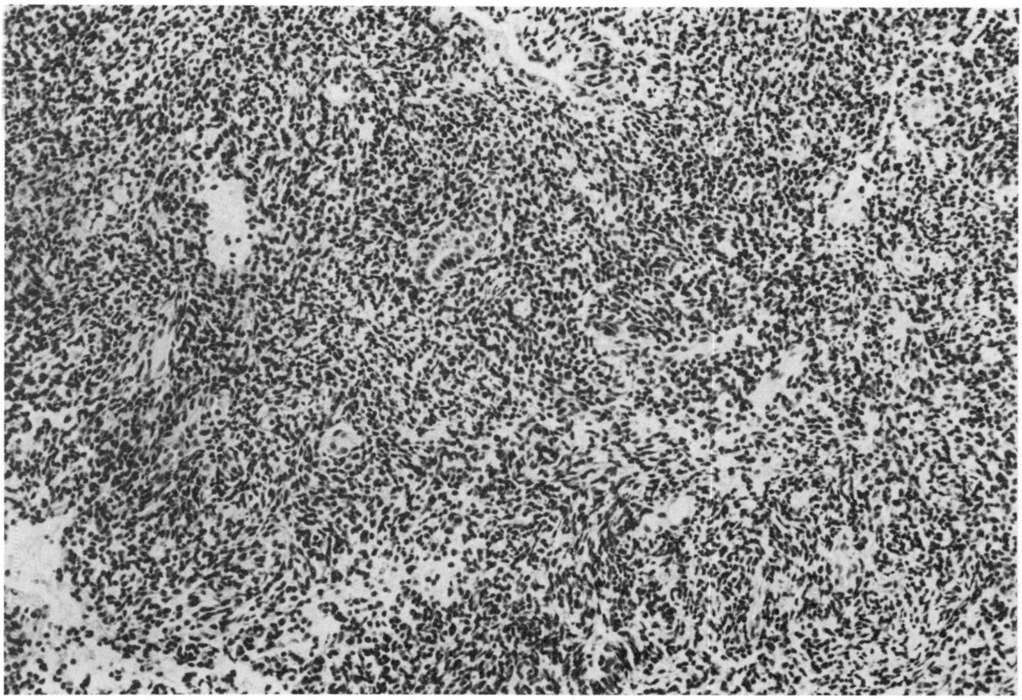

FIGURE 22.12 Synovial sarcoma. H&E X 170

spindle cell sarcomatous component. In general, the more highly anaplastic tumors are more highly malignant than the better differentiated less anaplastic ones.

Surgical excision, radiotherapy and chemotherapy are all used in treatment.

Bibliography

Aegerter E, Kirkpatrick A Jr: *Orthopedic Diseases: Physiology, Pathology, Radiology,* 4th Ed. Philadelphia, W.B. Saunders, 1975.

Anderson WAD, Kissane JM (eds.): *Pathology,* 7th Ed. St. Louis, C.V. Mosby, 1977.

Dahlin DC: *Bone Tumors,* 3rd Ed. Springfield, IL, Charles C. Thomas, 1978.

Enzinger FM, Weiss SW: *Soft Tissue Tumors.* St. Louis, C.V. Mosby, 1983.

Huvos AG: *Bone Tumors: Diagnosis, Treatment and Prognosis.* Philadelphia, W.B. Saunders, Philadelphia, 1979.

Jaffe HL: *Tumors and Tumorous Conditions of the Bones and Joint.* Philadelphia, Lea and Febiger, 1958.

Lichtenstein L: *Bone Tumors,* 5th Ed. St. Louis, C.V. Mosby, 1977.

Miller FN Jr: *Peery and Miller's Pathology: A Dynamic Introduction to Medicine and Surgery,* 3rd Ed. Boston, Little, Brown and Co., 1978.

Mirra JM: *Bone Tumors: Diagnosis and Treatment.* Philadelphia, J.B. Lippincott, 1980.

Morehead RP: *Human Pathology: An Introduction to Medicine.* New York, The Blakiston Division, McGraw-Hill, 1965.

Robbins SL, Cotran RS: *Pathologic Basis of Disease,* 2nd Ed. Philadelphia, W.B. Saunders, 1979.

Rosai J: *Ackerman's Surgical Pathology,* 6th Ed. St. Louis, C.V. Mosby, 1981.

Spjut HJ, Fechner RE, Ackerman LV: *Tumors of Bone and Cartilage. Atlas of Tumor Pathology,* Fascicle 5, Second Series. Supplement. Washington, DC, Armed Forces Institute of Pathology, 1981.

Spjut HJ, Fechner RE, Ackerman LV: *Tumors of Bone and Cartilage. Atlas of Tumor Pathology,* Fascicle 5, Second Series. Washington, DC, Armed Forces Institute of Pathology, 1971.

Chapter 23

RHEUMATIC MANIFESTATIONS OF SYSTEMIC DISEASE

Elliott L. Semble, M.D. and Christopher M. Wise, M.D.

Many systemic diseases may be complicated by symptoms and signs that might otherwise be attributed to specific rheumatic diseases. The recognition of these syndromes is important, since diagnostic and therapeutic decisions may be influenced greatly by the knowledge that an apparent rheumatic complaint may represent a manifestation of a more generalized condition.

In this chapter, we will review rheumatic syndromes that occur in relationship to several categories of systemic diseases. These conditions will include endocrine diseases, hemoglobinopathies, sarcoidosis, lipid disorders, bleeding disorders, hemochromatosis, amyloidosis, and malignancies.

Rheumatic Manifestations of Endocrinopathies

Endocrine disorders may be associted with well-defined rheumatologic diseases or syndromes, or with nonspecific osteoarticular findings. This section will detail rheumatic manifestations of the major endocrinopathies.

Agromegaly

Patients with acromegaly may develop an arthropathy resembling osteoarthritis. A history of joint pain is generally elicited in acromegalic arthropathy, but may be absent. Large and small peripheral joints are usually affected. Physical examination may reveal coarse crepitation on joint motion. Synovial or periarticular thickening is often present, but joint effusions are uncommon. Synovial fluids are generally noninflammatory with low leukocyte counts (1,2). Radiographic findings include widened joint spaces, periosteal proliferation, marginal osteophyte formation, and bone remodeling (Figure 23.1).

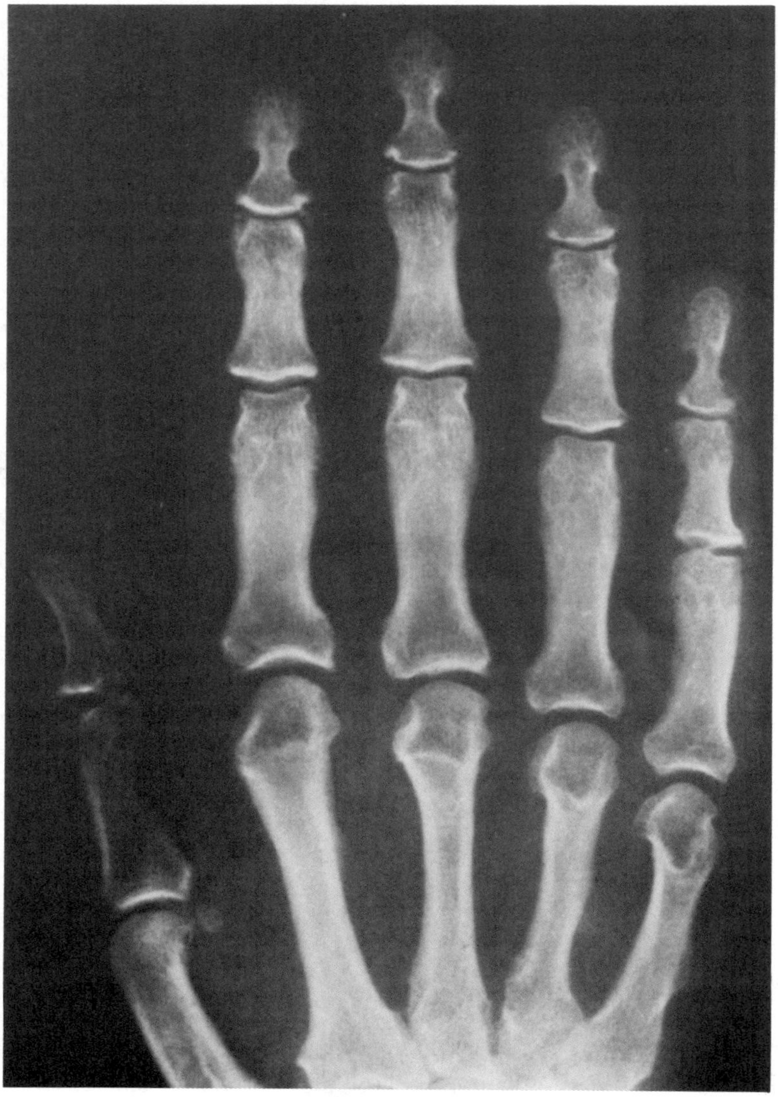

FIGURE 23.1 Radiograph of an acromegalic hand showing widened joint spaces, capsular ossification of distal interphalangeal joints, and remodeling of proximal phalanges. (From *Clinics in Rheumatic Diseases,* with permission of W.B. Saunders, and author Rodney Bluestone, M.D.)

Back pain is a common symptom in acromegaly. The lumbosacral spine is usually involved, but the cervical and thoracic spine may be affected. Hypermobility of the spine may occasionally be detected on joint examination. Radiographic features of spinal involvement in acromegaly include widened disc spaces, osteophyte formation at the anterior vertebral margins, and increased concavity at the posterior surfaces of the vertebral bodies (2).

Carpal tunnel syndrome and Raynaud's phenomenon may occur in patients with acromegaly (3). Carpal tunnel compression may be due to impingement of the carpal tunnel by proliferating bone and soft tissue or local swelling and hypertrophy of the median nerve. The mechanism of Raynaud's phenomenon in this disease is unknown, but thickening of the blood vessel walls may be important in the etiology of the digital vasospasm.

The treatment of the pituitary lesion in acromegaly does not prevent the progression of the peripheral or spinal joint disease (1). However, pituitary ablation generally results in a rapid improvement in carpal tunnel symptomatology. Nonsteroidal antiinflammatory drugs may be useful in controlling joint symptoms in acromegaly. Total joint replacement may be necessary if hips or knees have been destroyed by articular disease.

Hypothyroidism

Rheumatic manifestations of hypothyroidism are listed in Table 23.1.

Myxedematous arthropathy has an insidious onset with joint pain, stiffness, and swelling. The knees, ankles, hands, and feet are frequently involved. Physical examination may reveal synovial thickening with minimal pain and tenderness. Joint effusions are often present. Synovial effusions are extremely viscous with leukocyte counts in the noninflammatory range (4). Elevated erythrocyte sedimentation rates and increased serum uric acid concentration may also be seen (5). Radiologic findings are nonspecific and include generalized osteopenia, soft tissue swelling, and synovial effusions.

Chondrocalcinosis and pseudogout have been reported in patients with hypothyroidism (4). Carpal tunnel syndrome may also be seen in this disease and is occasionally associated with myxedematous arthropathy.

Patients with hypothyroidism often complain of muscle pain, stiffness, and weakness. Myxedema may be associated with a severe myopathy characterized by proximal muscle weakness, elevated serum creatine phosphokinase levels, and abnormal muscle biopsies.

Autoimmune (Hashimoto's) thyroiditis is a major cause of hypothyroidism. Rheumatologic syndromes associated with Hashimoto's thyroiditis include fibrositis and chest wall pain. Clinical studies in patients with Hashimoto's thyroiditis have suggested an increased incidence of coexisting rheumatic diseases (6), especially rheumatoid arthritis.

TABLE 23.1 Rheumatological Manifestations of Hypothyroidism

Myxedematous arthropathy
Chondrocalcinosis and pseudogout
Carpal tunnel syndrome
Myopathy
Fibrositis
Chest wall pain

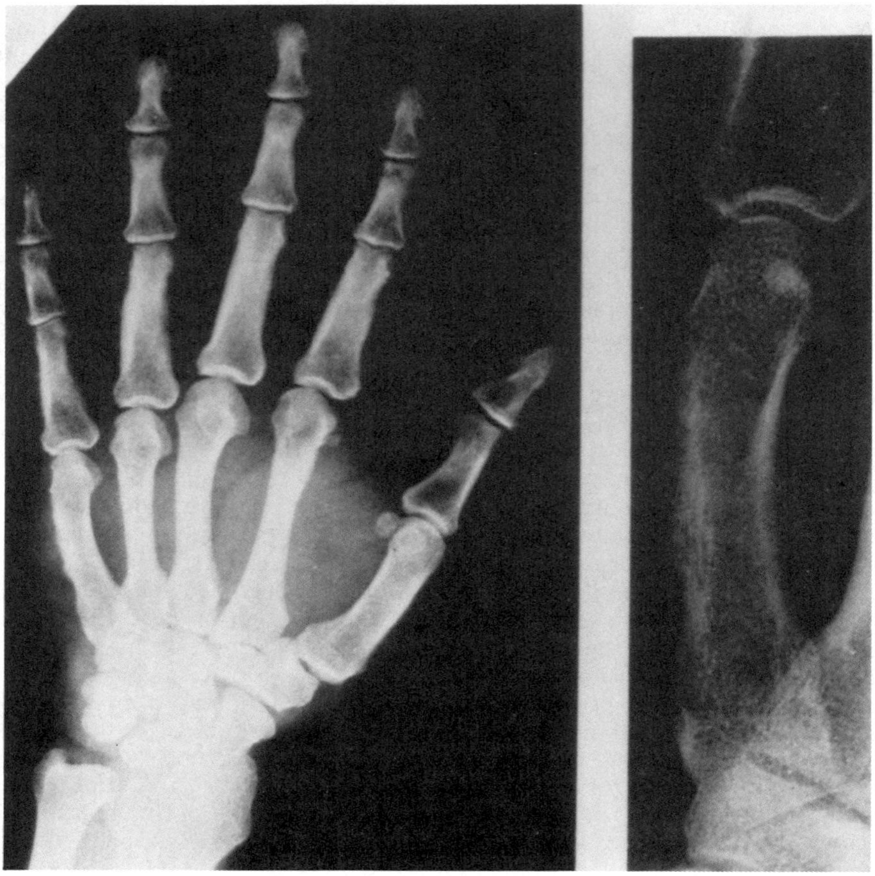

FIGURE 23.2 Radiograph of a hand showing the periostitis of thyroid acropachy. Note the irregular soft periosteal reaction most marked along the ulnar aspect of the fifth metacarpal (right). (From *Clinics in Rheumatic Diseases,* with permission of W.B. Saunders, and author Rodney Bluestone, M.D. and original source Leslie Preger, M.D.)

Myxedematous arthropathy, carpal tunnel syndrome, myopathy, and the soft tissue syndromes associated with Hashimoto's thyroiditis are usually improved by treatment with thyroid hormone.

Hyperthyroidism

Graves' disease is one of the major causes of hyperthyroidism. Thyroid acropachy, an unusual rheumatologic syndrome, may complicate Graves' disease. This syndrome is characterized by clubbing of the fingers and toes, and periostitis of the digits and distal extremities with soft tissue swelling (1,7). Radiological findings are shown in Figure 23.2. Thyroid acropachy is generally unresponsive to treatment.

Diabetes Mellitus

A variety of rheumatologic manifestations may complicate diabetes mellitus. These include neuropathic arthropathy, periarthritis of the shoulder, Dupuytren's contracture, and flexor tenosynovitis.

The typical patient with neuropathic arthropathy (Charcot joint) has long-standing diabetes mellitus with sensory neuropathy. The tarsal, tarsometatarsal, and metatarsophalangeal joints are usually affected, but the ankles, knees, and lumbar spine may also be involved.

The neuroarthropathic foot is characterized by edema, thicken tarsal soft tissues, minimal pain and tenderness, deformities, and callus formation over abnormal weight-bearing areas (1,8). Early radiographic changes include osteopenia and juxtaarticular cortical erosions in the phalanges or metatarsal heads (9). Later radiographic findings include cartilage loss, fragmentation and absorption of subchondral bone, and marginal osteophytes which tend to be bulky and bizarre in configuration (10) (Figure 23.3).

The therapy of neuropathic arthropathy involves prolonged nonweight-bearing to prevent further trauma to the involved area.

Periarthritis of the shoulder is more common in the diabetic population. It usually affects insulin-dependent diabetics over the age of 40 (8). Pain and disability may remit spontaneously or progress to a frozen shoulder. The treatment of periarthritis of the shoulder includes heat, analgesics, physical therapy, and local corticosteroid injection(s).

A group of soft tissue syndromes affecting the hands appears to be more frequent in diabetes mellitus. Dupuytren's contracture, a nodular or plaque-like thickening of the palmar fascia, is seen in approximately 8% of the diabetic population (1). Patients with diabetes may develop flexor tenosynovitis or trigger fingers (8). Juvenile diabetics may have an increased incidence of noninflammatory joint contractures (11).

Hyperparathyroidism

Hyperuricemia and gout are associated with primary hyperparathyroidism. The frequency of attacks of acute gouty arthritis in hyperparathyroidism varies from 3 to 45% (2). The mechanism(s) of hyperuricemia in hyperparathyroidism is unknown, but may be related to renal disease in some patients.

Patients with primary hyperparathyroidism have an increased incidence of calcium pyrophosphate deposition disease. Radiological evidence of chondrocalcinosis is often seen in primary hyperparathyroidism. Recurrent attacks of pseudogout have been well documented in this endocrinopathy and are often precipitated by parathyroidectomy.

Patients with secondary hyperparathyroidism in the clinical setting of chronic renal failure (renal osteodystrophy) may have attacks of acute periarticular inflammation in the soft tissues around joints and in tendon sheaths. These attacks may be related to calcium hydroxyapatite deposition. The therapy of these inflammatory episodes consists of nonsteroidal antiinflammatory agents or local injections of corticosteroids.

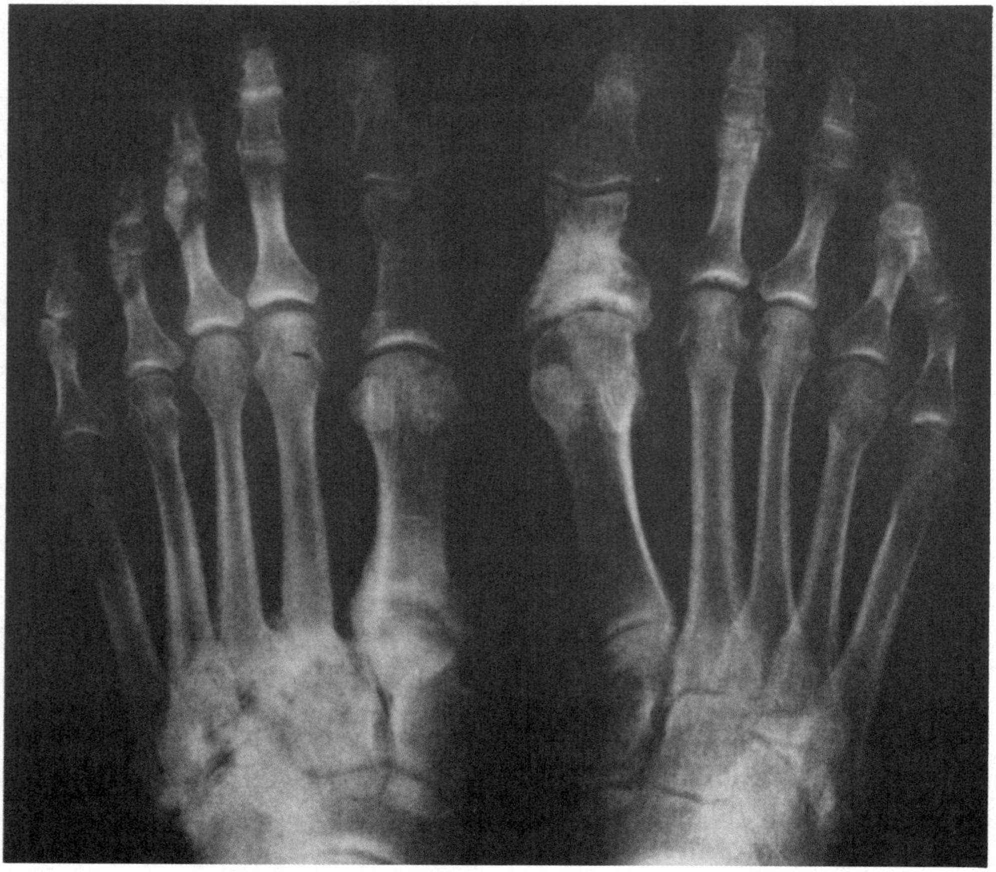

FIGURE 23.3 Neuropathic arthropathy involving the right first metatarsophalangeal joint and left tarsometatarsal joints of a 31-year-old woman who had developed diabetes mellitus at the age of 6. (Reprint from the *Primer of Rheumatic Diseases,* 8th Ed., copyright 1983, used by permission of the Arthritis Foundation.)

Arthritis Associated with Sickle Cell Disease and Other Hemoglobinopathies

Patients with sickle cell disease may develop hyperuricemia, osteomyelitis, septic arthritis, bone infarctions, avascular necrosis, or noninflammatory joint effusions (Table 23.2).

Hyperuricemia is often detected in patients with sickle cell disease, but gouty arthritis is rare. The mechanisms of hyperuricemia may be related to impaired renal function and/or overproduction of uric acid (12,13,14).

Bacterial infections are more common in sickle cell anemia. The frequency of osteomyelitis is more than 100 times that seen in normal controls (15). Septic arthritis may occur, but is much less frequent than osteomyelitis. Staphylococci, *Escherichia coli,* enterobacter, and salmonellae have been responsible for most joint infections (13).

TABLE 23.2 Rheumatological Manifestations in Sickle Cell Disease

Hyperuricemia and gout
Osteomyelitis
Septic arthritis
Bone infarction
Avascular necrosis
Noninflammatory joint effusions

Bone infarctions in sickle cell disease may be due to sickling and thromboses in small vessels. Avascular or aseptic necrosis refers to bone infarction at the joint margins resulting in the collapse of periarticular bone and cartilage. Avascular necrosis of the head of the femur is frequently seen in patients with sickle cell disease and may be disabling (13,14). The humeral head, radius, tibial condyles, and vertebral bodies may also be sites of avascular necrosis. Early treatment of avascular necrosis of the hips consists of prolonged nonweight-bearing. If pain and disability is persistent, total hip replacement may be necessary.

The crises of sickle cell anemia are characterized by fever, leukocytosis, and polyarthralgia. Joint effusions may occur during sickle crisis, usually involving the knees or ankles. These effusions are generally noninflammatory (16). Synovial biopsies have demonstrated evidence of microvascular thrombosis (13). Joint effusions are usually self-limited and require no specific therapy. The sickle cell crisis should be managed with analgesics, hydration, and supportive care.

Rheumatologic syndromes may also be found in hemoglobinopathies other than sickle cell disease. Bone infarctions and avascular necrosis may occur in SC disease and S thalassemia. Patients with beta thalassemia may develop ankle pain associated with tenderness and mild swelling (17). The articular findings in beta thalassemia appear to be related to underlying bone disease and are unresponsive to therapy.

Sarcoidosis

Sarcoidosis is a multisystem disease of unknown etiology characterized by the presence of noncaseating granulomas in involved organs. The major rheumatologic manifestations include sarcoid arthropathy and bony involvement.

Acute sarcoidosis is characterized by hilar adenopathy, fever, erythema nodosum, and articular findings (Löfgren's syndrome). Physical examination reveals pain, limitation of motion, and periarticular swelling of the knees, ankles, proximal interphalangeal joints, wrists, and elbows (18). Synovial effusions are usually minimal or absent. Synovial fluid analysis generally reveals noninflammatory effusions (19). The erythrocyte sedimentation rate is frequently elevated. Tests for serum rheumatoid factor are occasionally positive. Joint manifestations of acute sarcoidosis may last from several weeks to 4 months, but rarely progress to the chronic form. Acute sarcoid arthritis may occasionally be confused with rheumatoid arthritis, but the presence of bilateral hilar adenopathy and erythema nodosum differentiates sarcoidosis from rheumatoid disease.

Chronic sarcoid arthritis may begin early or late in the course of sarcoidosis (19). The knees and ankles are most often affected. Joint destruction and disability are uncommon, but may occur (20). Synovial fluid analysis usually reveals an inflammatory effusion (21). Synovial biopsy specimens from patients with chronic sarcoid arthritis occasionally demonstrate noncaseating granulomas (22). Rheumatoid factor is often detected in the serum of these patients.

Patients with sarcoidosis may be genetically predisposed to develop arthritis. An increased incidence of the HLA-B8 antigen has been reported in patients with sarcoid arthritis (23).

Many patients with mild symptoms require no treatment. Salicylates have been helpful in alleviating symptoms in moderately severe, acute sarcoid arthritis (19). Oral colchicine therapy has been reported to be beneficial in acute or chronic sarcoid arthritis of moderate severity (24). Prednisone in doses of 15-40 mg daily has been effective in suppressing joint symptoms in patients with severe symptomatic acute or chronic sarcoid arthritis, or in patients unresponsive to salicylates or colchicine (19). Prednisone should be tapered to the lowest effective maintenance dosage for long-term treatment. Methotrexate and azathioprine may be considered if patients are resistant to prednisone therapy.

Bony involvement occurs infrequently in sarcoidosis. The bone lesions are generally asymptomatic and occur most often in the hands and feet (25). Radiographic findings of osseus sarcoidosis involving the hands include cystic lesions of the phalanges, erosive changes of the metacarpal heads, and loss of bone substance of the distal phalanges (Figure 23.4). The diagnosis of bony sarcoidosis is usually not difficult, since abnormal chest radiographs and chronic skin lesions are present in the majority of these patients (25). Osseus sarcoidosis usually does not require treatment. However, if pain or disability occur prednisone therapy may be indicated.

Arthritis Associated with Hyperlipoproteinemia

Rheumatologic manifestations of the heritable forms of hyperlipoproteinemia include arthritis and tenosynovitis.

Familial Hyperlipoproteinemia or Type IIa Hyperlipoproteinemia

Familial hypercholesterolemia or type IIa hyperlipoproteinemia is characterized by elevated levels of plasma cholesterol, phospholipids, and low density lipoproteins. Clinical features include tendinous, cutaneous, and periosteal xanthomatosis, xanthelesma, corneal arcus, and a propensity for early atherosclerosis (26).

Achilles tendinitis, and tenosynovitis occasionally accompanying arthritis of the knee, are the most common presenting features in patients with heterozygous familial type IIa hyperlipoproteinemia (27,28). These findings usually first appear in the adolescent age group.

Patients with this disease usually have recurrent attacks involving one or both Achilles tendons or knees. These attacks generally last 2-3 days and may occur over long periods of time. The affected areas on physical examination are warm, erythematous, and tender. Joint deformity or loss of motion does not occur. Tendon xanthomas usually appear several years after the onset of these attacks.

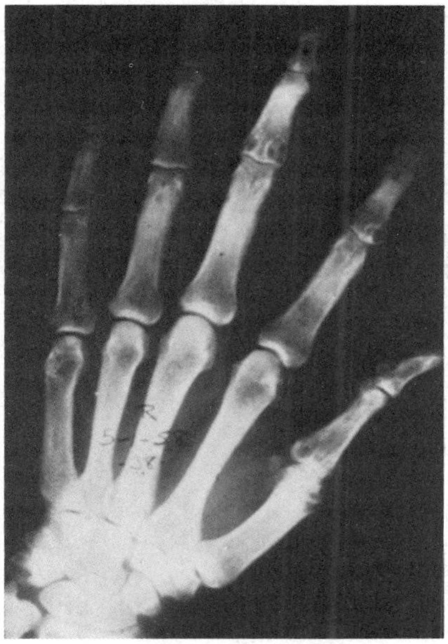

FIGURE 23.4 In this radiograph of a patient with sarcoidosis there are cystic changes involving the bases of the middle phalanges of the middle and index fingers; erosions are present in the first metacarpal head. The terminal tuft of the distal phalanx of the index finger shows loss of bone substance. (Reprinted from the Revised Clinical Slide Collection on the Rheumatic Diseases, copyright 1981, used by permission of the Arthritis Foundation.)

Recurrent attacks of a migratory polyarthritis may develop in patients who are homozygous for type IIa hyperlipoproteinemia (26). Large peripheral joints are usually affected. These joint attacks may be mild or short-lived or severe with objective signs of inflammation lasting for as long as a month. These patients may have an early onset of xanthomatosis, often starting between 4 and 8 years of age (28).

The erythrocyte sedimentation rate may be elevated in type IIa hyperlipoproteinemia. Patients suspected of having this lipid disorder should have plasma cholesterol and triglyceride determinations. The plasma cholesterol concentrations are significantly elevated while triglyceride levels are normal.

The recognition of this lipid abnormality may permit appropriate therapy at an early age (28,29). Young children may be responsive to dietary manipulation. Cholestyramine resin and diet may be effective in normalizing plasma cholesterol low density lipoprotein levels in older children (27,29). It is expected that proper management of this disease will improve or prevent some of its clinical manifestations.

Type IV Hyperlipoproteinemia

Type IV hyperlipoproteinemia may be associated with a bilateral, asymmetrical arthritis affecting a few joints (30). Objective findings on physical examination include mild inflammation involving both small and large joints. Synovial effusions usually reveal mild inflammation with a predominance of mononuclear cells

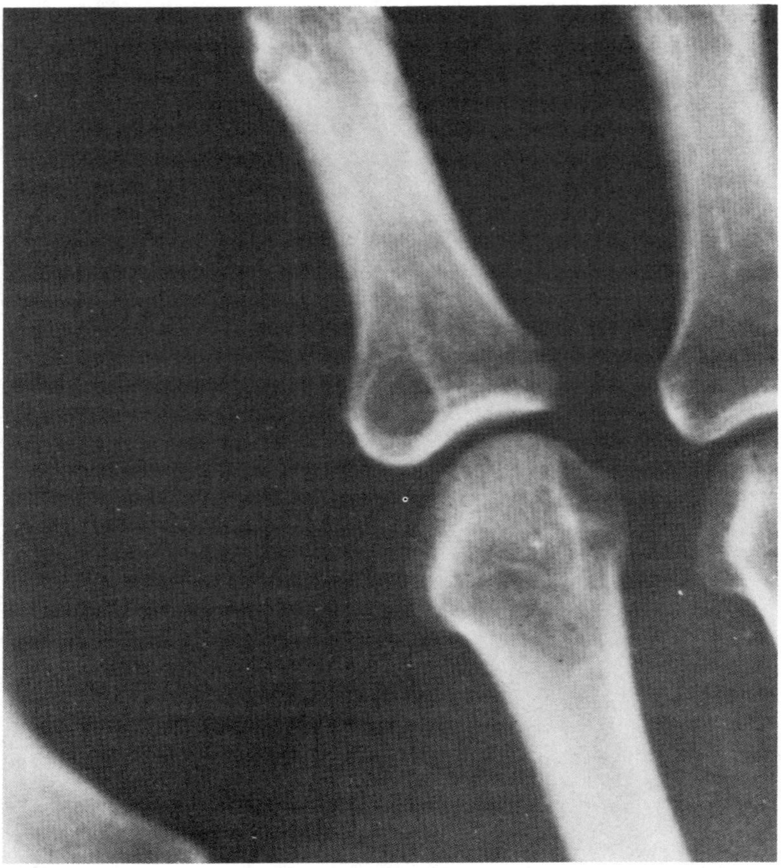

FIGURE 23.5 A typical bone cyst is seen in the second proximal phalanx of this patient with type IV hyperlipoproteinemia. (From *Textbook of Rheumatology,* with permission of the author Giles Bole Jr., and W.B. Saunders.)

(28,30). Biopsy specimens of synovium have demonstrated moderate hyperplasia of synovial lining cells and a mononuclear cell infiltration (28,30).

Laboratory findings include elevated serum triglyceride levels and normal or slightly increased concentrations of serum cholesterol. Lipoprotein electrophoresis reveals elevation in beta lipoproteins. Juxtaarticular osteopenia and cystic lesions may be noted on radiographs (Figure 23.5). Biopsies of these cysts usually show fibrous connective tissue and fat cells (30).

The treatment of type IV hyperlipoproteinemia consists of restricting carbohydrate, alcohol, and total calories in order to normalize plasma triglyceride levels. Joint findings may improve following this dietary manipulation.

Arthritis with Hemophilia

Although hemarthrosis has been described in most of the heritable coagulation disorders (with the exception of factor V deficiency), the functional deficiencies of clotting factor VIII (hemophilia A) and factor IX (hemophilia B) are the most common causes of recurrent hemarthrosis (31). These two conditions are seen almost exclusively in males, and are inherited in an X-linked recessive fashion. The frequency and severity of hemarthrosis correlates with the level of factor deficiency with levels under 1% associated with most severe disease (32,33). In addition to reports of hemarthrosis in other heritable factor deficiencies, this may also be seen in patients on anticoagulants (34), or with platelet disorders (35,36).

The reasons for the striking propensity for hemarthrosis in these disorders is uncertain, but it has been speculated that the availability of a relatively large space for uncoagulated blood plays a role (37). Progressive deterioration of joint structure and function appears to result from inflammatory reaction (pannus formation) due to the chronic presence of blood within the joint space (38). Cartilage destruction appears to be a secondary process, resulting from the action of enzymes produced by white cells or activated synovial cells (32,37).

Acute hemarthrosis may occur without any history of prior trauma. The most commonly involved joints, in order of decreasing frequency, are the knee, elbow, ankle, and shoulder, although sternoclavicular, hip, hand, and foot involvement has been reported.

After the initial episode of hemarthrosis, the joint is predisposed to further episodes by a combination of synovial proliferation and hypervascularity. Muscular atrophy results in compromise of joint protection and stability. Chronic recurrent hemarthrosis eventually results in a degenerative arthropathy in which abnormalities exist even between acute bleeding episodes. Chronic synovial thickening, small effusions, and mild flexion deformities and limitations are frequent (32,33). In end-stage hemophilic arthropathy, joint function is lost and motion is markedly restricted. Flexion deformity, subluxation, joint laxity, and malalignment are common. Ankylosis, when it occurs, tends to be fibrous and not bony.

Bleeding into muscle and soft tissues is common in hemophilia, and may sometimes closely resemble intraarticular bleeds. Iliopsoas hemorrhage may be associated with acute pain in the groin region, and the hip is held in flexion, but hip motion is not limited. Bleeding into the forearm and gastrocnemius muscles may cause contracture and deformities in these areas. On occasion, a periosteal pseudotumor may occur as a result of a suboptimally treated major hematoma becoming organized and vascular (32).

The activated partial thromboplastin time serves as a screening test for detecting heritable clotting factor abnormalities, and any abnormality in this test should be followed up with specific assays for activity levels of factor VIII, factor IX, or other factors. Individuals with less than 1% of normal factor activity are considered to have severe hemophilia, while those with greater than 5% are considered to have mild disease. Patients previously treated with replacement therapy should be evaluated for the presence or absence of acquired inhibitor antibodies against factor VIII or IX (32).

The earliest radiographic changes are those of joint capsule distention and increased soft tissue density. Epiphyseal overgrowth and irregularity may be seen in children. Chronically, marginal erosions, joint space narrowing, and subchondral bone irregularity may develop. Subchondral bone cysts frequently may be found and are often quite large. Osteophytes are common, but bony ankylosis is rare. End-stage disease is indistinguishable from primary osteoarthritis. Several other less usual but more characteristic findings have been described (32). These include widening of the intercondylar notch of the femur, squaring of the distal patella, and enlargement of the proximal radius. Hip involvement may resemble Legg-Perthes disease in childhood, and flattening of the talus and bony ankylosis may be seen in the ankle.

Patients with mild factor deficiencies rarely have disability resulting from chronic arthropathy. On the other hand, in one large Swedish series, over half of patients with severe hemophilia had marked or severe disability resulting from chronic arthropathy (39). In this group, 20% required crutches or other orthopedic appliances to ambulate, while 8% were wheelchair-bound. Although infections are a cause of death in up to 25% of patients, septic arthritis is an extremely rare complication of this disorder (37).

Hemophilia should be treated at the earliest symptoms suggestive of joint hemorrhage, long before the development of any physical findings. Bedrest, elevation of the affected limb, and ice packs to reduce pain and inflammation should be undertaken initially. Treatment of the underlying bleeding disorder with replacement of the missing factor is essential to successful management. Patients with hemophilia should have immediate access to factor replacement, either through an intensive program of home therapy, or through a medical center. Factor VIII (or, when appropriate, factor IX) infusion should begin as soon as possible. Initial infusion is usually calculated to obtain a factor VIII level of 30%, and 95% of acute episodes will be arrested by a single infusion to this level (32). Factor VIII is usually replaced either in the form of a relatively pure preparation or as frozen cryoprecipitate. Factor IX is available commercially in combination with factors II, VII, and X. Inhibitor antibodies develop in some patients chronically exposed to factor VIII, and this complication requires specialized treatment programs.

Although fever is frequently seen during acute hemarthrosis, infection is rare (37). Nevertheless, if suspicion exists, arthrocentesis should be performed to rule this out, but only after the infusion of missing factor has begun. Arthrocentesis with or without injection of corticosteroids is advocated for tense, extremely painful effusions (31).

Following the acute episode, chronic prophylactic factor replacement is recommended, usually to maintain a 5-10% level of factor activity. In addition, all hemophiliacs and their families should be involved in an intensive education program to recognize early symptoms requiring medical therapy.

Intensive physical therapy to strengthen muscles, surgical correction of flexion contractures, and splinting of affected joints should be part of the management of chronic hemophilic arthropathy. In advanced cases, synovectomy may be necessary if cartilage damage is minimal. Reconstructive hip and knee surgery has been successful in many patients, but must be preceded and followed by vigorous prophylactic replacement therapy. Because of the difficulties in controlling bleeding, elective surgery is not recommended for patients with factor VIII inhibitors.

Arthropathy with Hemochromatosis

The abnormal accumulation of iron in tissues occurs in a number of conditions. The term hemosiderosis is used when iron accumulates primarily in the cells of the reticuloendothelial system and relatively few organs, such as the liver and bone marrow. In hemosiderosis, there is no alteration of function or structure of involved organs and few if any pathologic changes. Hemochromatosis implies the chronic, excessive deposition of iron in multiple organs, resulting in functional and structural impairment. This disorder may be associated with cirrhosis, diabetes mellitus and other endocrinologic dysfunction, and myocardial disease. Primary idiopathic hemochromatosis is a familial form of iron overload which results from a lack of control of iron absorption. Secondary hemachromatosis may result from multiple transfusions for chronic anemia, or increased iron absorption resulting from chronic refractory anemia or preexisting cirrhosis (40). Idiopathic hemochromatosis affects men more often than women, and usually presents between the ages of 40 and 60 with symptoms related to cirrhosis, bronze discoloration of the skin, diabetes, hypopituitarism, and may be associated with a characteristic arthropathy.

Although hemochromatosis is a familial disease, the exact mode of inheritance has not been established. Recent studies have shown an association between HLA antigens A3 and B14 and hemochromatosis (41). The exact molecular basis for the accumulation of excess iron and hemosiderin in tissues in primary hemochromatosis is not completely defined, but most evidence suggests an abnormal increase in absorption of intestinal iron (42).

The exact mechanism by which joint damage occurs is unclear, but several mechanisms have been hypothesized, including the inhibition by ferrous ion of synovial fluid pyrophosphatase, the alteration of mucopolysaccharide complexes within cartilage, or the increase of lipid peroxidation by iron (40).

Joint disease may be seen in 40-50% of all patients with idiopathic hemochromatosis (43,44). The onset of the arthritis most often occurs along with other systemic manifestations, but joint symptoms occasionally predate other clinical manifestations (45,46). In general, though, patients with arthropathy tend to be older and have more chronic disease than those without joint manifestations.

The characteristic arthropathy of hemochromatosis was initially described by Schumacher in 1964 (43). The small joints of the hands, especially the second and third metacarpal phalangeal (MCP) joints are the earliest and most frequently involved. Pain, stiffness, swelling, and loss of flexion are seen. As the disease progresses, bony enlargement and degenerative changes may occur. A generalized degenerative arthropathy also occurs involving the wrists, shoulders, elbows, and occasionally the hips, knees, ankles, and spine. Approximately one-half of patients have superimposed episodes of acute inflammation, possibly related to the deposition of calcium pyrophosphate dihydrate crystals (pseudogout).

The most useful screening test is the measurement of plasma iron and total iron binding capacity (40). The vast majority of symptomatic patients with primary hemochromatosis have elevated plasma iron concentration and transferrin saturation over 75%. Serum ferritin is elevated in most patients. Total body iron stores may be estimated using a chelating agent, such as deferroxamine, and measuring iron in a 24-hour urine sample (42). Hypouricemia is often seen in hemochromatosis and may serve as a diagnostic clue (47). However, the definitive diagnostic test for primary hemochromatosis is liver biopsy, with quantitation of parenchymal iron.

Synovial biopsy may demonstrate thickening of the synovium, but there is usually very little or no inflammation present. There is usually an increase in hemosiderin within lining cells, but this is not specific for this disorder, and may be seen in rheumatoid arthritis as well (48). Calcium pyrophosphate dihydrate deposition has been observed in both synovium and cartilage, and hemosiderin is present within the cartilage and in chondrocytes. The cartilage is otherwise quite similar pathologically to that seen in typical osteoarthritis.

The characteristic radiographic features in primary hemochromatosis are loss of articular cartilage, subchondral cystic changes and sclerosis, and articular chondrocalcinosis (43,44,46). These features are quite similar to other forms of degenerative arthropathy, but cystic lesions with sclerotic margins of the MCP joints suggest primary hemochromatosis.

Hemochromatosis is usually a fatal disease, with death occurring as a result of a combination of hepatic, cardiac, and endocrine dysfunction. The arthropathy does not usually improve with therapy of the underlying condition. A chronic indolent degenerative arthropathy, with superimposed acute flares of pseudogout, is the usual pattern in the early stages. The arthritis may cause suprisingly few symptoms, and tends to be relatively benign and slowly progressive. However, hip involvement may cause significant disability.

The therapy of the arthritis is mainly palliative. Salicylates or other nonsteroidal antiinflammatory drugs may be helpful in controlling symptoms of chronic arthropathy. Acute episodes of pseudogout may be treated with joint drainage, intraarticular corticosteroids, and nonsteroidal antiinflammatory drugs or colchicine. Surgical intervention in chronic arthropathy may be helpful in selected cases and prosthetic hip and knee replacements have been performed with some success.

The treatment of choice of the underlying disease is the removal of excess body iron, usually by phlebotomy in which 500 ml of blood is removed once or twice weekly.

Amyloidosis

Amyloidosis is a syndrome characterized by the deposition of an insoluble amorphous material in the extracellular matrix of one of several organs (49). In 1854, Virchow first used the term "amyloid" to describe the starch-like staining properties of this substance with iodine and acid. Since then, much has been learned about the structure of what is actually protein.

Various schemes of classification of amyloidosis have evolved over the years. Currently, amyloidosis is classified in five major categories, with certain important subgroups (50,51) (see Table 23.3). Primary amyloidosis occurs without any evidence of underlying disease. Amyloidosis associated with multiple myeloma is included in this group, because of similar clinical and biochemical characteristics. Secondary amyloidosis may occur with a large number of chronic infectious or inflammatory diseases (see Table 23.4). Familial amyloidosis is a group including several familial syndromes in Portuguese, Japanese, and Swedish groups, as well as familial mediterranean fever. Localized amyloidosis occurs in local deposits without systemic disease. Senile amyloidosis describes the syndrome associated with aging.

The recent advent of more sophisticated immunochemical methods has allowed more exact characterization of the proteins causing tissue damage in amyloidosis (52). The two major amyloid proteins deposited in tissues are protein AA, found in secondary amyloidosis and also associated with familial mediterranean fever, and protein AL, occurring in primary amyloidosis and with multiple myeloma. Other chemical types have been shown to exist in localized, familial (AF), and senile (AS) amyloidosis. Protein AA is chemically related to a serum protein SAA, an acute phase reactant that can be found in the sera of normal patients, but appears to be elevated in certain types of infection and inflammation. Protein AL is composed primarily of fibrils which have similarities to the variable portion of kappa light chains of immunoglobulin molecules (Bence Jones protein). It is not known whether these light chain components are newly synthesized or represent degradation products of light chains.

TABLE 23.3 Classification of Amyloidosis

Primary Generalized Amyloidosis
Without underlying disease
Associated with multiple myeloma
Secondary Generalized Amyloidosis
Familial Amyloidosis
Portuguese, Japanese, Swedish, etc.
Familial Mediterranean Fever
Localized Amyloidosis
Senile Amyloidosis

TABLE 23.4 Diseases Associated with Secondary Amyloidosis

Rheumatoid Arthritis	
Juvenile Rheumatoid Arthritis	
Other Chronic Inflammatory Diseases	
Ankylosing spondylitis	Scleroderma
Reiter's syndrome	Polymyositis
Psoriatic arthritis	SLE
Infections	
Tuberculosis	
Leprosy	
Chronic decubitus ulcers	
Osteomyelitis	
Chronic pyelonephritis	
Neoplasms	
Hypernephroma	
Hodgkin's disease	
Others	

The clinical syndrome of amyloidosis results from the deposition of these proteins in vital organs and subsequent dysfunction of these organs. Several factors may be important in this deposition, including overproduction of these proteins as well as abnormalities in catabolism of amyloid fibrils. Some evidence suggests that tissue phagocytes in patients with amyloidosis do not degrade precursors properly, and that this may be related to lack of elastase, collagenase, or other degradative enzymes (50).

TABLE 23.5 Clinical Manifestations of Primary Generalized Amyloidosis

Neuropathy
Peripheral
Sensorimotor
Autonomic
Cardiomyopathy
Restrictive
Purpura
Arthropathy
Macroglossia
Hemorrhagic diathesis
Nephrotic syndrome
Carpal tunnel syndrome

Primary Generalized Amyloidosis

This condition occurs most often in older individuals. Although it has been reported as early as the second decade, it is rarely seen under the age of 40, and the mean age at diagnosis is in the range of 55-65 years (49,50). Men are affected more often than women, and whites more often than nonwhites. Weakness, fatigue, and weight loss are the most common initial symptoms. The characteristic clinical manifestations of primary amyloidosis are listed in Table 23.5. In addition to these characteristic findings, hepatomegaly is present in about one-third of patients. The vast majority of patients (80-90%) will demonstrate a monoclonal protein in serum or urine.

Myeloma Associated Amyloidosis

Amyloidosis occurs in 10-15% of patients with multiple myeloma. By definition, all of these patients will demonstrate monoclonal proteins in serum, and many also in urine. The epidemiology, clinical manifestations, and clinical syndrome are virtually indistinguishable from those seen in primary generalized amyloidosis, although anemia and bone pain are more common with myeloma.

Secondary Generalized Amyloidosis

This can occur as a result of a wide variety of chronic infectious, inflammatory, or neoplastic conditions (see Table 23.4). Rheumatoid arthritis is considered by many the most frequent cause of secondary amyloidosis in this country today. Past studies have suggested that this occurs in 10-20% of patients with rheumatoid arthritis, although more recently, this figure has declined to roughly 3% (51). Juvenile rheumatoid arthritis may also be complicated by amyloidosis. Chronic infections are particularly important in causing secondary amyloidosis on a worldwide basis. Tuberculosis and leprosy are among the most common associated infections. In addition, patients with chronic paraplegia may develop amyloidosis as a result of chronically infected decubitus ulcers, osteomyelitis, and chronic pyelonephritis. Neoplasms, such as hypernephroma and Hodgkin's disease, are most often associated with amyloidosis, although it has been recognized with a large number of other malignancies.

Proteinuria, nephrotic syndrome, and massive hepatomegaly are the chief manifestations of secondary amyloidosis. Although cardiac abnormalities are found in some patients, these can usually be attributed to other causes, and any amyloid infiltration found on autopsy studies is rarely responsible for clinical abnormalities.

Familial Amyloidosis

A large variety of familial amyloid syndromes have been described. Various combinations of neuropathic features as well as other manifestations such as renal disease, cardiac and hepatic disease, and cutaneous changes have been described, with each syndrome having a characteristic pattern. In addition, a familial cardiopathic syndrome has been described in a Danish kinship (49).

Amyloidosis with Familial Mediterranean Fever

Familial mediterranean fever (FMF) was first recognized in 1945 and is characterized by idiopathic recurring, self-limited attacks of fever often associated with serositis and synovitis or an erythematous rash (53). It occurs mainly in people of Mediterranean ancestry, particularly sephardic Jews, Armenians, and Arabs. Symptoms usually begin during childhood, and generalized amyloidosis complicates the picture, often before the age of 40. Clinical manifestations of the amyloidosis of FMF are similar to those of secondary amyloidosis, and protein AA is demonstrable in tissue deposits. Acute attacks may result in considerable morbidity, but unless complicated by amyloidosis, FMF is not associated with increased mortality. This syndrome is unique in that colchicine appears to be effective in treating the acute attacks and may be helpful in preventing amyloidosis.

Localized Amyloidosis

Various types of amyloidosis have been described that seem to be localized to a given organ or tissue. Several varieties limited to the skin have been described. Other localized amyloid deposition syndromes have been described associated with medullary carcinoma of the thyroid, insulinoma, pituitary tumors, and concretions in the prostate, lung, and liver.

Senile Amyloidosis

The existence of this clinical syndrome and its relationship to other forms of amyloidosis have been subjects of much controversy (51). Infiltration of the heart with a particular type of amyloid (ASc) is frequently seen in elderly patients in autopsy studies. It is not always associated with clinical symptoms and is not often a cause of death. In cases of clinically significant senile cardiac amyloidosis, a congestive cardiomyopathy associated with intractable congestive heart failure may be seen. Widespread organ involvement is not seen in this syndrome and diagnosis is difficult to make antemorten.

Organ System Involvement

Cutaneous Disease

The skin is most frequently involved in primary and myeloma-associated amyloidosis. There appears to be a preference for deposition of amyloid in the face and upper trunk. Clinical findings include papules, purpura, or nodules. Marked skin thickening and even changes mimicking scleroderma may be seen. Purpura is frequent and can often be induced by gentle stroking of the skin; periorbital purpura may be induced by valsalva maneuver or proctoscopic examination (post-proctoscopic purpura).

Arthropathy

Joint involvement is most often seen in primary or myeloma-associated amyloidosis. The arthropathy can affect any joint and may resemble rheumatoid arthritis. Pain and stiffness are the usual initial symptoms. Soft tissue contractures may be an early finding. Joint swelling on examination is usually firm or gritty. Soft tissue swelling and induration of the shoulders may result in the "shoulder pad sign," a feature highly suggestive of amyloid arthropathy. Synovial fluid is usually noninflammatory, but bloody effusions have been described. X-rays show soft tissue swelling, osteoporosis, and occasional lytic lesions.

Neuropathy

Carpal tunnel syndrome is most often seen in primary or myeloma-associated amyloidosis, but can occur in certain familial types. Peripheral neuropathy occurs in many of the acquired and hereditary forms. The most common presentation in acquired cases is a sensory neuropathy affecting primarily pain and temperature. Motor dysfunction may develop later. Orthostatic hypotension and gastrointestinal disturbance may result from autonomic nerve abnormalities.

Nephropathy

The kidneys can be involved in most forms of amyloidosis, although pronounced renal involvement is more characteristic of secondary syndromes. Proteinuria may occur and often progresses to nephrotic syndrome and renal failure. Hematuria and cellular casts are seldom found. Hypertension occurs in about one-half of patients. The kidneys may be enlarged or of normal or small size, and renal biopsy is necessary for definitive diagnosis. The demonstration of amyloid fibrils in urinary sediment, initially thought to be helpful in diagnosing this syndrome, is probably nonspecific.

Cardiac Disease

The heart can be involved in most of the amyloid syndromes. Restrictive cardiomyopathy with signs and symptoms of right heart failure dominate the early picture. Early radiographs may demonstrate mild cardiomegaly. Electrocardiograms show low voltage, arrhythmias, or conduction disturbances. Echocardiographic studies show marked symmetrically increased wall thickness, hypokinesia, and a small or normal ventricular cavity. The treatment of cardiac amyloidosis is unsatisfactory at best. Amyloid cardiomyopathy typically is poorly responsive to digitalis, and such treatment has been associated with sudden death.

Respiratory Amyloidosis

Deposition of amyloid deposits within the respiratory tract has been described as an isolated syndrome or as part of primary amyloidosis. Isolated deposits, diffuse tracheal-bronchial infiltration, hilar adenopathy, isolated pulmonary nodules, and diffuse interstitial deposits have all been described.

Gastrointestinal Involvement

All levels of the gastrointestinal tract may be involved by amyloidosis, and GI disease has been described in most of the syndromes. Infiltration of the gingiva and tongue may lead to classic oral manifestations, including massive macroglossia that may interfere with speech, swallowing, or respiration. Upper esophageal deposition can result in swallowing abnormalities, while intestinal disease may cause diarrhea, constipation, malabsorption, hemorrhage, perforation, or ischemia. Liver involvement, either as hepatomegaly, or with biopsy evidence of amyloid deposition, is apparent in most cases of amyloidosis. Liver function tests are usually normal, and the clinical consequence of amyloid deposition in the liver is minimal.

The laboratory features of amyloidosis depend on the type of amyloidosis. In primary amyloidosis, mild anemia is seen in about 10–20% of cases and a majority of patients show a mild to marked elevation of erythrocyte sedimentation rate. As noted previously, all cases of myeloma-associated amyloidosis and 80–90% of cases of primary generalized amyloidosis will show a monoclonal paraprotein when both serum and urine are screened (49,50,52). Forty percent of all patients will have abnormal serum protein electrophoresis, 68% will have abnormalities on immunoelectrophoresis, and 72% will show monoclonal light chains in adequately concentrated urine specimens (50).

The deposition of amyloid material in vital organs gives a characteristic stain. On light microscopy, eosinophilic staining of amorphous deposits may be seen. Most of these deposits have an affinity for staining with congo red. The most useful histologic procedure for detecting amyloid deposits is by examination of a congo red-stained specimen under polarized microscopy. This will produce a characteristic apple green birefringence, which is diagnostic.

Amyloidosis may be diagnosed by demonstrating the typical deposits on biopsy specimens from involved organs. Renal and liver biopsies are often useful, but fatal hemorrhage has been reported after liver biopsy, so this should be done with extreme caution. Rectal biopsy is positive in a majority of patients, and bone marrow, small bowel, skin, or synovial biopsies may be diagnostic. Subcutaneous fat aspiration may be useful (54).

The natural history of amyloidosis depends on the type. Primary generalized amyloidosis is a rapidly fatal condition with a median survival of 12–14 months. Patients presenting with congestive heart failure and orthostatic hypotension appear to have a particularly poor prognosis, while those presenting with carpal tunnel syndrome or peripheral neuropathy may have a better outcome. The most common cause of death is related to cardiac disease, with renal disease next most frequent. Myeloma-associated amyloidosis has an even worse prognosis, with median survival being approximately 5 months. In secondary amyloidosis, the nature of the underlying illness dictates the prognosis. Several cases of recovery from secondary amyloidosis have been noted when the underlying disease is controlled.

There is no specific uniformly effective therapy available for amyloidosis. In patients with primary generalized amyloidosis, the treatment of a presumed underlying plasma cell disorder is usually attempted. Cytotoxic agents, such as melphalan, in combination with prednisone have been used, and have produced temporary remission in some patients.

Colchicine in divided doses of 1.0-1.5 mg/day has been shown to decrease the frequency and severity of acute febrile attacks in familial mediterranean fever (53). Although this is recommended for all patients with this disorder, there is no evidence as yet that this will prevent amyloidosis. Some authors also suggest a trial of colchicine for secondary generalized amyloidosis. Dimethylsulfoxide (DMSO) has been shown to produce disappearance of amyloid deposits in animal models, although no definite efficacy has been shown in humans. Corticosteroids are not indicated unless as part of the therapy of the underlying condition.

Supportive measures, such as mild diuretics for cardiac disease, treatment of malabsorption syndromes with broad spectrum antibiotics, hemodialysis, and occasionally transplantation have been helpful as supportive measures for specific organ problems, although recurrence of amyloidosis in transplanted kidneys has been reported.

Malignancy and Rheumatologic Syndromes

The signs and symptoms of malignancy are not always related to the affected organs. It has been estimated that over one-half of patients with neoplastic disease will have some remote effect not related to the primary tumor or metastases (55). In this section, we will discuss rheumatologic syndromes that result from the direct and remote effects of malignant disease.

Direct Associations

Direct involvement of bone, muscle, and joints by neoplastic cells may cause musculoskeletal symptoms. Bony metastases may be found in all types of neoplasms, but most particularly in lung cancers. These occur almost exclusively in large proximal bones, but small peripheral metastases have been described. In addition, peripheral bony metastases may be associated with an adjacent synovitis, and direct metastases to synovium have been described. Nonpulmonary neoplasms may also be associated with peripheral bony metastases, but less often.

Acute leukemia is frequently associated with pain in the joints and bones. This is particularly true during childhood, where the clinical presentation may be confused with rheumatic fever or juvenile rheumatoid arthritis. Most of these manifestations in leukemia are thought to be due to direct leukemic infiltration of synovial tissue, periarticular bone, and other structures (56). Arthritis in acute leukemia tends to involve large peripheral joints and is often asymmetric and polyarticular. Pain may be severe and seem out of proportion compared to the degree of apparent synovitis. Synovial fluid may show a mild inflammatory response or marked inflammation with several hundred thousand white blood cells; occasionally, leukemic cells are identified. Radiologic evaluation may be normal, but will often show lytic bone lesions, osteoporosis, or periosteal or epiphyseal radiolucency. The arthritis associated with acute leukemia may respond temporarily to salicylates or nonsteroidal antiinflammatory medications.

Chronic leukemia is less often complicated by arthritis. This arthritis may be more frequently asymmetric, and usually occurs later in the disease. Direct leukemic infiltration is thought to be the mechanism of involvement, and radiographic findings are similar to those seen in acute leukemias. Recently, several patients with bone and joint involvement with hairy cell leukemia have been reported (57,58).

Lymphomas usually cause bone pain through direct skeletal involvement, although rarely a true arthritis has been described. Lesions showing mixed osteolysis and osteosclerosis have been shown. Synovial reaction, when it occurs, is usually due to adjacent bone disease.

Indirect Associations

Polymyositis and Dermatomyositis

There has long been noted an association between inflammatory muscle disease and neoplasia. It is estimated that approximately 5-10% of all patients with myositis will have an underlying malignancy, usually involving lung, ovary, stomach, and breast. Neoplasms seem to be more common in those patients that have dermatomyositis, and the frequency seems to be increased in those over the age of 40 and in males. Treatment of the underlying neoplasm may occasionally result in marked improvement of the muscle disease. Further discussion of polymyositis and dermatomyositis can be found in Chapter 16.

Hypertrophic Osteoarthropathy

Hypertrophic osteoarthropathy (HOA) is a clinical syndrome including chronic proliferative periostitis of the long bones, clubbing of the fingers and/or toes, and oligo- or polyarthritis (59). This disorder has been described both in a primary form and associated with a number of underlying diseases (see Table 23.6), but the most frequently seen associations are with pulmonary disease and various types of neoplasm. Virtually any intrapulmonary process can be associated with this syndrome, with the most common causes being bronchogenic carcinoma, bronchiectasis, or lung abscess.

A primary familial form exists, also known as pachydermoperiostosis. In addition, idiopathic and familial forms of clubbing, without the full-blown syndrome of HOA exist. Clubbing of the fingers may also be associated with many other underlying disease processes, without the other characteristic features of HOA (see Table 23.6).

The exact cause and mechanism of this syndrome are unknown. Reversal of the syndrome by vagotomy in certain cases suggests a neurogenic mechanism. Other studies suggest a role for circulating components, such as immune complexes, from the underlying neoplasm. Increased vascularity appears to play a pathogenic role, as do endocrine abnormalities. Nevertheless, exact mechanisms for all this are still unknown.

Symptoms of hypertrophic osteoarthropathy usually begin insidiously and tend to progress more rapidly in secondary forms than in primary forms. Periostitis is manifest by acute or subacute severe deep and burning pain, usually in the extremities. The pain characteristically is worsened by dependent position and relieved by elevation. Because of this, several authors have described unusual attempts to relieve pain, such as elevating the feet above the head or even standing on the head. On examination of these painful areas, warmth, tenderness, and trophic skin changes, such as thickening, perspiration, or erythema may be

TABLE 23.6 Classification of Hypertrophic Osteoarthropathy

- Primary
  - Pachydermoperiostosis
  - Idiopathic
- Secondary
  - Pulmonary disease
    - neoplasm
    - infection - TB, bronchiectasis, abscess
    - other
  - Cardiovascular
    - cyanotic congenital heart disease
  - Gastrointestinal
    - neoplasm
    - hepatic (neoplasm, cirrhosis, primary biliary cirrhosis)
    - inflammatory (infection, Crohn's, ulcerative colitis)
  - Other neoplasm
    - lymphoma, mesothelioma

observed. Clubbing in the fingers and toes rarely causes pain and discomfort, but is usually noticed by the patient. Clinically, there is fluctuance and softening of the nail bed with loss of the normal angle between the nail and cuticle. Fragility of the nail tends to be accentuated and hardening or loosening may follow. In severe forms, the fingers and toes develop a "drumstick" appearance (Figure 23.6). The arthritis of hypertrophic osteoarthropathy is often a symmetrical polyarthritis resembling rheumatoid arthritis. Warmth, tenderness, and swelling may be present in the more symptomatic joints, but other joints may have little or no inflammatory changes. The most frequently involved joints are the knees and ankles with wrists and small joints being next most common. Synovial fluid analysis usually reveals a clear noninflammatory fluid, and this may be helpful in differentiating the syndrome from rheumatoid arthritis.

Most routine laboratory studies are normal, although mild elevations of the erythrocyte sedimentation rate and alkaline phosphatase have been noted in some patients. X-rays of the long bones show periosteal thickening along the shaft, usually in the distal diaphyseal regions (Figure 23.7) (60). Similar findings may be seen in the phalanges as well. On occasion, the periosteal changes may show some separation from the bony cortex. Bone scanning is abnormal in most cases, with increased uptake along the shafts of bone as well as in the affected joints demonstrated. Pathologically, the periosteal reaction represents the formation of new subperiosteal cancellous bone. Synovial histology may be normal, or may resemble that seen in rheumatoid arthritis.

Management of hypertrophic osteoarthropathy begins with treatment of the underlying condition in most cases. Dramatic relief of pain and resolution of symptoms are often reported after removal of the primary tumor or correction of the underlying disease. Vagotomy has been successful in some patients. Aspirin and other nonsteroidal antiinflammatory drugs may be beneficial symptomatically.

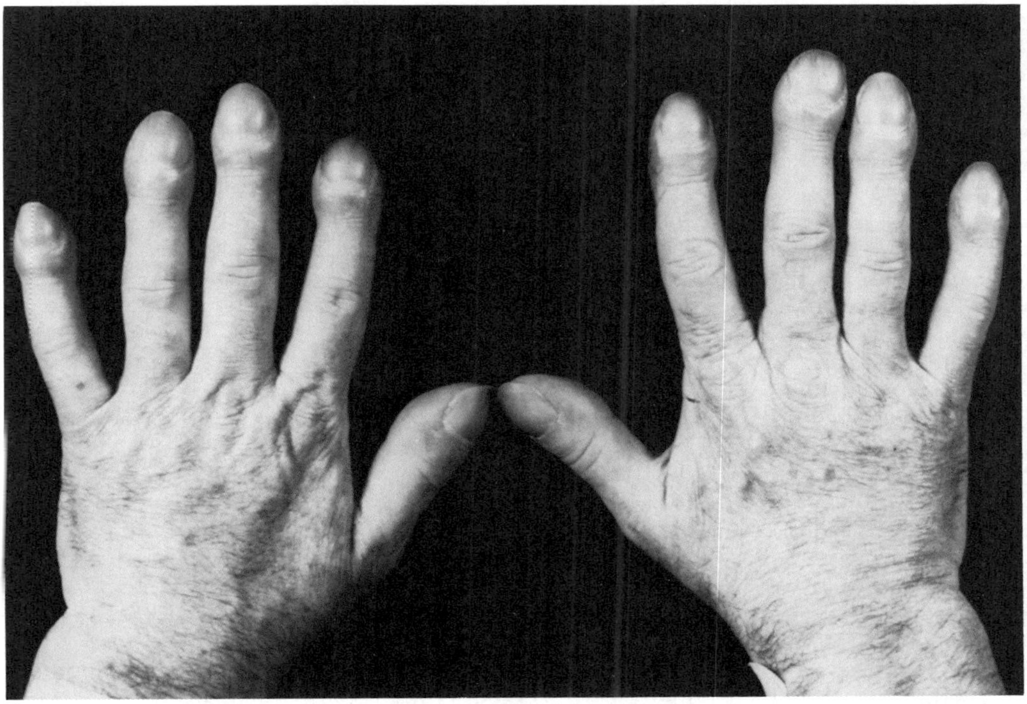

FIGURE 23.6 Classical clubbing of the fingers in a patient with carcinoma of the lung.

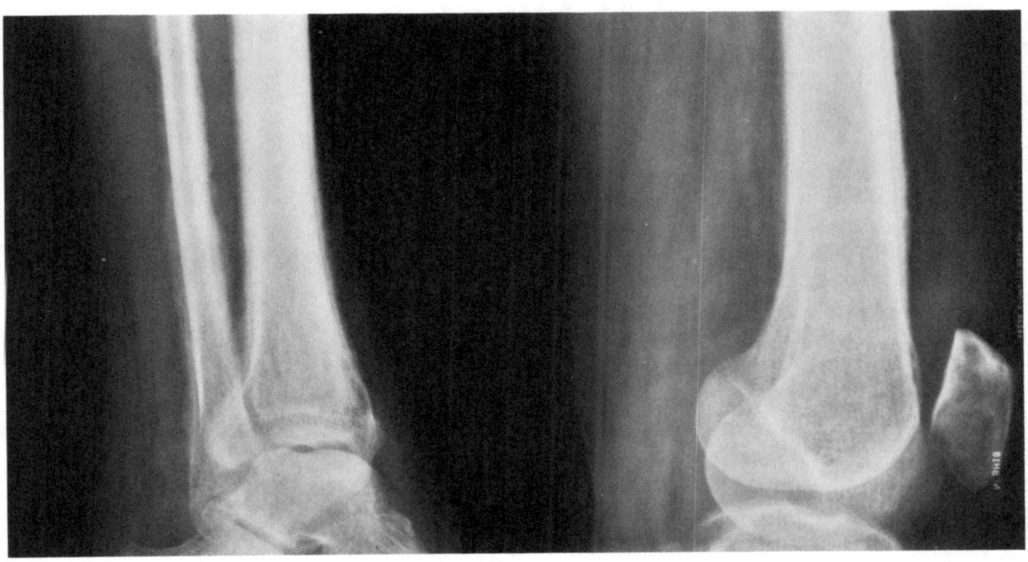

FIGURE 23.7 Typical periosteal thickening (periostitis) of the distal femur and tibia, from a patient with hypertrophic osteoarthropathy associated with carcinoma of the lung.

Carcinoma Polyarthritis

A syndrome of polyarthritis associated with underlying malignancy has been termed carcinoma polyarthritis (61). It is often confused with rheumatoid arthritis. However, carcinoma polyarthritis tends to occur in older individuals and joint involvement is more likely to be asymmetric than in rheumatoid arthritis. The onset may be explosive, and the lower extremities are more often involved. Rheumatoid factor is negative in most cases. Thus, an older individual with an asymmetric, seronegative polyarthritis should be carefully investigated for underlying malignancy. Breast carcinoma appears to be the most frequently associated neoplasm, but lymphomas, gastrointestinal cancer, or any other malignancy may be seen. The pathogenesis of this syndrome is unknown, but autoimmune phenomena related to cross-reactivity with neoplastic tissue have been speculated as a possible mechanism.

Lupus Syndromes

Several patients with underlying malignancy have been reported to develop a characteristic lupus-like syndrome associated with polyarthritis, pleural and pulmonary involvement, and positive antinuclear antibodies. Rarely, such a syndrome may actually preceed the recognition of the neoplasm. In addition, serologic overlap between various malignancies and connective tissue syndromes has been reported. Approximately 10-15% of patients with leukemia and 5% of lymphomas have been reported as having positive tests for antinuclear antibodies (56). The frequency of rheumatoid factors and elevated levels of measurable circulating immune complexes may even be higher.

Vasculitic Syndromes

Several vasculitic syndromes have been described in association with various types of neoplasms (62). Systemic necrotizing vasculitis (polyarteritis nodosa) has been described in several patients with hairy cell leukemia, and is often associated with arthralgias and arthritis (63). Other vasculitic syndromes have been described in patients with lymphomas or other sarcomas. Granulomatous vasculitis has been reported with Hodgkin's disease, and hypersensitivity vasculitis has been seen with a large variety of neoplasms, including Hodgkin's disease, other lymphomas, multiple myeloma, and carcinoma.

Other Associations

A wide variety of other rheumatologic syndromes have been described in small number of patients with underlying malignancies. Reflex sympathetic dystrophy has been seen, not only in central nervous system and pulmonary tumors, but also with intraabdominal neoplasms. Sclerodermatous syndromes have been described, particularly with adenocarcinomas and carcinoid tumors. Polymyalgia rheumatica has rarely been associated with malignancy, and more often is confused diagnostically. Panniculitis and subcutaneous fat necrosis are occasionally found in patients with pancreatic carcinoma.

References

Endocrinopathies

1. Bluestone R: Arthropathies associated with endocrine disorders. In WN Kelley, ED Harris, S Ruddy, CB Sledge (eds.), *A Textbook of Rheumatology.* Philadelphia, W.B. Saunders, 1981, pp. 1622-1636.

2. Persellin RH, Rutstein JE: Rheumatic aspects of endocrinopathies. In DJ McCarty (ed.), *Arthritis and Allied Conditions,* 9th Ed. Philadelphia, Lea and Febiger, 1979, pp. 1318-1334.

3. Bluestone R, Bywaters EGL, Hartog M, Holt PJL, Hyde S: Acromegalic arthrography. *Ann Rheum Dis* 30:243-258, 1971.

4. Dorwart BB, Schumacher HR: Joint effusions, chondrocalcinosis and other rheumatic manifestations in hypothyroidism. A clinicopathologic study. *Am J Med* 59:780-790, 1975.

5. Bland JH, Frymoyer JW: Rheumatic syndromes of myxedema. *N Engl J Med* 282:1171-1174, 1970.

6. Becker KL, Ferguson RH, McConahey WM: The connective-tissue diseases and symptoms associated with Hashimoto's thyroiditis. *N Engl J Med* 268: 277-280, 1963.

7. Ford PM: Thyroid acropachy. *Proc R Soc Med* 63:284-285, 1970.

8. Gray RG, Gottlieb NL: Rheumatic disorders associated with diabetes mellitus: Literature review. *Semin Arthritis Rheum* 6:19-34, 1976.

9. Clouse ME, Gramm HF, Legg M, Flood T: Diabetic osteoarthropathy: Clinical and roentgenographic observations in 90 cases. *Am J Roentgenol Radium Ther Nucl Med* 121:22-34, 1974.

10. Rodnan GP, Schumacher HR: *Primer on the Rheumatic Diseases.* Atlanta, Arthritis Foundation, 1983, pp. 108-110.

11. Grgic A, Rosenbloom AL, Weber FT, Giordano B, Malone JI, Shuster JJ: Joint contracture - Common manifestation of childhood diabetes mellitus. *J Pediatr* 88:584-588, 1976.

Hemoglobinopathies

12. Ball GV, Sorensen LB: The pathogenesis of hyperuricemia and gout in sickle cell anemia. *Arthritis Rheum* 13:846-848, 1970.

13. Schumacher HR: Arthritis associated with sickle cell disease and other hemoglobulinopathies. In WN Kelley, ED Harris, S Ruddy, CB Sledge (eds.), *A Textbook of Rheumatology.* Philadelphia, W.B. Saunders, 1981, pp. 1614-1621.

14. Rodnan GP: Arthropathies associated with hematologic disorders, storage, storage diseases and dysproteinemias. In DJ McCarty (ed.), *Arthritis and Allied Conditions,* 9th Ed. Philadelphia, Lea and Febiger, 1979, pp. 925-952.

15. Barrett-Conner E: Bacterial infection and sickle cell anemia: An analysis of 250 infections in 166 patients and a review of the literature. *Medicine* 50:97-112, 1971.

16. Schumacher HR, Andrews R, McLaughlin G: Arthropathy in sickle cell disease. *Ann Intern Med* 78:203-211, 1973.

17. Gratwick GM, Bullough PG, Bohne WHO, Markenson AL, Peterson CM: Thalassemic osteoarthropathy. *Ann Intern Med* 88:494-501, 1978.

Sarcoidosis

18. Spilberg I, Siltzbach LE, Mc Ewen CE: The arthritis of sarcoidosis. *Arthritis Rheum* 12:126-137, 1969.

19. Arnold WJ: The rheumatic manifestations of sarcoidosis. In WN Kelley, ED Harris, S Ruddy, CB Sledge (eds.), *A Textbook of Rheumatology.* Philadelphia, W.B. Saunders, 1981, pp. 1531-1537.

20. Bjarnason DF, Forrester DM, Swezey RL: Destructive arthritis of the large joints: A rare manifestation of sarcoidosis. *J Bone Joint Surg* 55: 618-622, 1973.

21. Siltzbach LE, Duberstein JL: Arthritis in sarcoidosis. *Clin Orthop Rel Res* 57:31-50, 1968.

22. Sokoloff L, Bunim JJ: Clinical and pathological studies of joint involvement in sarcoidosis. *N Engl J Med* 260:841-847, 1959.

23. Brewerton DA, Cockburn C, James DC, James DG, Neville E: HLA antigens in sarcoidosis. *Clin Exp Immunol* 27:227-229, 1977.

24. Kaplan H: Further experience with colchicine in the treatment of sarcoid arthritis. *N Engl J Med* 268:761-764, 1963.

25. Neville E, Carstairs LS, James DG: Bone sarcoidosis. *Ann NY Acad Sci* 278:475-487, 1976.

Hyperlipoproteinemia

26. Khachadurian AK: Migratory polyarthritis in familial hypercholesterolemia (type II hyperlipoproteinemia). *Arthritis Rheum* 11:385-393, 1968.

27. Glueck CJ, Levy RI, Fredrickson DS: Acute tendinitis and arthritis. A presenting symptom of familial type II hyperlipoproteinemia. *JAMA* 206: 2895-2897, 1968.

28. Bole GG: Arthritis associated with hyperlipidemia and hypercholesterolemia. In WN Kelley, ED Harris, S Ruddy, CB Sledge (eds.), *A Textbook of Rheumatology.* Philadelphia, W.B. Saunders, 1981, pp. 1638-1646.

29. Shapiro JR, Fallat RW, Tsand RC, Glueck CJ: Achilles tendinitis and tenosynovitis. A diagnostic manifestation of familial type II hyperlipoproteinemia in children. *Am J Dis Child* 128:486-490, 1974.

30. Buckingham R, Bole GG, Bassett DR: Polyarthritis associated with type IV hyperlipoproteinemia. *Arch Intern Med* 135:286-290, 1975.

Hemophilia

31. Rodnan GP: Arthritis associated with hematologic disorders, storage diseases and dysproteinemia. In DJ McCarty (ed.), *Arthritis and Allied Conditions,* 9th Ed. Philadelphia, Lea and Febiger, 1979, pp. 925-952.

32. Mainardi CL, Levine PH: Hemophilia and arthritis. In WN Kelley, ED Harris, S Ruddy, CB Sledge (eds.), *A Textbook of Rheumatology,* 1st Ed. Philadelphia, W.B. Saunders, 1981, pp. 1605-1613.

33. Duthie RB, Rizza CR: Rheumatological manifestations of the haemophilias. *Clin Rheum Dis* 1:53-93, 1975.

34. Wild JH, Zvaifler NJ: Hemarthrosis associated with sodium warfarin therapy. *Arthritis Rheum* 19:98-102, 1976.

35. Siame JL, DuQuesnoy B, Theuenon A et al.: Hemarthrosis and thrombocythemia. *J Rheumatol* 8:521-522, 1981.

36. Klofkorn RW, Lightsey AL: Hemarthrosis associated with Glanzmann's thrombasthenia. *Arthritis Rheum* 22:1390-1393, 1979.

37. Isenberg DA, Shoenfeld Y: The rheumatologic complications of hematologic disorders. *Semin Arthritis Rheum* 12:348-358, 1983.

38. Roy S, Ghadially FN: Ultrastructure of synovial membrane in human hemarthrosis. *J Bone Joint Surg* 49A:1636-1646, 1967.

39. Ahlberg A: Hemophilia in Sweden VII. Incidence, treatment and prophylaxis of arthropathy and other musculoskeletal manifestations of hemophilia A and B. *Acta Orthop Scand* 77:5-132, 1965.

Hemochromatosis

40. Fox IH: Arthropathy with iron storage disease. In WN Kelley, ED Harris, S Ruddy, CB Sledge (eds.), *A Textbook of Rheumatology,* 1st Ed. Philadelphia, W.B. Saunders, 1981, pp. 1538-1548.

41. Simon M, Bourel M, Genetet B, Fauchet R: Idiopathic hemochromatosis: Demonstration of recessive transmission and early detection by family HLA typing. *N Engl J Med* 297:1017-1021, 1977.

42. Polycove M: Hemochromatosis. In JB Stanbury, JB Wyngaarden (eds.), *The Metabolic Basis of Inherited Disease,* 4th Ed. New York, McGraw-Hill, 1978, pp.

43. Schumacher HR: Hemochromatosis and arthritis. *Arthritis Rheum* 7:41-50, 1964.

44. Dymock IW, Hamilton EBP, Law JW, Williams R: Arthropathy of hemochromatosis. *Ann Rheum Dis* 29:469-476, 1970.

45. Hamilton E, Williams R, Barlow KA, Smith PM: The arthropathy of idiopathic hemochromatosis. *Quart J Med* 37:171-182, 1967.

46. Askari AD, Muir WA, Rosner IA et al.: Arthritis of hemochromatosis. Clinical spectrum, relation to histocompatability antigens, and effectiveness of early phlebotomy. *Amer Jour Med* 75:957-965, 1983.

47. Rosner IA, Askari AD, McLaren GD, Muir A: Arthropathy, hypouricemia and normal serum iron studies in hereditary hemochromatosis. *Amer Jour Med* 70:870-874, 1981.

48. Schumacher HR: Ultrastructure of the synovial membrane in idiopathic hemochromatosis. *Ann Rheum Dis* 31:465-473, 1972.

Amyloidosis

49. Ignaczak TF: Amyloidosis. In WN Kelley, ED Harris, S Ruddy, CB Sledge (eds.), *A Textbook of Rheumatology,* 1st Ed. Philadelphia, W.B. Saunders, 1981, pp. 1511-1530.

50. Kyle RA, Greipp PR: Amyloidosis (AL). Clinical and laboratory features in 229 cases. *Mayo Clin Proc* 58:665-683, 1983.

51. Wright JR, Calkins E: Clinical-pathologic differentiation of common amyloid syndromes. *Medicine* 60:429-448, 1981.

52. Glenner GG: Amyloid deposits and amyloidosis. *N Engl J Med* 302:1283-1292, 1333-1343, 1980.

53. Meyerhoft J: Familial mediterranean fever: Report of a large family, review of the literature, and discussion of the frequency of amyloidosis. *Medicine* 59:66-77, 1980.

54. Libbey CA, Skinner M, Cohen AS: Use of abdominal fat tissue aspirate in the diagnosis of systemic amyloidosis. *Arch Int Med* 143:1549-1552, 1983.

Malignancy

55. Caldwell DS: Musculoskeletal syndromes associated with malignancy. *Semin Arth Rheum* 10:198-222, 1981.

56. Isenberg DA, Shoenfeld Y: The rheumatologic complications of hematologic disorders. *Semin Arth Rheum* 12:348-358, 1983.

57. Sattar MA, Cawley MID: Arthritis associated with hairy cell leukemia. *Ann Rheum Dis* 4:289-291, 1982.

58. Quesada JR, Keating MJ, Libshitz HI, Llamas L: Bone involvement in hairy cell leukemia. *Amer Jour Med* 74:228-231, 1983.

59. Altman RD, Tenenbaum J: Hypertrophic osteoarthropathy. In WN Kelley, ED Harris, S Ruddy, CB Sledge (eds.), *A Textbook of Rheumatology,* 1st Ed. Philadelphia, W.B. Saunders, 1981, pp. 1647-1657.

60. Schumacher HR: Articular manifestations of hypertrophic pulmonary osteo-arthropathy in bronchogenic carcinoma. *Arthritis Rheum* 19:629-635, 1976.

61. Sheon RP, Kirsner AB, Tangsintanapas P, Samad F, Garg ML, Finkel RI: Malignancy in rheumatic disease. Interrelationships. *J Am Ger Soc* 25: 20-27, 1977.

62. Cupps TR, Fauci AS: *Vasculitis and Neoplasm, The Vasculitides,* Philadelphia, W.B. Saunders, 1981, pp. 116-122.

63. Weinstein A: Editorial. Systemic vasculitis and hairy cell leukemia. *J Rheumatol* 9:349-350, 1982.

INDEX

INDEX

Abdominal pain
in Schölein-Henoch purpura, 548
in SLE, 392
Acetaminophen, in osteoarthritis, 283
Acetic acid derivatives, 134-135
Acetylsalicylic acid, *see* Aspirin
Achilles tendon and tendonitis, 27, 301
378, 379, 642
Acromegalic arthropathy, 270, 635-637
Acromioclavicular joint, 16, 356
Acromionectomy, 218
Acute arthritis, 30-32
Acute phase proteins, 39-41
Adhesive capsulitis, 355-356
Adson test, 13, 357
Alcohol
in gout, 327, 333
myopathy from 467
Alkaptonuria, 568
Allergic granulomatosis and angitis,
498-500
asthma in, 499
diagnosis, 499
eosinophilia in, 499
management, 449
pathology, 498
Allopurinol, 146-148, 332-333
Alopecia, 391
Amphotericin B for fungal arthritis, 607
Amyloidosis, 648-654
classification of, 649
diagnosis, 653
familial, 651
laboratory in, 653
myeloma associated, 650
primary, 650
secondary, 649, 650
senile, 651
treatment, 654
Amyotrophic lateral sclerosis, 468
ANA, *see* Antinuclear antibodies
Anemia, autoimmune hemolytic, *see* Hemolytic anemia
Aneurysmal bone cyst, 619
Ankle and subtalar joint, 26-27, 377-378
bracing, 224
in rheumatoid arthritis, 242
surgery, 224
Ankylosing hyperostosis, *see* Diffuse idiopathic skeletal hyperostosis (DISH)
Ankylosing spondylitis, 287-299
cardiac complications, 294
cauda equina syndrome in, 295
clinical presentation, 289
diagnosis, 290-293
in enteropathic arthritis, 314
epidemiology, 288
etiology, 288
eye disease in, 295
hip involvement in, 293
historical aspects, 287-288
HLA-B27 in, 288, 289, 290
IgA nephropathy in, 295
juvenile onset, 295, 530, 537-538
Klebsiella in, 288
laboratory features, 296
management, 298-299
natural history, 298
pathology, 296-297
peripheral arthritis in, 293-294
pharmacotherapy, 299
in psoriasis, 311
pulmonary involvement, 294
radiology in, 80, 89, 90, 91, 93, 108-110,
297-298
secondary, 292-293
spinal fractures in, 293
spondylodiscitis in, 293
surgery in, 217, 299
in women, 295
Anserine bursa, 26, 374
Anterior compartment syndrome, lower
leg, 376
Anterior uveitis, *see* Uveitis
Anticentromere antibody in PSS, 430
Anticonvulsant drugs
drug induced SLE from, 402
osteopenia from, 581-584

Antimalarial drugs, 139-140, 256, 407, 490, 535
myopathy from, 467
Antinuclear antibodies (ANA), 43-48, 405, 430-431, 452, 468, 529, 532
patterns and disease associations, 46
Anti-seizure drugs, *see* Anticonvulsant drugs
Aortitis
in ankylosing spondylitis, 294
in Reiter's syndrome, 305
Apatite crystal deposition, *see* Hydroxy-apatite deposition disease
Arachidonic acid, metabolism, 126-127
role in rheumatoid arthritis, 239
Arachnodactyly in Marfan's syndrome, 28
Arthritis mutilans, 310
Arthrocentesis, 33-34
Arthrodesis, 216
of ankle, 224
of hip, 223
of knee, 223
Arthroplasty, 215
hip, 223
infection after, 217
in JRA, 534
knee, 224-225
Arthroscopy, 215
Articular cartilage, biology of, 265
Aschoff body in rheumatic fever, 556
Aseptic necrosis of bone, *see* Avascular necrosis
Aspirin, 125-130, 253, 535, 557
enteric coated, 130
hypersensitivity, 127
pharmacology of, 125-126
toxicity, 127-129
Assistive devices in arthritis, 168-171
Atlas, 13
Atlantoaxial joint involvement, 79, 84
in rheumatoid arthritis, 241
surgery, 226, 227
Auranofin, 141
Aurothioglucose, *see* Gold compounds
Avascular necrosis of bone, 111, 113, 388, 641
Axial arthritis, differential diagnosis of, 31, 33
Axis, 13
Azathioprine, 142, 256, 307, 313, 407-408, 473, 497

Back pain, 14-16, 366-370
in ankylosing spondylitis, 289
management of, 366-367
Bacterial arthritis, 591-602
after arthroplasty, 217
in children, 600-602
laboratory, 592
management of, 595-596
pathogenesis, 592
radiology of, 61, 593
in sickle cell disease, 640
synovial fluid in, 38, 593

Balanitis, *see* Circinate balanitis
Baker's cyst, 26
Bamboo spine in ankylosing spondylitis, 290
Bechterew disease, *see* Ankylosing spondylitis
Bechet's disease, 512-515
diagnosis, 515
epidemiology, 513
genital ulcers in, 514
management, 515
oral ulcers in, 514
pathology, 514
skin lesions in, 514
uveitis in, 514
Benoxaprofen, 133
Biceps tendon, 16, 355
Biliary cirrhosis, relationship to PSS, 416
Bleomycin-induced fibrosis, scleroderma and, 435
Bone cysts, 619
Bone infarction in sickle cell disease, 641
Bone remodeling and metabolism, 570-571
Bone disease, metabolic, 570-589
Bone scan in reflex sympathetic dystrophy, 343
Bone tumors, 613-628
benign, 614-621
malignant, 621-628
Bouchard's nodes, 23, 271, 274
Boutonniere deformity in rheumatoid arthritis, 23
Bracking, ankle, 224
Buerger's disease, *see* Thromboangiitis obliterans
Bulge sign, 26
Bursitis, 341, 355, 358-359, 374
infectious, 358-359
Butterfly rash in SLE, 388, 390
Bypass surgery for obesity, ârthritis following, 315

C-reactive protein (CRP), 40-41
Caisson disease, *see* Avascular necrosis of bone
Calcific periarthritis, apatite crystals in, 335
Calcific tendonitis of shoulder, 353
Calcinosis, 417, 463, 543, 589
Calcitonin, 575, 588
Calcium metabolism and homeostasis, 572-576
Calcium, for osteoporosis, 582
Calcium oxalate deposition, 336
Calcium pyrophosphate dihydrate (CPPD) deposition disease, 333-336
associated diseases, 334
clinical patterns, 333-334
diagnosis, 333, 334
in hemochromatosis, 647
hereditary forms, 334
hyperparathyroidism, 639
hypothyroidism and, 637
management, 335
pharmacotherapy, 335

CPPD (Continued)
radiology in, 69, 95, 96, 97, 123, 335
synovial fluid in, 37-38, 334-335
Campylobacter arthritis, 316, 317
Caplan's syndrome, 245
Carcinoma polyarthritis, 658
Cardiac involvement, *see* specific diseases
Carditis in rheumatic fever, 554
Carotidynia, 351
Carpal tunnel syndrome, 21-22, 244, 362, 637, 638, 652
surgical therapy for, 221
Cartilage, 265
Cauda equina syndrome, 295
Causalgia, *see* Reflex sympathetic dystrophy syndromes
Cervical nerve root syndromes, 352, 353
Cervical spine
examination of, 13
in juvenile rheumatoid arthritis, 533
in osteoarthritis, 275-276
in rheumatoid arthritis, 241
surgery, 226-227
Cervical strain, 351-352
Cervical traction, 352
Charcot joints, *see* Neuropathic arthropathy
Chemonucleolysis for lumbar disc herniation, 368
Chest wall pain syndromes, 364-365
CH50, *see* complement
Childhood, rheumatic diseases of, 522-561
Chlamydia in Reiter's syndrome, 300
Chlorambucil, 407-408
Chloroquine, *see* Antimalarial drugs
Cholesterol crystals, in synovial fluid, 38, 336
Choline magnesium salicylate, 128, 130, 253
Chondroblastoma, 620
Chondrocalcinosis, 93, 270, *see also* Caldium pyrophosphate dihydrate (CPPD) deposition disease
Chondroitin sulfate, 265
Chondromalacia patellae, 26, 263, 373
Chondromyxoid fibroma, 620
Chondromatosis, synovial, 630-631
Chondrosarcoma, 623
Chordoma of bone, 628
Chorea, 554
Chrysotherapy, *see* Gold compounds
Churg-Strauss vasculitis, *see* Allergic granulomatosis and angiitis
Chymopapain injection, *see* Chemonucleolysis
Circinate balanitis in Reiter's syndrome, 302, 304
Circulating immune complexes, 50-53
Cirrhosis, primary biliary, 416
Clubbing, 655, 657
Coccygodynia, 372
Codman's tumor, 620
Colchicine, 146, 331, 335, 642, 654
Collagen, metabolism of, 562-565
Complement, measurement of, 48-50, 405, 488
Complement deficiencies, inheritied, 399, 401
Compression fractures, vertebral, 369
Congenital heart block, in SLE offspring, 393
Conjunctivitis in Reiter's syndrome, 302
Corticosteroids, 137-138
in JRA, 535
in MCTD, 490
myopathy from, 467
in polymyositis, 472
in rheumatic fever, 557
in rheumatoid arthritis, 254-255
in SLE, 407
in Sjögren's syndrome, 445
in vasculitis syndromes, 497, 499, 504, 506, 510-511, 512, 515
Cranial arteritis, *see* Giant cell arteritis
CREST syndrome, *see* Progressive systemic sclerosis
Crithidia luciliae assay for antibodies to DNA, 48
Crohn's disease, arthritis in, 313, 315, 317-318
Cryoglobulinemia, *see* Mixed cryoglobulinemia
Crystal-induced synovitis, 323-338
synovial fluid in, 38
Cushing's syndrome, myopathy in, 467
osteoporosis in, 580
Cutaneous vasculitis, *see* Hypersensitivity angiitis
Cutis laxa, 566
Cyclooxygenase, inhibition by NSAIDs, 126-127
Cyclophosphamide, 142, 407-408, 473, 497, 502
Cytoplasmic staining (on ANA testing), 45, 46
Cytotoxic drugs, *see* Specific drugs, Azathioprine; Cyclophosphamide; Chlorambucil; Methotrexate

Dactylitis in Reiter's syndrome, 302
Deformity, 11
Degenerative joint disease, *see* Osteoarthritis
deQuervain's tenosynovitis, 22, 360
Depression, 158
Dermatomyositis (DM), *see* Polymyositis
Diabetes mellitus rheumatic manifestations of, 639
adhesive capsulitis and, 356, 639
amyotrophy in, 467
osteoporosis in, 580
Diet in arthritis, *see* Nutrition
Diffuse idiopathic skeletal hyperostosis (DISH), 263, 277, 280, 290
Diflunisal, 131, 253
Dimethyl sulfoxide, 142, 654
Diphenylhydantoin, 402, 581, 584

Diphosphonates in Paget's disease, 588
Discharge planning, 164
Discoid lupus erythematosis (DLE), 388, 391
Disseminated gonoccal infection (DGI), 593, 595-599
  diagnosis, 597-599
  management of, 599
  pathogenesis, 598
  skin lesions in, 597, 598
  synovial fluid in, 38
DNA, native, antibodies to, in SLE, 47-48, 405
D-penicillamine, 141, 255, 440
  myopathy from, 467
"Drawer" test, 26
"Drop arm" sign for rotator cuff tear, 354
Drug-induced lupus, 399, 402, 403
Dupuytren's contracture, 22, 361-362, 639
Dysentery, arthritis and, *see* Enteropathic arthritis

Effusions, radiology of, 56, 71
Ehlers-Danlos syndrome, 28, 565-567, 569
Elastin, 568-569
Elbow, 18, 357-359
  in rheumatoid arthritis, 241
  surgery of, 219
Electromyography, 342, 469
Enchondroma, 617-618
Endocrine diseases, rheumatic manifestations, 635-639
Energy conservation, in managing arthritis, 171-172
Enteropathic arthritis, 313-317
  juvenile onset, 538
  peripheral arthritis in, 314
  radiology of, 90, 91
  spondylitis in, 314
Enthesopathy, 294
  radiology, 93-94
Entrapment neuropathies, *see* Nerve entrapment syndromes
Eosinophilic faciitis, 413, 434
  aplastic anemia in, 435
Eosinophilic myositis, 468
Epicondylitis, 18, 20, 357-358
Epimyoepithelial islands, in Sjögren's syndrome, 453
Epstein-Barr virus (EBV) and rheumatoid arthritis, 238
Erosions, radiology of, 56-81
Erosive osteoarthritis, 263, 272
Erythema chronicum migrans in Lyme arthritis, 604
Erythema marginatum in rheumatic fever, 555
Erythema nodosum
  in Behcet's disease, 514
  in sarcoidosis, 641

Erythrocyte sedimentation rate (ESR), 39-40
Esophageal hypomotility in PSS, 424-425, 429
Essential mixed cryglobulinemia, 506
Etidronate in Paget's disease, 588
Ewing's sarcoma, 624-625
Examination for musculoskeletal disease, 9-29
Exercise therapy, 173-174, 298
  for back pain, 366-368
Extractable nuclear antigen (ENA), 47

Fabere test, 25
Familial hypophosphatemic rickets, 585
Familial Mediterranean fever, 651, 654
Family history, 9
Fascia lata syndrome, 372
Fatigue, 158
Felty's syndrome in rheumatoid arthritis, 245, 529
Femoral epiphysis, slipped capital, 572
Fenamic acid derivatives, 137
Fenoprofen, 132-133, 254
Fibroma, 615-616
  ossifying, 617
Fibromyalgia, *see* Fibrositis
Fibrosarcoma of bone, 625
Fibrositis, 28, 182-183, 201, 343-350
  clinical features, 345
  diagnosis, 346-348
  epidemiology, 343
  hypothyroidism and, 637
  laboratory in, 348
  management, 349-350
  natural history, 349
  personality in, 344
  primary, 343
  pharmacotherapy, 350
  psychological aspects, 344, 350
  secondary, 343
  sleep disturbance in, 344
  trigger points in, 345-347
Fibrous dysplasia, 588, 616-617
Finkelstein test, 22, 360
Flat foot, 380
Flexion exercises for back pain, 366-368, 369
Focal nodular myositis, 468
Foot, 26-28, 379-381
  in rheumatoid arthritis, 242
  surgery, 225-226
Forestier's disease, *see* Diffuse idiopathic skeletal hyperostosis
Frozen shoulder, *see* Adhesive capsulitis
Functional disability, assessment of, 184-188
Fungal arthritis, 607
Fusion of joints, *see* Arthrodesis

Gallium scan, in PSS pulmonary disease, 426
Ganglion cysts, 21, 362-363, 631-632
Garrod, description of rheumatoid arthritis, 237

Genital ulcers in Behcet's disease, 514
Genu, varus, 26
    recurrent, 26
    valgus, 26
Giant cell arteritis, 507-511
    diagnosis, 510
    epidemiology, 507
    headache in, 508
    jaw claudication in, 509
    laboratory in, 509
    management, 510-511
    pathology of, 507-508
    polymyalgia rheumatica in, 509-510
    visual manifestations, 508
Giant cell tumors of bone, 627-628
Glenohumeral joint, 16, 356
Glomerulonephritis in SLE, 394-396
Glucocorticoids, *see* Corticosteroids
Glucose-6-phosphatase deficiency, 330
Gold compounds, 140-141, 255
    in JRA, 535
    in psoriatic arthritis, 313
Golfer's elbow, 20, 357
Gonococcal arthritis, *see* Disseminated gonococcal infection
Gottron's papules, in dermatomyositis, 461
Gout, 38 323-333
    acute arthritis in, 323
    alcohol consumption in, 327, 333
    diagnosis, 329, 330
    epidemiology, 324-326
    fever in, 324
    historical aspects, 323-324
    hyperparathyroidism and, 639
    hyperuricemia in, 324-325, 330
    laboratory features, 330
    management, 331-333
    obesity in, 327, 333
    pathologic findings, 331
    pharmacotherapy of, 144-148, 331-333
    podagra, 324
    prognosis, 331
    and pseudogout, 327-334
    radiology of, 62, 78, 121-122, 331
    renal disease in, 328
    synovial fluid in, 329, 330
    tophaceous, 327-329
Graft-versus-host disease, 413
Gram-negative bacilli, infectious arthritis from, 594
Granulomatous myositis, 468
Granulomatous vasculitis, *see* Wegener's granulomatosis
Graves' disease, 638
Grip strength assessment, 12, 22

Hallux rigidus, 380
Hallux valgus, 380
Hammer toe, 380
Hand, 20-23
    in osteoarthritis, 273-274
Hand (Continued)
    in rheumatoid arthritis, 240
    surgery of, 221-222
Hashimoto's thyroiditis, 416, 484, 637
HbsAg, *see* Hepatitis B virus surface antigen
Heart block in neonatal SLE, 393
Heat, local therapy, 174
Heberden's nodes, 23, 271, 274
Heliotrope rash in dermatomyositis, 461-462
Hemangioma of bone and joints, 619, 631
Hemarthrosis, 37, 645
Hemochromatosis, 270, 334, 646-648
Hemodialysis, chronic, arthropathy in, 336
Hemoglobinopathies, arthritis in, 640-644
Hemolytic anemia in SLE, 404
Hemophilic arthropathy, 645-646
    psychological intervention in, 196
Hemosiderosis, 647
Henoch-Schönlein purpura, 504-505, 548-550
Hepatitis associated with arthritis, 602-603
Hepatitis B virus surface antigens
    in mixed cryglobulinemia, 506
    in polyarteritis nodosa, 498
Heredofamilial amyloidosis, 651
Heritable disorders of connective tissue, 562-569
Hidradenitis suppuritiva, and arthritis, 311
Hip, 23-25, 370-373
    in ankylosing spondylitis, 293
    in osteoarthritis, 274-275
    in rheumatoid arthritis, 241
    surgery of, 222
History taking, 5-9
HLA antigens, 54-56, 288-289, 300, 307, 387, 446, 507, 532
Hoffman procedure, 226
Homogenous pattern ANA, 44, 46
Homocystinuria, 568
Hydralazine-induced lupus, 399
Hydroxyapatite deposition, 335-336, 639
Hydroxychloroquine, *see* Antimalarial drugs
Hyperlipidemia, *see* Hyperlipoproteinemia
Hyperlipoproteinemias, arthritis in, 642-644
Hypermobility of joints, 28, 239, 272
Hyperparathyroidism, 334, 579, 639
Hypersensitivity angiitis, 503-506
    cutaneous manifestations, 504
    diagnosis, 504
    management, 504
    pathogenesis, 503
    pathology, 503
    subgroups, 504-506
Hyperthryoidism, 638
    myopathy in, 467
    osteoporosis in, 579
Hypertrophic osteoarthropathy (HOA), 655-657
Hyperuricemia, 311, 324-327, 330
    in sickle cell disease, 640
Hypocomplementemia, 50, 405
Hypocomplementemic vasculitis, 505

Hypogonadism, osteoporosis in, 579
Hypokalemia, myopathy in, 467
Hypomagnesemia, myopathy in, 467
Hypopituitarism, osteoporosis in, 579
Hypothyroidism, 334, 348, 637-638
    myopathy in, 467, 637
Hypoxanthine-guanine-phosphoribosyl transferase deficiency, 330

Ibuprofen, 131-133, 254
Ice, local therapy, 174
Iliopectineal bursa, 23, 372
Iliotibial band syndrome, 375
Immune complexes
    in MCTD, 488
    in polyarteritis nodosa, 495
    in SLE, 387
    testing for, 50-53
Immunomodulating agents in rheumatoid arthritis, 138, 142
Immunosuppressive drugs, 141-142, *see also,* Azathioprine; Chlorambucil; Cyclophosphamide; Methotrexate
Indoles, 134-135
Indomathacin, 134-135, 254, 307, 332
    toxicity from, 135, 332
Infectious arthritis, 591-607, *see also,* Bacterial; Viral; Tuberculous; Fungal arthritis
    in children, 600-602
Infectious bursitis, 358-359
Infectious myositis, 465-467
Inflammatory bowel disease, *see* Entero-pathic arthritis arthropathy
Infrapatellar bursitis, 374
Infrapatellar tendonitis, 374
Intestinal bypass arthritis, 315, 317
Intestinal diseases associated arthritis, *see* Enteropathic arthritis
Intraarticular injection, 33-34
Iridocyclitis, *see* Uveitis
Ischiogluteal bursa, 23, 373
Isoniazid-induced SLE, 403
Ixodes dammini, Lyme disease and, 605-605

Jaccoud's syndrome, 115, 554
Jo-1 antigen, antibodies in polymyositis, 468
Joint
    classification of, 9
    examination, 9-29
Joint protection, principles of, 168-169
Joint replacement, *see* Arthroplasty
Joints, tumors of, 629-633
    benign, 629-632
    malignant, 632-633
Jones criteria in diagnosis of rheumatic fever, 553-555
JRA, *see* Juvenile rheumatoid arthritis
Jumper's knee, 374
Juvenile rheumatoid arthritis, 522-536
    antinuclear antibodies in, 529, 532
    diagnosis, 523, 530, 532
    epidemiology, 523
    etiology, 523
Juvenile rheumatoid arthritis (Continued)
    fever in, 523, 527
    growth failure in, 523
    laboratory in, 532
    management, 534-536
    pathogenesis, 523
    pathology of, 526, 534
    pauciarticular, 529-530
    pharmacotherapy of, 127, 135, 143, 535-536
    polyarticular, 528-529
    prognosis, 534
    psychosocial effects, 182, 184, 188
    radiology of, 65, 87, 88, 533
    rheumatoid factor in, 529, 532
    subgroups, 524-526
    surgery in, 534
    synovial fluid in, 534
    systemic onset of, 524-527
    uveitis in, 529-530, 535

Kawasaki disease, 551-552
Keller procedure, 226
Keratan sulfate, 265
Keratodermia blenorrhagica, 302-303
Keratoconjunctivitis sicca, 447
Klebsiella in ankylosing spondylitis, 288
Knee, 25-26, 373-375
    in osteoarthritis, 274
    in rheumatoid arthritis, 242
    surgery, 223-225

La antigen antibodies to, *see* SSB
Laminectomy, 368
Latex fixation test, *see* rheumatoid factor
LE cell phenomenon, 43, 386
Lead intoxication, hyperuricemia and, 327
Leg cramp, 376
Leg pain, 375-377
Lesch-Nyhan syndrome, 324, 327
Leukemia arthritis and, 654
    hairy cell and vasculitis, 658
Leukopenia in SLE, 404
Leukotrienes, 128
Levamisole, 142
Libman-Sacks endocarditis in SLE, 393
Ligament strains and sprains, 341
Lipoma, synovial, 631
Lipoxygenase, role in aspirin sensitivity, 128
Livedo reticularis, 496
Liver disease in rheumatoid arthritis, 246
Liver toxicity
    from indomethacin, 135
    from salicylates, 129, 535
Löfgren's syndrome, 641
Low back pain, *see* Back pain
Lumbar disc disease, 367, 368
Lumpar spine in osteoarthritis, 276-279
Lumbar stenosis, 277, 278, 369
Lumbrosacral strain, 366-367
Lupus, see Discoid lupus erythematosus; drug induced lupus; Systemic lupus erythematosus
Lupus anticoagulant, 404
Lupus band test, 406

Lyme arthritis, 604-605
Lymphadenopathy in rheumatoid arthritis, 246, 250
Lymphoid irradiation, 256
Lymphoma
in bone, 627
in Sjögren's syndrome, 451, 455

Macroglossia in amyloidosis, 653
Magnesium salicylate, 253
Malignancy, rheumatologic syndromes and, 654-658
Malignant fibrous histiocytoma, 625
Marfan's syndrome, 28, 568, 569
Marie-Strumpell's disease, see Ankylosing spondylitis
MCTD, see Mixed connective tissue disease
Meclofenamate, 137, 254
Mefenamic acid, 137
Melorheostosis, 434
Meningococcal arthritis, 599
Meniscus, 25
cyst of, 632
Menke's syndrome, 568
Meralgia paresthetica, 373
Metabolic bone disease, 576-589
Metatarsalgia, 28, 379
Methotrexate, 141, 307, 313, 473, 497
"Milwaukee shoulder," 336, 356
Mixed connective tissue disease (MCTD), 115, 399, 413, 477-493
antinuclear antibodies in, 485
arthritis in, 482, 490
cardiac involvement, 484, 490
diagnosis, 479-480, 485
epidemiology, 480
esophageal manifestations, 483, 491
gastrointestinal manifestations, 483, 489
immunologic abnormalities in, 478
juvenile onset, 542
laboratory findings in, 485-486
management, 489-491
myositis in, 463, 482-483, 490
neurologic manifestations, 484, 491
pathogenesis, 478
pharmacotherapy, 489-491
prognosis, 489
pulmonary disease in, 481, 483-489, 490
radiology in, 488-489
Raynaud's phenomenon in, 481, 482, 490
renal disease in, 484
telangectasia in, 482
Mixed cryoglobulinemia, 506
Monoarthritis, differential diagnosis of, 30, 31
Mononeuritis multiplex in polyarteritis nodosa, 496
Monosodium urate crystals in gout, 38, 327, 330
Morning stiffness, 7
Morton's neuroma, 28, 379, 381
Mucin clot test, 38
Mucocutaneous lymph node, *see* Kawasaki's disease
Multiple myeloma, amyloidosis associated with, 650
Multipurpose arthritis centera (MAC's), 154
Muscle function, assessment, 11, 12
Muscle involvement, in rheumatoid arthritis, 246
Muscle strain, 341
Muscular dystrophy, similarity to polymyositis, 468
Musculoskeletal complaints, differential diagnosis of, 29, 30
Musculoskeletal examination, 9-29
Myasthenia gravis, 466, 467
Myeloma, plasma cell of bone, 626-627
Mycobacteria arthritis, 606
Myocarditis
in rheumatoid arthritis, 245
in SLE, 392
Myopathy, drug induced, 467
Myxedema, *see* Hypothyroidism

Nail involvement
in psoriatic arthritis, 307-308
in Rieter's syndrome, 302
Nailfold changes in PSS, 431, 434
Naproxen, 132, 133, 535
Native DNA, antibodies to in SLE, 47, 48, 405
Neck pain, 351-352
Necrotizing arteritis, *see* Polyarteritis nodosa
Necrotizing vasculitis, *see* Polyarteritis nodosa
Neisseria gonorrhoeae, infectious arthritis from, *see* Disseminated gonococcal infections
Neonatal systemic lupus erythematosus, 393
Neoplasms
of bone and joints, 611-634
classification, 611-613
Nephritis, *see* Glomerulonephritis
Nephrolithiasis in gout, 328
Nerve conduction tests, 342
Nerve entrapment syndromes, 341, 359, 373, 380-381
Neuropathic arthropathies, 269, 273, 334
in diabetes, 639, 640
New Zealand mice, model for SLE, 387
Nonacetylated salicylates, *see* Salicylates
Nonadherance, 190, 201-202
Nonarticular rheumatism, 339-385
Nonsteroidal antiinflammatory drugs (NSAIDs), 125-137, 143-144, 253-254, 283, 307, 312, 332, 335
Nuclear ribonucleoprotein (RNP), 47, 405, 478, 479, 485-487
Nucleolar pattern ANA, 44, 46, 430
Nurse specialist in rheumatology, 154, 156-157

Nutrition, 160-162

Obesity and osteoarthritis, 283
Occupational therapist, role of, 168-172, 283, 534
Ochronosis, 270, 334
Olecranon bursitis, 18, 358, 359
Ollier's disease, 618
Onycholysis, 302, 307-308
Oral contraceptives in SLE, 406
Oral lesions
  in Behcet's disease, 514
  in Reiter's syndrome, 302
  in SLE, 389
Osgood-Schlatter disease, 376
Ossifying fibroma, 617
Osteitis condensans ilii, 291, 370
Osteitis deformans, *see* Paget's disease of bone
Osteitis pubis, 370
Osteoarthritis, 261-286
  aging and, 266
  articular disease, patterns, 271, 273-281
  cartilage changes in, 265-268
  diagnosis, 281
  epidemiology, 261, 264-265
  erosive, 263, 272
  historical aspects, 262
  laboratory features, 281-282
  management of, 282-284
  pathogenesis, 265-270
  pharmacotherapy, 143-144, 283-284
  primary, 262, 263, 271
  prognosis, 282
  radiology of, 70, 116-120, 282
  secondary, 262, 263, 269-270, 272, 273
  surgery in, 284
  synovial changes in, 269
  synovial fluid in, 281
  trauma and, 269, 273
Osteoarthrosis, *see* Osteoarthritis
Osteoblast, 570
Osteoblastoma, benign, 619
Osteochondritis dissecans, 98
Osteochondroma, 614-615
Osteogenesis imperfecta, 28, 565-566
Osteogenic fibroma, 617
Osteogenic sarcoma, 587, 617-623
Osteoid osteoma, 618
Osteomalacia, 583-587
  from anticonvulsant therapy, 584-585
  drug related, 586
  in hypophosphatemia, 585
  therapy, 586
Osteomyelitis in sickle cell disease, 640
Osteonecrosis, 270, 273, 274
Osteopenia, 60, 576
Osteophytes, 88
Osteoporosis, 576, 583
  in Cushing's syndrome, 580
  in diabetes, 580
Osteoporosis (Continued)
  drug related, 581
  in hyperparathyroidism, 579
  in hyperthyroidism, 579
  in hypogonadism, 579
  in hypopituitarism, 579
  involutional, 581
  with immobilization, 581
  nutritional, 580
  postmenopausal, 577-579
  in pregnancy, 580
  treatment of, 582
Osteosarcoma, *see* Osteogenic sarcoma
Osteosclerosis, 588-589
Osteotomy, 215
  of hip, 222
  of knee, 223
Overlap diseases, 477-493
Oxicam derivatives, 137

Paget's disease of bone, 273, 292, 587-588
  osteogenic sarcoma in, 587, 623
Pain, 6, 157-158, 183-184
P-aminobenzoate, in PSS, 440
Pannus formation, 249
Parathyroid hormone (PTH), 572
Parotitis in Sjögren's syndrome, 453
Patient education, 159-160
Patrick test, 24
Pauciarticular onset JRA, 529 -530
Pelligrini-Stieda syndrome, 375
Pelvic girdle pain, *see* Hip
"Pencil-in-cup," 312
Penicillamine, *see* D-Penicillamine
Penicillin
  in Lyme arthritis, 605
  in rheumatic fever, 557
Pentazocine-induced fibrosis, scleroderma and, 512
Periarteritis nodosa, *see* Polyarteritis nodosa
Pericarditis
  in PSS, 426
  in rheumatoid arthritis, 244
  in SLE, 392
Periostitis, 81, 85, 656
Peripheral pattern ANA, 45, 46
Peroneal tendonitis, 378
Personality in rheumatoid arthritis, 179-180
Phalen's sign, 21-22, 362
Phenobarbital, *see* Anticonvulsant drugs
Phenylbutazone, 136, 254, 299, 307, 332
Photosensitivity, 388
Physical examination, joints, 9-29
Physical therapy, 173-175, 283, 534
"Piano-key" sign, 22
Pigmented villonodular synovitis, 629-630
Piroxicam, 137, 254
Plantar fasciitis, 301, 379
Plasmacytoma, malignant of bone, 626
Plasmapheresis, 256, 407, 408, 473
Pleuritis
  in rheumatoid arthritis, 245

Pleuritis (Continued)
in PSS, 425
in SLE, 391
Plica syndrome, knee pain in, 375
PM-1 antigen, antibodies to in polymyositis, 468
Pneumatosis intestinalis, in MCTD, 483
Podagra, 326
Polyarteritis nodosa, 494-498
angiography in, 497-498
arthritis in, 496
cardiac disease, 497
diagnosis, 497
epidemiology, 495
juvenile onset, 550-551
management, 497
neuropathy in, 496
pathogenesis, 495
pathology, 495-496
renal disease in, 497
Polyarthritis, differential diagnosis of, 31
Polyarthritis in carcinoma, 658
Polyarticular onset JRA, 528-529
Polymyalgia rheumatica, 348, 468, 509-510
Polymyositis (PM), 458-476
adult, 460-461
antinuclear antibodies in, 468
arthritis in, 463
aspiration pneumonia, 471
calcinosis in, 463, 543
cardiac disease in, 464
childhood onset, 463, 542-544
dermatomyositis, 461-462, 542-544
diagnosis, 464
electromyography in, 469-470
epidemiology, 458-459
etiology, 459
immunologic abnormalities in, 459-460
juvenile onset, 463, 542-544
laboratory features, 468
malignancy and, 462-463, 655
management, 471-473
in MCTD, 463
muscle enzymes in, 469
pathogenesis, 459
pathology in, 469-472
pharmacotherapy, 472-473
prognosis, 471
in PSS, 428, 463
radiology of, 99, 115
in rheumatoid arthritis, 463
in SLE, 388, 463
in Sjögren's syndrome, 463
toxoplasma and, 460, 467
vascular abnormalities in, 460, 463, 464, 469, 543
viral associations, 460, 465
Porphyria cutanea tarda, and PSS, 435
Popliteal tendonitis, 375
Prednisolone, *see* Corticosteroids
Pregnancy, aspirin during, 129
indomethacin during, 135
in MCTD, 489
in SLE, 398-399
Prepatellar bursa, 26, 374
Primary biliary cirrhosis, 416
Probenecid, 148, 332
Procainamide-induced lupus-like syndrome, 403
Progressive systemic sclerosis, (PSS, scleroderma, 411-444
animal models, 420
antinuclear antibodies in, 430-431
articular disease in, 429-430, 440
bleomycin-induced, 435
calcinosis in, 417
cardiac involvement, 426-427, 432, 439
cellular immunity in, 418
classification, 412-413
colon involvement in, 427
CREST syndrome, 414
diagnosis, 414-415, 433-434
diffuse, 414
eosinophilic fasciitis, 413, 434
epidemiology, 417
esophageal disease in, 424-425, 439
etiology, 417
fibroblast activity in, 420
graft vs. host disease, 413, 435
humoran immunity in, 418
juvenile onset, 547
linear, 434, 445-456
localized, 413, 434, 544-546
malabsorption in, 427, 439
management, 437-440
morphea, 413, 434, 545-546
muscle disease in, 428, 440, 463
pathology, 432-433
pathogenesis, 418-420
pericarditis in, 426
prognosis, 436
pulmonary involvement in, 425-426, 432, 440
radiology of, 63, 114, 431
Raynaud's phenomenon in, 414, 422-423, 437-438
renal involvement in, 427-429, 433
scleredema, 413, 416, 435
Sjögren's syndrome in, 430
Skin involvement in, 423, 424, 433, 434, 440
small bowel involvement, 427, 439
telangectasia in, 414, 423
thyroid disease in, 430
vascular abnormalities in, 420
vinyl chloride and, 435
Pronator syndrome, elbow, 359
Priopionic acid derivatives, 131-133, 254
Prostaglandins, 126-127
Proteoglycans, 265
PRPP (5-phosphoribosyl-1-pyrophosphate)

PRPP (Continued)
    synthetase, 330
Pseudoarthrosis in ankylosing spondylitis, 293
Pseudogout, *see* Calcium pyrophosphate dihydrate deposition disease
Pseudolymphoma in Sjögren's syndrome, 451-455
Pseudoxanthoma elasticum, 568-569
Psoriasis, 308
Psoriatic arthritis, 307-313
    arthritis, patterns of, 308-311
    epidemiology, 307
    etiology, 308
    HLA typing in, 307
    hyperuricemia, 311
    juvenile onset, 539
    management, 312, 313
    nail changes in, 307-308
    natural history, 312
    pathology of, 312
    pharmacotherapy of, 312-313
    radiology of, 59, 66, 76, 77, 82, 108, 312
    spondylitis in, 311
PSS, *see* Progressive systemic sclerosis
Psychogenic rheumatism, 347
Psychological aspects of arthritis, 178-213
Psychological therapy, 175, 193-205
Psychosis in SLE, 396-398
Psychosocial factors, 162-163, 181-193
Pubis, osteitis of, 370
Pulmonary involvement
    in ankylosing spondylitis, 294
    in MCTD, 483
    in PM, 464
    in PSS, 425-426
    in rheumatoid arthritis, 245
    in Sjögren's syndrome, 448
    in SLE, 393-394
Pulseless disease, *see* Takayasu's arteritis
Purine metabolism, 324-326
Purpura in amyloidosis, 652
Pustulotic arthroosteitis, 311
Pyriformis syndrome, 373
Pyrazolon derivatives, 136, 254

Quinidine-induced SLE, 403
Quinine for leg cramp, 376

RA cells, 38
Radial tunnel syndrome, 359
Radiology in the rheumatic diseases, 58-123
Ragocyte, *see* RA cells
Range of motion, assessment of, 11
Raynaud's phenomenon, 391, 414, 422-423, 450, 481-482, 516, 637
Reactive arthropathies, 315-316, 539
Reflex sympathetic dystrophy syndromes, 342-343, 357, 377, 582, 658

Reiter's syndrome, 300-307
    antibiotics in, 306
    arthritis in, 301
    cardiac involvement, 305
    cutaneous manifestations, 302-303
    diagnosis, 303-304
    enthesopathy in, 301
    epidemiology of, 300
    etiology, 300
    historical aspects, 300
    HLA typing in, 289, 300
    infectious agents in, 300
    juvenile onset, 538
    laboratory findings, 305
    management, 306-307
    mucous membrane involvement, 302
    natural history, 306
    neurologic involvement, 305
    ocular disease in, 302, 305
    pathology in, 306
    pharmacotherapy of, 307
    pulmonary involvement, 305
    radiology of, 66, 85, 92, 94, 111, 112, 306
    spondylitis in, 305
    synovial fluid, 305
    urethritis in, 301
Renal involvement
    in ankylosing spondylitis, 294
    in MCTD, 484
    in PSS, 427-429, 433
    in Sjögren's syndrome, 449
    in SLE, 394-396, 407, 408
Renal stones in gout, 328
Renal toxicity
    gold, 140
    nonsteroidal antiinflammatory drugs, 129, 135
Renal tubular acidosis in Sjögren's syndrome, 449
Restless leg syndrome, 376
Rest, role in therapy, 174
Retinopathy from antimalarial drugs, 140
Rheumatic diseases
    classification, 3
    prevalence, 4, 153
Rheumatic fever, 552-557
    arthritis in, 554
    carditis in, 554
    chorea in, 554
    diagnosis, 552, 553, 555
    epidemiology, 552
    etiology, 553
    laboratory in, 556
    management, 557
    nodules in, 555
    pathology of, 556
    prognosis, 556
    radiology of, 115
Rheumatism, defined, 3
Rheumatoid arthritis (RA), 237-260
    anemia in, 245, 248

Rheumatoid arthritis (Continued)
articular features, 240-242
cardiac involvement, 244-245
diagnosis, 246-248
epidemiology, 237-238
Epstein-Barr virus and, 238
etiology, 283
extra-articular, 242-246
Felty's syndrome in, 245
Hashimoto's thyroiditis and, 637
HLA antigens in, 238
laboratory features, 248
management, 252-256
neuropathy in, 244
nodules in, 241, 250
ocular complications, 246
pathogenesis, 239-240
pathologic findings, 249-250
personality and stress in, 179-180
pharmacotherapy of, 124-142, 253-256
prognosis, 252
psychological effects, 181-193
psychological intervention in, 196-201
pulmonary disease in, 245
radiology of, 64, 66, 67, 68, 72, 73, 74, 75, 79, 83, 84, 86, 100-107, 251
surgery in, 214-234
synovial fluid in, 38, 249
vasculitis in, 242-244, 250, 506
Rheumatoid factor, 41-42, 247, 405, 431, 452, 487, 495, 529, 532
Rheumatoid nodules, 241, 250, 391, 529
Rheumatoid pannus, 249
Rheumatoid pneumoconiosis, *see* Caplans syndrome
Rheumatoid spondylitis, *see* Ankylosing spondylitis
Rheumatology, defined, 3
Rib-tip syndrome, 365
Ro antigen, antibodies to, *see* SSA
Rose Bengal staining in Sjögren's syndrome, 451
Rotator cuff, 16, 352-354
Rotes-Querol disease, *see* Diffuse idiopathic skeletal hyperostosis (DISH)
RNR, *see* Nuclear ribonucleoprotein antigen
Rubella infection, arthritis associated with, 603-604

Sacroiliac joints, 16, 79, 80, 281, 290, 305
Salicylates, 125-131, 253, *see also* Aspirin
serum levels, 128
uric acid excretion and, 148
Salmonella
arthritis after infection, 315, 317, 539
role in Reiter's syndrome, 300
Salmonella osteomyelitis in sickle cell anemia, 640
Salsalate, 128, 131, 253
Sarcoidosis, arthritis in, 641-642
Scheuremann's disease, thoracic spine, 365
Schirmer test in Sjogren's syndrome, 447-448
Schober test for lumbar flexion, 15, 289
Schönlein-Henoch purpura, 504-505, 548-550
Sciatica, 369
Scl-70 antigen in PSS, 430
Scleredema, 413, 416, 435
Scleredema adultorum of Büschke, *see* Scleredema
Sclerodactyly in PSS, 423
Scleroderma, *see* Progressive systemic sclerosis
Scleromalacia perfornas in rheumatoid arthritis, 246
Sedimentation rate, *see* Erythrocyte sedimentation rate
Septic arthritis, *see* Infectious arthritis
Seronegative spondylarthropathies, 287-322
Serum sickness, *see also* Hypersensitivity angiitis, 550
Sexual concerns in arthritis, 163-164, 188-189, 203
Sheep cell agglutination test (SCAT), *see* Rheumatoid factor
Shigella arthritis, 315, 317, 539
Shigella flexneri in Reiter's syndrome, 300
Shin splints, 375
Shoulder, 16-18, 352-357
surgery of, 217-219
Shoulder-hand syndrome, *see* Reflex sympathetic dystrophy
"Shoulder pad" sign in amyloidosis, 652
Sialography in Sjögren's syndrome, 451
Sicca complex in Sjögren's syndrome, 447
Sickle cell disease, arthritis in, 640-644
Sjögren's syndrome, 445-447
animal models, 447
antinuclear antibodies in, 452
arthritis in, 448
cutaneous manifestations, 449
definition, 445
diagnosis, 451-452
etiology, 446
gastrointestinal manifestations, 449
graft vs. host disease and, 451
HLA typing in, 446
immunologic abnormalities in, 446
infectious agents and, 446
in juvenile rheumatoid arthritis, 529
laboratory features, 452
liver abnormalities in, 449
lymphoproliferation in, 451-455
management, 454-455
myositis in, 463
neurologic involvement in, 449
ocular manifestations, 447
oral manifestations, 447
pathogenesis, 446-447
pathology in, 453
polymyositis and, 451
primary, 445

Sjögren's syndrome (Continued)
prognosis, 454
in progressive systemic sclerosis, 416, 430, 450
pulmonary manifestations, 448
Raynaud's phenomenon in, 450
renal involvement in, 449
in rheumatoid arthritis, 246, 445, 450
Rose bengal staining, 451
salivary gland biopsy in, 451-453
Schirmer test in, 447-448
in systemic lupus erythematosus, 398, 450
thyroid disease in, 449
vasculitis in, 450
SLE, *see* Systemic lupus erythematosus (SLE)
Sleep disturbance, 189, 344
Slipping rib syndrome, *see* Rib-tip syndrome
Sm antigen, 47, 405, 487
Social worker, in health care team, 175
Snapping hip, 372
Sodium salicylate, 125, 128
Solitary bone cyst, 619
Speckled pattern ANA, 44, 46
Spinal stenosis, *see* Lumbar stenosis
Spirochetal infection and arthritis, *see* Lyme arthritis
Splenomegaly
in juvenile rheumatoid arthritis, 524
in rheumatoid arthritis, 245
Splinting, 171-173
for carpal tunnel syndrome, 362
Spondylarthropathies, 287-322
Spondylitis, *see* Ankylosing spondylitis
Spondylodiscitis in ankylosing spondylitis, 293
Spondylolisthesis, 369
Spondylosis, 275
Sprains, 341
SSA, antibodies to, 47, 405, 452
SSB, antibodies to, 47, 405, 452
Staphylococcus aureus, infectious arthritis from, 594
Steinberg, thumb sign of, 28
Steroids, injection of, 33-34, 138, 255, 284, 307, 312, 353, 355-362, *see also* Arthrocentesis; Corticosteroids; Drugs inflammation following, 336
Stiffness, 7, 158
Still's disease, 524-527
Sternalis syndrome, 365
Sternoclavicular joint, 16, 356
Sternocostoclavicular hyperotosis, 311
Streptococcal infection
in rheumatic fever, 553
spetic arthritis form, 594
Stress, role in rheumatoid arthritis, 180
Subcutaneous nodules, 241, 250, 391, 529, 555
Subtalar joint, 26
Sudeck's atrophy, *see* Reflex sympathetic dystrophy syndromes
Sulfinpyrazone, 148, 332
Sulfonamides
in rheumatic fever, 557
in SLE, 406
Sulindac, 135, 254, 332
Suprapatellar bursa, 374
Supraspinatus tendonitis, *see* Rotator cuff
Surgical management of arthritis, 214-234, 284
for lumbar disease, 368-369
Swan-neck deformity, 23, 82
Swelling, 7, 10, 58, 59
Sydenham, description of rheumatoid arthritis, 237
Syndesmophytes, 88-92
Synarthrodial joints, 9
Synovenctomy, 215
of knee, 223
Synovial chondromatosis, 630-631
Synovial chondrometaplasia, 630-631
Synovial cyst, 631
Synovial fluid analysis
in calcium pyrophosphate dihydrate, 33, 36-38
deposition disease, 334
in gout, 329-330
in JRA, 534
in osteoarthritis, 281
in PSS, 430
in Reiter's syndrome, 305
in rheumatoid arthritis, 249
in SLE, 388
Synovial sarcoma, 632-633
Synovium and synovial joints, 9
Syphilis, false positive serology for in SLE, 404
Syringomyelia and neuropathic arthropathy, 273
Systemic lupus erythematosus (SLE), 386-410, 416
abdominal pain, 392, 398
alopecia in, 391
"ANA-negative", 390, 399
anemia in, 404
animal models, 387
antinuclear antibodies (ANA) in, 405
arthritis in, 388
cardiac involvement in, 392-393
coagulation abnormalities in, 404
congenital heart block and, 393
cutaneous disease in, 388-391
diagnosis, 399-400
discoid lesions in, 388, 390
drug-induced, 399, 402, 403
epidemiology, 387
etiology, 387
genetic factors, 387
hemolytic anemia in, 404
HLA typing in, 387
hormonal factors in, 387
immune complexes in, 387
juvenile onset, 539-542
laboratory features, 404-405

SLE (Continued)
leukopenia, 404
Libman-Sacks endocarditis, 393
liver abnormalities, 398
malar rash, 388, 391
in malignancies, 658
management, 406-408
myopathy in, 388, 463
neonatal, 393
neurologic involvement, 396-398, 405, 407, 408
nodules in, 391
ocular manifestations, 395
oral ulcers, 389
pathology in, 405-406
pathogenesis, 387
pericarditis in, 392
pharmacotherapy, 406-408
photosensitivity in, 388
pleural disease in, 391
pregnancy in, 398-399
prognosis, 406
psychiatric disease in, 396-398
pulmonary involvement, 393-394
radiology of, 111, 113
Raynaud's phenomenon, 391
renal disease in, 394-396, 407
Sjögren's syndrome, 398
synovial fluid in, 388
syphilis, serology in, 404
thrombocytopenia in, 404
thrombosis in, 404
vasculitis in, 389, 506
Systemic onset juvenile rheumatoid arthritis, 524-527
Systemic necrotizing vasculitis, *see* polyarteritis nodosa

Tabes dorsalis and neuropathic arthropathy, 273
Takayasu's arteritis, 511-512
arteriography in, 512-513
diagnosis, 512
epidemiology, 511
management, 512
pathology in, 511
Tarsal tunnel syndrome, 28, 380
Tartrazine, and aspiring sensitivity, 128
Telangiectasia, 414, 423, 482
Temperature, assessment of, 11
Temporal arteritis, *see* Giant cell arteritis
Temporomandibular joint (TMJ), 12, 351
Tender points in fibrositis, 345-347
Tenderness, assessment, 8-9
Tendinitis, *see* Tendonitis
Tendonitis, 341, 378
Tennis elbow, 20, 357
Tenosynovitis, 22, 341, 360
Tetracycline in Lyme arthritis, 605
Thoracic disc disease, 365
Thoracic outlet syndrome, 357
Thromboangiitis obliterans, 515-517
diagnosis, 516
epidemiology, 515
management, 517
smoking in, 516
Thrombocytopenia in SLE, 404
Thrombocytosis, in rheumatoid disease, 248
Thrombophlebitis in SLE, 404
in Behcet's disease, 515
Thumb, surgery, 222
Thyroid acropachy, 638
Thyroid disease associated with rheumatic disease, 637-638
Thyroid fibrosis in PSS, 430
Thyroiditis, *see* Hashimoto's thyroiditis
Tietze's syndrome, 365
Tinel's sign, 21-22, 362
Tinnitus from aspirin, 128-129
Tolmetin, 135, 254, 535
Tophaceous gout, 327-329
Tophi, 327-329
Toxoplasma, antibodies to in PM/DM, 460, 467
Traction, cervical, 352
Traumatic arthritis, 269, 273
Triamcinolone, *see* Corticosteroids injection of
Trichinosis, 467
Trigger finger, 360
Trigger points, in fibrositis, 28, 345-347
Trochanteric bursa, 23, 372
Tropical pyomyositis, 465
Tuberculous arthritis, 606
Tumoral calcinosis, 589
Tumor of bone and joints, 611-634

Ulcerative colitis, arthritis in, 313, 314, 317
Ulnar nerve entrapment, 359
Urate crystals, *see* Monosodium urate crystals
Urethritis in Reiter's syndrome, 301
Uric acid, metabolism of, 144-146, 324-326
Uricosurics for hyperuricemic gout, 148, 332
Uveitis, 295, 302, 314, 529-530, 535

Varni treatment protocol, in hemophilic arthropathy, 196-198
Vasculitis, 494-521, *see also* specific types
classification, 494-495
juvenile onset, 548-552
in malignancies, 658
in rheumatoid arthritis, 242-244, 250, 506
Villonodular synovitis, 629-630
Vinlychloride disease, scleroderma and, 435
Viral arthritis, 602-604

Viscosity of synovial fluid, 37
Vitamin C deficiency, 568
Vitamin D, 568, 573-575, 583-584
Vocational rehabilitation counselor, 175
von Bechterew's disease, *see* Ankylosing spondylitis

Waaler-Rose test, *see* Rheumatoid factor
Walker and Murdoch, wrist sign of, 28
Weakness, *see* Muscle function
Wegener's granulomatosis, 500-502
  diagnosis, 501
  epidemiology, 500
  management, 502
  pathology of, 500
  pulmonary disease in, 501-502
  renal disease in, 500
  upper respiratory sedimentation rate, 39
Westergren sedimentation rate, 39
Whipple's disease, 316, 317
Williams' flexion exercises, *see* Flexion exercises
Wilson's disease, 270, 334
Wrist, 20-23, 359-360
  in rheumatoid arthritis, 240-241
  surgery of, 219-221

Xerophthalmia, 445
Xerostomia, 445, 447
Xiphoidalgia, 365

Yersinia enterocolitica, in REiter's syndrome, 300
Yersinial arthritis, 314, 315, 539

Zomepirac, 135